Pearls and Tricks in Pediatric Surgery

Martin Lacher · Shawn D. St. Peter · Augusto Zani
Editors

Pearls and Tricks in Pediatric Surgery

Springer

Editors
Martin Lacher
Department of Pediatric Surgery
University of Leipzig
Leipzig, Germany

Augusto Zani
Division of General and Thoracic Surgery,
The Hospital for Sick Children
University of Toronto
Toronto, ON, Canada

Shawn D. St. Peter
Department of Surgery
Children's Mercy Hospital
Kansas City, USA

ISBN 978-3-030-51066-4 ISBN 978-3-030-51067-1 (eBook)
https://doi.org/10.1007/978-3-030-51067-1

This Springer imprint is published by the registered company Springer Nature Switzerland AG
The registered company address is: Gewerbestrasse 11, 6330 Cham, Switzerland

Foreword by Benno Ure

Dramatic improvements and expansions in the field of pediatric surgery have been achieved during the last decades. As a consequence, many textbooks have been released dealing with established concepts, new technology and refinements of surgery in newborns, children and adolescents. However, numerous aspects concerning indications, details of operations and their advantages and disadvantages are still controversially discussed within the pediatric surgical community.

The present book *Pearls and Tricks in Pediatric Surgery* adds essential information to this discussion using an exceptional format. Experts answer to questions and thus present their opinion on nearly all relevant issues of pediatric surgery. Their subjective answers are not only valuable information. They also demonstrate that a considerable number of recommendations on dealing with a specific pediatric surgical problem are still under discussion.

The list of authors of this book is extensive and somehow reads like a Who is Who in pediatric surgery. These authors meet the need of opinions on pediatric surgical concepts when evidence for decision making is limited. The pediatric surgical community may be grateful to the editors Martin Lacher, Shawn St. Peter and Augusto Zani as well as the authors for their great work. This book will assist pediatric surgical trainees and experienced clinicians in their daily work.

Benno Ure, M.D.
Editor-in-Chief, European Journal
of Pediatric Surgery
Chairman and Professor of Pediatric Surgery
Hannover Medical School
Hannover, Germany

Foreword by George W. Holcomb

The editors have done an excellent job collating a large amount of available knowledge into a concise, easy-to-read book that will be helpful to all who care for the surgical conditions in infants and children. As in previous editions of this book, the title of the book is really a misnomer. In reality, there are few, if any, secrets in the care of our patients. Rather, this book provides up-to-date knowledge from authors who have a great deal of experience and expertise in their topic. Although I feel the book is directed to the more inexperienced caregiver for infants and children, I think all of us can benefit from the information in this book.

The editors are to be congratulated on a wonderful effort!

George W. Holcomb, III MD, MBA
Editor-in-Chief, Journal of Pediatric Surgery,
Children's Mercy Kansas City
Nashville, USA

Foreword by Agostino Pierro

This comprehensive and innovative book contributes to the dissemination of knowledge that is essential to improve and guide the surgical treatment of children. Drs. Lacher, St. Peter and Zani have finalised a book characterized by comprehensiveness and innovation.

Several chapters have been included covering a magnitude of clinical problems highly relevant to the work of pediatric surgeons as well as trainees in surgery, nurses and other caregivers. The editors have obtained important contributions from a multitude of world class experts working in various countries and in different health systems.

The book is innovative as it is based on questions and answers, therefore highlighting practical problems in the surgical care of neonates and children and reporting the options favoured by the experts. Its value is pivotal for the daily care of these children as well as for the training of a new generation of pediatric surgeons.

Pediatric Surgery is a young specialty which has made enormous progress during the last decades. The outcome of the diseases covered in the book should be further improved, and this book can contribute to refining the surgical management of the children affected. *Pearls and Tricks in Pediatric Surgery* will provide a rapid and detailed reference to clinical problems while discussing the way of managing them. I am expecting that this book will produce a positive impact in Pediatric Surgery and will be utilised by many worldwide.

On behalf of the international community of pediatric surgeons, I would like to express gratitude to Drs. Lacher, St. Peter and Zani for having produced such important contribution in Pediatric Surgery.

Agostino Pierro
Co-Editor in Chief of Pediatric Surgery International
Professor of Surgery, University of Toronto
Toronto, Canada

Preface

Pearls and Tricks in Pediatric Surgery encompass the wide range of complex pediatric surgical issues.

The content presented in this book should be considered as an additional core knowledge not only for the surgeon but also the pediatrician, the gastroenterologist, the neonatologist, the nurse, the surgical trainee, and the medical student.

The scope of this book is not to replace the information in a regular pediatric surgical textbook but to supplement it. Developed from the learner´s standpoint, the questions and answers include clinical presentation of the diseases, essentials of pathophysiology, treatments, and possible outcomes.

Pearls are formed inside a shell as a defense mechanism against a potentially threatening irritant. The pearls of knowledge provided in this book should help all caretakers improve the care provided by enhancing their defense mechanisms against complex pediatric surgical issues.

A trick is an effective or quick way of doing something. This book uses the question–answer teaching strategy as an effective vehicle to facilitate learning. It is an old strategy developed by the famous philosopher Socrates who considered the question as the key to all educative activities above the habit-skill level. Its strategy is focused on to achieve the cognitive objectives and bring knowledge to the conscious level.

The authors of the various chapters provide state-of-the-art knowledge based on the current literature, evidence, and personal experience. The quality of the chapters reflects their interest, enthusiasm, and true dedication to learning and teaching the medical school classes and surgical residencies in their institutions. It is an honor, privilege, and a continuing stimulus to be a part of this group of dedicated colleagues. We want to thank them for their excellent job.

We could not have completed this project without the support and understanding of our families with their tireless support and devotion.

Leipzig, Germany	Martin Lacher M.D.
Kansas City, USA	Shawn D. St. Peter M.D.
Toronto, Canada	Augusto Zani M.D.

Contents

1 **Evaluation of the Pediatric Surgical Patient** 1
Scott S. Short and Michael D. Rollins

2 **Nutrition, Fluids and Electrolytes for the Pediatric Surgical Patient** 7
Simon Eaton

3 **Chest Wall Deformities** 13
Marcelo Martinez-Ferro, Luzía Toselli and Gaston Bellia-Munzon

4 **Congenital Diaphragmatic Hernia** 25
Louise Montalva and Augusto Zani

5 **Esophageal Atresia With or Without Tracheoesophageal Fistula** 35
Christina M. Bence and Dave R. Lal

6 **Gastroesophageal Reflux Disease** 41
Charlene Dekonenko and George W. Holcomb III

7 **Caustic Ingestion of the Esophagus** 47
Rashmi Kabre

8 **Esophageal Foreign Bodies** 53
Dan C. Little and A. Justin Malek

9 **Congenital Lung Malformations** 59
Shaun M. Kunisaki

10 **Acquired Lung and Pleural Disease** 65
Shawn D. St. Peter

11 **Tracheobronchial Foreign Bodies** 69
Paolo Campisi

12 **Pediatric Surgical Diseases of the Larynx, Trachea, and Bronchi** 77
Elizabeth F. Maughan, Colin Butler, Richard Hewitt, and Paolo De Coppi

13 **Mediastinal Masses** 89
Arnaud Bonnard

14 **Congenital Cardiac Anomalies** 95
William Gibson and James E. O'Brien Jr.

15 **Hemangiomas and Vascular Malformations** 101
Jo Cooke-Barber and Roshni Dasgupta

16 **Umbilical Problems** 109
Jeffrey J. Dehmer

17 **Hernias—Epigastric, Inguinal and Incisional** 113
Jill Sutherland Quirt and Annie Fecteau

18 **Abdominal Wall Defects, Gastroschisis and Omphalocele** 125
Kevin Johnson and Saleem Islam

19 **Exstrophy-Epispadias Complex** 131
Abdulrahman E. Alshafei and Raimondo Maximilian Cervellione

20 **Prune Belly Syndrome** 139
A. J. Pomajzl and Gwen M. Grimsby

21 **Normal Embryology, Anatomy, and Physiology of the Gastrointestinal Tract** 147
Faten Al Rubian and Richard Keijzer

22 **Small Intestinal Obstruction** 155
Justin L. Hunter and Hanna Alemayehu

23 **Intestinal Atresia and Webs** 161
Raphael H. Parrado and Daniel J. Ostlie

24 **Malrotation and Midgut Volvulus** 169
R. Ellen Jones, Jordan S. Taylor, and Matias Bruzoni

25 **Gastrointestinal Surgical Aspects of Cystic Fibrosis** 179
Ross M. Beckman and Samuel M. Alaish

26 **Necrotizing Enterocolitis (NEC)** 185
Xiaoyan Feng and Martin Lacher

27 **Meckel's Diverticulum & Vitelline Duct Remnants** 191
R. Cartland Burns and Matthew P. Landman

28 **Appendicitis** 195
Tomas Wester and Jan F. Svensson

29 Intussusception 201
Alexander T. Gibbons, Alejandra M. Casar Berazaluce, Rachel E. Hanke, and Todd A. Ponsky

30 Small Left Colon Syndrome (SLCS) 207
Colleen M. Fitzpatrick

31 Disorders of Colonic Motility/Hirschsprung Disease 211
Rebecca M. Rentea and Marc A. Levitt

32 Inflammatory Bowel Disease 219
Sebastian King

33 Gastrointestinal Bleeding 227
Aaron T. Scott and Julia Shelton

34 Anorectal Malformations 233
Hira Ahmad and Marc A. Levitt

35 Anorectal Complaints (Proctology): Hemorrhoids, Fissures, Abscesses, Fistulae 247
Brian C. Gulack, Justyna M. Wolinska, and Sharifa Himidan

36 Biliary Atresia 257
Federico Scottoni and Mark Davenport

37 Choledochal Cyst 265
Omid Madadi-Sanjani and Claus Petersen

38 Pediatric Gallbladder Disease 271
Anna Elizabeth West and Matthew SClifton

39 Portal Hypertension 275
Alexander Dzakovic and Riccardo Superina

40 Disorders of the Spleen 281
Jacob C. Langer

41 Pancreas 287
Elke Zani-Ruttenstock and Agostino Pierro

42 Pearls for Pediatric Head and Neck Masses 295
Julie L. Wei

43 Thyroglossal Duct Cysts and Sinuses 301
Priscilla P. L. Chiu

44 Branchial Clefts and Arch Anomalies 305
Reto M. Baertschiger and Lourenço Sbragia

45 Torticollis 313
Jill M. Arganbright and Jason R. Brown

46 Renal Cystic Diseases 319
Alexandra Rehfuss, Christina Ching, Daniel DaJusta, and Molly Fuchs

47 Obstructive Uropathy 325
Alexandra Rehfuss, Molly Fuchs, Daniel DaJusta, and Christina Ching

48 Vesicoureteral Reflux (VUR) 331
Xiaoyan Feng, Prem Puri and Martin Lacher

49 Circumcision and Disorders of the Penis 339
Bristol B. Whiles and Alonso Carrasco Jr.

50 Testicular Problems and Varicocele 351
Karen Milford and Armando Lorenzo

51 Gynaecological Problems 359
Tazim Dowlut-McElroy

52 Disorders/Differences of Sex Development (DSD) 367
Kathleen van Leeuwen

53 Trauma–General Considerations 373
Christian J. Streck Jr

54 Pediatric Traumatic Brain Injury and Cervical Spine Injuries 379
Matthias Krause

55 Thoracic Trauma 387
Maeve O'Neill Trudeau, Joshua Ramjist, and Paul W. Wales

56 Abdominal Trauma 393
Raphael H. Parrado and David M. Notrica

57 Soft Tissue Injuries 401
Aaron T. Scott and Bindi Naik-Mathuria

58 Orthopedic Trauma and Sports Injuries 409
Kevin H. Latz

59 Pediatric Burns 415
Eduardo I. Gus, Joel Fish, and Charis Kelly

60 Neuroblastoma 425
Jochen Hubertus and Dieterich von Schweinitz

61 Wilms Tumor 431
Denis A. Cozzi and Silvia Ceccanti

62 Hepatic Tumors 437
Michael Berger and Dietrich von Schweinitz

63 Endocrine Tumors 443
Mary Brandt

64 Germ Cell Tumors 449
Andrea Doud and Mary E. Fallat

65 Miscellaneous Tumors 455
Andrew J. Murphy and Andrew M. Davidoff

66 Pediatric Radiology 465
Abdullah Alshabanat, Ailish Coblentz, and Alan Daneman

67 Transplantation in Children 477
Michael Berger

68 The Neonatal Surgical Patient 485
Francesco Morini, Patrizia Bozza, and Pietro Bagolan

69 Pediatric Endocrine Diseases 497
Jason D. Fraser

70 Pediatric Anesthesia 501
Nan Gai and Jason Maynes

71 Fetal Surgery 507
Seyed Arshia Arshad and KuoJen Tsao

72 How to Become a Pediatric Surgeon? 515
Sara Mahler and Oliver J. Muensterer

73 Evidence Based Medicine Concepts/Clinical Research 521
Peter C. Minneci and Katherine J. Deans

74 Short Bowel Syndrome 527
Annika Mutanen and Mikko P. Pakarinen

75 Evidence in Minimally Invasive Surgery 535
Rim Kiblawi, Benno Ure, and Jens Dingemann

Index 543

Chapter 1
Evaluation of the Pediatric Surgical Patient

Scott S. Short and Michael D. Rollins

Abstract This chapter provides a brief introduction to the nuances and challenges associated with the surgical evaluation of the pediatric patient.

Keywords Surgery · Pediatric · Neonate

1.1 Introduction

It is often stated that children are not small adults. This aphorism simplifies the complexity involved with assessment of the pediatric patient. Not only do children manifest surgical conditions differently than their adult counterparts they have conditions which are specific to periods of development. Further, common conditions can manifest in a variety of ways dependent upon the child's physiologic and psychological development. The "contrast to adult life is greatest in infancy and becomes progressively less until" they have progressed through puberty [1].

1. **How are pediatric patients different from adults?**

Childhood can be divided into different time periods: neonatal, infant, toddler, child, and adolescent. Each of these developmental periods impart different physiologic and psychosocial features.

S. S. Short (✉)
Division of Pediatric Surgery, Department of Surgery, University of Utah Health/Primary Children's Hospital, 100 N. Mario Cappecchi Dr., Suite #3800, Salt Lake City, UT 84113, United States
e-mail: Scott.Short@hsc.utah.edu

M. D. Rollins
University of Utah School of Medicine, Primary Children's Hospital, Salt Lake City, Utah, United States

M. Lacher et al. (eds.), *Pearls and Tricks in Pediatric Surgery*,
https://doi.org/10.1007/978-3-030-51067-1_1

a. The neonatal period (<30 days of life) is characterized by unique fluid, electrolyte, metabolic, and thermoregulatory requirements. These factors are further influenced by gestational age, birth weight, prenatal factors, and co-morbid conditions. Examples include high resting energy expenditure and glucose requirements, which not only change during the 1st week of life but are directly affected by size and gestation. Clear understanding of these issues as well as unique neonatal conditions (e.g. duodenal atresia, necrotizing enterocolitis) is required by the surgeon.
b. Infancy (30 days to 1 year of life) is characterized by a period of rapid growth and developmental change. Children often double their birth weight by 6 months of life and see progressive development of motor and social skills. This period is also characterized by unique surgical conditions (e.g. pyloric stenosis).
c. Toddler (1–3 years) is one of the most challenging periods as communication with the child is difficult and fear of medical personnel often prevents a reliable physical exam. Unique conditions such as intussusception may be seen in this period.
d. Childhood (4–12 years) reflects continued development towards adulthood. Psychosocial implications of surgery can be quite distressful and many children may experience anxiety and/or regression of developed skills.
e. Adolescents (>12 years) more commonly have adult type conditions but psychosocial aspects must be considered to develop healthy physician-patient relationships to foster trust, and treatment compliance.

2. **What about the parents?**

Parents and providers of children are critical in understanding the child's history, presentation, and context of their condition. Young children are non-verbal or often unable to effectively communicate their problems. Older children may not share important information and be resistant to interacting with providers. It is therefore, critical to develop a relationship with the parent not only to understand the clinical problem but to alleviate or address the concerns of the parents themselves. Parental anxieties are known to exacerbate anxiety in the child. Having a sick or injured child is stressful for caregivers and the surgeon must consider their needs in addition to the patient's needs.

3. **What do I need to know? What are the important aspects of the history?**

In the young child an understanding of the prenatal period is critical. It is important to understand details surrounding the pregnancy (prenatal care, known anomalies, maternal medication use, maternal infections, maternal co-morbid conditions), birth (gestational age, meconium present, rupture of membranes, APGAR scores), and early perinatal course.

Beyond the perinatal period much of the assessment is similar. A complete evaluation of the history of present illness, past medical/surgical history, prior anesthesia history, a family history, social history and physical examination appropriate for the clinical scenario.

Children may present with rare or unusual conditions that may require multidisciplinary discussion to fully understand the complete picture and to ensure adequate components of the history have been obtained.

Caveats: The family history may be more impactful in some patients and may clue the provider into disease process with known genetic or heritable components. Example: A 2 y.o. girl with a cystic lung lesion. It is important to assess the family for other lesions such cystic nephroma, multinodular goiter, mesenchymal hamartoma of the liver, etc. to evaluate risk for DICER1 mutations. If positive, one would be concerned that the cystic lung lesion could represent pleuropulmonary blastoma.

4. **How do I examine a child? How is this different?** [2]

   a. The assessment:

      i. Child life resources with toys and electronics to distract young children may be helpful in performing an assessment.
      ii. Garnering parental/caregiver support and involvement may not only be necessary but may also allow for a more complete physical examination.
      iii. It is important to try to make the child feel comfortable and safe. This may include examining the child while a parent holds them and/or actively engages them in the assessment. It is also helpful to let the child know what you are going to do next.
      iv. Occasionally, adequate assessment requires an evaluation in the operating room. Examples include: the developmentally delayed child who is too large to safely restrain to adequately evaluate a perianal lesion or a teenage girl who may be too uncomfortable to relax for evaluation of a pelvic straddle injury.

   b. The child's size, age, and disease process may affect the exam. Example:

      i. In young infants suspected inguinal hernias can be quite difficult to appreciate on exam. There are many cases where one cannot identify the hernia on exam but the history remains highly suspicious. In these cases of uncertainty, obtaining photos of the hernia can provide confidence before proceeding to surgical repair.

5. **What are requirements/considerations for children undergoing surgical procedures?**

   a. Fasting recommendations: [3]

      i. Clear liquids 2 hours
      ii. Breast milk 4 hours
      iii. Infant formula 6 hours
      iv. Full meal 8 hours.

   b. If tasked with intubation how do I decide on the appropriate sized endotracheal tube?

    i. Rule of thumb (Child>2 years): ETT size=(Age +16)/4

  c. Do children have different physiologic considerations important to surgery?

    i. Yes, Cardiac output varies by age:

      1. Neonate: 350 ml/kg/min, infant 150 ml/kg/min, Adult 75 ml/kg/min.

    ii. Yes, they have increased oxygen consumption and alveolar ventilation

      1. Preterm infants may have 3 fold increase in oxygen consumption and children have increased respiratory rates compared to adult counterparts.

    iii. Yes, they have increased vagal sensitivity

      1. More frequent bradycardic events with airway stimulation.

  d. Premature infants can have apneic events. How long do they need to be observed?

    i. Premature infants (<37 weeks) who are 60 weeks or less post menstrual age require overnight observation
    ii. Term infants<44 weeks post menstrual age require observation in a monitored bed at least 4 hours
    iii. Term infants>44 weeks with no history of neonatal apnea can be discharged after meeting discharge criteria.

6. **Is routine laboratory evaluation required?**

The majority of healthy children undergoing routine outpatient procedures do not require pre-operative laboratory evaluation. For children with medical co-morbid conditions, surgical judgement should be used to decide relevant laboratory values to guide management and limit procedures on children. Examples include obtaining metabolic panels to evaluate the chloride, bicarbonate, and potassium levels on children prior to pyloromyotomy for pyloric stenosis, evaluation of hemoglobin S component on children with known sickle cell disease, and obtaining pregnancy tests in adolescent girls prior to surgery.

7. **The parents are worried about anesthesia risk and surgery. How safe is it?**

Overall mortality rates have been estimated at less than 1 in 45,000 and many of these occur in children with ASA scores of three or higher [4].

8. **How do I effectively communicate surgical planning with a difficult family?**

  a. Find a private area for discussion and where distractions can be limited
  b. Discuss the indications, risks, and benefits in a way the family can understand.

    i. **Don't be rushed**

ii. It may be helpful to set aside extended time for challenging families (e.g. last clinic patient of the day).

c. Involve partners and colleagues in the decision making process. “We discussed this as a group and this is what we think will best help your child” or “I spoke to several of my colleagues at other centers and they support the recommendation”.
d. Utilization of pictures, diagrams, or slides may be helpful in getting the family to understand the proposed procedure. An example may be a PowerPoint slide to illustrate the Nuss procedure for pectus excavatum.
e. Ask the family (and **patient**) what concerns they have and what they think may help.
f. Offer a second visit to review ongoing concerns or questions.
g. Offer to facilitate a 2nd opinion from another provider.

References

1. Bolling RW. Surgery of childhood. New York: Appleton; 1928. p. 1928.
2. Lerwick JL. Psychosocial implications of pediatric surgical hospitalization. Semin Pediatr Surg. 2013;22(3):129–33.
3. Practice guidelines for preoperative fasting and the use of pharmacologic agents to reduce the risk of pulmonary aspiration: application to healthy patients undergoing elective procedures: an updated report by the American Society of Anesthesiologists task force on preoperative fasting and the use of pharmacologic agents to reduce the risk of pulmonary aspiration. Anesthesiology. 2017;126(3):376–93.
4. Flick RP, Sprung J, Harrison TE, Gleich SJ, Schroeder DR, Hanson AC, et al. Perioperative cardiac arrests in children between 1988 and 2005 at a tertiary referral center: a study of 92,881 patients. Anesthesiology. 2007;106(2):226–37; quiz 413–4.

Chapter 2
Nutrition, Fluids and Electrolytes for the Pediatric Surgical Patient

Simon Eaton

Abstract Nutritional care of surgical infants and children is of major importance. This is for several reasons: (i) body stores are often smaller and more precarious; (ii) infants and children not only require energy for maintenance, but also for growth; and (iii) as in adults, recovery from surgery is faster in those patients who are adequately nourished. Surgery for congenital and acquired gastrointestinal anomalies often results in a period during which enteral feeds are not tolerated or absorbed, and provision of parenteral nutrition is often necessary in these patients. However, parenteral nutrition is associated with complications, and should be given only until infants and children are able to tolerate enteral feeds. Fluid and electrolyte balance of surgical infants and children is similarly crucial, because growth and physiological changes in body composition may mask dehydration, edema and electrolyte imbalances exacerbated by losses from the gastrointestinal tract.

Keywords Growth · Nutrition · Parenteral nutrition · Sodium · Stoma

1. **How do energy stores in the body alter with age?**

Energy stores are only adequate for ~2 days at 24–25 weeks gestation, increase to ~20 days at term as glycogen and fat stores increase and are in excess of 50 days in the adult, hence the urgent need for adequate caloric intake in preterm infants after birth. Full-term neonates have higher content of endogenous fat (approximately 600 g) and therefore can tolerate a few days of undernutrition.

S. Eaton (✉)
UCL Great Ormond Street Institute of Child Health,
30 Guilford Street, London WC1N 1EH, UK
e-mail: s.eaton@ucl.ac.uk

M. Lacher et al. (eds.), *Pearls and Tricks in Pediatric Surgery*,
https://doi.org/10.1007/978-3-030-51067-1_2

2. **What is the optimum nutritional route for infants?**

The optimum nutritional route is oral enteral feeding. However, artificial enteral feeding or parenteral nutrition (PN) may be required if adequate oral feeds cannot be tolerated. The basic principle underlying choice of feeding routes is that the most physiological route that is safely possible should be used: oral preferred over tube feeding, gastric feeds are preferred over jejunal feeds, enteral feeds are preferred over parenteral feeds etc.

3. **How should the nutrition of surgical infants and children be monitored?**

Effectiveness of nutrition should be assessed. Growth of all paediatric surgical patients, especially those receiving artificial nutritional support, should be monitored longitudinally using appropriate charts. Although measurement of weight, height/length, and head circumference is important, it is essential that these are monitored serially, and plotted on centile charts., which are often available on a national basis, or if not, are available from the World Health Organization. It is especially important to also consider hydration, as over- or under- hydration can be an important contributor to weight change.

4. **Why can't premature infants be fed orally?**

The swallowing reflex is not fully developed in premature infants so they should be fed by naso- or oro- gastric tubes until the swallowing reflex is developed and it is safe to give oral feeds.

5. **Why are gastric enteral feeds preferred over jejunal feeds?**

Gastric feeding is preferable to intestinal feeding because it allows for a more natural and complete digestive process i.e. allows action of salivary and gastric enzymes and the antibacterial action of stomach acid, in addition to the use of the stomach as a reservoir. Gastric feeding is associated with a larger osmotic and volume tolerance and a lower frequency of diarrhea and dumping syndrome. Thus, transpyloric feeds are usually restricted to infants or children who are either unable to tolerate naso- or oro- gastric feeds, at increased risk of aspiration; or who have anatomical contra-indications to gastric feeds.

6. **Why is long-term nasogastric or orogastric feeding not recommended?**

In infants requiring gastric tube feeding for extended periods (e.g. more than 6–8 weeks) it is advisable to insert a gastrostomy, to decrease the negative oral stimulation of repeated insertion of nasal or oral tubes.

7. **When should cow's milk protein allergy be considered?**

Cow's milk protein allergy can be acute (IgE-mediated) or delayed (non-IgE mediated). Gastrointestinal symptoms are usually present (reflux, colic, constipation etc.), and intolerance in the absence of anatomical reasons may be a manifestation of Cow's milk protein allergy. It can be present even in exclusively breast-fed infants, as bovine antigens may be passed from the mother.

8. **What are the advantages of minimal enteral (trophic) feeding?**

Minimal feeds may prevent gut mucosal atrophy, increase intestinal blood flow, improve activity of digestive enzymes and thus 'prime' the gut for subsequent higher volume, nutritive feeds. In addition, oral stimulation may prevent later oral aversion.

9. **If infants and children are tolerating full feeds, should weight monitoring cease?**

Tolerance is not the same as absorption, as infants and children may require a significant period of time for intestinal adaptation to allow complete absorption of administered feeds. Growth monitoring should continue and be checked against centile charts at outpatient follow-up.

10. **What might explain poor growth in an infant with a stoma?**

Sodium is essential for growth, so that infants with a stoma may have inadequate sodium intake. Low urinary sodium with normal serum sodium suggests active sodium conservation, and sodium supplementation may be appropriate [1].

11. **When should parenteral nutrition (PN) be given to a surgical infant or child?**

PN is given when enteral feeding is impossible, inadequate, or hazardous, but should be given for the shortest period of time possible and the proportion of nutrition given enterally increased as tolerated. Energy reserves are such that stable term infants can tolerate 3–4 days without enteral feeds, and older children 7–10 days, before starting PN, if it is anticipated that enteral nutrition may be resumed within this time. Premature neonates have smaller energy reserves and the time before introducing PN is much shorter. The most frequent indications in paediatric surgery are intestinal obstruction due to congenital anomalies, although acquired conditions such as post-operative ileus, necrotizing enterocolitis, short-bowel syndrome, gastroenterological indications, and respiratory co-morbidity may require PN for variable lengths of time.

12. **Why should PN not be administered peripherally?**

Peripheral administration gives significant risk of complications from hyperosmolar glucose, which can cause vascular irritation or damage and thrombosis. PN should be administered via centrally placed catheters (including peripherally inserted central catheters (i.e. PICC lines), surgically placed central catheters or centrally-placed umbilical catheters) dependent on the vascular access already available and the length of time that PN is anticipated to be needed for [2].

13. **Which are the components of PN that should be considered as making up the energetic requirements?**

The caloric requirements for PN are provided by carbohydrate [3] and lipid [4]. Protein is required for growth and is not used as a source of calories. The ideal

PN regimen therefore, should provide enough amino acids for protein turnover and tissue growth [5], and sufficient calories to minimize protein oxidation for energy.

14. **What lipid emulsions should be used in PN of infants and children?**

Although pure soybean lipid emulsions can be used short-term, composite lipid emulsions with or without fish oils should be used for PN lasting more than a few days, as this is thought to help prevent cholestasis, one of the major complications of PN [4].

15. **Are the energy requirements on PN similar to EN?**

No, energy requirements are approximately 10% lower because calorie losses in stool etc. are minimal.

16. **Why does weight often drop in the first few days after birth?**

This is a normal physiological change in fluid compartments, resulting in diuresis and weight loss of 5–10%.

17. **How are hyponatremia and hypernatremia defined?**

Hyponatremia is a serum sodium less than 128 mEq/L in the neonate and less than 135 mEq/L in children; hypernatremia is a serum sodium greater than 150 mEq/L.

18. **Why are post-operative infants and children at risk of hyponatremia?**

Anti-diuretic hormone is secreted for several days in response to operative stress, which can lead to hyponatremia. In addition, gastrointestinal fluid losses also lead to electrolyte losses. Isotonic rather than hypotonic fluids should be administered to decrease risk of hyponatremia, and gastrointestinal electrolyte losses measured and replaced.

19. **Which neonatal acquired emergency of term infants is typically accompanied by dehydration and electrolyte disturbances?**

Pyloric stenosis typically presents with dehydration together with hyponatremia, hypokalemia, and metabolic alkalosis, so that appropriate resuscitation and correction of electrolyte balance are essential before surgery is performed.

20. **How are respiratory and metabolic acidosis/alkalosis differentiated?**

In respiratory acidosis/alkalosis, PaCO2 is >45 mmHg (acidosis) or <35 mmHg (alkalosis) and treatment is via appropriate respiratory support. In metabolic acidosis/alkalosis, bicarbonate <21 mmol/l (acidosis) or>26mmmol/l (alkalosis). In metabolic acidosis it is useful to check the anion gap [$=Na+-(Cl-+HCO_3-)$, which is normally 12 ± 2 mEq/l] to understand the underlying cause and correct the existing deficits. It is also important, before treatment with sodium bicarbonate bolus, to check the volemic status because of this condition can be due to a tissue hypo perfusion.

21. **When should hypotonic fluids be administered?**

Hyponatremia at admission, or post-operatively is relatively common in children, so administration of hypotonic fluids should be reserved only for those with a demonstrated hypernatremia >145–150 mEq/L.

References

1. Mansour F, Petersen D, De Coppi P, Eaton S. Effect of sodium deficiency on growth of surgical infants: a retrospective observational study. Pediatr Surg Int. 2014;30(12):1279–84.
2. Kolacek S, Puntis JWL, Hojsak I, ESPGHAN/ESPEN/ESPR/CSPEN working group on pediatric parenteral nutrition. ESPGHAN/ESPEN/ESPR/CSPEN guidelines on pediatric parenteral nutrition: venous access. Clin Nutr. 2018;37(6 Pt B):2379–91.
3. Mesotten D, Joosten K, van Kempen A, Verbruggen S, ESPGHAN/ESPEN/ESPR/CSPEN working group on pediatric parenteral nutrition ESPGHAN/ESPEN/ESPR/CSPEN guidelines on pediatric parenteral nutrition: carbohydrates. Clin Nutr. 2018;37(6 Pt B):2337–43.
4. Lapillonne A, Fidler Mis N, Goulet O, van den Akker CHP, Wu J, Koletzko B, et al. ESPGHAN/ESPEN/ESPR/CSPEN guidelines on pediatric parenteral nutrition: lipids. Clin Nutr. 2018;37(6 Pt B):2324–36.
5. van Goudoever JB, Carnielli V, Darmaun D, Sainz de Pipaon M, ESPGHAN/ESPEN/ESPR/CSPEN working group on pediatric parenteral nutrition. ESPGHAN/ESPEN/ESPR/CSPEN guidelines on pediatric parenteral nutrition: amino acids. Clin Nutr. 2018;37(6 Pt B):2315–23.

Chapter 3
Chest Wall Deformities

Marcelo Martinez-Ferro, Luzía Toselli and Gaston Bellia-Munzon

Abstract Chest wall malformations include excavated deformities or pectus excavatum (PEX) and carinated deformities or pectus carinatum (PC). These deformities can be mixed defects and they may also be a part of a congenital syndrome such as the Currarino Silverman syndrome. The development in the field of chest wall malformations has been steep in the three last decades and both adult and pediatric surgeons have become specialized in the subject pushing even forward the baggage of knowledge. We aim to introduce the reader in the different aspects related to pectus deformities.

Keywords Pectus excavatum · Pectus carinatum · Chest wall deformities · MIPRE · Minimally invasive surgery · Dynamic compression system · Vacuum bell

1. **What are the typical chest wall deformities?**

The most common are the caved in sternum or pectus excavatum (PEX) and the protruding sternum or pectus carinatum (PC). When these defects coexist in the same patient they are called mixed deformities. Also, deformities may be asymmetric or part of a syndrome such as the Currarino Silverman syndrome, which is

M. Martinez-Ferro (✉) · L. Toselli · G. Bellia-Munzon
Capital Federal, Av. Crámer 4602. C1429AKL, Buenos Aires, Argentina
e-mail: m.martinezferro@gmail.com

L. Toselli
e-mail: luzia79@hotmail.com; dra.luzia.toselli@gmail.com

G. Bellia-Munzon
e-mail: gastonbellia@gmail.com

M. Martinez-Ferro · L. Toselli · G. Bellia-Munzon
Fundacion Hospitalaria Mother and Child Medical Center, Buenos Aires, Argentina

M. Lacher et al. (eds.), *Pearls and Tricks in Pediatric Surgery*,
https://doi.org/10.1007/978-3-030-51067-1_3

characterized by a congenital cardiac malformation and pectus arcuatum, a wide, non-articulated, short sternum.

2. **What are the demographic characteristics of pectus excavatum (PEX)?**

The incidence of PEX has been traditionally described as 1 in 1000, and comprises 80% of all the pectus deformities. However, and probably due to the rise of non-operative approaches to PC, there has been an increase in referrals of PC patients to pectus clinics in the last decades with a shift in the relative incidences in favor of PC resulting in a ratio of 1:1. The sex distribution is predominantly male, with a 4:1 ratio. A family history is common and connective tissue diseases are more frequently associated with pectus deformities.

3. **How is PEX classified?**

PEX can be classified as typical and atypical. The typical forms can be classified as localized or diffuse, shallow or deep, and as symmetric or asymmetric (Fig. 3.1). The atypical forms include mixed deformities and the Poland syndrome.

4. **How is a patient with PEX studied?**

The physical examination will provide information regarding the type of PEX and the probability of success with a non-surgical approach. A vacuum bell connected to a vacuometer can predict how much pressure is necessary to correct the excavation and if the vacuum bell may be effective (Fig. 3.2). We follow our patients with photos taken from 6 predetermined angles at diagnosis and follow-up.

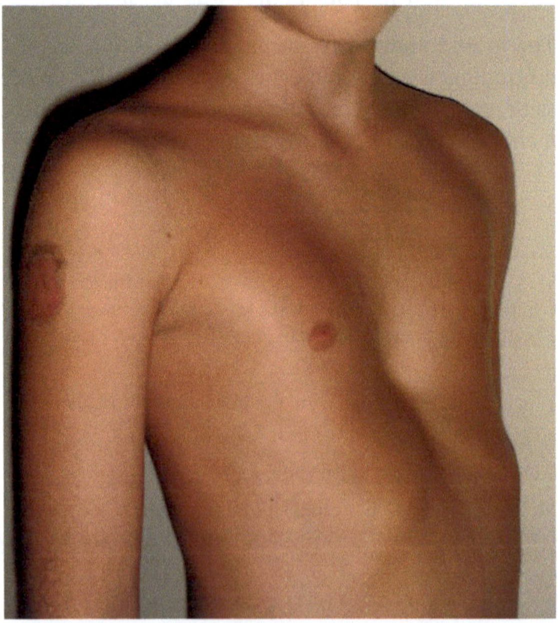

Fig. 3.1 The concept of pectus excavatum (PEX) comprises a wide variety of excavated deformities with typical and atypical presentations. In this figure a deep, localized, symmetric deformity is depicted

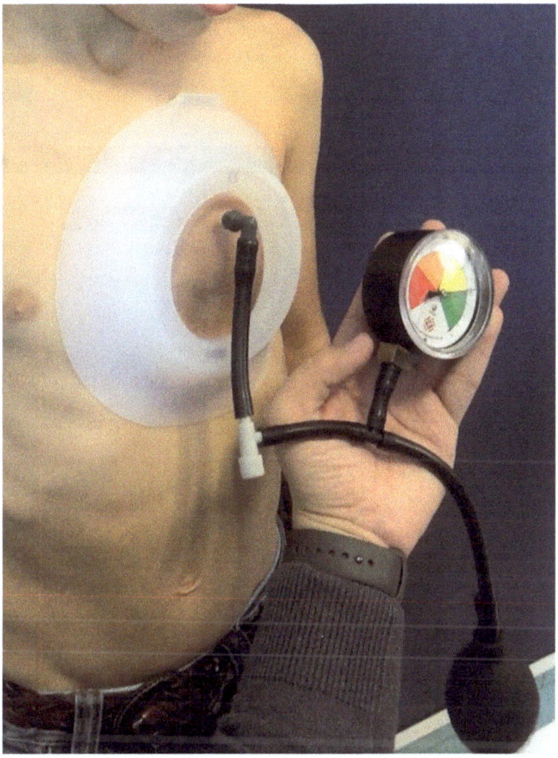

Fig. 3.2 A vacuometer is used to determine objectively the degree of negative pressure necessary to correct the excavated chest wall deformity. This is an indirect way to evaluate the rigidity/elasticity of the deformity

In surgical candidates, a CT scan is performed to quantify the depth of the defect. Physiologic testing may include stress echocardiography as well as a dynamic cardiac magnetic resonance imaging. A history of metal allergy should be inquired and if uncertain, a nickel allergy test has to be performed to determine the patient will tolerate a steel bar. If not, a titanium bar will be needed.

We generally employ a 3D scanning system with virtual reconstruction for diagnosis and follow-up with a visual color-scale that varies according to its depth (Fig. 3.3).

5. **What indices are most commonly used to measure the severity of PEX?**

The Haller index is the original measure, and it results from the ratio between the lateral distance and the anteroposterior distance between the sternum and the spine, calculated by means of a chest CT scan at the point of maximum sternal depth. This index was not originally validated and it is highly variable depending on sex, symmetry, the shape of the thorax, and the respiration phase in which the study is acquired. Nowadays, the Correction Index has received validation and is more precise to discriminate affected from non-affected subjects.

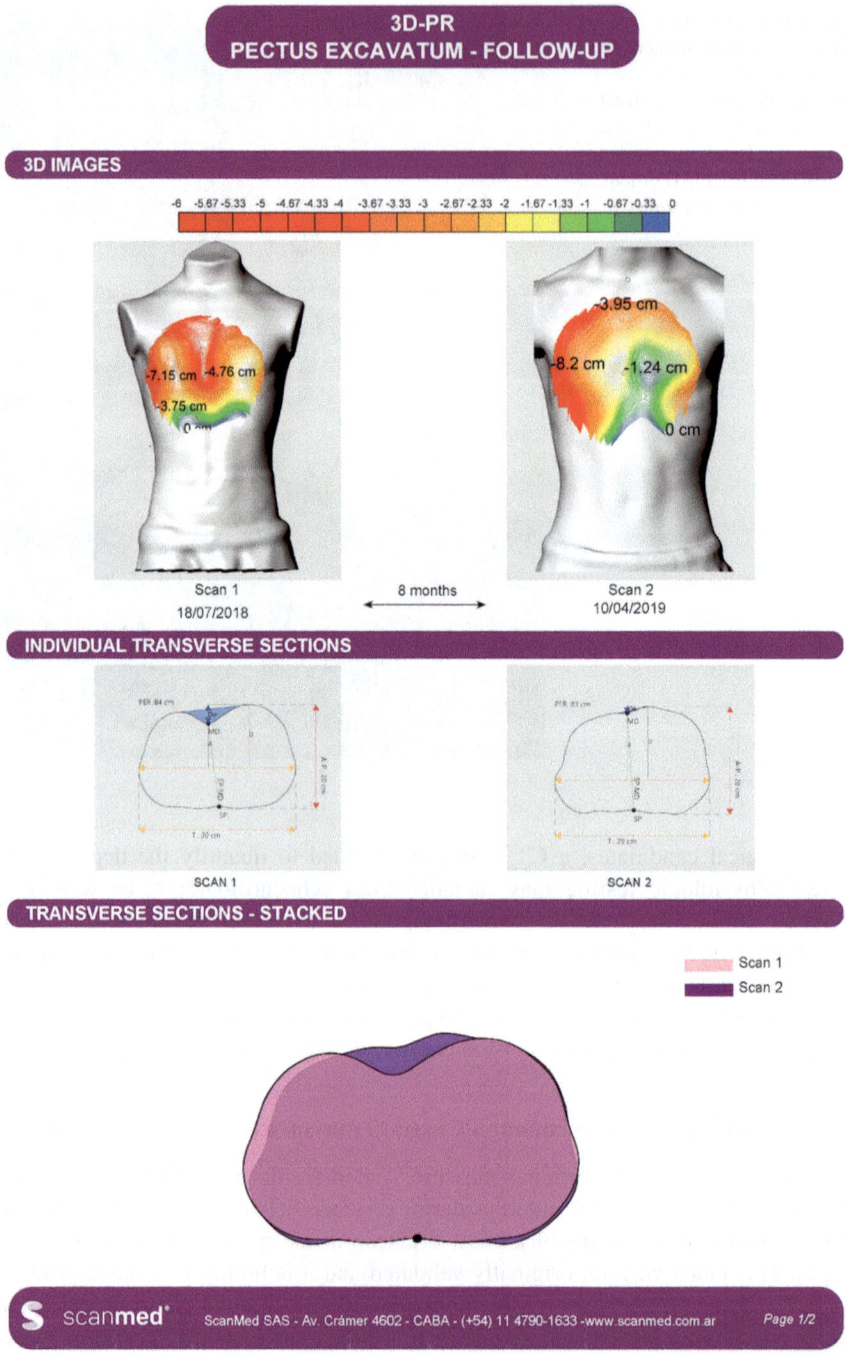

Fig. 3.3 A 3D scanner is used for follow-up. This tool is non-invasive, it does not require radiation, is available at the office and relatively inexpensive when compared to other imaging methods. In this example, this comparative report shows the difference between pre and postoperative transverse section of the chest at the site of maximum depression. Different indexes are determined. In a virtual reconstruction of the anterior chest wall, colours allow an easy interpretation of the geometry of the chest

6. **What is the impact of PEX in the cardiopulmonary function?**

In echocardiographic studies, functional alterations can be found such as ventricular dysfunction during exercise. Employing dynamic cardiac magnetic resonance, 76% of the patients with PEX have shown some degree of right ventricular compression. Recently, reports have demonstrated a relationship between sternal torsion and cardiac compression as well. Normalization of cardiac function and structure has been reported after PEX repair. More studies are currently underway.

7. **What strategies are there for the treatment of PEX?**

There are operative and non-operative treatments for patients with PEX. In most cases, chest wall flexibility determines whether surgery will be necessary to solve the deformity. Chest wall flexibility can be determined manually or utilizing a vacuometer. However, some patients have very dysplastic sternums or rib cages that may require an operation no matter the flexibility they may have.

8. **What is the non-operative treatment for PEX?**

Since the first report in 2005, the use of a Vacuum Bell has become an option for patients with flexible rib cages [1]. This device is usually appropriate for patients under 11 years old with pectus depth less than 1.5 cm and with good compliance, who wear the device as many hours per day as possible. It is noteworthy that an adjustment period of approximately 6 months of the presternal soft tissue is usually needed to avoid local lesions.

9. **In patients with an indication of surgery, what approaches can be used?**

Donald Nuss reported the minimally invasive placement of a retrosternal bar in the '90 s. While many variants are described, open resection of costal cartilages is rare today and is generally reserved for extremely asymmetric or mixed deformities.

10. **What safety measures should be applied during PEX surgery?**

Thoracoscopic guidance is most commonly employed to decrease the possibility of undetected cardiac lacerations when introducing the tunnel dissector. Upward traction on the sternum by vacuum bell or even a crane can be used (Fig. 3.4). A subxiphoid finger can also be used to guide the bar and protect the heart [2].

11. **What is the role of cryoanalgesia in pain control of PEX?**

Cryoanalgesia has recently become a promising strategy for pain control during and after PEX repair. Thoracic cryoanalgesia consists of the transitory demyelination of the 3rd to the 7th intercostal nerves by the application of a cryoprobe for 2 minutes each at −70 degrees Celsius (Fig. 3.5). Randomized trials have demonstrated that cryoanalgesia is superior to thoracic epidural and patient controlled analgesia in terms of length of stay and requirement of complementary opioids.

12. **How long does the bar stay in?**

Usually 2.5–3 years.

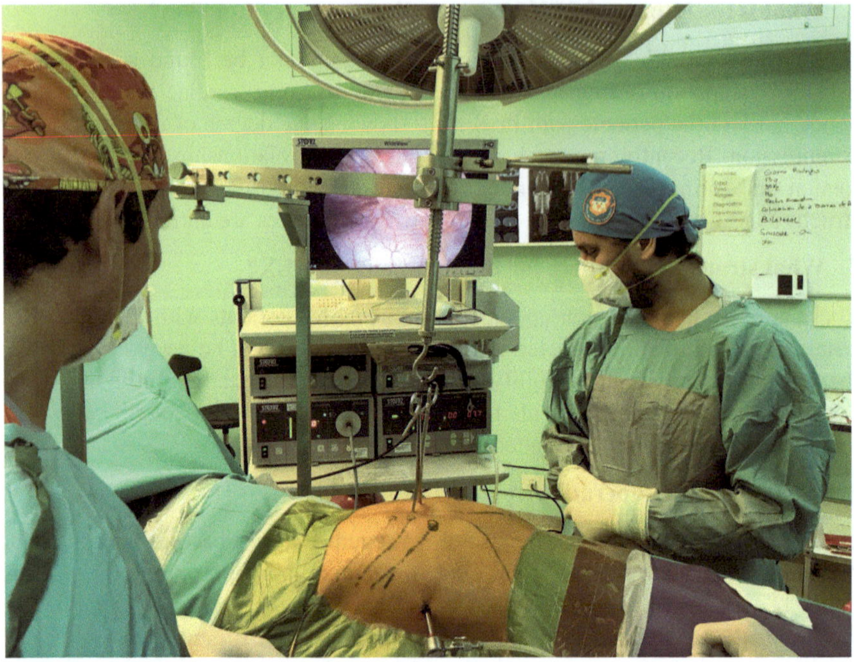

Fig. 3.4 A crane is our preferred option to lift the sternum prior to retrosternal passage of the dissector. This strategy increases the retrosternal space decreasing the possibility of tears to the pericardium or lacerations to the heart. The sternum is pulled-up via a Lewin surgical clamp exerting traction through small lateral incisions

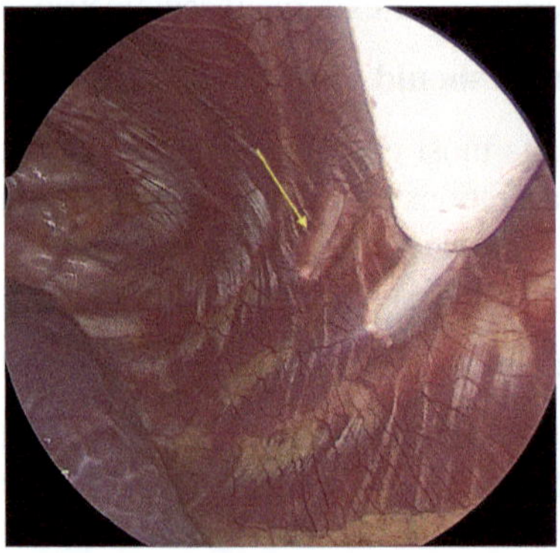

Fig. 3.5 Cryoanalgesia is becoming one of the most interesting strategies for pain control during and after PEX repair. A cryoprobe is introduced to each hemithorax under thoracoscopic guidance. Selective ventilation is performed and the posterior aspect of the intercostal spaces are exposed. The cryoprobe is applied for 2 minutes each space at −70 degrees Celsius. Note the yellow arrow pointing at the previous site of cryoablation

13. **What complications may be found during follow-up?**

Pneumothorax, pleural effusion, and metal allergy. The more serious complications are bar infection and displacement of the implant. The worst complications are related to cardiac or aortic injury during or after PEX repair.

14. **How is Pectus Carinatum (PC) classified?**

PC is classified in chondrogladiolar and chondromanubrial types (Fig. 3.6). If the protrusion involves the caudal third of the sternum, it is called chondrogladiolar, the most frequent variant. The chondromanubrial type is a protrusion of the proximal segment of the sternum and frequently comprises a pectus arcuatum, an atypical variant consisting of a wide, short, unsegmented sternum. If it is associated with a cardiac anomaly it is called Currarino Silverman Syndrome. Also, PC may be classified in symmetrical, asymmetrical and mixed.

15. **How is a patient with PC studied?**

The evaluation of a patient with PC consists of a physical examination with medical photography destined for diagnosis and follow up. CT scans or X-rays are reserved for special cases in which association with skeletal malformations are suspected.

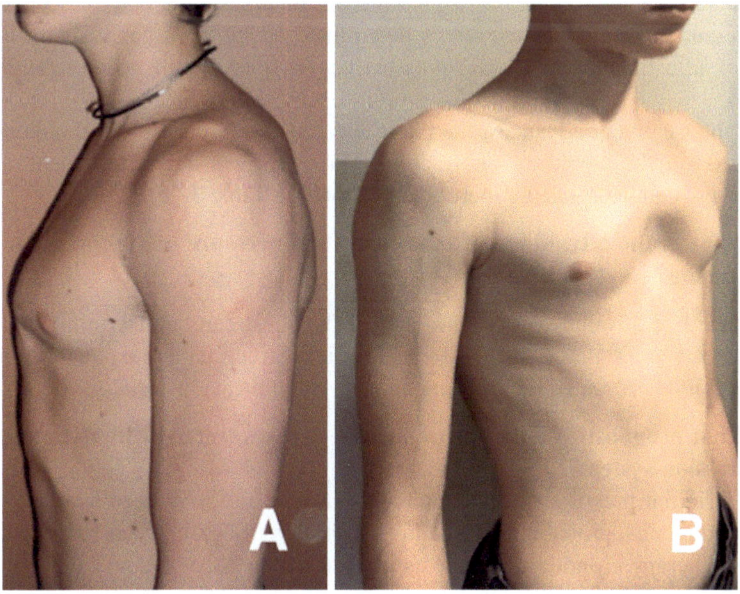

Fig. 3.6 The two most frequent variants of pectus carinatum (PC) are shown. **a** is a teenager with a chondrogladiolar PC in whom the protrusion involves the lower third of the sternum. **b** shows a teenager with a chondromanubrial PC or pectus arcuatum, a very severe form of carinated deformity

In the last years, 3D scanning has become a relevant, radiation-free tool for the workup of chest wall malformations. We perform 3D scans in all patients with PC at the moment of initial diagnosis, during, and after corrective treatments (Fig. 3.7).

16. **What is the impact of PC in the health of patients?**

PC is not an isolated protrusion of a segment of the sternum. Rather, PC consists of a dysplastic rib cage as a whole with posterior asymmetry, disproportionate shoulders, sternal rotation, chondro-costal anomalies, and scoliosis and kyphosis. No cardiopulmonary anomalies are associated. However, the psychosocial impact of PC includes shame, shyness, anguish, anxiety, depression, difficulties with social interactions and sports.

17. **What is the non-operative treatment for PC?**

Bracing is the treatment of choice for most patients. In 2008, we developed and reported the usefulness of a dynamic compressor and a pressure measuring device for this purpose (Fig. 3.8). This device provided objectivity to the amount of pressure to be applied to the chest to correct the protrusion for the first time (pressure of initial correction) and how much pressure to be applied during the different stages of treatment (pressure of treatment).

18. **How are patients with dynamic compression systems followed-up?**

A scheme of gradual increase of pressure of compression is determined. At first, the pressure of initial correction is determined to set up a goal. Then, the first stage of adjustment with a lower pressure begins for 6 months to avoid soft tissue lesions.

As the treatment advances, the chest becomes more elastic and this is evident by a drop in the pressure of correction. Thus, the pressure of treatment and the time of use can be gradually increased as shown in Table 3.1.

19. **What is the advantage of measuring the pressure of compression while bracing?**

There are two advantages: the elasticity of the chest can be determined precisely at diagnosis determining the pressure of initial correction, and damage to the soft tissues can be prevented by avoiding excessive compression initially.

20. **What prognostic factors favor success in cases treated with dynamic compression systems?**

A lower initial pressure of correction and younger age have been associated with improved results, probably due to a higher chest wall flexibility. A longer duration of brace therapy is another variable associated with a good outcome and one of the most important limiting factors of success is the lack of compliance among teenagers [3].

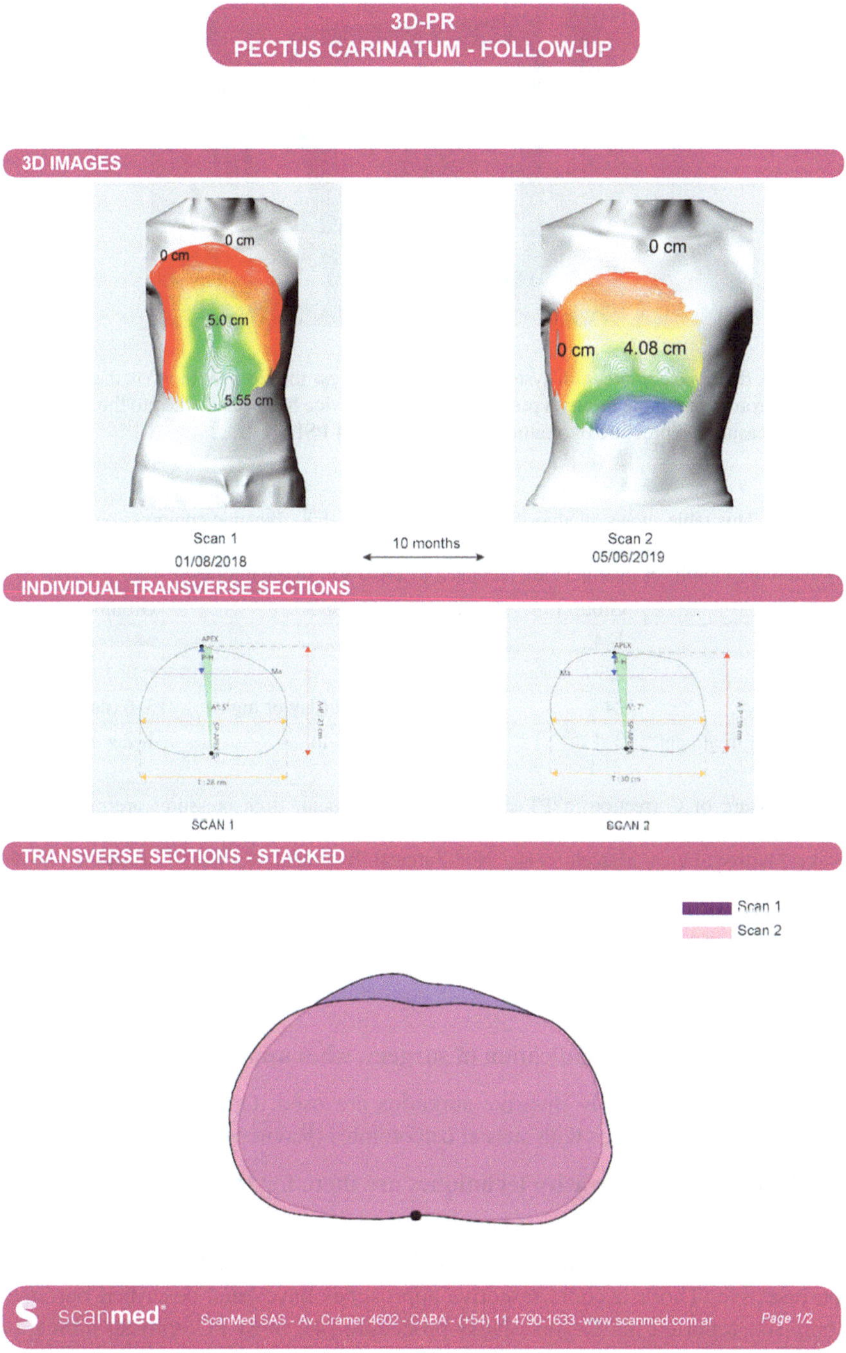

Fig. 3.7 As in PEX, PC cases are followed-up by means of scan 3D. This figure is an example of the variation in the pre and post treatment results of a non-invasive 10 months application of a dynamic compression system

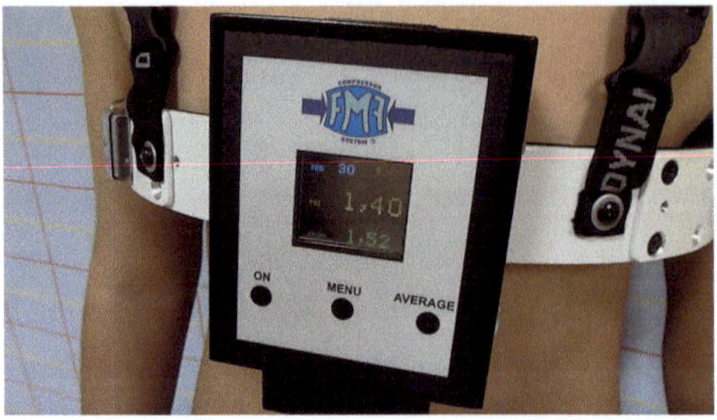

Fig. 3.8 A dynamic compression system is used to compress the sternum in PC at the site of maximal protrusion. In the figure, a pressure measuring device has been docked to the brace in order to measure the pressure of treatment (in this case, 1.4 PSI)

Table 3.1 This table shows an algorithm of use of the FMF® dynamic compression system for PC. As the chest is more rigid, more pressure is necessary to correct the deformity, less hours per day and more months of treatment are indicated to avoid soft tissue injuries

	Group 1	Group 2	Group 3	Group 4
PC*	1–4	4–6	6–8	>8
PT**	2,5	2	1,5	1
Use [hs/day]	24	12 to 24	6–12 (day or night)	3–6 (day or night)
Duration of treatment (approx.)	2–4 m	4–8 m	8–12 m	1–2 y

*PC = Pressure of Correction; **PT = Pressure of Treatment. Both pressures are measured in [PSI-FMF]

Source Martinez-Ferro, Marcelo et al. "Non-Surgical Treatment of Pectus Carinatum with the FMF® dynamic compressor system". *Journal of Visualized Surgery* 2 (2016): 57–57. Publication authors have granted use consent to PAMPAMED S.R.L. Although this Table is a general guideline, treatment can be customized by the physician for each patient considering, amongst other things, individual tolerance, characteristics of the defect, skin status and age

21. **In patients with an indication of surgery, what approaches can be used?**

Both open and minimally invasive surgeries are used. Open techniques involve resecting costal cartilages with sternal osteotomies (Ravitch procedure).

22. **What minimally invasive techniques are there for the operative treatment of PC?**

Minimally invasive techniques for PC can be classified in resective and non-resective. Thoracoscopic resective approaches have been described but since Abramson reported the Reverse-Nuss procedure [4], most PC with an indication of surgery have been resolved with non-resective operations. These last operations aim to remodel the chest wall by means of the introduction of a pre-sternal implant

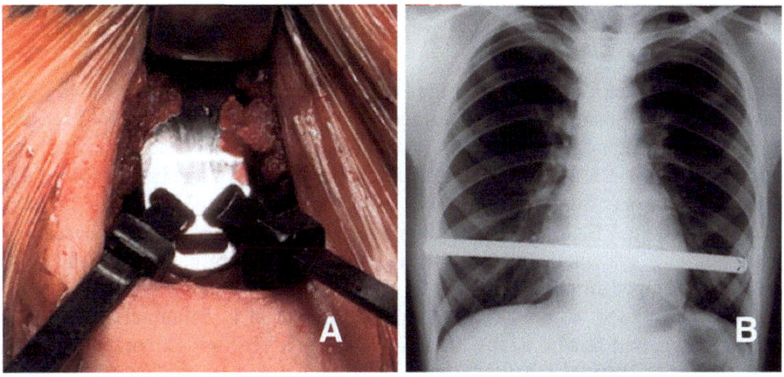

Fig. 3.9 The Zip-back technique is a minimally invasive technique for the treatment of PC. Special features of this operation are represented in (**a**), a magnification of the stabilization mechanism of the implant with zip-ties fixed to the ribs, and (**b**), a chest x-ray showing the implant at place and the absence of lateral stabilizers and wire for fixation

through a subcutaneous tunnel. This implant is stabilized to the ribs by a metal device fixed with wire. There have been several modifications to this technique like the Yüksel technique [5] with a special design of implants and lateral stabilizers depending on the characteristics of the deformity and the Zip-back technique with pre-molded implants, the intraoperative use of a sternal compressor, and the avoidance of lateral stabilizers by employing polymer zip-ties to fix the implants to the ribs (Fig. 3.9). All these modifications are intended to avoid displacement and complications at the time of bar removal.

For asymmetrical PC, Park and Kim have described the Sandwich technique which consists in the utilization of an internal and external bar thus treating at the same time carinatum and excavatum deformities.

23. **How is postoperative follow up done and what complications should be closely looked for?**

The patient is seen at one and two weeks postoperatively, at 1, 2, 4, 6 months and then yearly. Chest x-rays are done by 1 week, 1 month, 4 months, and then yearly.

The implant is removed at 2 or 3 years postoperatively and a 3D scan is done in the immediate preoperative month.

Complications include metal allergy, pleural effusion, foreign body reaction, wound infection, and bar displacement.

24. **What are the future directions in the evolution of diagnosis and treatment of chest wall deformities?**

Defining the cardiopulmonary impact of PEX in the long term is one of the most interesting challenges in the field. In the evolution of the treatment of chest wall deformities, the development of 3D based implants are the next step.

Bibliography

1. Haecker F-M. 15 years clinical application of the vacuum bell for conservative treatment of pectus excavatum—lesions we have learned. J Soc Mech Eng. 2019;121(1201):45. https://doi.org/10.1299/jsmemag.121.1201_45.
2. Nuss D, Obermeyer RJ, Kelly RE Jr. Pectus excavatum from a pediatric surgeon's perspective. Ann Cardiothorac Surg. 2016;5(5):493–500. https://doi.org/10.21037/acs.2016.06.04.
3. de Beer SA, Blom YE, Lopez M, de Jong JR. Measured dynamic compression for pectus carinatum: a systematic review. Semin Pediatr Surg. 2018;27(3):175–82. https://doi.org/10.1053/j.sempedsurg.2018.06.001.
4. Abramson H, Aragone X, Blanco JB, Ciano A, Abramson L. Minimally invasive repair of pectus carinatum and how to deal with complications. J Vis Surg. 2016;2:64–64. https://doi.org/10.21037/jovs.2016.03.111.
5. Yuksel M, Lacin T, Ermerak NO, Sirzai EY, Sayan B. Minimally invasive repair of pectus carinatum. Ann Thorac Surg. 2018;105(3):915–23. https://doi.org/10.1016/j.athoracsur.2017.10.003.

Chapter 4
Congenital Diaphragmatic Hernia

Louise Montalva and Augusto Zani

Abstract Congenital diaphragmatic hernia (CDH) is characterized by the herniation of abdominal organs into the fetal chest through a diaphragmatic defect. The mortality and morbidity rates of babies with CDH remain high, and are directly related to the degree of pulmonary hypoplasia (lung underdevelopment) and the severity of pulmonary hypertension. CDH is typically diagnosed antenatally and observed/expected lung-to-head ratio is a common prenatal prognostic marker of pulmonary hypoplasia. Newborns with CDH often have life-threatening respiratory distress for which immediate intubation at birth is recommended. Moreover, they are usually managed with gentle ventilation, which allows permissive hypercapnia and aims to provide adequate tissue oxygenation, while avoiding barotrauma. Some patients are managed with extracorporeal membrane oxygenation (ECMO) that provides rest to the hypoplastic lungs, allowing them to grow and avoiding ventilation-induced barotrauma. When the neonate is clinically stable, the diaphragmatic repair is performed either from the abdomen (laparotomy or laparoscopy) or from the chest (thoracotomy or thoracoscopy). Large defects that cannot be closed primarily are closed with a synthetic or natural patch. CDH is associated with short- and long-term morbidities; the latter are better addressed in a dedicated multidisciplinary clinic.

Keywords Bochdalek hernia · LHR · ECMO · FETO

L. Montalva · A. Zani
Division of General and Thoracic Surgery, Department of Surgery, The Hospital for Sick Children, University of Toronto, Toronto, Canada

A. Zani (✉)
Division of General and Thoracic Surgery, The Hospital for Sick Children, 1524C-555 University Ave, Toronto, ON M5G 1X8, Canada
e-mail: augusto.zani@sickkids.ca

M. Lacher et al. (eds.), *Pearls and Tricks in Pediatric Surgery*,
https://doi.org/10.1007/978-3-030-51067-1_4

1. **What are the different types of congenital diaphragmatic defects?**

   – Congenital diaphragmatic hernia (CDH), characterized by a defect that is postero-lateral (*Bochdalek hernia*) or anterior (*Morgagni hernia*).
   – Diaphragmatic eventration, characterized by an abnormal elevation of one or both intact hemidiaphragms.

2. **How does the diaphragm form?**

Four structures give rise to the diaphragm between week 4 and 8 of gestation (Fig. 4.1):

– septum transversum (forms the tendinous part of the diaphragm);
– pleuroperitoneal folds;
– thoracic body wall mesenchyme (both from the muscular part of the diaphragm);
– esophageal mesentery (forms the crura).

Bochdalek CDH occurs when a pleuroperitoneal fold fails to close the pleuroperitoneal canal. Morgagni CDH is characterized by a retrosternal herniation through the sternocostal triangle.

3. **What causes CDH to occur?**

The etiology is poorly understood, but CDH seems to be due to a combination of genetic, developmental, and environmental factors.

4. **What is the prevalence of CDH?**

2.3 in 10,000 livebirths.

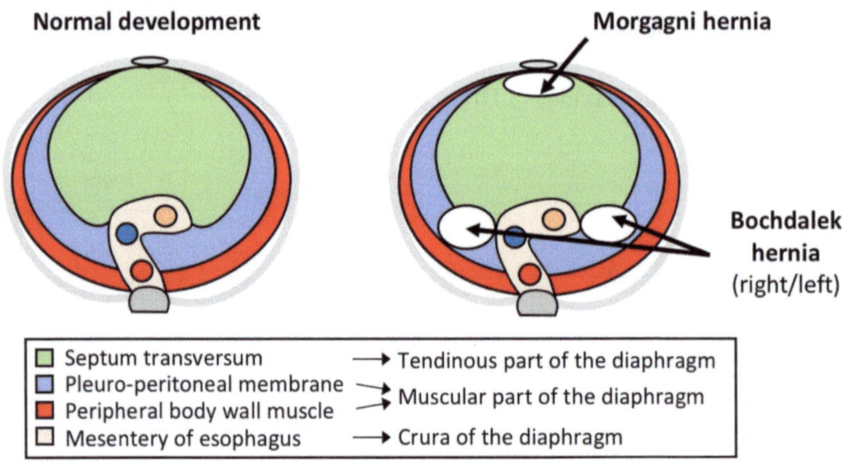

Fig. 4.1 Embryology of the diaphragm

5. **What anomalies can be associated with CDH?**

50% of babies with CDH have at least one associated anomaly.
10–35% have chromosomal abnormalities (trisomy 13, 18, and 21).
Most common anomalies are:

- congenital heart disease (15%)
- defects of the urogenital system (5%)
- musculo-skeletal system (5%)
- central nervous system (5%).

6. **What are the main syndromes associated with CDH?**

Bochdalek CDH

- Pallister-Killian syndrome (mosaic tetrasomy 12p): central nervous system anomalies, short limbs, coarse facial features, and intellectual impairment.
- Fryns syndrome: facial dysmorphism, clefts, hypertelorism, genitourinary, and cardiovascular anomalies.

Morgagni CDH can be part of the pentalogy of Cantrell, characterized by:

- midline supraumbilical abdominal wall defect (exomphalos)
- lower sternum anomaly
- Morgagni hernia
- congenital intracardiac anomalies
- ectopia cordis.

7. **What are the main determinants of morbidity and mortality in babies with CDH?**

- *Pulmonary hypoplasia* (decreased number of alveoli and thickened mesenchyme)
- *Pulmonary hypertension*, due to fetal vascular remodeling (decreased number of vessels and increased muscularization of distal pulmonary vessels).

Prenatal Work-Up

8. **How is CDH prenatally diagnosed and worked-up?**

Around 60–70% of cases are diagnosed prenatally at the anatomy scan (18–20 weeks of gestation), that may show:

- polyhydramnios
- absence of an intra-abdominal stomach
- intra-thoracic abdominal organs
- mediastinal shift.

Additional prenatal evaluations include:

- detailed fetal ultrasound scan
- fetal echocardiography
- amniocentesis.

In some centers, a prenatal magnetic resonance imaging is also performed.

9. **What are the prenatal markers to evaluate prognosis of a fetus with CDH?**

- *Lung-to-head ratio* (LHR), expressed as observed/expected LHR, as it correlates to the degree of pulmonary hypoplasia and to predicted survival (Table 4.1)
- Liver or stomach herniation
- Associated anomalies, such as congenital heart defects
- Chromosomal anomalies (fetal karyotype or microarray).

10. **After prenatal diagnosis, what is the current prenatal management of fetuses with CDH?**

It is expectant, with ultrasound surveillance for fetal growth and development, parental counseling, and maternal steroids only if at risk of preterm delivery.

11. **When and where should a baby with prenatally diagnosed CDH be delivered?**

Scheduled full term delivery in a tertiary center at early term (37–38 weeks).

12. **What treatment can be offered prenatally?**

Surgical repair in utero was proven to be associated with increased fetal demise. Currently, the only available prenatal intervention for fetuses with predicted severe pulmonary hypoplasia is the fetoscopic endo-tracheal occlusion (FETO), which entails the intra-tracheal deployment of a small balloon under fetoscopy at 26–28 weeks of gestation. The balloon avoids the egression of the pulmonary fluid and keeps the lungs expanded. At around 34 weeks of gestation, the balloon is removed. Experimentally, FETO has been reported to improve lung growth and it is currently being evaluated by a randomized controlled trial (TOTAL trial).

Table 4.1 Correlation of the observed/expected lung-to-head ratio (O/E LHR) with the degree of pulmonary hypoplasia and predicted survival

O/E LHR (%)	Degree of pulmonary hypoplasia	Predicted survival (%)
<15	Extreme	0
15–25	Severe	20
26–45	Moderate	30–60
>45	Mild	>75

Nonetheless, FETO is associated with the risk of premature rupture of membranes and preterm birth.

Postnatal Management

13. **What is the postnatal management of a newborn with CDH?**

- Immediate intubation with sedation for assisted ventilation to all neonates with prenatal/postnatal diagnosis CDH. No mask ventilation as it distends the herniated stomach/intestine [1]. Deep sedation and neuromuscular blockade should be avoided.
- Intravenous access + arterial line (preferably into the right radial artery), with a restrictive fluid management in the first 24 hours of life (40 ml/kg/day) [2].
- Nasogastric tube placement for gastrointestinal decompression.
- Thorough physical exam looking for associated anomalies.
- Chest x-ray (two views).
- Echocardiography in the first 48 hours of life (to be repeated at 2–3 weeks of life) to assess cardiac anatomy, severity of pulmonary hypertension, presence/direction of ductal and intracardiac shunting, and left and right ventricular function.
- Parenteral feeding [2].

Use of surfactant is not recommended in term CDH neonates.

14. **What are the postnatal markers of prognosis?**

Several clinical prediction models have been developed, and contain variables such as:

- Birth weight
- Apgar score
- Blood gases, such as highest PaO2, lowest PaCO2, and best oxygenation index (BOI) on day1 that is calculated as follows:

$$\text{BOI (d1)} = \frac{\text{FiO}_2\text{\% x MAP(cmH}_2\text{O)}}{\text{PaO}_2\text{ (kPa)}}$$

(where MAP is the mean arterial pressure)

- Pulmonary hypertension
- Chromosomal and major cardiac anomalies.

15. **What is the recommended ventilation strategy?**

CDH neonates are managed with gentle ventilation ("gentilation"), which allows permissive hypercapnia and aims to provide adequate tissue oxygenation, while avoiding barotrauma. The recommended initial ventilator settings are [3]:

- peak inspiratory pressure (PIP): <25 cm H_20;
- positive end-expiratory pressure (PEEP): 2–5 cm H_20 with a frequency of 40–60/min

Oxygen is administered with the goal of a preductal $SaO_2 > 85\%$ and arterial pCO_2 45–60 mmHg (permissive hypercapnia) [4]. If conventional ventilation fails, high frequency oscillatory or jet ventilation are used [3].

16. **What hemodynamic support can be provided in case of poor systemic perfusion and/or pulmonary hypertension?**

Poor perfusion and low systemic blood pressure can be managed with crystalloid infusion (not exceeding 20 mL/kg), inotropes (dopamine or epinephrine), and hydrocortisone. If poor perfusion continues, the cardiac function should be assessed by echocardiography and central venous saturation.

Pulmonary hypertension can be managed by various therapies, such as:

- Oxygen.
- Inhaled nitric oxide (iNO) should be considered for patients with severe suprasystemic pulmonary arterial hypertension, preserved left ventricular function, and adequate lung recruitment. However, in case of no clinical or echocardiographic improvement, iNO should be discontinued.
- Sildenafil is a phosphodiesterase-5 inhibitor that can be considered in case of refractory pulmonary hypertension with no response to iNO or when weaning from iNO.
- Milrinone is a phosphodiesterase-3 inhibitor that can be considered in case of cardiac dysfunction associated to refractory pulmonary hypertension as it can improve ventricular function and blood gas parameters.
- Prostacyclin, a potent vasodilator, and its analogues (e.g. treprostinil) can be used in case of refractory pulmonary hypertension. Prostaglandin E1 can be used to maintain ductus arteriosus patency and reduce right ventricular afterload.
- Extracorporeal membrane oxygenation (ECMO).

17. **What is the role of ECMO in babies with CDH?**

ECMO functions as a heart-lung bypass, with the rationale to provide rest to the hypoplastic lungs, allowing them to grow and avoiding ventilation-induced barotrauma. However, the indication for and use of ECMO are center-dependent and available evidence shows that survival for neonates with CDH is not affected by the use of ECMO.

Possible candidates for ECMO are CDH babies with refractory hypoxemia (preductal $SaO_2 < 85\%$, postductal $SaO_2 < 70\%$), oxygenation index ≥ 40 for at least 3 h, persistent acidosis (lactate > 5 mmol/L; pH < 7.2), persistent hypercapnia ($pCO_2 > 70$ mmHg, with FiO_2 100%) and/or hypotension resistant to fluid and inotrope therapy [2]. Relative contraindications include weight < 2 kg, gestational age < 34 weeks, intraventricular hemorrhage (grade $\geq$ 2), or bleeding disorders [2].

Surgical Treatment

18. **When is the optimal timing for CDH repair?**

- CDH is not considered a surgical emergency and preoperative stabilization before surgery is essential.
- Most surgeons would not perform CDH repair during the first day of life, as some babies may be in a "honeymoon period" of clinical stability before developing a pulmonary hypertensive crisis.
- Nonetheless, timing for CDH repair remains controversial, as it does not influence survival after adjusting for disease severity.

19. **What are the possible surgical approaches for CDH repair?**

Diaphragmatic repair can be performed from the abdomen (laparotomy or laparoscopy) or from the chest (thoracotomy or thoracoscopy) (Table 4.2). The most commonly used approach is laparotomy [5].

Table 4.2 Surgical approaches for CDH repair

	Advantages	Disadvantages
Open approach		
Laparotomy	- Good visualization - Diagnosis ± correction of associated malrotation - Inspection of reduced organs - Excision of hernia sac if present	- Cosmesis - Postoperative pain - Risk of adhesive small bowel obstruction
Thoracotomy	- Main indication for right CDH - Useful in hernia recurrence	- Cosmesis - Postoperative pain - No bowel inspection - Difficult reduction
Minimally-invasive approach		
Laparoscopy	- Cosmesis - Pain control - Less risk of adhesions	- Longer operating time - Learning curve - Less widely used - Difficult organ visualization - Difficult organ reduction
Thoracoscopy	- Cosmesis - Pain control - Less risk of small bowel obstruction	- Learning curve - Longer operating time - Higher recurrence rate - Intra-operative acidosis and hypercapnia

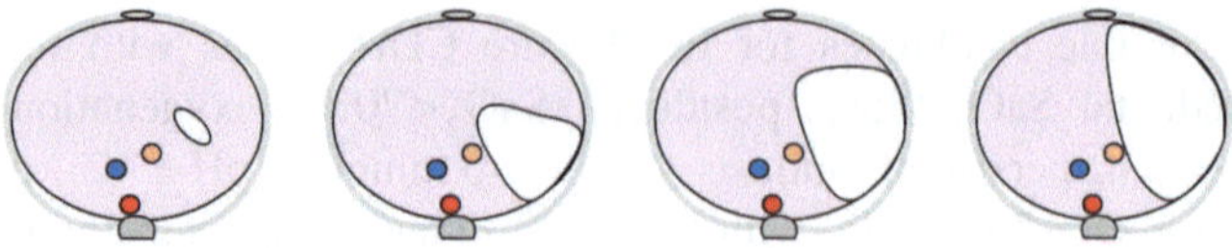

CDHSG stage	A	B	C	D
Size of defect (% of hemi-diaphragm)	<10%	<50%	>50%	agenesis
Incidence	14%	40%	33%	13%
Mortality	<1%	5%	23%	46%
Early recurrence	1.1%	1.2%	3.2%	4.4%

Fig. 4.2 Defect size and associated survival rates (CDH Study Group classification—[6])

20. **What are the main steps of CDH surgery?**

(1) Gentle and cautious reduction of the hernia contents back into the abdomen. Division of the umbilical vein and falciform ligament allows the liver rotation and reduction (especially in right-sided CDH with liver herniation, where hepatic veins and inferior vena cava are at risk of kinking).
(2) Assessment of hernia defect for *size* (Fig. 4.2) [6], presence of sac (in 20% of cases), and diaphragmatic tissue available for repair (the pericostal rim might not be present and needs to be developed to allow repair).
(3) Surgical repair with non-absorbable sutures:

   a. Small defects—primary repair with interrupted non-absorbable sutures on the edge of the diaphragm
   b. If muscle edges can be approximated, avoid a tight closure (high recurrence risk)
   c. Large defects—repair with a natural or synthetic patch (the commonest is GoreTex®, made of polytetrafluoroethylene) or autologous muscle flap (the commonest is the transversus abdominis).

The placement of a chest tube is not recommended.

Postnatal Management

21. **How should a neonate with CDH be managed after surgery?**

- gradually de-escalate mechanical ventilation
- no evidence for postoperative paralysis
- enteral feeding can be started when postoperative ileus is resolved, and antireflux therapy should be started.

22. **What are the main surgical complications?**

Short-term

- Infection/sepsis
- Bleeding (mainly neonates treated with ECMO at the time of surgery)

- Early recurrence (2%, higher risk in defects size C and D, and cases repaired with minimally invasive surgery) [6]
- Chylothorax (5%, higher risk following patch repair and in neonates treated on ECMO)
- Pleural effusion (common, rarely requiring a drain as it will resolve with lung expansion)
- Abdominal compartment syndrome.

Long-term

- CDH recurrence (7–15%, higher risk after patch repair, in right-sided CDH, and in infants treated with ECMO)
- Adhesive small bowel obstruction (20%, higher risk after patch repair; the majority requires surgery)

23. **What long-term morbidities can affect children born with CDH?**

Respiratory

– Long-term pulmonary dysfunction (50%, secondary to pulmonary hypoplasia and prolonged ventilation).

Digestive

– Gastro-esophageal reflux (10–20% require fundoplication)
– Failure to thrive (1/3 of survivors<5 percentile at one year of age, 20% requiring tube feeds).

Musculo-skeletal

– Chest wall or spinal deformities (1/3 of survivors has scoliosis, pectus excavatum, chest asymmetry).

Neurodevelopmental

– Impairment affects 25% survivors (neuromuscular hypotonia, hearing and visual impairment, neurobehavioral issues, and learning difficulties).

To address CDH morbidities, a dedicated multidisciplinary (surgery, neonatology, pulmonology, gastroenterology, nutrition, neurology, audiology, orthopedics) follow-up is recommended.

References

1. Canadian Congenital Diaphragmatic Hernia Collaborative, Puligandla PS, Skarsgard ED, Offringa M, Adatia I, Baird R, Bailey M, Brindle M, Chiu P, Cogswell A, Dakshinamurti S, Flageole H, Keijzer R, McMillan D, Oluyomi-Obi T, Pennaforte T, Perreault T, Piedboeuf B, Riley SP, Ryan G, Synnes A, Traynor M. Diagnosis and management of congenital diaphragmatic hernia: a clinical practice guideline. CMAJ. 2018;190(4):E103–12.
2. Snoek KG, Reiss IK, Greenough A, Capolupo I, Urlesberger B, Wessel L, Storme L, Deprest J, Schaible T, van Heijst A, Tibboel D; CDH EURO Consortium. Standardized Postnatal

Management of Infants with Congenital Diaphragmatic Hernia in Europe: The CDH EURO Consortium Consensus—2015 Update. Neonatology. 2016;110(1):66–74.
3. Puligandla PS, Grabowski J, Austin M, Hedrick H, Renaud E, Arnold M, Williams RF, Graziano K, Dasgupta R, McKee M, Lopez ME, Jancelewicz T, Goldin A, Downard CD, Islam S. Management of congenital diaphragmatic hernia: a systematic review from the APSA outcomes and evidence based practice committee. J Pediatr Surg. 2015;50(11):1958–70.
4. Jancelewicz T, Brindle ME, Guner YS, Lally PA, Lally KP, Harting MT; Congenital Diaphragmatic Hernia Study Group (CDHSG); Pediatric Surgery Research Collaborative (PedSRC). Toward standardized management of congenital diaphragmatic hernia: an analysis of practice guidelines. J Surg Res. 2019;243:229–35.
5. Zani A, Zani-Ruttenstock E, Pierro A. Advances in the surgical approach to congenital diaphragmatic hernia. Semin Fetal Neonatal Med. 2014;19(6):364–9.
6. Harting MT, Lally KP. The congenital diaphragmatic hernia study group registry update. Semin Fetal Neonatal Med. 2014;19(6):370–5.

Chapter 5
Esophageal Atresia With or Without Tracheoesophageal Fistula

Christina M. Bence and Dave R. Lal

Abstract Esophageal atresia with or without tracheoesophageal fistula is a congenital anomaly resulting from abnormal embryonic development of the foregut. It is frequently associated with other congenital anomalies and genetic syndromes, most commonly congenital heart disease. Prior to the advent of surgical repair in 1941, EA was a universally fatal diagnosis. Current management strategies have now improved survival of EA to over 90%. This chapter reviews the diagnostic workup, associated comorbidities, operative considerations, and common postoperative complications related to esophageal atresia with or without tracheoesophageal fistula.

Keywords Esophageal atresia · Tracheoesophageal fistula · VACTERL

Content:

1. **How common is esophageal atresia (EA) with or without tracheoesophageal fistula (TEF)?** [1]

The worldwide prevalence of EA is estimated at 2–3 per 10,000 births, and 70–90% are associated with TEF. Spontaneous intrauterine fetal demise occurs in ~3% of cases.

C. M. Bence
Division of Pediatric Surgery, The Medical College of Wisconsin, Milwaukee, WI, USA
e-mail: cbence@mcw.edu

D. R. Lal (✉)
Division of Pediatric Surgery, The Medical College of Wisconsin, 999 North 92nd Street, Suite CCC 320, Milwaukee, WI 53226, USA
e-mail: dlal@mcw.edu

M. Lacher et al. (eds.), *Pearls and Tricks in Pediatric Surgery*,
https://doi.org/10.1007/978-3-030-51067-1_5

2. **What is the etiology of EA?** [1]

EA is a congenital anomaly that results from abnormal embryonic development of the foregut. The exact mechanisms are unknown, yet the process likely involves a combination of genetic, environmental, and biomechanical factors.

3. **Which genetic syndromes and other congenital anomalies are associated with EA/TEF?** [1, 2]

The most common congenital anomalies associated with EA/TEF involve the Vertebral, Anorectal, Cardiac, TEF, Renal and Limb abnormality (VACTERL) spectrum of disorders (Table 5.1). Nearly 70% of infants with EA will have at least one other associated anomaly, most commonly cardiac (~35%), with many patients having multiple. Associated chromosomal abnormalities include trisomies 18 and 21, as well as CHARGE syndrome.

4. **What are the relationships between prematurity, low birth weight, and EA/TEF?** [3]

Up to one-third of patients with EA are born prematurely, likely due to associated polyhydramnios. Low birth weight infants with EA have a higher risk of mortality than their normal weight counterparts, and often surgical repair is delayed until infants reach 1,500–2,000 g to lower the risk of operative morbidity.

5. **What is the mortality associated with EA/TEF?** [2]

Prior to the first successful EA/TEF repair in 1941, mortality of this disorder was 100%. Survival has steadily increased over time and is currently>90%. Mortality is primarily related to the associated comorbidities of congenital heart disease and prematurity.

6. **How is EA classified?** [1, 2, 4]

The most widely used classification system for EA/TEF is the Gross classification, which includes types A–E (Fig. 5.1). As is shown in Fig. 5.1, the most common malformation is Gross Type C, which involves EA associated with a distal TEF. Gross Type E has no atresia but instead an isolated, or "H-type" TEF.

Table 5.1 Other congenital anomalies associated with esophageal atresia and their respective incidences

Associated anomaly	Incidence (%)
Cardiac	35
Renal	23
Vertebral	22
Anorectal	20
Limb	14
Chromosomal	11

From Lal D, et al. Perioperative management and outcomes of esophageal atresia and tracheoesophageal fistula. *J Pediatr Surg.* 2017;52(8):1245–1251

7. **How is EA diagnosed?** [1, 3]

Prenatal diagnosis of EA is about 20% in patients with EA/TEF and over 50% in patients with isolated EA. Prenatal imaging findings that are indicative of EA include polyhydramnios, a small or absent stomach bubble, and a dilated upper esophageal pouch ("pouch sign"). The sensitivity and specificity of prenatal diagnosis are significantly improved with MRI over ultrasound.

After birth, infants with EA commonly present with early feeding intolerance and increased oral secretions that can lead to respiratory compromise. The diagnosis of EA is confirmed with failed attempts at orogastric tube placement followed by an abdominal x-ray demonstrating coiling of the enteric tube within the proximal esophageal pouch. The presence of an associated distal TEF is indicated by the finding of gas within the stomach and/or intestine.

8. **What further clinical workup is recommended following the diagnosis of EA/TEF?**

Further workup is aimed at determining EA type, evaluating for the presence of a TEF, estimating esophageal gap length (distance between the proximal and distal esophageal pouches), and assessing for other anomalies (VACTERL). An x-ray of the chest and abdomen can diagnose a TEF if intestinal gas is present, estimate the length of the proximal esophageal pouch by placing gentle downward traction on the oral-esophageal (OE) tube, and identify vertebral anomalies. Preoperative laryngotracheobronchoscopy is used to assess for coexisting laryngeal clefts and to

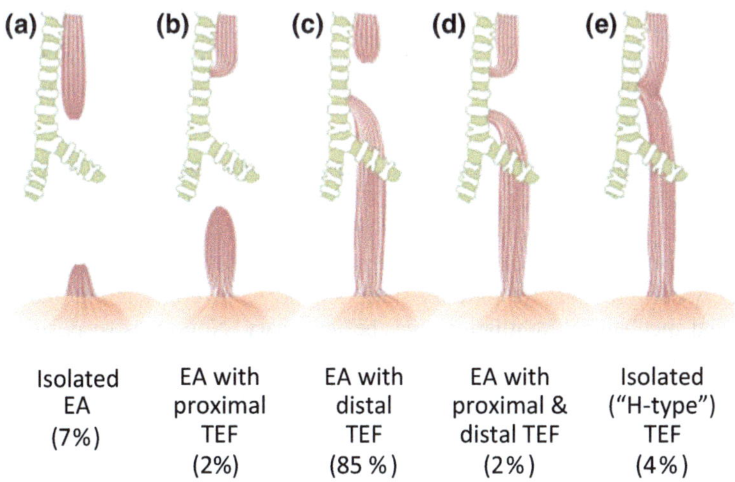

Fig. 5.1 Gross classification of esophageal atresia (EA) with or without tracheoesophageal fistula (TEF), including overall incidence (%) of each type (adapted from van der Zee DC, et al. Esophageal atresia and tracheo-esophageal fistula. *Semin Pediatr Surg*. 2017; 26(2):67–71.)

identify the location of a TEF. Occasionally pre-operative fluoroscopy is utilized to diagnose EA and determine EA type and gap length.

Echocardiogram is essential prior to EA repair to identify congenital heart disease and to determine the side of the aortic arch. Approximately 5% of EA/TEF patients will have a right sided aortic arch, and this may alter the decision regarding which side the surgical repair should be performed on. Lastly, renal ultrasound and anorectal exam are performed to evaluate for renal anomalies and anorectal malformations.

9. **How is long gap atresia defined and what is its impact on management?** [1]

The term "gap length" refers to the distance between the proximal and distal esophageal pouches, and primary EA repair can be difficult or impossible to achieve if the gap is long. There is no consensus on the specific definition of long gap EA, however it is often described by the number of vertebral bodies present between the two ends of esophagus (typically 2–5), the gap length in centimeters (typically 2–5 cm), or based on a surgeon's intraoperative gestalt.

10. **How can one assess esophageal gap length preoperatively?**

Gap length can be evaluated preoperatively by plain film or fluoroscopy. The length of the proximal pouch is estimated by placing gentle downward traction on the OE tube while an x-ray is taken. In patients with Type C or D EA/TEF, the esophageal length can be estimated by using the carina on x-ray as a landmark for the proximal extent of the distal pouch. Therefore, esophageal gap length can be predicted by the distance between the distal extent of the proximal pouch and the carina on x-ray. In patients with Type A or B EA that have a gastrostomy tube in place, fluoroscopy can be utilized to determine the length of the distal pouch either via contrast administration alone or by inserting a guidewire, endoscope, or metal probe retrograde through the g-tube site and advancing into the distal pouch.

11. **What are the important aspects of preoperative management in the setting of EA/TEF?**

Immediately following a diagnosis of EA, the patient should be positioned in reverse-Trendelenburg position and an OE tube placed to continuous suction with its tip located just above the distal end of the proximal esophageal pouch. Adequate decompression of the proximal pouch is essential to prevent aspiration and further respiratory compromise. Respiratory status should be carefully monitored as intubation and mechanical ventilation may be necessary. Non-invasive positive pressure strategies should be avoided as they can result in significant gastric distention when a TEF is present. If severe gastric distention occurs and impedes ventilation, emergent percutaneous decompression of the stomach using a large-bore needle can be lifesaving. Other options for management of severe gastric distention include placing a gastrostomy tube, advancing the endotracheal tube past the fistula in intubated patients, and finally ligating and dividing the TEF if all else fails.

12. **When should initial TEF ligation be considered prior to definitive EA repair?**

TEF ligation may be necessary prior to definitive EA repair if the fistula is causing physiologic compromise and EA repair is delayed due to patient size, long gap length, or other reasons.

13. **How do outcomes of thoracoscopic versus standard thoracotomy approaches compare for EA/TEF repair?** [5]

A recent meta-analysis comparing open and thoracoscopic approaches to esophagoesophagostomy for EA/TEF repair found no differences in outcomes including anastomotic leak rate, esophageal stricture rate, pulmonary complications, time to first oral feeding, or blood loss. Thoracoscopic repair was found to decrease postoperative ventilation time and length of stay, though operative times were significantly longer compared to open repair.

14. **What are surgical options for long gap EA if primary esophagoesophagostomy is not possible?**

The least invasive option is placement of a gastrostomy tube followed by delayed primary repair, generally after waiting a period of ~12 weeks. This theoretically allows the esophageal pouches to lengthen from somatic growth as well as a combination of pooled oral secretions (proximal pouch) and gastroesophageal reflux (distal pouch). Other options for esophageal lengthening include circular or spiral myotomy, the Kimura extrathoracic lengthening procedure, and the Foker staged suture-traction method. Finally, esophageal replacement with a stomach, colon, or small bowel interposition graft may be required if esophageal preservation is not feasible.

15. **What postoperative complications are most common following EA/TEF repair?** [6]

Over 60% of patients undergoing EA/TEF repair will have a post-operative complication, with the most common being anastomotic stricture (>40%). Other common complications include anastomotic leaks (~20%), recurrent fistulas (~5%), and vocal cord paralysis (~5%). Recent research has found associations between the use of transanastomotic esophageal tubes with increased rates of anastomotic stricture, as well as placement of prosthetic material between the esophageal and tracheal suture lines with increased rates of anastomotic leak.

16. **What long-term comorbidities are associated with EA following repair?** [1]

Dysphagia, esophageal dysmotility, gastroesophageal reflux (GERD) and respiratory conditions such as wheezing and recurrent infections are common problems that persist following EA/TEF repair and must be managed over a lifetime.

17. **Are there guidelines for the management of GERD and subsequent screening for Barrett esophagus and malignancy later in life?** [1]

Due to the nearly 4-fold increased risk of Barrett esophagus identified in adults with repaired congenital EA and the relative lack of reported GERD symptoms in this population, current guidelines recommend performing lifelong endoscopic surveillance (with multistaged biopsies) starting before the age of 15 years. Further, fundoplication should be considered in the setting of recurrent esophageal stricture, respiratory complications, or medically refractory GERD.

18. **What is known about the quality of life (QOL) for individuals who were born with EA?**

Though there is relatively little data regarding QOL in older patients born with EA, overall adult survivors report their health-related QOL to be equivalent to that of the general population.

References

1. Van Lennep M, Singendonk MMJ, Dall'Oglio L, et al. Oesophageal atresia. Nat Rev Dis Primers. 2019;5(1):26.
2. Lal DR, Gadepalli SK, Downard CD, et al. Perioperative management and outcomes of esophageal atresia and tracheoesophageal fistula. J Pediatr Surg. 2017;52(8):1245–51.
3. Sfeir R, Bonnard A, Khen-Dunlop N, et al. Esophageal atresia: Data from a national cohort. J Pediatr Surg. 2013;48(8):1664–9.
4. van der Zee DC, Tytgat SHA, van Herwaarden MYA. Esophageal atresia and tracheo-esophageal fistula. Semin Pediatr Surg. 2017;26(2):67–71.
5. Wu Y, Kuang H, Lv T, Wu C. Comparison of clinical outcomes between open and thoracoscopic repair for esophageal atresia with tracheoesophageal fistula: a systematic review and meta-analysis. Pediatr Surg Int. 2017;33(11):1147–57.
6. Lal DR, Gadepalli SK, Downard CD, et al. Challenging surgical dogma in the management of proximal esophageal atresia with distal esophageal fistula: outcomes from the midwest pediatric surgery consortium. J Pediatr Surg. 2018;53(7):1267–72.

Chapter 6
Gastroesophageal Reflux Disease

Charlene Dekonenko and George W. Holcomb III

Abstract Gastroesophageal reflux disease (GERD) results from persistent gastroesophageal reflux (GER) leading to bothersome symptoms and/or complications. Certain pediatric patient populations are at increased risk for GERD, such as those with certain congenital defects and those with neurologic impairment. While studies can be used to aid in characterizing reflux, diagnosis is clinical. Treatment options include non-pharmacological, pharmacologic, and surgical approaches. Pediatric surgeons must be able to recognize symptoms of GERD and determine when surgical management is the optimal method of treatment.

Keywords Gastroesophageal reflux disease · Fundoplication · Transient lower esophageal sphincter relaxations · Esophagitis

1. **What is the difference between GER and GERD?**

GER: involuntary retrograde passage of gastric contents into the esophagus with/without regurgitation or vomiting.

GERD: persistent troublesome symptoms and/or complications of GER that affect quality of life (QOL).

C. Dekonenko · G. W. Holcomb III (✉)
Children's Mercy Kansas City, 2401 Gillham Road, Kansas City, MO 64108, United States
e-mail: gholcomb3@outlook.com

C. Dekonenko
e-mail: cdekonenko@cmh.edu

M. Lacher et al. (eds.), *Pearls and Tricks in Pediatric Surgery*,
https://doi.org/10.1007/978-3-030-51067-1_6

2. **What are the normal physiologic defense mechanisms to the development of GERD?**

Prevention of reflux: 12–25 mmHg resting LES pressure, acute angle of His, intra-abdominal esophagus length, relative increased intra-abdominal pressure.

Limitation of injury: saliva, decreased gastric acid, pepsin, trypsin, and bile acid levels.

Clearance of refluxate: saliva, esophageal peristalsis, effect of gravity [1].

3. **Describe the physiology of normal neonatal reflux**

Transient lower esophageal sphincter relaxations (TLESRs) occur independent of swallowing and last 5–30 seconds, allowing gastric refluxate to contact the esophageal mucosa. Neonates also have a short esophagus and lack coordination of esophageal contractions which can cause inadequate clearance of refluxate.

4. **How do symptoms of GERD vary by age?**

Neonates: breath holding, sneezing, coughing, choking, back arching, grimacing, swallowing/feeding difficulties, failure to thrive (FTT), aspiration pneumonia, apparent life-threatening events (ALTE).

Infants: vomiting, chronic respiratory problems, sleeping problems, apnea, inconsolable crying/irritability, poor weight gain, food refusal.

Adolescents: retrosternal/epigastric pain, chronic cough, bronchitis, dysphagia, hoarseness, sore throat, hematochezia/melena from gastritis, esophagitis, ulcers.

5. **What congenital anomalies are associated with an increased incidence of GERD?**

The incidence of GERD is ≈30% in children with abdominal wall defects. It is higher in children with larger defects and those with omphalocele compared to gastroschisis.

GERD complicates repair of esophageal atresia in 40–65% with up to 90% receiving some kind of treatment for GERD after repair. Up to 30% may require an anti-reflux procedure.

6. **What is the incidence of GER in patients who are neurologically impaired?**

Up to 75% of neurologically impaired (NI) patients have GER, likely due to the dysregulation of aerodigestive reflexes and increased spasticity. Retching and poor swallowing mechanisms lead to gagging and/or choking that increase abdominal pressure, potential development of a hiatal hernia, predisposing them to GERD.

7. **Does a gastrostomy for feeding increase the risk of GERD?**

Gastrostomy can widen the angle of His causing loss of the natural protective mechanism at the gastroesophageal junction. Open gastrostomy is more likely to result in the need for subsequent fundoplication compared to percutaneous gastrostomy. Laparoscopic gastrostomy has been shown to improve gastric emptying which reduces GER, and the subsequent need for fundoplication.

8. **Describe outcomes of surgically treated GERD in NI children?**

Mortality and major complications are more common in NI children, but may be due to the underlying neurological disease or other comorbidities. There are no differences in early complications, recurrence, or parent satisfaction following the fundoplication in comparison to non-NI patients. QOL is improved after fundoplication compared to prior to fundoplication in NI patients.

9. **How is GERD diagnosed in children?**

There are low levels of evidence for the accuracy of diagnostic tests for GERD in children. Reflux on an upper gastrointestinal series doesn't always correlate with reflux symptoms. It can be useful to rule out other diagnoses, or to evaluate the integrity/location of the fundoplication wrap in the setting of post-surgical symptoms.

An esophagogastroduodenoscopy (EGD) has a low negative predictive value. It can be used to rule out eosinophilic esophagitis, Crohn disease, or Barrett esophagus.

pH monitoring with multiple intraluminal impedance (MII) can distinguish acid from non-acid, antegrade versus retrograde flow, and liquid versus gas versus mixed content of refluxate. Its limitations include a weak association between the study findings and the need for fundoplication [2].

Diagnosis is clinical via a thorough history and physical exam. A trial of acid suppression medication is not recommended in infants, but can be trialed in older children and adolescents with classic symptoms.

10. **What are the pathologic findings on EGD and bronchoscopy in a patient with GERD?**

Evidence of erosive esophagitis manifests as visible mucosal breaks, ulcers, and metaplasia. On biopsy, one may find H. pylori, eosinophils, papillary lengthening, and basal cell hyperplasia. Bronchoscopy and laryngoscopy may show generalized erythema, ulceration, and/or pseudopolyps.

11. **How is radionucleotide scintigraphy useful in patients with GERD?**

Radionucleotide tracer seen in bronchi suggests aspiration from oropharyngeal aspiration of the tracer or from refluxed contents. It is helpful when GERD is non-responsive to treatment, if delayed gastric emptying (DGE) is suspected, or to evaluate for failure and/or transmigration of a wrap.

12. **Describe the non-medical approaches for the treatment for GER in infants.**

Thickening feeds, administration of a reduced volume of feeds, a 2–4 week trial of extensively hydrolyzed protein/amino acid formula, and positional therapy with head of bed elevation and/or left lateral positioning in older children.

13. **What are the pharmacologic agents used for the treatment of GERD?**

Proton pump inhibitors used for 4–8 weeks are first-line. H2 antagonists are second-line. Prokinetic agents such as metoclopramide, domperidone, and erythromycin are not recommend due to limited evidence of effectiveness and side effects [2].

14. **What are the surgical indications for GERD?**

Recurrent aspiration pneumonia, apneic episodes, bradycardia, ALTEs, bronchopulmonary dysplasia, severe vomiting, FTT, esophagitis, stricture, and failed medical therapy.

15. **What other disease processes present similarly to GERD?**

Hypertrophic pyloric stenosis, tracheoesophageal fistula, achalasia, intussusception or other intestinal obstructive diseases like Hirschsprung disease.

16. **What is the Nissen fundoplication and how does it control symptoms of GERD?**

Following creation of a retroesophageal window, the stomach is brought posteriorly around the esophagus above the GEJ, resulting in a 360° 2–3 cm length wrap oriented at the 11 o'clock position. A bougie diameter size relative to the patient's weight is used to prevent narrowing of the lower esophagus.

A fundoplication increases LES baseline pressure, decreases the number of TLESRs, decreases the nadir pressure during swallow-induced relaxation, increases the length of the intra-abdominal esophagus, accentuates the angle of His, and fixes a hiatal hernia if present.

17. **What other surgical options besides a Nissen fundoplication can be used for children with GERD?**

Partial wraps: Dor (anterior 180° wrap), Thal (anterior 270° wrap), Toupet (posterior 270° wrap).

Gastrojejunostomy has been performed in NI children.

Total esophagogastric disconnection with an esophagojejenual anastomosis has been considered a rescue procedure for NI patients with failed fundoplication. Gastric feeds are given via a gastrostomy in the remnant stomach, but without the risk of reflux.

Transpyloric/jejunostomy feeding is considered an alternative, but has a high rate of complications [3].

18. **Are there differences in patient outcome based on a partial versus complete wrap?**

No superiority in symptom control has been found between partial and complete wraps. A complete wrap may lead to more post-operative dysphagia requiring endoscopic dilation. Most surgeons prefer the Nissen fundoplication as it is a more straight-forward technique and easier to perform laparoscopically than the Thal [3].

19. **How effective is fundoplication for control of symptomatic GERD?**

The overall success rate is around 95% for typical symptoms, if no complications develop. Significant improvements in respiratory symptoms and QOL have also been reported [4, 5].

20. **What are the complications of fundoplication?**

Dysphagia from a wrap that is too tight, retching, gas bloat syndrome, wrap breakdown, hiatal herniation, slipped wrap, and recurrence of reflux.

21. **What is the recurrence rate of GERD following fundoplication? What are the risk factors for recurrence?**

Recurrence is <10–20% over 10–20 years. Risk factors include younger age at surgery, preoperative hiatal hernia, post-operative retching, need for post-operative esophageal dilations, certain underlying disorders (esophageal atresia), and re-do fundoplication. Minimal esophageal mobilization in laparoscopic Nissen fundoplication decreases post-operative wrap transmigration and the need for a re-do fundoplication.

References

1. Holcomb III GW. Gastroesophageal reflux. Holcomb and ashcraft's pediatric surgery, 7th Ed. Elsevier Inc.;2020. p. 460–77.
2. Rosen R, Vandenplas Y, Singendonk M, et al. Pediatric gastroesophageal reflux clinical practice guidelines: joint recommendations of the North American Society for pediatric gastroenterology, hepatology, and nutrition and the European Society for pediatric gastroenterology, hepatology, and nutrition. J Pediatr Gastroenterol Nutr. 2018;66:516–54.
3. Jancelewicz T, Lopez ME, Downard CD, et al. Surgical management of gastroesophageal reflux disease (GERD) in children: a systematic review. J Pediatr Surg. 2017;52:1228–38.
4. St. Peter SD, Barnhart DC, Ostlie DJ, et al. Minimal versus extensive esophageal mobilization during laparoscopic fundoplication: a prospective randomized trial. J Pediatr Surg. 2011;46:163–8.
5. Desai AA, Alemayehu H, Holcomb III GW, et al. Minimal vs. maximal esophageal dissection and mobilization during laparoscopic fundoplication: long-term follow-up from a prospective, randomized trial. J Pediatr Surg. 2015;50:111–4.

Chapter 7
Caustic Ingestion of the Esophagus

Rashmi Kabre

Abstract Children represent up to 80% of the population globally who are exposed to caustic ingestion injury. Caustic injury to the esophagus may be caused by alkalis and acids, both producing very different injury patterns. Initial management should prioritize respiratory and cardiovascular stability. Upper gastrointestinal endoscopy and endoscopic grading of esophageal injury remains the mainstay of diagnosis and may aid management decisions. Further studies are necessary as there continues to be minimal evidence for the use of adjuvant medical therapy including antacids, antibiotics, and steroid use. Sequelae such as esophageal strictures may be managed initially with esophageal dilation, with surgical management reserved for failure of dilations. Long-term endoscopic screening is necessary for the development of esophageal cancer, which may occur decades later from the injury.

Keywords Caustic ingestion · Caustic injury · Corrosive ingestion · Caustic strictures · Esophageal injury · Esophageal strictures

1. **What are the substances ingested by children that may cause caustic injury?**

Most corrosive substances are divided into either alkalis or acids. Alkaline substances constitute the majority of ingested matter in Western countries, while acidic material is more common in developing countries [1].

R. Kabre (✉)
Ann and Robert H. Lurie Children's Hospital of Chicago, Northwestern University Feinberg School of Medicine, Chicago, United States
e-mail: rkabre@luriechildrens.org

M. Lacher et al. (eds.), *Pearls and Tricks in Pediatric Surgery*,
https://doi.org/10.1007/978-3-030-51067-1_7

2. **Do acid and alkaline injuries differ?**

Yes. Acids cause coagulation necrosis with eschar formation. This may limit the tissue penetration and depth of the injury. Since they are usually less viscous, injury is typically more distal in the esophagus. In contrast, alkali agents combine with tissue proteins and cause liquefactive necrosis and saponification. The higher viscosity and longer contact times produce deeper tissue penetration.

3. **What age groups are at risk for caustic ingestion?**

Presentation occurs in a bimodal distribution with the first peak in children under five years old. Ingestions in this age group are typically accidental. The second peak occurs in adolescents and are more often related to intentional suicide attempts.

4. **What is the clinical presentation of caustic ingestion in children?**

Symptoms may vary depending on the type of substance, amount of exposure, time of presentation, depth and location of the injury. Reported symptoms may include hoarseness, wheezing, dyspnea, and stridor, which may be indicative of potential respiratory compromise. Common gastrointestinal symptoms may include drooling, dysphagia, odynophagia, epigastric/chest pain, and hematemesis. More severe initial presentations may include tracheoesophageal fistula and cardiovascular collapse.

5. **What is the first step in evaluation of a child with caustic injury?**

Initial management should include establishing an airway and hemodynamic stabilization. Ongoing airway edema may cause airway obstruction and present the need for emergent airway management.

6. **Should vomiting be induced when a child has ingested a caustic substance?**

No—this is actually contraindicated as regurgitation may cause repeat injury and also places the child at risk for aspiration pneumonia. Similarly, gastric lavage, milk, and activated charcoal are also contraindicated.

7. **What is included in the diagnostic work-up for a child with known caustic ingestion?**

An initial chest x-ray may reveal pneumoperitoneum, pneumomediastinum, pneumothorax or pleural effusion—all indicative of full-thickness injury. A water contrast esophagram may confirm any question of full-thickness injury, evaluate the extent, and guide further care. Endoscopy to grade the severity of injury is indicated and best done within the first 12–48 hours. The endoscopy is typically limited to the first level of injury to avoid perforation. A CT scan may show the extent of inflammation and will diagnose perforation.

8. **How is the severity of injury from caustic ingestion graded endoscopically?**

Grade	Description
0	Normal
1	Edema and hyperemia of mucosa
2a	Superficial injury with friability, hemorrhage, erosion, or blisters
2b	Conditions in 2a plus limited areas of deeper or circumferential injury
3a	Scattered area of necrosis or brown/black/gray discoloration
3b	Extensive necrosis
4	Perforation

9. **Should a nasogastric tube be placed to assist in management of caustic injury?**

Nasogastric tubes are not mandatory, but may be placed to prevent emesis, allow feeding past the esophageal injury, and serve as a stent in circumferential burns. These should not be placed blindly due to risk of esophageal perforation.

10. **What is the typical management of the patient taking into account the endoscopic appearance of the caustic injury?**

Patients who are grade 1 and 2a may be allowed oral intake and discharged after a limited in-hospital observation. Grades 2b and higher require longer hospital observation with adequate nutritional support and will need monitoring for stricture formation during follow-up.

11. **What is the role of antacid therapy and mucosal protection in caustic injury of the esophagus?**

H2 blockers, intravenous proton pump inhibitors and sucralfate are often initiated to theoretically allow faster mucosal healing, prevent stress ulcers and provide mucosal protection. The efficacy of gastric acid suppression with H2 blockers or proton-pump inhibitors has not yet been proven although a small prospective study in adults has shown significant endoscopic healing after IV omeprazole infusion. [2] Sucralfate has been shown in a small randomized controlled study to decrease the frequency of stricture formation in advanced corrosive esophagitis, however efficacy has not been established in a larger sample of patients [3].

12. **What is the role of corticosteroids in the prevention of stricture formation?**

There is conflicting evidence regarding systemic corticosteroid administration. Due to this, current recommendations are to avoid use, especially since they also increase the risk of infectious complications. Several meta-analyses have suggested limiting the use of steroids to those patients with established respiratory tract edema. Intralesional steroid injections (triamcinolone 40–100 mg/session) have been utilized although no consensus exists regarding appropriate dosage and frequency [4, 5].

13. **What is the role of antibiotics in caustic esophageal injury?**

No data support routine use of antibiotic prophylaxis. The use of antibiotics is advised if corticosteroids are initiated, lung involvement is identified, or in the setting of systemic infection and perforation [1].

14. **What are the indications for immediate surgical intervention?**

Patients with clinical or radiological evidence of perforation may require immediate laparotomy, or possible thoracotomy, esophagectomy, cervical esophagostomy, gastrectomy, or gastrostomy/jejunostomy tube placement.

15. **How does ingestion of a button battery result in caustic injury of the esophagus?**

A button battery discharges electrical current, which hydrolyzes water and generates hydroxide. This creates focal injury to the tissue at the level of impaction.

16. **Is button battery ingestion a surgical emergency?**

Yes. Serious burns can occur within as little as two hours. It is imperative that one be able to identify the difference between a radiopaque coin and the double ring sign of the button battery on anteroposterior and lateral chest x-ray. A button battery is a surgical emergency and may rapidly cause ulceration, perforation, mediastinitis, or tracheoesophageal fistula, which a surgeon must be prepared to manage at the time of battery removal.

17. **What are late sequelae of caustic ingestion of the esophagus?**

Stricture incidence may be as high as 70% in grade 2b and up to 100% in grade 3 esophageal injuries. Esophageal dysmotility may accompany this, in addition to intractable pain, gastric outlet obstruction, mucosal metaplasia and development of esophageal carcinoma [1].

18. **What are the options for management of esophageal strictures?**

Balloon or bougie dilation starting at three weeks after ingestion and occurring at an interval varying from 1–3 weeks may help in achieving a good outcome. Delayed presentation, as well as delayed dilations are both associated with a worse prognosis and more closely associated with future esophageal replacement [1].

19. **Is there a role for esophageal stenting in children in the setting of caustic ingestion?**

Stent use during the acute phase is not recommended. There is not enough data to support the routine use of esophageal stents in children.

20. **What are the indications and surgical options for esophageal replacement?**

If esophageal dilations fail or if the esophagus cannot be salvaged, surgical options include gastric pull-up, and colonic or small intestinal interposition. No surgical technique has established clear superiority over the others.

21. **What is the incidence of development of esophageal neoplasms?**

The reported incidence ranges from 2–30% and may occur anytime between 10 and 30 years after ingestion. These risks may be 1000–3000 times higher than normal [1].

22. **When should endoscopic surveillance for esophageal cancer indicated?**

Endoscopic surveillance is mandatory. Evaluation should be started at age 20 and repeated every 1–3 years depending on findings.

References

1. Contini S, Scarpignato C. Caustic injury of the upper gastrointestinal tract: a comprehensive review. World J Gastroenterol. 2013;19(25):3918–30.
2. Çakal B, Akbal E, Köklü S, Babalı A, Koçak E, Taş A. Acute therapy with intravenous omeprazole on caustic esophageal injury: a prospective case series. Dis Esophagus. 2013;26(1):22–6.
3. Gümürdülü Y, Karakoç E, Kara B, Taşdoğan BE, Parsak CK, Sakman G. The efficiency of sucralfate in corrosive esophagitis: a randomized, prospective study. Turk J Gastroenterol. 2010;21:7–11.
4. De Lusong MAA, Timbol ABG, Tuazon DJS. Management of esophageal caustic injury. World J Gastrointest Pharmacol Ther. 2017;8(2):90–8.
5. Fulton JA, Hoffman RS. Steroids in second degree caustic burns of the esophagus: a systematic pooled analysis of fifty years of human data: 1956–2006. Clin Toxicol (Phila). 2007;45:402–8.

Chapter 8
Esophageal Foreign Bodies

Dan C. Little and A. Justin Malek

Abstract Esophageal foreign bodies represent a common clinical challenge for pediatric surgeons. These children often present with chest pain, dysphagia, and inability to swallow. Both rigid and flexible esophagoscopy are acceptable techniques. Recent investigative work has focused on cost of care and consideration for advancement of the foreign body into the stomach. Most of these cases are performed under general anesthesia. The anesthesia team should be alerted to the increased possibility of tooth injury or accidental endotracheal tube dislodgement during the procedure. Complications are increased with children suffering from esophageal food impaction or button battery ingestion. These children are best served with early intervention. Surgeons should have a host of techniques available for successful intervention.

Keywords Esophageal foreign body · Foley balloon extraction · Button battery

1. **What are the most common esophageal foreign bodies?**

In the United States, coins represent the most common esophageal foreign bodies; however fish bones are more common worldwide.

2. **What are the most common sites for esophageal foreign body impaction?**

There are three areas of anatomical narrowing in the esophagus that could serve as potential areas of impaction. These include the cricopharyngeus sling (70%),

D. C. Little (✉)
McLane Children's Hospital, Texas A&M College of Medicine, 1901 SW HK Dodge Loop, Temple, TX 76502, Unites States
e-mail: dlittle@sw.org

A. Justin Malek
Department of Surgery, Texas A&M Health Science Center, 2401 S 31st Street, Temple, TX 76508, Unites States

M. Lacher et al. (eds.), *Pearls and Tricks in Pediatric Surgery*,
https://doi.org/10.1007/978-3-030-51067-1_8

the level of the aortic arch in the mid esophagus (15%), and the lower esophageal sphincter (15%).

3. **Should contrast examinations be *routinely* used to localize an esophageal foreign body?**

A contrast examination should not be performed routinely primarily because of the risk of aspiration and secondarily because coating of the foreign body and esophageal mucosa compromises subsequent esophagoscopy.

4. **Describe the workup for suspected radiopaque and radiolucent foreign bodies**

Radiopaque objects can easily be detected with routine chest x-ray; however radiolucent ones may require additional imaging. Contrast esophagram is an option in select patients who can protect their airway. Injected volume should be limited. A high index of clinical suspicion for a radiolucent foreign body combined with appropriate physical findings such as drooling may mandate esophagoscopy.

5. **How commonly will lodged esophageal coins pass spontaneously?**

Coins pass naturally in up to 20 to 30% of children within 24 hours. Criteria that may influence passage including child's age, time of esophageal lodging, and type of coin are unpredictable. Distal esophageal coins pass more commonly than proximal coins. Thus a period of observation in select patients and consideration of a repeated x-ray is warranted prior to an invasive procedure [1, 2].

6. **Are sharp esophageal foreign bodies managed differently than smooth?**

Smooth foreign bodies, with the exception of button batteries, rarely cause significant esophageal problems. Interestingly, small sharp objects and straight pins can be managed conservatively in the majority of cases. Larger sharp esophageal foreign bodies such as nails, needles, screws, and bones have a risk of perforation of 15–35% and thus should be managed with endoscopic retrieval [3].

7. **What options exists for removal of an esophageal foreign body?**

A successful endoscopist must have competence in several techniques when approaching a child with an esophageal foreign body. Foley balloon extraction, flexible and rigid esophagoscopy (using various graspers), direct laryngoscopy, and push esophagoscopy are commonly described techniques.

8. **Describe the technique for Foley balloon extraction**

This technique requires the fluoroscopic placement of a Foley catheter just distal to the foreign body. Once catheter position has been confirmed, contrast is placed in the Foley balloon. The catheter is then slowly withdrawn until the foreign body is expressed or readily visualized in the oral pharynx. Children should be restrained, but sedatives are not required. Resuscitation equipment should be readily available.

9. **What is the success rate for Foley balloon extraction of esophageal foreign bodies?**

Foley balloon extraction with fluoroscopy has been shown to have an 80% success rate [4].

10. **What are the fiscal benefits of Foley balloon extraction of esophageal foreign bodies?**

Published data suggest significant potential cost savings for Foley balloon extraction compared to standard endoscopy under general anesthesia. Cost for Foley balloon extraction averaged $1231 versus $3615 for standard endoscopy [5].

11. **What techniques can be used for very proximal esophageal foreign bodies lodged at the cricopharyngeus sphincter?**

At times, especially in a young child, an esophageal foreign body can be lodged in the most proximal portion of the esophagus making standard esophagoscopy, whether rigid or flexible, more challenging. In these cases, practitioners may opt to use a Miller direct laryngoscope blade to expose the proximal esophagus and Magill forceps to retrieve the foreign body. Straight laparoscopic graspers are helpful if the Magill forceps prove to bulky for a small mouth.

12. **How are esophageal coins differentiated from esophageal button batteries?**

Both esophageal coins and button batteries have a similar look on initial plain film. They share a similar size and are smooth and round. However, with closer inspection, one will note the double lucency shadow consistent with button batteries (Figs. 8.1 and 8.2). This key finding is critical to detect and will influence timing of surgery and possible complications.

13. **Why are button batteries treated with more urgency than other esophageal foreign bodies?**

Esophageal button battery ingestion should be treated as a true pediatric surgical emergency. Standard NPO guidelines do not apply. Button battery ingestions are associated with increased morbidity secondary to rapid tissue injury that occurs through leakage of alkali solution. Liquefaction necrosis of the esophageal mucosa and muscularis can advance rapidly. Experience suggests that initial mucosal injury may occur with contact time as little as one hour.

14. **Describe alternative management for esophageal button battery impaction if the battery cannot be retrieved via standard esophagoscopy**

Button batteries can be pushed into the stomach where most can successfully pass throughout the gastrointestinal tract without consequence. Alternatively, a basket can be used to retrieve the gastric button battery at the time of esophagoscopy or if the patient manifests postoperative signs or symptoms of injury to the gastrointestinal tract. Surgeons should consider retrieving button batteries larger than

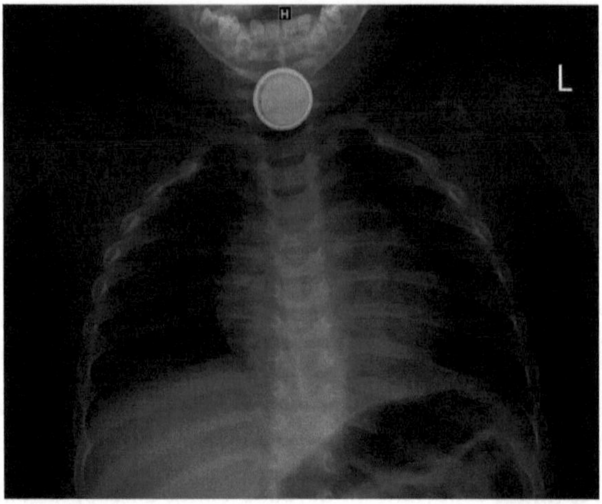

Fig. 8.1 10-month-old AP XRAY with esophageal button battery showing double lucency sign

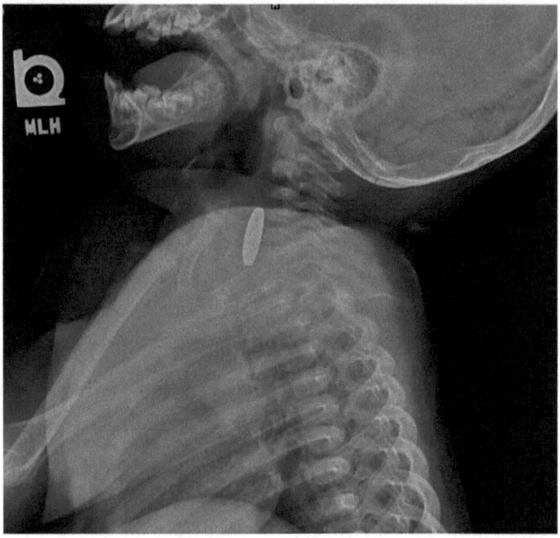

Fig. 8.2 Same child with lateral projection

20 mm diameter that remain in the stomach greater than 48 hours as determined by x-ray. Emetics are not beneficial in the management of disk battery ingestions, and cathartics and acid suppression have no proven role in treatment of battery ingestion [6].

15. **Are special studies required following esophageal button battery removal?**

This depends on the assessment of the esophageal mucosa at the time of button battery removal. If concern exists, then an intraoperative esophagram or formal esophagram in the radiology department is warranted. Mucosal irregularities and contained perforations are possible. When concern exists, placement of a distal nasogastric feeding tube is helpful to allow direct enteral feeds while the esophageal mucosal injury heals. In the absence of progressive symptoms, repeated esophagram in one week is recommended.

16. **Describe the short and long term complications of button battery impaction**

Short term complications include mucosal injury and possible full thickness injury with esophageal contained perforation or even free rupture. Long term complications include tracheoesophageal fistula, stricture, and death.

17. **What techniques are available to manage esophageal food impaction?**

Both flexible and rigid esophagoscopy are practiced. One benefit of rigid open channel esophagoscopy includes the use of internal extraction forceps to remove larger chunks of food (often chicken or hot dogs) or other debris without having to remove the rigid scope. With patience, the job can also be accomplished with flexible techniques using the coin grasper or other grasping forceps. However larger pieces cannot be removed *inside* the flexible scope. The scope must be removed multiple times as small pieces are extracted. With repeated withdrawals and advancements of the flexible scope, one must be very attentive not to cause an accidental dislodgement of an endotracheal tube.

18. **Can the esophageal foreign body simply be advanced into the stomach and be allowed to pass naturally?**

Historically, "pull techniques" have been favored over "push techniques." Recent data suggests that both techniques are safe and have similar success rates at 65% and 68% respectively [7]. If one technique is not successful, conversion to the other is the next move. Of note, in children with previous esophageal surgery the practitioner must be aware of a possible distal esophageal stricture.

19. **How do you recognize and manage incidental extubation during esophagoscopy?**

Most pediatric anesthesiologists require endotracheal intubation prior to attempted removal of an esophageal foreign body. Security of the endotracheal tube should be paramount. In less experienced hands or in cases of repeated placement of the esophagoscope, dislodgement can occur. Oxygen desaturation and loss of end tidal CO_2 are early indicators for accidental extubation. The surgeon should immediately withdraw the esophagoscope and allow the child to receive positive pressure ventilation and repeated intubation.

20. **Are tooth injuries common during esophagoscopy?**

Generally speaking, tooth injuries in children should be uncommon. However, the exploring nature of children often coincides when they may be losing their deciduous teeth. Inspection of the oral cavity and documentation of loose teeth is recommended before proceeding. Use of an endoscopic mouth guard is recommended with flexible esophagoscopy. When rigid esophagoscopy is employed, mindful attention to not rear back or rest the scope of the upper teeth is prudent.

References

1. Dedhia K, Chang Y-F, Leonardis R, Chi DH. Is there a need for repeat radiologic examination of children with esophageal coin foreign body? Otolaryngol-Head Neck Surg. 2017;156(1):173–9.
2. Soprano JV, Fleisher GR, Mandl KD. The spontaneous passage of esophageal coins in children. Arch Pediatr Adolesc Med. 1999;153(10):1073–6.
3. Wahbeh G, Wyllie R, Kay M. Foreign body ingestion in infants and children: location, location, location. Clin Pediatr. 2002;41(9):633–40.
4. Little DC, Shah SR, St Peter SD, Calkins CM, Morrow SE, Murphy JP, et al. Esophageal foreign bodies in the pediatric population: our first 500 cases. J Pediatr Surg. 2006;41(5):914–8.
5. Gonzalez KW, Reddy SR, Mundakkal AA, Peter SDS. The financial impact of flipping the coin. J Pediatr Surg. 2017;52(1):153–5.
6. Eisen GM, Baron TH, Dominitz JA, Faigel DO, Goldstein JL, Johanson JF, et al. Guideline for the management of ingested foreign bodies. Gastrointest Endosc. 2002;55(7):802–6.
7. Kriem J, Rahhal R. Safety and efficacy of the push endoscopic technique in the management of esophageal food bolus impactions in children. J Pediatr Gastroenterol Nutr. 2018;66(1):e1–5.

Chapter 9
Congenital Lung Malformations

Shaun M. Kunisaki

Abstract This chapter discusses the major pearls and tricks in the diagnosis and management of congenital lung lesions, which include congenital pulmonary airway malformations, bronchogenic cysts, bronchopulmonary sequestrations, and congenital lobar emphysema. Collectively, congenital lung malformations can be uniquely challenging for pediatric surgeons in part because they are rarely encountered in most clinical practices and often require multi-disciplinary expertise, including maternal-fetal medicine specialists, neonatologists, and pediatric radiologists. Moreover, lung lesions can have highly variable clinical presentations and unclear natural histories. The current standard of care for the most common clinical scenarios is discussed, and specific areas of controversy are highlighted.

Keywords Lung malformation · Bronchopulmonary sequestration · Lobar emphysema · Bronchogenic cyst

1. **What are the four major types of lung malformations?**

The four major types of lung malformations are [1] congenital pulmonary airway malformation (CPAM), formerly congenital cystic adenomatoid malformation; [2] bronchopulmonary sequestration (BPS); [3] congenital lobar emphysema (CLE); and [4] bronchogenic cyst [1].

2. **What are the main differences between congenital pulmonary airway malformations (CPAM) and bronchopulmonary sequestrations (BPS)?**

CPAMs communicate with airways of the native lung and have a vascular supply derived from the pulmonary circulation. In contrast, BPS lesions are non-aerated

S. M. Kunisaki (✉)
Johns Hopkins Children's Center, 1800 Orleans Street, Suite 7353, Baltimore, Maryland, MD 21287, USA
e-mail: skunisa1@jhmi.edu

M. Lacher et al. (eds.), *Pearls and Tricks in Pediatric Surgery*,
https://doi.org/10.1007/978-3-030-51067-1_9

lung tissue that has a large systemic arterial blood supply, often coming directly off of the aorta.

3. **What are the two major types of bronchopulmonary sequestrations and how do you tell the difference between them on postnatal cross-sectional imaging?**

BPS lesions are classified as intralobar (75%) or extralobar (25%). Intralobar BPS is entirely invested with the visceral pleura with venous drainage usually to the pulmonary venous system. In contrast, extralobar BPS represents accessory pulmonary lung tissue that is invested in its own pleural lining that is completely separate from normal lung parenchyma. Extalobar BPS usually has both a systemic arterial and venous blood supply.

4. **What is the most common anatomic locations for each of the lung malformations?**

Most CPAM and BPS lesions are located in one of the lower lobes of the lung. CLE most commonly involves the left upper lobe. The second most common site is the right middle lobe. Bronchogenic cysts tend to be centrally located within the mediastinum in the paratracheal or subcarinal regions.

5. **What are hybrid lung lesions?**

Hybrid lung lesions have characteristics of at least two different types of lung malformations. The most common hybrid lesion is a CPAM with a systemic arterial blood supply. This is seen in approximately 9–25% of all resected lung malformations.

6. **How common are congenital lung malformations?**

Recent reports suggest that the incidence has been increasing and may be approximately 1 in 2,500 live births. The increasing incidence is likely secondary to widespread prenatal screening by ultrasound as well as improvements in sonographic image quality.

7. **How are CPAMs usually diagnosed?**

Lung malformations can have a highly variable clinical presentation. However, the majority of CPAM and BPS lesions (>75%) are now diagnosed during fetal life as an echogenic lung mass.

8. **How can congenital lung malformations affect the developing fetus?**

Large lung malformations can compress the esophagus, resulting in impaired fetal swallowing and polyhydramnios. Analogous to the situation in congenital diaphragmatic hernia, mass effect may also lead to pulmonary hypoplasia and pulmonary hypertension. Rarely, the mass can impair venous return to the heart and lead to hydrops, in which fluid accumulates in body cavities in conjunction with generalized skin edema. In severe cases of hydrops, placentomegaly and right heart failure are signs of impending fetal demise.

9. **Are fetal lung lesions associated with other birth defects?**

In greater than 90% of cases, a fetal lung malformation is an isolated finding, and screening for karyotype anomalies is not indicated.

10. **You are asked to counsel a pregnant woman carrying a 21-week fetus with a lung malformation identified on ultrasound. What imaging information are most important in terms to determining the potential morbidity of the lesion at birth?**

The most important characteristic is its relative size, most often measured in terms of the CVR (CPAM volume ratio). Serial monitoring of the CVR is required because many of these lesions increase in size until 26 weeks. Fetuses with lesions with a CVR less than 0.9 are usually born asymptomatic and can be delivered at the birthing center of the family's choosing. However, lesions with a CVR greater than 0.9 are at increased risk for respiratory symptoms at birth, and these fetuses should probably be delivered at a tertiary care referral center with pediatric surgery coverage. Other characteristics on ultrasound that may influence the delivery plan include the presence of mediastinal shift and macrocystic disease [2].

11. **What is the Stocker classification?**

The Stocker classification scheme was the original description of CPAMs based on pathologic specimens. Type I lesions have macrocysts, and type III lesions are solid or microcystic. Type II lesions have a mixed of both microcysts and macrocysts.

12. **A pregnant woman is carrying a 23-week fetus with a microcystic lung malformation. The ultrasound shows a CVR of 2.5, and there is ascites. What are some potential management options for this fetus?**

Lesions with a CVR greater than 1.6 are at increased risk for hydrops. The first line of therapy is the administration of maternal betamethasone. Other options include fetal resection, which is uncommonly performed and associated with high mortality. If the lesion has a large, dominant macrocyst, fetal thoracocentesis or thoracoamniotic shunting can be helpful to reduce the mass effect of the lesion. In near-term fetuses, another option is to resect the lesion while still on placental support, otherwise known as ex utero intrapartum treatment (EXIT)-to-resection.

13. **Can fetal CPAMs regress in size prior to delivery? What about postnatal regression of a CPAM identified on CT?**

Many CPAMs regress in size during the third trimester of pregnancy. Other microcystic CPAMs can become isoechoic with the adjacent lung tissue by ultrasounds after 32 weeks of gestation. Therefore, these lesions can be difficult to visualize in utero but are usually subsequently identified on postnatal cross-sectional imaging. For this reason, all fetal lung malformations, regardless of whether they have "disappeared" on subsequent fetal sonograms, should undergo postnatal chest CT, usually at 2–3 months of age [3]. Postnatal regression of a CPAM is a controversial topic, but most investigators believe that complete regression after a child is born is extremely rare.

14. **You are called to the neonatal intensive care unit to see a 6-hour old neonate in respiratory distress. Chest x-ray shows mediastinal shift to the right hemi-thorax and a hyperlucent left chest. How would you manage this patient?**

This child has a left upper lobe CLE and should go to the operating room in an expeditious manner in preparation for a thoracotomy and left upper lobectomy. If the baby is *in extremis*, a bedside thoracotomy with exteriorization of the affected lung can be a life-saving maneuver. Intubation should generally be avoided because positive pressure can exacerbate air trapping.

15. **Describe the basic steps involved in a neonatal lung resection for a CPAM.**

A thoracotomy with formal lobectomy represents the standard of care in neonates. Lung isolation is not required. Since most of these lesions involve one of the lower lobes, the inferior pulmonary ligament is divided. If this is a hybrid lesion, any systemic feeding vessels are identified and controlled with clips, energy devices, or ligatures. The pulmonary arteries and veins are identified and controlled in similar fashion. The bronchus to the affected lobe is taken last using clips, staplers, or ligatures. A chest tube is left in place to help with lung re-expansion and to evacuate pleural fluid.

16. **A newborn with a prenatally diagnosed lung malformation was born several hours ago. She appears to be in no respiratory distress and has a normal physical exam. What are the next steps?**

This patient can be discharged in 24–48 hours. Plain film radiographs of the chest are often performed as a baseline study. However, even if the plain film is completely normal, a chest CT is indicated because of the low sensitivity of plain films. Most referral centers do not perform a chest CT until a child is at least 2 months old in order to obtain the best images for preoperative planning purposes. MRI avoids the ionizing radiation of CT, but is not the preferred imaging modality because it requires sedation to minimize motion artifacts and gives inferior resolution of the lung parenchyma.

17. **A four-month old healthy child with a small, asymptomatic CPAM on CT comes to your office. Would you recommend surgical resection? If so, why and when would this be performed? If not, why not?**

Although there are no well-designed, prospective studies on the natural history of CPAMs, early surgical resection of a CPAM has been the preferred management strategy in the USA. The median age at resection is about 5–6 months of age. The rationale for prophylactic lung resection is to prevent pneumonia and other complications. Earlier resection has also been embraced since the resection may be easier given that subclinical infection and inflammation have yet to occur. Early resection may also allow for maximal compensatory lung growth. Other pediatric surgeons cite a small, but defined risk for malignant degeneration. Finally, the optimal frequency and best imaging approach to monitor unresected CPAMs has not been defined.

Opponents of early surgical resection argue that the risk of pneumonia in selected CPAMs may be as low as 5%. Since some lesions may regress and most may never become symptomatic, it may be difficult to justify performing an operation that can have its own complications, including massive hemorrhage and prolonged air leak. Moreover, the cancer risk is believed to be very small, especially in prenatally diagnosed lesions. There are also concerns about the possible long-term neurotoxic effects of anesthesia in younger children.

18. **What is pleuropulmonary blastoma?**

Pleuropulmonary blastoma (PPB) is a rare malignant primary cancer of the lung. Type 1 PPB presents at a mean age of about 9 months and can be confused with macrocystic CPAM by chest CT. As a result, many surgeons strongly urge resection of all CPAMs for fear of inadvertently observing PPB. The treatment of PPB involves a gross total resection and chemotherapy. Roughly a third of PPB lesions are associated with the DICER1 mutation, a gene defect with increased susceptibility to ovarian and kidney tumors [4].

19. **What is the best operative approach for an asymptomatic congenital lung malformation in an infant?**

There remains debate on the best operative approach. The traditional operative approach in infants is an open (thoracotomy) incision, which is safe, well-tolerated, and associated with a three day hospital stay. A muscle-sparing approach has been adopted by many pediatric surgeons to help minimize musculoskeletal morbidity, including scoliosis. More recently, minimally invasive (thoracoscopic) approaches have gained traction since they result in smaller scars and obviate the need for an epidural catheter to attain good postoperative pain control. However, thoracoscopic surgery necessitates effective lung isolation, is associated with a relatively steep learning curve despite ongoing refinements in surgical instrumentation, and has generally longer operative times. Hospital lengths of stay are similar or only marginally shorter after thoracoscopic resection [5].

20. **Is there a role for segmentectomy or wedge resection in the surgical management of CPAM?**

Yes, there is a small and limited role for lung preserving resections in selected patients with lung malformations. Routine use of segmental or wedge resections has generally been discouraged because of increased risk of parenchymal leak from the cut surface of the lung as well as concerns regarding leaving residual disease behind. However, those with bilateral disease (1–2%) or CPAMs involving multiple lobes on the same side might benefit from segmental or wedge resection. Those with lung function that is already compromised (e.g., bronchopulmonary dysplasia) may also be ideal candidates.

21. **How do you manage a child with an intralobar BPS?**

Children with intralobar BPS are at increased risk for pneumonia and high-output cardiac failure because of chronic shunting of blood through a large systemic feeding artery. For these reasons, surgical resection is indicated.

22. **How do you manage a child with a small extralobar BPS?**

The management of small extralobar BPS lesions is controversial given that they are not contiguous with the native lung and therefore less likely to become infected. Opinions on management vary amongst pediatric surgeons and range from observation to catheter embolization to thoracoscopic resection.

23. **What are the histologic features of bronchogenic cysts? How would you manage a child with an asymptomatic bronchogenic cyst identified by CT scan?**

Bronchogenic cysts contain cartilage and ciliated columnar epithelium. Most should be excised before complications (e.g., airway obstruction, abscess) ensue. If complete surgical excision is not possible without causing damage to adjacent mediastinal structures, then other options include sclerotherapy or de-epithelialization.

References

1. Kunisaki SM, Saito JM, Fallat ME, St Peter SD, Lal DR, Johnson KN, et al. Development of a multi-institutional registry for children with operative congenital lung malformations. J Pediatr Surg. 2019.
2. Ehrenberg-Buchner S, Stapf AM, Berman DR, Drongowski RA, Mychaliska GB, Treadwell MC, et al. Fetal lung lesions: can we start to breathe easier? Am J Obstet Gynecol 2013;208(2):151 e1–7.
3. Kunisaki SM, Ehrenberg-Buchner S, Dillman JR, Smith EA, Mychaliska GB, Treadwell MC. Vanishing fetal lung malformations: Prenatal sonographic characteristics and postnatal outcomes. J Pediatr Surg. 2015;50(6):978–82.
4. Nasr A, Himidan S, Pastor AC, Taylor G, Kim PC. Is congenital cystic adenomatoid malformation a premalignant lesion for pleuropulmonary blastoma? J Pediatr Surg. 2010;45(6):1086–9.
5. Kunisaki SM, Powelson IA, Haydar B, Bowshier BC, Jarboe MD, Mychaliska GB, et al. Thoracoscopic vs open lobectomy in infants and young children with congenital lung malformations. J Am Coll Surg. 2014;218(2):261–70.

Chapter 10
Acquired Lung and Pleural Disease

Shawn D. St. Peter

Abstract Although there are a large variety of acquired conditions affecting the lung and pleura, the most common disease process that requires surgical engagement is the spectrum of parapneumonic effusions. This chapter focuses on this spectrum with focus on empyema particularly the management of these patients. In addition, other potential surgical conditions of the lung and pleural will be exposed.

Keywords Parapneumonic effusion · Empyema

1. **What is empyema?**

Empyema is derived from the Greek word *empyein* which means to 'put pus in'. In general medical care, it refers to purulence within the pleural space.

2. **What is the cause of empyema?**

This occurs most commonly secondary to pneumonia; however, other sources such as infected hematoma or extension of mediastinal, retropharyngeal, or paravertebral infections.

3. **What are the stages of parapneumonic pleural effusion?**

The exudative stage is a simple parapneumonic effusion which is clear and free flowing pleural with a low white cell count. The fibrinopurulent stage is a complicated parapneumonic effusion or empyema with septations and fibrin strands appear. The most advanced state is termed the organization stage when a thick peel is present.

S. D. St. Peter (✉)
Children's Mercy Hospital, Gillham Rd 2401, Kansas City, MO 64108, United States
e-mail: sspeter@cmh.edu

M. Lacher et al. (eds.), *Pearls and Tricks in Pediatric Surgery*,
https://doi.org/10.1007/978-3-030-51067-1_10

4. **Does Degree of Illness Progress with these stages?**

No, patients may be quite systemically ill early in the course of severe pneumonia but stabilize by the time thicker material develops.

5. **What are the Light Criteria?**

As the stages advance, the chemistry of the parapneumonic fluid changes where glucose decreases, pH decreases and lactate dehydrogenase rises. The Light criteria for complicated parapneumonic effusion include pH < 7.2, lactate dehydrogenase > 1000 units, glucose < 40 mg/dl or < 25% blood glucose, Gram stain or culture positive and with loculations or septations proven with imaging.

6. **What is the best imaging to diagnose empyema?**

US should be the first step to identify septations and loculations. Sometimes it can help differentiate between parenchymal and pleural based processes. CT with intravenous contrast can delineate the degree of necrotic lung and quantify pleural space disease which can be helpful if operative planning is being considered.

7. **How do you manage simple parapneumonic effusion?**

If there is free-flowing effusion with no solid components or signs of frank pus, the intervention will depend on size and symptoms. Symptoms precipitating intervention are generally poor feeding tolerance, tachypnea, and increasing oxygen requirements. Drainage is then indicated by a chest tube. This should be a tube that can be used to treat empyema if that were to evolve, or if empyema were diagnosed while placing the tube by the presence of frank pus. This is generally a 12F chest tube (Thal-Quick Chest Tubes, Cook Critical Care, Bloomington, Indiana, USA).

8. **How is empyema managed?**

The pleural space can be cleared of solid material surgically via the minimally invasive approach, video-assisted thoracoscopy (VATS), or chemically with fibrinolytic agents. Three prospective, randomized trials have been conducted comparing fibrinolysis to VATS upon diagnosis of empyema in children, all of which found no difference in outcomes. Since these patients can be treated without an operation, fibrinolysis is recommended as first line therapy.

9. **How is fibrinolysis performed?**

The simple published algorithm is 4 mg of tissue plasminogen activator mixed into 40 ml of saline placed through the chest tube every 24 hours for 3 rounds. Each round includes a dwell time of 1 hour by clamping the chest tube. While this has been shown to be effective first line therapy, there are no good comparative studies with other regimen.

10. **What if the patient is still ill after fibrinolysis?**

While VATS has been used after failure of fibrinolysis in the trials according to the protocols, however, surgeons should be cautious because the ongoing illness is most frequently to persistent pneumonia or parenchymal necrosis. Therefore, being patient with either another round of fibrinolysis or observation with continued antibiotic therapy can result in the rare need for VATS. Further ongoing illness should not be considered fever, but poor oral intake or oxygen requirements. These patients should be imaged if further intervention is considered to define ongoing pleural disease versus parenchymal disease.

11. **What if the imaging shows pulmonary necrosis?**

Don't touch it.

12. **How do you treat a pulmonary abscess without empyema?**

In general, an operation should be avoided as abscesses can be treated to resolution with antibiotics only as was the historical standard. If the lesion is peripheral, not associated with airway connection then image guided drainage or catheter placement is feasible.

13. **What if the abscess has a solid appearing ball inside of it?**

This is a fungal infection and it present a unique challenge. Resection is usually necessary, by thoracoscopic wedge resection or lobectomy. These are usually more central and not visible on the surface so wedge resection often requires wire localization.

14. **What is bronchiectasis?**

Bronchiectasis s defined as a permanent dilatation of segmental airways. This is not a pathophysiologic process, but architectural abnormalities resulting from any pathologic processes causing persistent pulmonary inflammation leading to the damage. The damaged tissue includes muscle and connective tissues leading to narrowing and dilated segments of airway. Decreased epithelial and mucociliary integrity results in poor airway clearance leading to predisposition for further infections.

15. **Why does the pediatric surgeon care about bronchiectasis?**

Children with cystic fibrosis can develop bronchiectasis resulting in a lobar pneumonia that can't be cleared with protracted medical management requiring a lobectomy. These are difficult cases due to inflammation, lymphadenopathy and a bulky solid lobe that will not decompress.

16. **What is chylothorax?**

Chylothorax is a chylous effusion or the presence of lymphatic fluid within the pleural space.

Chyle typically demonstrates a total fat content greater than 400 mg/dL, triglycerides greater than 200 mg/dL, or a specific gravity greater than 1.012. It usually contains >90% lymphocytes and chylomicrons.

17. **How is chylothorax managed?**

First level is fat restricted diet rich in medium-chain fatty acids. The next level of management would be nothing by mouth and total parenteral nutrition. Finally, if no resolution, thoracic duct ligation. As many as 80% of patients respond to conservative management.

References

1. Bradley JS, Byington CL, Shah SS, et al. Executive summary: the management of community acquired pneumonia in infants and children older than 3 months of age: clinical practice guidelines by the Pediatric Infectious Disease Society and the Infectious Disease Society of America. Clin Infect Dis. 2011;53:617–30.
2. Islam S, Calkins CM, Goldin AB, Chen C, Downard CD, Huang EY, Cassidy L, Saito J, Blakely ML, Rangel SJ, Arca MJ, Abdullah F, St Peter SD; APSA Outcomes and Clinical Trials Committee, 2011–2012. The diagnosis and management of empyema in children: a comprehensive review from the APSA Outcomes and Clinical Trials Committee. J Pediatr Surg. 2012;47(11):2101–10.

Chapter 11
Tracheobronchial Foreign Bodies

Paolo Campisi

Abstract This chapter presents useful pearls and tricks that facilitate the management of children with tracheobronchial foreign bodies. Specifically, the epidemiology, clinical presentation, anesthetic and surgical principles associated with the diagnosis and successful retrieval of tracheobronchial foreign bodies will be reviewed. An overview of the most common foreign bodies and their physical properties is presented.

Keywords Foreign · Tracheobronchial · Choking · Dyspnea · Peanut

1. **How common are tracheobronchial foreign bodies?**

The aspiration of tracheobronchial foreign bodies is fortunately not common. However, asphyxiation caused by an inhaled laryngeal or tracheobronchial foreign bodies is one of the leading causes of accidental death in children under the age of 4 years in many countries.

In Europe, a retrospective study of 19 European countries was undertaken to determine the incidence of airway foreign bodies between 2000 and 2002 [1]. Cases were identified using hospital discharge records and International Classification of Disease (ICD-9) codes. During this time period, 170 cases of laryngeal of pharyngeal foreign bodies (ICD 933) and 552 cases of tracheobronchial foreign bodies (ICD 934) were identified.

P. Campisi
Department of Otolaryngology—Head and Neck Surgery, University of Toronto, Toronto, Canada

P. Campisi (✉)
Hospital for Sick Children, 555 University Avenue, 6th Floor Burton Wing, Toronto, ON M5G 1X8, Canada
e-mail: paolo.campisi@sickkids.ca

M. Lacher et al. (eds.), *Pearls and Tricks in Pediatric Surgery*,
https://doi.org/10.1007/978-3-030-51067-1_11

In the United States, non-choking rates were reviewed by the Morbidity and Mortality Weekly Report [2]. In 2001, approximately 17,537 children aged 14 years or less were treated in emergency departments for choking related episodes. This incidence corresponds to a rate of 29.9 per 100,000 population. The rates were reported for specific age groups.

2. **What is the age distribution of tracheobronchial foreign bodies?**

In a European study, there was a higher reported incidence of tracheobronchial foreign body aspiration in males (63%) and the median age at presentation was 2 years [1]. In a review of cases presenting at a tertiary care center in Eastern India, 82 cases were identified between 2001 and 2008 [3]. The most common age at presentation was between 1 and 3 years (56.4%).

In the US, the highest rates of non-fatal choking events were found for infants aged<1 year (140.4 per 100,000 population) [2]. Overall, 82.3% of all cases were in children 0–4 years of age. As found in the European study, most of the cases were in males (55%).

In a more recent review of the English literature, 12,979 children with suspected (11,145 cases confirmed) foreign body aspiration were reported between 2000 and 2010 [4]. Most of the children were under the age of 3 years. The median age range was 1–2 years and the mean age range was 2.1–3.8 years.

It should be noted that foreign body aspiration is also reported in adolescents. In these instances, the adolescent is commonly neurodevelopmentally delayed or incapacitated by alcohol or drug use. In this age group, non-food foreign bodies are more common (pins, coins, pen caps, etc.).

3. **Why are tracheobronchial foreign bodies most common in very young children?**

There are several factors that predispose very young children to accidental foreign body aspiration [5]. A major factor is their inherent oral curiosity. Infants typically explore their environment by placing objects in their mouth. This behaviour can be particularly problematic when they begin to crawl or walk and gain access to many objects. Young children lack molars to grind food adequately and prematurely swallow large food boluses. Choking on food substances can occur when the children are given unsuitable foods such as nuts or raw vegetables by an unsuspecting parent or young sibling. Young children typically demonstrate active behaviours while eating which may also predispose to accidental choking. Finally, young children have very small airways that are susceptible to complete blockage of the airway by foods with a round shape such as uncut grapes and hotdogs.

4. **What is the mortality associated with tracheobronchial foreign bodies?**

The mortality associated with tracheobronchial foreign bodies is not precisely known. However, national mortality data related to choking have been reported in the United States. In 2000, 160 children aged 14 years or less died from obstruction of the respiratory tract as a result of an inhaled or ingested foreign body (ICD

W79–W80, 10th Edition) [2]. Death was more commonly caused by a non-food substance (59%) than a food substance (41%).

In a review of the English literature, mortality data was reported in 26 of the 30 articles included in the review [4]. There were 43 deaths among 10,236 children with aspirated foreign bodies giving an overall mortality rate of 0.42%. It should be noted that many of the reported deaths occurred either during the treatment bronchoscopy or due to a complication of the procedure. The reported mortality rate is likely an underestimate of the true death rate as the review does not include deaths that occurred prior to reaching medical care.

5. **What are the most common tracheobronchial foreign bodies encountered?**

It is clear from the literature that the nature of foreign bodies encountered varies according to geographical and cultural food preferences.

In a European study, the most common foreign bodies were nuts, seeds, berries, corn and beans [1]. In an Indian study, food materials such as seeds and beans were encountered in 48.8% of cases [3].

In the United States MMWR report, 59.5% of reported cases involved food substances, 31.4% non-food substances and in 9% of cases the nature of the foreign body was not reported [2]. The most common food substances were "solid food" which included cookies, chips/crackers, popcorn, nuts/seeds, bones, bread, meats, fruit, pasta/rice/cereals and candy/gum. Common non-food foreign bodies encountered were coins, toys, marbles, balloons, puzzle pieces, paper, pen caps, tape, and screws.

6. **What are the most dangerous tracheobronchial foreign bodies?**

It should be emphasized that all tracheobronchial foreign bodies are dangerous as they can cause immediate life-threatening airway compromise and serious longer-term complications such as pneumonia and lung collapse. However, there are several food and non-food foreign bodies that pose an added risk of injury, long term complication and death. The foreign bodies that fall into this category are summarized in Table 11.1.

7. **What are the most common clinical presentations associated with tracheobronchial foreign bodies?**

A patient that presents to the emergency department with a history of a witnessed choking event should be considered to have a tracheobronchial foreign body until proven otherwise. The suspicion should remain high even if the patient does not have any signs or symptoms suggestive of a foreign body aspiration.

If the choking event was not witnessed, children typically present with a recent onset of unexplained cough, wheezing, and shortness of breath. If the choking event occurred remotely, the patient may present with 'atypical asthma' that is not responsive to treatment with bronchodilators, chronic cough, or recurrent or non-resolving pneumonia.

Table 11.1 This table summarizes the foreign bodies, their physical characteristics and the associated airway implications

Foreign body	Characteristic	Implications
Balloons, rubber gloves	Inflatable	Complete blockage of airway lumen
Marbles, rocks, balls	Round, hard, smooth surface	Complete blockage of lumen, unable to be grasped, cannot be broken
Medications (e.g. iron, potassium tablets)	Dissolve causing pain and inflammatory reaction	Inflammation or perforation of airway lumen
Sharp objects (e.g. pins, needles)	Sharp edge	Perforation of the airway lumen
Button batteries	Caustic, heavy metals	Severe caustic burn of the airway lumen
Nuts, seeds	Secrete oils	Inflammation and granulation tissue in airway
Grapes, hotdogs	Round, smooth	Complete blockage of airway lumen

8. **What are the most common presenting clinical signs associated with tracheobronchial foreign bodies?**

The clinical signs of a tracheobronchial foreign body in children may range from acute airway distress to subtle chest findings. A child with acute airway distress may demonstrate nasal flaring, preference for an upright posture, tracheal and subcostal indrawing, tachypnea, tachycardia, cyanosis and sialorrhea. Careful inspection of the eyes may reveal multiple scleral hemorrhages. If the foreign body is lodged in the larynx, the child will also present with stridor, dysphonia or aphonia. Aphonia should alert the treating physician to the possibility of a laryngeal foreign body and the need for immediate intervention as laryngeal foreign bodies are associated with a very high risk of death.

Foreign bodies in the lower airway are more commonly associated with diminished breath sounds in a unilateral lung field, ronchi, or wheezing. These clinical findings are more likely to be detected in the right lung field. Foreign bodies are more likely to migrate to the right main bronchus given its orientation which is more in line with the trachea.

9. **What are the most common and useful imaging modalities to assess a patient with a suspected tracheobronchial foreign body?**

The chest radiograph is the most useful imaging modality for the initial assessment of a child with a suspected tracheobronchial foreign body. It is particularly useful for the detection and localization of radio-opaque foreign bodies. However, the chest radiograph may not be helpful with food substances or with objects that are typically non-radio-opaque. In several reported case series, chest radiographs were reported as normal in 17% of cases of confirmed FB aspiration [4].

In some instances, the chest radiograph may detect segmental collapse, atelectasis, hyperinflation of the affected infiltrate or deviation of the mediastinum.

Lateral, inspiratory/expiratory, and lateral decubitus views may be required to detect air trapping caused by a foreign body.

Computed tomography scans and virtual bronchoscopy are other useful imaging modalities to detect tracheobronchial foreign bodies. These investigations are more sensitive, especially for non-radio-opaque foreign bodies, when the diagnosis is equivocal, or if the patient presents with persistent symptoms after bronchoscopy. However, there are concerns with using computed tomography as a first-line investigation such as unnecessary radiation exposure to children, cost and availability. Most importantly, this should not be performed in an unstable or uncooperative patient especially if the imaging equipment is in a remote location or if the child requires sedation. In these instances, the patient should proceed directly to bronchoscopy.

10. **How should patients with tracheobronchial foreign bodies be prioritized for treatment?**

Children with confirmed or a high suspicion of a tracheobronchial foreign body should be assigned the highest priority for treatment, especially if the patient is presenting with concerning clinical signs. For most institutions, the highest priority indicates that the procedure should be performed within 1 hour. With severe airway compromise, fasting rules may be compromised.

An airway foreign body may lead to acute airway compromise, hypoxia and death. The most serious complications associated with delayed treatment of tracheobronchial foreign bodies include pneumothorax, pneumomediastinum, hypoxic brain injury, post-obstructive pulmonary edema, need for tracheostomy, cardiac arrest and death.

Unrecognized and therefore delayed treatment of tracheobronchial foreign bodies may result in pneumonia and loss of lung function.

11. **How are tracheobronchial foreign bodies removed?**

Tracheobronchial foreign bodies are removed under general anesthesia and bronchoscopy [6]. In most pediatric medical centres, tracheobronchial foreign bodies are removed with rigid ventilating bronchoscopes. A full range of ventilating rigid bronchoscopes, rigid telescopes and optical grasping forceps are required equipment. A variety of grasping forceps are commercially available that are designed for specific types of foreign bodies (Fig. 11.1). A thorough description of the tools, and methods to remove foreign bodies is beyond the scope of this chapter (see references). Foreign bodies can also be removed by flexible bronchoscopes with side ports that allow the introduction of grasping forceps. They are particularly useful for very distal foreign bodies that are beyond the reach of rigid bronchoscopes.

12. **When should a tracheostomy be performed to manage a tracheobronchial foreign body?**

A tracheostomy is not usually required for the management of tracheobronchial foreign bodies. However, if the foreign body is firmly lodged at the glottic level, is

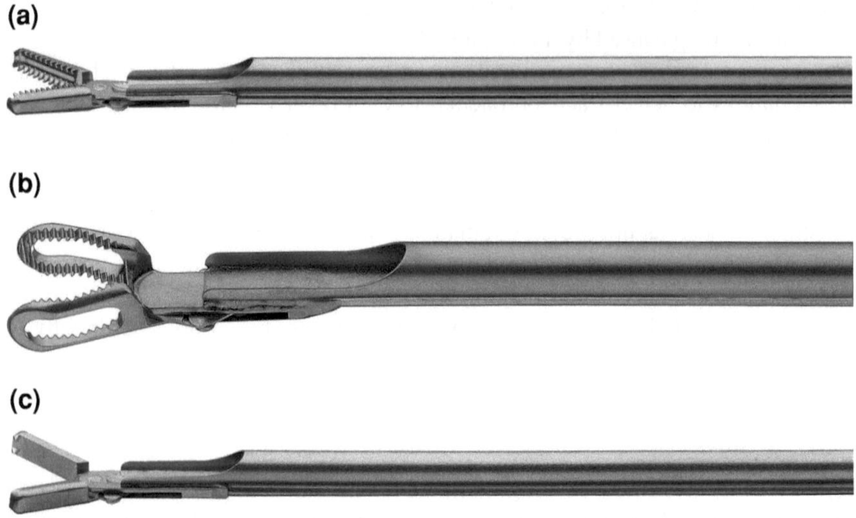

Fig. 11.1 This figure demonstrates a variety of optical grasping forceps commercially available to retrieve foreign bodies. **a** Alligator forceps. **b** Peanut forceps. **c** Coin forceps (photos courtesy of © KARL STORZ SE & Co. KG.)

causing severe airway obstruction, and cannot be easily removed, a tracheostomy may be required.

A temporary tracheostomy may be required for large or irregularly shaped foreign bodies that cannot be withdrawn through the vocal folds. In these rare instances, the foreign body is removed through the tracheostomy.

It should be noted that tracheostomies are not helpful with foreign bodies in the distal trachea or bronchi and therefore should not be performed.

13. **What are the important anaesthetic principles that should be considered when treating a child with a tracheobronchial foreign body?**

Children undergoing rigid bronchoscopy for a tracheobronchial foreign body require a general anesthetic [4]. Anesthesia is induced and maintained by either inhalational agent, intravenous medication or a combination of the two modalities. An intravenous agent may be needed if the airway obstruction is severe and absorption of inhalational agent is compromised. Regardless of the agent used, it is preferable that the induction of anesthesia be gradual so that the patient can maintain spontaneous ventilation throughout the procedure. Spontaneous ventilation avoids dislodging a proximal airway foreign body and minimizes the hyperinflation of the involved lung and therefore the risk of pneumothorax.

Patience must be exercised to allow the patient to achieve the ideal plane of anesthesia to avoid coughing, bucking, desaturation and injury to the airway lumen. Topicalization of the larynx and carina may facilitate rigid bronchoscopy by blunting the stimulation caused by the procedure. In severe cases, the surgeon may need to proceed expeditiously to relieve the airway obstruction and therefore forego an ideal anesthetic plane.

The anesthesiologist should consider the use of anticholinergic medications to decrease the airway secretions and prevent bradycardia, and steroids to minimize glottic and subglottic edema caused by the procedure.

It must be emphasized that rigid bronchoscopy for tracheobronchial foreign bodies requires excellent communication between surgeon and anesthesiologist for an uneventful procedure and best patient outcomes.

14. **What are the important surgical principles that should be considered when treating a child with a tracheobronchial foreign body?**

The surgeon must develop and communicate the plan for the procedure with the anesthetist and nursing team prior to the start of the procedure. A detailed 'time-out' with the team will ensure that the necessary equipment and contingency plans are in place if there is difficulty with maintaining a safe airway during the procedure.

The team should have at their disposal a wide array of laryngoscopes, bronchoscopes and optical grasping forceps to deal with any food and non-food foreign body [6]. The equipment should be well organized, easily accessible and familiar to the nursing team. In many institutions, a dedicated 'airway room' is established to manage tracheobronchial foreign bodies and other airway emergencies.

15. **What is the recommended post-operative care after removal of a tracheobronchial foreign body?**

Infants and young children are typically admitted following a rigid bronchoscopy to remove tracheobronchial foreign bodies. A unit with monitored beds is advisable for the early detection of airway complications. A postoperative chest radiograph is considered if the procedure was prolonged, challenging or if there was injury to the airway lumen.

Patients with signs of airway inflammation, granulation or purulent secretions during bronchoscopy may require systemic antibiotics and inhalational steroids as adjuvant treatment.

Patients with persistent symptoms after bronchoscopy may require a repeat bronchoscopy or computed tomography imaging if residual foreign body fragments are suspected.

16. **Are there choking prevention programs available to physicians and parents?**

There are several established choking prevention programs in North American that provide useful information to physicians and caregivers. The names and websites of available programs is presented below.

American Academy of Pediatrics (www.healthychildren.org/English/health-issues/injuries-emergencies/Pages/Choking-Prevention.aspx).

Canadian Paediatric Society (www.cps.ca/en/documents/position/preventing-choking-suffocation-children).

University of British Columbia (https://dontchoke.ubc.ca).

References

1. Gregori D, Salerni L, Scarinzi C, Morra B, Berchialla P, Snidero S, Corradetti R, Passali D. The ESFBI Study Group: Foreign bodies in the upper airways causing complications and requiring hospitalization in children aged 0-14 years: Results from the ESFBI study. Eur Arch Otorhinolaryngol. 2008;265:971–8.
2. Centers for Disease Control and Prevention (CDC). Nonfatal choking-related episodes among children—United States, 2001. MMWR Morb Mortal Wkly Rep. 2002;51:945–948.
3. Jaswal A, Jana U, Maiti PK. Tracheo-bronchial foreign bodies: a retrospective study and review of literature. Indian J Otolaryngol Head Neck Surg. 2014;66(Suppl 1):S156–60.
4. Fidkowski CW, Zheng H, Firth PG. The anesthetic considerations of tracheobronchial foreign bodies in children: a literature review of 12,979 cases. Anesth Analg. 2010;111:1016–25.
5. Rimell FL, Thome A, Stool S, Reilluy JS, Rider G, Stool D, Wilson CL. Characteristics of objects that cause choking in children. JAMA. 1995;274:1763–6.
6. Campisi P, Forte V. Rigid endoscopy of the airway—basic technique. In: Najmaldin A, editor. Operative endoscopy and endoscopic surgery in infants and children. London: Edward Arnold Ltd.; 2005. p. 53–60.

Chapter 12
Pediatric Surgical Diseases of the Larynx, Trachea, and Bronchi

Elizabeth F. Maughan, Colin Butler, Richard Hewitt, and Paolo De Coppi

Abstract The larynx, trachea and bronchi have separate embryological development and as such a variety of congenital anomalies are possible. In addition, improvements in neonatal intensive care have led to increased numbers of children with secondary airway pathology. Our preference is for conservative or endoscopic management for the majority of cases, but severely stenotic or defective airways may require immediate or open correction in the neonatal period.

Keywords Laryngomalacia · Subglottic stenosis · Vocal cord palsy · Laryngeal cleft · Congenital tracheal stenosis · Tracheobronchomalacia

1. **How do the larynx, trachea and bronchi develop?**

The larynx, trachea/oesophagus, bronchi and lungs have individual embryological developmental patterns [1]. The laryngotracheal groove, or sulcus, appears in the proximal foregut in the 3rd week of gestation and progresses caudally to form a tracheoesophageal septum which separates primitive airway and digestive tracts, and complete separation of the trachea and oesophagus has usually occurred by the 6th week. The bronchial primordia develop in parallel as asymmetric tracheal tip buds. The cartilaginous and muscular components of the trachea and bronchi are detectable from the 10th week and are derived from proliferating coelomic cavity cells. At birth the tracheal length is approximately 3 cm in length and 5 mm in diameter. It continues to grow around 5 mm a year, reaching full adult dimensions of around 15 cm in length and 20 mm in diameter by the age of 16 years.

These separate embryological developments account for the diversity in congenital anomalies that can be found in the respiratory tree [1], as possible

E. F. Maughan · C. Butler · R. Hewitt · P. De Coppi (✉)
Great Ormond Street Hospital Tracheal Service, London, UK
e-mail: p.decoppi@ucl.ac.uk

M. Lacher et al. (eds.), *Pearls and Tricks in Pediatric Surgery*,
https://doi.org/10.1007/978-3-030-51067-1_12

malformations exist on a spectrum of severity and can affect any portion of the upper respiratory tract from face to bronchi.

2. **What surgical pathologies are classically seen in the pediatric airway?**

The common surgical pathologies of the larynx and trachea are shown in Table 12.1, and can represent either:

- narrowing of the airway caliber (i.e. subglottic stenosis or congenital tracheal stenosis);
- structural deficiency of the airway (i.e. laryngomalacia, tracheobronchomalacia or laryngeal cleft); or
- problems with functional mobility (i.e. vocal cord palsy).

The severity and symptoms can vary greatly for each condition, and can all be congenital, secondary or due to a mixture of etiologies. It should be noted that, with the exception of laryngomalacia, most conditions are uncommon or rare in the general population, and as such there should be a low threshold for management of these children in a tertiary pediatric center.

3. **How are pediatric airway problems assessed?**

Clinical evaluation should include a history that is focused on airway symptoms, which will be dependent on the location and severity of disease. Characteristic symptoms include dysphonia, abnormal cry and dysphagia. There may be a history of increasing respiratory distress, shortness of breath (related to exertion/feeding) and accompanying stertor or stridor. Cyanotic episodes are a notable feature that should expedite clinical investigations. Recurrent unexplained aspiration

Table 12.1 Common airway pathologies in children and their reported incidence [1–7]

Condition	Incidence/Prevalence
Laryngomalacia	Prevalence: 60% of all infants with stridor
Recurrent respiratory papillomatosis	Incidence 0.5-1.0/100,000 whole population.
Subglottic stenosis	Primary: Secondary to intubation: Up to 2% of NICU graduates, 11% of PICU graduates
Vocal cord palsy	4-8% of infants post-cardiac surgery
Tracheobronchomalacia	1:2100 births
Laryngeal cleft	1:20,000 births Up to 8% of MLBs for unexplained chronic aspiration
Tracheoesophageal fistula*	* Chapter 5 discusses this condition in more detail.
Congenital tracheal stenosis	1:64,500 live births

episodes or lower respiratory tract infections should raise clinical suspicions of abnormal communications between the airway and esophagus.

Direct evaluation of the airway is typically performed through endoscopy. Flexible nasendoscopy will allow evaluation of the nasopharynx, pharynx and larynx, and can be performed in the awake child. Laryngomalacia can typically be diagnosed by this method, and the child's inevitable cry during examination is of a characteristic quality. In a severely affected infant, the risk of a second, more distal, airway lesion may be as high as 50% [2], so clinicians should maintain a high index of suspicion and a low threshold for full evaluation of the large airways by microlaryngoscopy and tracheobronchoscopy (MLB) under general anesthesia (Fig. 12.1). This investigation is performed with a child self-ventilating, provides some dynamic information of the airway and enables evaluation from the larynx to the first bronchial division. Alternative evaluation can also be performed through flexible bronchoscopy and allows for distal evaluation of the airway.

Radiological assessment includes computed tomography (CT) particularly when evaluating for external (vascular) compression. Other radiological investigations include bronchography (Fig. 12.1), which provides dynamic evaluation of the airway particularly related to malacia. Increasingly 4D CT is being used to evaluate the airway in the appropriate child.

4. **What is laryngomalacia and how is it assessed?**

Laryngomalacia is a congenital condition whereby the supraglottic component of the larynx partially or completely collapses on inspiration. It is the most common cause of congenital stridor [3], but its precise pathophysiology is unclear. A clinical history will typically be characterized by a high-pitched inspiratory stridor present shortly after birth. Stridor will often be exacerbated when the infant is active or cry, and symptoms resolve when settled or asleep. The natural history of

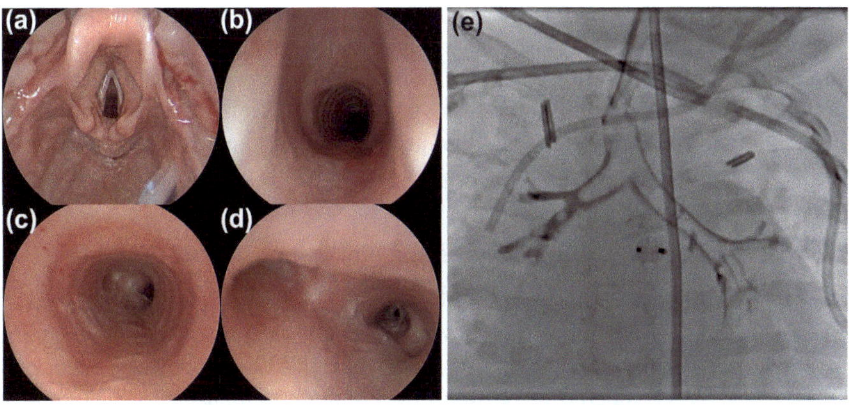

Fig. 12.1 Assessment with microlayrngoscopy and bronchoscopy (A–proximal to distal: supraglottis, subglottis, mid trachea and carina) combined with bronchography (E)

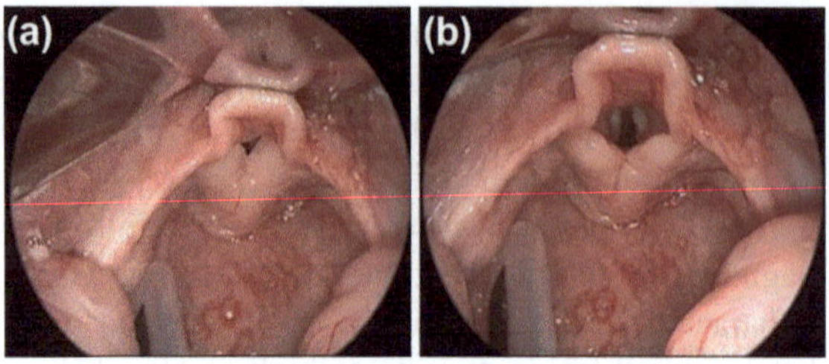

Fig. 12.2 Characteristic endoscopic appearance of laryngomalacia during inspiration (**a**) and expiration (**b**), demonstrating shortened aryepiglottic folds and tall prolapsing arytenoids during inspiration leading to airway obstruction

the disease is such that symptoms are at their peak at 9 months and then resolve after 12–18 months.

Evaluation would include evaluating a child's weight and continued growth according to their birth centile, as well as a history of respiratory distress or decompensation in times of illness, and a flexible nasendoscopy can be performed in an outpatient clinic. Features seen on endoscopy will included a long and curled epiglottis (omega shaped) and aryepiglottic folds that are tall and bulky. The aryepiglottic folds will tend be short in anteroposterior direction or tether to the epiglottis. With significant respiration, a soft epiglottis and/or the redundant mucosa of the aryepiglottic folds may be seen to collapse into the airway (Fig. 12.2).

5. **How is laryngomalacia managed?**

As with most pediatric airway conditions, the management of laryngomalacia is primarily guided by the degree of symptoms experienced. Babies with otherwise asymptomatic stridor or mild difficulties with feeding should be managed conservatively as long as the child is gaining weight appropriately. Adjustments to sleeping and feeding strategies (i.e. front sleeping and bottle-feeding) may be necessary to support this.

If a child is failing to thrive or gain weight, or has evidence of ongoing or recurrent respiratory distress, endoscopic assessment and surgical management is required. Surgery is performed according to the areas of the supraglottis that are seen to be causing excessive obstruction under spontaneous ventilation, and classically involve partial or complete division of the aryepiglottic folds (aryepiglottoplasty) and/or trimming of excess prolapsing arytenoid mucosa. Given the inevitable improvement in the condition as the child ages, an extremely conservative approach to removing tissue is always preferable to prevent the likelihood of swallow compromise.

6. **What is respiratory papillomatosis and how is it managed?**

Recurrent respiratory papillomatosis (RRP) is a condition caused by infection of the upper airway by the human papilloma virus (HPV) strains 6 and 11, whereby exophytic outgrowths occur in the airway. HPV11 is the more aggressive viral strain. They are considered to be the most common benign laryngeal tumor to occur in children. In children, the virus is thought to be transmitted from mother to child at the time of delivery, although it is still rare even in neonates born to

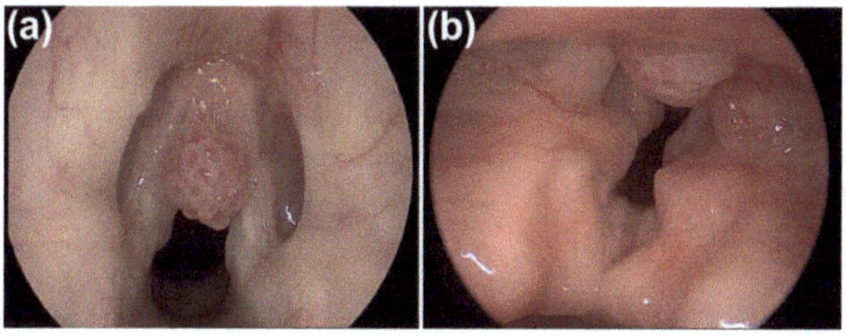

Fig. 12.3 Characteristic endoscopic appearance of RRP in two children with laryngeal disease demonstrating active laryngeal disease. **a** Respiratory papillomatous lesion at the anterior commissure occupying the glottis. **b** More diffuse laryngeal disease predominantly in the supraglottis

HPV-positive mothers. RRP can occur at any age, but pediatric cases are associated with a more aggressive course. Patients generally experience hoarseness and depending on the degree and location of these papillomata, severe cases may also develop subacute airway obstruction. Lesions are most commonly seen at the level of the glottis and/or supraglottis, but papillomata may extend along the entire length of the trachea (Fig. 12.3).

Treatment to clear established papillomatous disease is primarily surgical, with the utmost care taken to preserve the underlying structures. The biggest revolution in recent years in this condition has been the introduction of population-level HPV vaccination in North America, UK and Australia, which has already started showing demonstrable reductions in annual incidence levels. The vaccine may also have a role in treatment, by increasing average time intervals between surgical procedures. Other new medical treatments for established disease may include monoclonal antibody therapy such as Bevacizumab (Avastin) which targets VEGF receptors.

7. **What are the main causes for subglottic stenosis and how is it assessed?**

Subglottic stenosis (SGS) may be a primary, classically oval-shaped, pathology or may be a sequela of prolonged or traumatic intubation. Given general improvements in the prognosis of neonatal and pediatric intensive care graduates, post-intubation subglottic stenosis is growing in incidence [4]. SGS can also be found in association with syndromes such as Down's.

Children classically present with subacute respiratory distress (as the child outgrows their fixed subglottic airway diameter) with signs of decompensation during times of higher respiratory demand (i.e. feeding or concurrent illness). Recurrent croup episodes requiring hospital admission should therefore raise suspicion of an underlying stenosis and this presentation requires endoscopic evaluation. A classical presentation of secondary SGS would be an evolving difficulty in intubating an infant with an endotracheal (ET) tube of an age-appropriate diameter (Fig. 12.4).

At the time of MLB, the surgeon sizes the subglottis relative to endotracheal tubes of an age-appropriate size (calculated as (age in years+4)/4). If an 'age-appropriate' tube does not pass, smaller tubes are passed with a stepwise increase in size until an ET tube size that just passes with a leak of air around it.

Table 12.2 Cotton-Myer classification. The grading system for subglottic stenosis is based on percent of stenosis. (A) The degree of obstruction can be classified by the percent of obstruction. (B) This can be calculated using an endotracheal tube to size the stenosis which can then be compared to the expected size of the airway for different ages of the child. Figures and tables from Ann Otol Rhinol Laryngol 1994;103(4 Pt 1):319–323

(a)

Classification	From	To
Grade I	No obstruction	50% obstruction
Grade II	51% obstruction	70% obstruction
Grade III	71% obstruction	99% obstruction
Grade IV	No Detectable Lumen	

(b)

Percent airway obstruction based on endotracheal tube size									
Age	ETT	2	2.5	3	3.5	4	4.5	5	5.5
Pre-term	No detectable lumen	40%							
Pre-term		58%	30%			No obstruction			
0-3mo.		68%	48%	26%					
3-9mo.		75%	59%	41%	22%				
9mo-2yr		80%	67%	53%	38%	20%			
2yr		84%	74%	62%	50%	35%	19%		
4yr		86%	78%	68%	57%	45%	32%	17%	
6yr		98%	81%	73%	64%	54%	43%	30%	16%
	Grade IV	Grade III			Grade II		Grade I		

The Cotton-Myer system is also commonly used to convert this ET tube size to a percentage of airway obstructed (Table 12.2).

8. **What are the management options for subglottic stenosis?**

Management of mild SGS can be conservative with a watch-and-wait policy as the child grows. Gastroesophageal reflux disease may be a contributing factor to the formation of post-traumatic stenosis and should be managed closely. Temporary relief can be obtained with endoscopic balloon dilatation of the subglottis. A cricoid split can be considered in an acute scenario for more immediate management.

In symptomatic cases that have failed repeated endoscopic management, surgical augmentation of the cricoid may be necessary via laryngotracheal reconstruction (LTR). In the procedure, the cricoid ring is split in the anterior midline and a 'boat-shaped' cartilage rib autograft inserted to augment its diameter. In more severe or oval-shaped cases, a straight posterior graft may also be used (Fig. 12.4).

9. **How are vocal cord palsies assessed and managed in pediatrics?**

The intrinsic muscles of the larynx responsible for vocal cord movement are supplied by the recurrent laryngeal nerves (the notable exception being the cricothyroid muscle, responsible for pitch regulation, which is innervated by the external laryngeal nerves). Sensation is supplied by superior laryngeal nerves. Vocal cord palsies may be primary (idiopathic) or secondary and may one or both cords. In adults, the risk of neuropraxia or more permanent damage to the recurrent laryngeal nerves during thyroid surgery is well-documented, but this is a rare surgical pathology in children where the left recurrent laryngeal nerve is more commonly at risk during cardiac surgery, particularly patent ductus arteriosus ligation or aortic arch repairs. Symptoms generally include an impact on voice/cry and a history of an unsafe swallow with overt or silent aspiration leading to recurrent chest infections. Movement and sensation can be affected independently. Impaired sensation is often inferred from a history of recurrent chest infections or by videofluoroscopic examination demonstrating silent aspiration without a reliable cough reflex.

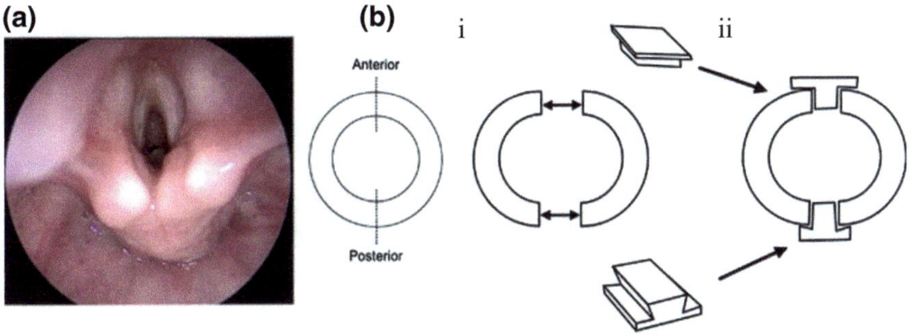

Fig. 12.4 Subglottic stenosis and typical surgical management with laryngotracheal augmentation. **a** Post intubation laryngotracheal stensosis. **b** Reconstruction for subglottic stenosis through laryngotracheal reconstruction with anterior and posterior grafts. (i) The airway is exposed and the cricoid is split via a laryngofissure allowing access to the posterior cricoid plate which can also be divided vertically in the midline (ii) An anterior graft can be inserted in isolation or combined with a posterior graft depending on the airway stenosis widening the diameter. A rib cartilage is typically fashioned to fill the space anterior and posteriorly. Anterior grafts are fashioned as diamond with flanges and the posterior graft is fashioned as "T-shape" graft

Children can usually compensate extremely well for a unilateral vocal cord palsy both in terms of voice and swallow function, and the mainstay of treatment should be speech and language therapy. Bilateral vocal cord palsies are far more likely to be symptomatic, and the symptoms experienced are related to the position of the cord. The non-functional cord(s) may lie in either adducted or abducted positions. Cords in the midline can lead to respiratory obstruction necessitating tracheostomy with the potential for a relatively preserved voice and swallow, whereas bilateral cord palsies in more abducted positions will lead to aspiration problems and aphonia.

Laryngeal innervation is increasingly considered for permanent vocal cord paralysis, and whilst full function is unlikely to be obtained, regaining muscle tone alone can lead to appreciable functional benefits as a salvage treatment option.

10. **What are the causes and management options for tracheobronchomalacia?**

Tracheobronchomalacia (TBM) remains an exceedingly difficult condition to manage successfully in the paediatric population, as evidence for diagnosis, classification and management is limited. It is arbitrarily defined by the excessive (>50%) collapse in the cross-sectional luminal area of the large airways during the normal physiological pressures of quiet respiration [5] (such that life-threatening cardiopulmonary events can occur. TBM may occur in isolation (potentially due to failure of the coelomic cavity cells responsible for cartilage formation to populate the trachea), or secondary to other local or general tracheal disease. Extrinsic compression by aberrant vasculature (such as pulmonary artery slings, aberrant aortic morphology or innominate artery compression) or other mediastinal structures may also lead to localised segments of TBM. Diagnosis is usually made on MLB and/or flexible bronchoscopy (Fig. 12.5), but other dynamic techniques such as

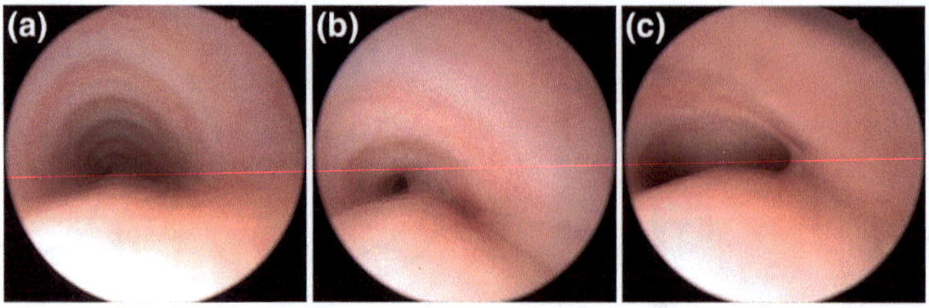

Fig. 12.5 Endoscopic appearance of tracheobronchomalacia

bronchography and CT may also show the condition. External compression from vascular structures is identified from a suspicious endoscopic appearance of the luminal tracheal shape and confirmed with a CT angiogram.

Management is largely related to the underlying cause. Respiratory support, if required, is generally given as continuous positive airway pressure via face mask or tracheostomy. Medical treatments include bronchodilators, mucolytics, antibiotics and chest physiotherapy. Surgical options are also targeted to the underlying area of structural weakness but can include aortopexy or posterior tracheopexy, resection of affected segments if short, internal stents or consideration of external splinting [5].

Although disease severity usually decreases after the first year or two of life in most primary non-syndromic cases as the child's airway cartilage matures, respiratory failure and resultant severe infections often require intensive therapy during infancy.

11. **What are laryngeal clefts and how do they present?**

Laryngeal clefts are a congenital posterosuperior defect in the posterior larynx and trachealis, caused by the failure of the tracheoesophageal septum to develop appropriately. This leads to an aberrant connection of variable size and length between the larynx/trachea and the esophagus. The spectrum of congenital abnormality is diverse and they are often associated with esophageal atresia (EA—see Chap. 5), tracheoesophageal fistulae, vocal cord palsies and malacia or other abnormalities including cardiac defects (ASD and VSD), gastrointestinal and genitourinary anomalies. They are also associated with midline malformation syndromes. Whilst mainly sporadic in inheritance there are reports of autosomal dominant pattern. The most commonly used classification system is by Benjamin and Inglis which classifies clefts into 4 types (Fig. 12.6):

- Type 1: the cleft involves the supraglottic inter-arytenoid region but no further than the level of true vocal cords;
- Type 2: the cleft extends beyond the true vocal cords into the cricoid (but not completely through it);
- Type 3: the cleft extends through the cricoid and into cervical trachea;
- Type 4: the cleft extends into the posterior wall of the thoracic trachea as far as the carina.

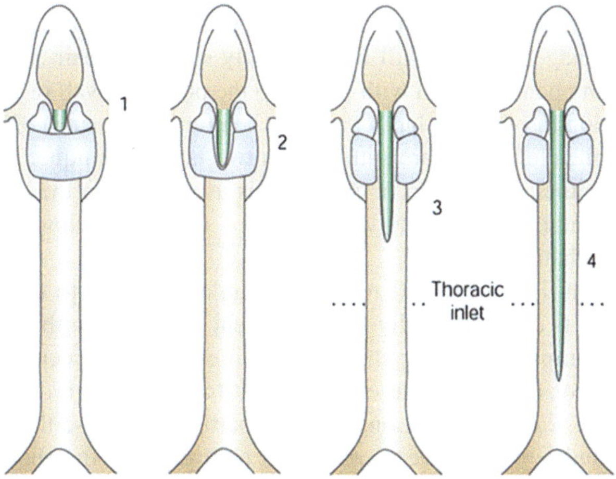

Fig. 12.6 Benjamin Inglis classification of laryngeal clefts. Type I: the cleft involves the supraglottic inter-arytenoid region but no further than the level of true vocal cords; Type II: the cleft extends beyond the true vocal cords into the cricoid (but not completely through it); Type III: the cleft extends through the cricoid and into cervical trachea; Type IV: extends into the posterior wall of the thoracic trachea as far as the carina. Reproduced from Benjamin B, Inglis A. Minor congenital laryngeal clefts: diagnosis and classification. Ann Otol Rhinol Laryngol. 1989;98(6):417–420. https://doi.org/10.1177/000348948909800603 with permission from SAGE publishing

A large laryngeal cleft (long Grade III and Grade IV) will present with acute respiratory distress on delivery. Intubation may be difficult as the endotracheal tube (ETT) is likely to displace posteriorly into the oesophagus through the cleft. Most children with Grades II and III will also be identified in the neonatal period with acute or subacute airway obstruction, recurrent chest infections, swallowing and/or feeding difficulties. However, smaller Grade I and II clefts can be missed and subsequently found in the older child. These children will present with a history of poor swallow and/or recurrent chest infections or intractable cough due to aspiration. A high index of suspicion is required to identify the underlying cause. Specialist paediatric swallow assessment is helpful in diagnosis, aspiration assessment and monitoring surgical success. A video fluoroscopic swallow study (VFSS) will show contrast penetrating the posterior aspect of the glottis. Formal identification of the extent of the cleft is performed on MLB by careful and thorough probing of the interarytenoid region and posterior tracheal wall.

12. **How are laryngeal clefts managed?**

The decision to use either endoscopic or open repair techniques is largely dependent on the cleft length. Small clefts may be initially treated with the use of thickened feeds and anti-reflux medication prior to surgical correction. Endoscopic repair is usually performed on type I and II clefts and involves excising the edges of the cleft with closure either as a single layer or two-layer technique.

Larger clefts (type III and type IV) will not usually tolerate a trial period of conservative management and will need an early surgical repair. This is typically performed by an open approach with access to the posterior wall of the trachea via a midline incision through the larynx and trachea (laryngofissure). Excess mucosa is excised and the cleft edges are sutured in a two-layer technique. In some cases, graft material (either periosteum or cartilage) is used between the layers for additional support. Intubation is usually required for 1 week to allow for the cleft to heal prior to extubation.

Outcomes from laryngeal cleft repair are similarly related to the length of the cleft. Type I and II clefts generally have excellent prognosis with almost all leading to symptom improvement for children identified at risk of recurrent aspiration. Other complications include failure of the cleft to close which can be related to dehiscence at the site of repair. Longer clefts, particularly those that extend to the thoracic inlet and beyond, have a protracted recovery due to inherent structural malacia associated with the cleft. There is also often a degree of oesophageal dysmotility and the need for a gastrostomy is not uncommon.

13. **How is congenital tracheal stenosis (CTS) classified and managed?**

Congenital tracheal stenosis (CTS) is typically classified as either short segment or long segment (spanning over 1 cm in the newborn and 1.5 cm in the infant, or affecting over 50% of the total tracheal length in older children). Primary CTS is due to the presence of complete tracheal rings rather than the normal 'C'-shape cartilage morphology, although it may also occur secondary to extrinsic pressure from nearby structures—60% of children born with CTS have other associated malformations, most commonly mediastinal and cardiovascular anomalies. It is usually the combination of both airway and cardiovascular disease that leads to life threatening compromise. The trachea may also demonstrate an abnormal branching pattern, often with downstream regions of associated malacia.

Infants with moderate or mild disease may not be diagnosed until later in childhood when their gas exchange demands start to outstrip the flow of air through the narrowed tracheobronchial section. At the other end of the spectrum, severely affected infants may need extracorporeal membrane oxygenation until definitive surgery can be performed. The slide tracheoplasty procedure has revolutionised the surgical treatment of children with CTS [6] (Fig. 12.7). In our patient series, one of the largest in the world, it has been shown to be both safe and reliable for short segment and acquired CTS with low associated morbidity and mortality.

14. **What is the CHAOS syndrome and how is it managed?**

Presentation and diagnosis of obstructing laryngeal and high tracheal birth defects usually occurs following routine prenatal ultrasound scanning with confirmation by in utero MRI, but can present later with immediate respiratory distress at birth. Obstructive lesions can be intrinsic, i.e. the so-called Congenital high airway obstruction syndrome (CHAOS) infant, but are more commonly caused by extrinsic compression by pharyngeal, cervical or thoracic mass lesions such as teratomas or cystic hygromas. In cases of intrinsic lesions, it is likely that failure of

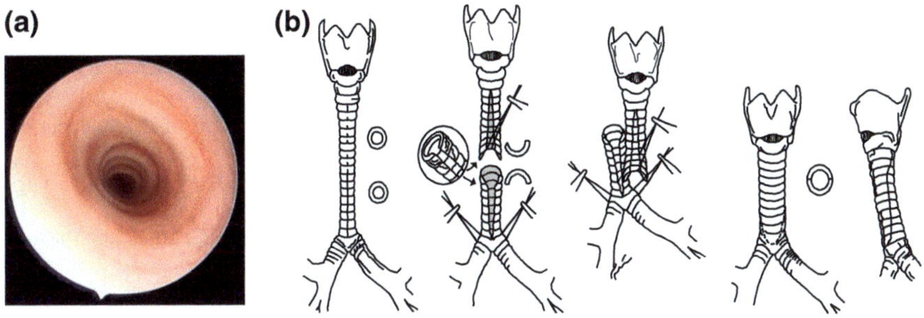

Fig. 12.7 Complete Tracheal stenosis and surgical management. **a** Tracheobronchoscopy demonstrating congenital complete trachea rings. **b** Figurative diagram demonstrating a standard slide tracheoplasty. The trachea is transected midstenosis and divided vertically over the anterior distal trachea and posterior proximal trachea. The proximal and distal segments are 'slid' over each other to augment the airway diameter and sutured in position.
Reproducted from Grillo HC, Wright CD, Vlahakes GJ, MacGillivray TE. Management of congenital tracheal stenosis by means of slide tracheoplasty or resection and reconstruction, with long-term follow-up of growth after slide tracheoplasty. J Thorac Cardiovasc Surg. 2002; 123(1):145–152 with permission from Elsevier

the laryngeal epithelial lamina to recanalize properly underlies cases of laryngeal webs or cysts, near-total stenosis or complete laryngeal atresia.

Without immediate surgical intervention, the congenital lack of a patent proximal airway is unsurvivable unless a bypassing pathway exists for intubation of the bronchi via associated fistulae with the esophagus distal to the obstruction. Careful discussion with parents must be conducted as to their wishes for treatment, especially given that primary laryngeal obstruction has a strong association with other congenital abnormalities such as Fraser syndrome. Prolonged obstruction to the respiratory tree throughout gestation may also lead to unsurvivable lung malformation. If parents are still in favor of continuing with the pregnancy, a planned delivery is possible via the *ex utero* intrapartum treatment (EXIT) procedure, where the precarious neonatal airway may be salvaged or established de novo via anesthetic techniques or tracheostomy, prior to cutting off oxygenation via the umbilical cord [7], followed by definitive airway establishment depending on the nature of the lesion.

Typical features of tracheomalacia is seen with anteroposterior compression of the airway. (A–C proximal trachea, mid trachea and carina).

References

1. Adamiec E, Dzieciolowska-Baran E, Czerwinski F, Miklaszewska D, Teul I. Prenatal development of the human trachea. Folia Morphol (Warsz). 2002;61:123–5.
2. Dickson JM, Richter GT, Meinzen-Derr J, Rutter MJ, Thompson DM. Secondary airway lesions in infants with laryngomalacia. Ann Otol, Rhinol Laryngol. 2009;118:37–43.

3. Holinger LD. Etiology of stridor in the neonate, infant and child. Annals of Otology, Rhinology & Laryngology. 1980;89:397–400.
4. Walner DL, Loewen MS, Kimura RE. Neonatal subglottic stenosis—incidence and trends. The Laryngoscope. 2001;111:48–51.
5. Wallis C, Alexopoulou E, Antón-Pacheco JL, et al. ERS statement on tracheomalacia and bronchomalacia in children. Eur Respir J. 2019;54:1900382.
6. Elliott M, Hartley BEJ, Wallis C, Roebuck D. Slide tracheoplasty. Curr Opin Otolaryngol Head Neck Surg. 2008;16:75–82.
7. Liechty KW. Ex-utero intrapartum therapy. Seminars in fetal and neonatal medicine. Elsevier; 2010, p. 34–9.

Chapter 13
Mediastinal Masses

Arnaud Bonnard

Abstract A variety of mediastinal masses may present in children. In the anterior mediastinum, germ cell tumors and thymomas are the main diagnoses. The need for thymectomy in a context of myasthenia will be discussed. In the middle mediastinum, hematologic diseases (lymphomas) are the most common. An appropriate imaging is necessary. Biopsies under general anesthesia need special precautions as the upper airways can collapse. Finally, in the posterior mediastinum three types of foregut duplication cysts may be diagnosed: bronchogenic cysts, esophageal duplication cysts, and neuroenteric cysts. Also, neurogenic tumors frequently occur in this anatomic compartment. Foregut duplication cysts are generally not a surgical problem. Thoracoscopy, whenever possible, should be used and favored over open surgery.

Keywords Mediastinum · Thymoma · Neurogenic tumors · Lymphoma · Thoracoscopy

1. **Which anatomic structures are located in the mediastinum and how is it divided?** [1]

The mediastinum is located in the chest and delimited laterally by the pleura of the right and the left lung. It is bordered superiorly by the thoracic inlet, inferiorly by the diaphragm, anteriorly by the sternum and posteriorly by the vertebra. Division of the mediastinum into specific anatomic compartments is mandatory to develop a differential diagnosis for a mediastinal mass identified on imaging. In the anterior mediastinum the thymus and heart are located. The trachea, carina, vena cava and aorta are part of the middle mediastinum. In the posterior mediastinum

A. Bonnard (✉)
Robert Debre Children University Hospital, APHP and Paris cité University,
48 Boulevard Sérurier, 75019 Paris, France
e-mail: arnaud.bonnard@aphp.fr

M. Lacher et al. (eds.), *Pearls and Tricks in Pediatric Surgery*,
https://doi.org/10.1007/978-3-030-51067-1_13

esophagus, sympathetic ganglia chain, thoracic duct, vagus nerve and descending aorta are the main structures.

2. **What is the most frequent localization of a pediatric mediastinal mass?**

Posterior mediastinal masses are most frequent. In a series of 120 cases, 44% tumors were located in the posterior mediastinum, 31% in the anterior and 25% in the middle mediastinum [2].

3. **How many % of mediastinal masses are malignant in children?**

50%. If a malignancy is suspected a collaboration with an oncologist is mandatory.

4. **What masses are typical for each part of the mediastinum?** [3, 4]

In the anterior mediastinum, the most common tumors include thymomas and teratomas followed by thymic cysts. In the middle mediastinum, malignant hemopathies such as lymphoblastic tumors, Hodgkin disease, or mediastinal large cell non-Hodgkin's lymphomas can develop. Because of the surrounding structures, respiratory symptoms can occur related to the compression of the carina and/or trachea. In the posterior mediastinum, neurogenic masses such as neuroblastomas or gangliomas are the most important tumors. Foregut duplication cysts deriving from the esophagus or bronchus and even rare masses like lymphangiomas can be found.

5. **What kind of mediastinal masses are diagnosed prenatally?**

Cystic masses. These can be foregut duplication cysts, lymphangiomas and rarely neuroenteric cysts. Infrequently, fetal mediastinal teratomas can be diagnosed compromising the airway or presenting with pericardial effusion which can lead to fetal demise. Parents need to be counselled before delivery. A CT scan or MRI needs to be performed postnatally to plan surgery.

6. **What is the role of the Ex Utero Intra Partum (EXIT) procedure in the management of prenatally diagnosed mediastinal mass?**

Mediastinal teratomas can compress intrathoracic structures and present with non-immune fetal hydrops and/or respiratory distress in the newborn. EXIT allows to secure the airway after delivery. Planning an EXIT requires a thorough planning with a multidisciplinary team.

7. **How do mediastinal masses present?** [1]

Many mediastinal masses are an incidental finding on chest radiographs and asymptomatic. The most common symptoms at presentation are dyspnea, cough, fever, aching pain. Children may also present with recurrent pulmonary infections. Malignant tumors are most likely to be symptomatic with dyspnea, orthopnea and cough. They are usually located in the anterior mediastinum. Rarely, Horner´s syndrome and superior vena cava syndrome are reported in relation with malignant lesions in the posterior or middle mediastinum.

8. **Which mediastinal masses have a rapid versus slow/chronic onset?**

A rapid onset of symptoms is suggestive for lymphoblastic non-Hodgkin's lymphoma, an intermediate onset Hodgkin's disease or mediastinal large cell non-Hodgkin's lymphoma, and a chronic onset is typical for slow growing tumors such as teratoma. In older patients, a mediastinal mass can develop in relation to malignant adenopathy deriving from a non-seminomatous germ cell tumor.

9. **How does the diagnostic workup for a mediastinal mass look like?** [1]

Imaging is the first step to accurately diagnose a mediastinal mass. It should be guided by a well conducted clinical exam looking for palpable lymph nodes, Horner's or superior vena cava syndrome, respiratory distress, wheezing or stridor consistent with a compression of the trachea. Incidental findings are usually discovered on a chest x-ray done for repeated and chronic respiratory symptoms. A CT scan needs to be performed to further workup the suspected diagnosis. Posterior mediastinal cystic masses are very well described (bronchogenic cysts, intestinal duplications as well as neurogenic tumors). For these cases MRI is useful to assess the extension to the intervertebral foramina. In anterior mediastinal masses, multiple enlarged lymph nodes on CT are the most frequent additional finding. FDG-PET/CT has become the modality of choice for staging most lymphomas and is more accurate in detecting both intranodal and extranodal disease than CT.

10. **What are the typical radiologic features of a mediastinal teratomas on MRI?**

A cystic or mixt cystic and solid lesion and containing fat, soft tissue and calcifications.

11. **Do all mediastinal masses require a biopsy?**

No. A cystic lesion arising in the posterior mediastinum doesn't need a needle or a surgical biopsy and primary surgical resection is indicated. For most of the other lesions, either posterior or anterior, a biopsy should be obtained to obtain a definite diagnosis.

12. **Can it be dangerous to biopsy a mediastinal mass under general anesthesia?**

Yes. The respiratory status of the patient need to be carefully assessed since the intra tracheal ventilation for general anesthesia can be difficult due to sudden airway and cardiovascular collapse. Of note, signs and symptoms of airway compression and cardiovascular instability may be absent prior to anesthesia. However, the possibility of life-threatening collapse of the airway or cardiovascular obstruction has to always be taken into consideration by both the surgeon and the anesthesiologist.

13. **What are the alternatives to a direct biopsy under general anesthesia?**

Whenever possible, an alternative biopsy site/specimen should be chosen and the tissue harvested under local anesthesia. This can be pleural effusion, peripheral blood smear for leukemia or Bone Marrow aspiration (BMA). If palpable lymph nodes are present, these may be easily removed and send for histology. Finally, if nothing but a biopsy under general anesthesia is doable, a mediastinoscopic biopsy should be considered as a safe technique in children.

14. **What biological workup should be done for a mediastinal mass?**

Cystic masses of the posterior mediastinum do not need any specific test. In contrast, solid lesions require tests such as Vanillylmandelic Acid, Homovanillic Acid, and Catecholamines in a urine sample. In case of an anterior mediastinal mass, α-FP and HCG for suspected teratomas. If the diagnosis is in favor of hematologic disease LDH, blood formula, peripheral blood smear or BMA should be obtained.

15. **What is the prognosis of a thoracic neuroblastoma compared to another localisation?** [5]

In a large neuroblastoma cohort of 1180 cases, primary tumors that arose from the adrenal gland ($N=646$) were associated with inferior outcomes in comparison to primary thoracic tumors ($N=118$), including reduced event-free (EFS; $P=0.006$) and overall (OS; $P<0.001$) survival.

16. **Do all mediastinal masses have to be surgically resected?**

No. Non Hodgkin Lymphoma and Lymphoma type B are treated medically; sometimes, even before the biopsy with steroids to avoid any complication related to a compromised airway.

17. **What is the association between myasthenia gravis and thymoma?**

In patients with myasthenia gravis (MG) a thymoma is associated in 8.5 to 15% of cases. MG affects about 30 to 40% of patients with thymoma and is the most common paraneoplastic syndrome. These patients are usually 10 years younger than those presenting with thymoma without MG.

18. **What is the classic differential diagnosis of a thymoma?**

Thymus hyperplasia. which can be differentiated on CT or MRI.

19. **What is the indication for thymectomy in patients with MG?**

Presence of thymoma is an absolute indication for thymectomy irrespective of the severity of MG. In contrast, indication for thymectomy in case of thymus hyperplasia is mainly dependent on the severity of the neurologic disease.

20. **What is the risk to develop MG after thymectomy?** [6]

The risk is estimated to be 1 to 3%, mainly related to a positive preoperative anti–acetylcholine receptor antibody level.

21. **What is the preferable surgical approach to a mediastinal mass?**

Whenever possible, a thoracoscopic approach should be used. Complication rates are similar to open techniques. It may require fewer blood transfusions, and shorter thoracic drainage and hospital stay. Correct imaging needs to be obtained prior to surgery to select the best candidate for this approach. A huge tumor involving great vessels, or with unclear limits should not approached minimal invasive. Foregut duplication cysts and thymus masses are the most reported procedures in the literature.

22. **Is there a place for robotic surgery in treating mediastinal masses?**

To date, there are only few reports on robotic surgery for mediastinal masses. The main issue is the size and the length of the equipment used. With the da Vinci Xi system, 8 mm instruments are used. Thus, the age of the patient is a crucial point. Other key issues include the loss of tactile feedback, and the cost of the robotic system itself. Nevertheless, robotic surgery is reported to be a safe and effective method for resecting mediastinal masses in children. Dissection might be facilitated by the articulating robotic instruments and the 3D visualization.

References

1. Carter BW, Benveniste MF, Madan R, Godoy MC, de Groot PM, Truong MT, Rosado-de-Christenson ML, Marom EM. ITMIG classification of mediastinal compartments and multidisciplinary approach to mediastinal masses. Radiographics. 2017;37:413–36.
2. Gun F, Erginel B, Ünüvar A, Kebudi R, Salman T, Çelik A. Mediastinal masses in children: experience with 120 cases. Pediatr Hematol Oncol. 2012;29:141–7.
3. Jaggers J, Balsara K. Mediastinal masses in children. Thorac Cardiovasc Surg. 2004;2004(16):201–8.
4. Detterbeck F. Clinical approach to mediastinal masses. In: Kuzdal JML, Muller M, Papagiannopoulos K, et al., editors. ESTS textbook of thoracic surgery. Exeter, UK: European Society of Thoracic Surgeons; 2014.
5. Oldridge DA, Truong B, Russ D, DuBois SG, Vaksman Z, Mosse YP, Diskin SJ, Maris JM, Matthay KK. Differences in genomic profiles and outcomes between thoracic and adrenal neuroblastoma. J Natl Cancer Inst. 2019.
6. Zielinski M. Management of myasthenic patients with thymoma. Thorac Surg Clin. 2011;21:47–57.

Chapter 14
Congenital Cardiac Anomalies

William Gibson and James E. O'Brien Jr.

Abstract The incidence of congenital heart defects is approximately 9 per 1000 live births. Some are isolated cardiac defects but many patients have multiple systems involved. It is not uncommon for a pediatric surgeon to care for a congenital heart patient and vice versa. A broad understanding of the unique physiology as well as the treatment algorithms, surgical palliations and repairs is essential for those providing care for the congenital heart patient.

Keywords Congenital · Heart · Birth defect · Physiology · Palliation · Shunt · Fontan

1. **What is the incidence of congenital heart disease?**

There are approximately 9 new cases of congenital heart disease per 1000 live births annually and this number is relatively constant around the world [1].

2. **When does the heart develop?**

Cells in the lateral mesoderm begin to differentiate into pre-cardiac cells early in the 3rd week of gestation. After a complex process of folding and spiraling, cardiac development is essentially complete by about 7 weeks gestation [2].

W. Gibson · J. E. O'Brien Jr. (✉)
Ward Family Heart Center, Section of Cardiothoracic Surgery, Children's Mercy Kansas City, University of Missouri—Kansas City, Kansas City, MO, US
e-mail: jobrien@cmh.edu

M. Lacher et al. (eds.), *Pearls and Tricks in Pediatric Surgery*,
https://doi.org/10.1007/978-3-030-51067-1_14

3. **What are the 3 physiologic fetal shunts?**

The ductus venosus, foramen ovale and ductus arteriosus are the 3 fetal shunts that help facilitate the streaming of oxygenated placental blood to the cerebral and coronary circulation and deoxygenated blood to the lower body, viscera and placenta for re-oxygenation.

4. **What factors affect ductal (arteriosus) patency?**

In the fetus, ductal patency is maintained by low oxygen saturation and high levels of circulating prostaglandins. After birth, the rise in oxygen saturation inhibits prostaglandin synthase resulting in a decreased level of prostaglandin. COX-2 inhibition (NSAIDs) can cause ductal constriction.

5. **When is ligation of a patent ductus arteriosus (PDA) indicated in pre-term infants?**

For pre-term infants, closure is indicated in a hemodynamically significant PDA. Hemodynamic significance is demonstrated by excessive left to right ductal flow resulting in too much blood flow to the lungs and too little blood flow to the body. Unless contra-indicated, NSAID trials are attempted prior to surgical ligation.

6. **What are important anatomic landmarks to identify a ductus arteriosus?**

After left posterolateral thoracotomy, the 3rd or 4th interspace is entered and the lung is retracted anteriorly and inferiorly. Once the phrenic and left recurrent laryngeal nerves are identified, enough pleura is opened to clearly identify the left subclavian artery, distal aortic arch, descending aorta and PDA. The PDA may be safely ligated about 1 to 2 mm from its aortic end at that time [3].

7. **What hemodynamic changes should occur after a PDA is ligated?**

A rise in systemic blood pressure—diastolic greater than systolic—should be seen [4].

8. **What are the commonly seen and described vascular rings?**

The complete vascular rings are: double aortic arch, right aortic arch with aberrant left subclavian artery, right aortic arch with mirror image branching and ligamentum arteriosum arising from descending aorta. Incomplete rings are: left pulmonary artery sling (left pulmonary artery arising from right pulmonary artery), innominate artery compression syndrome and left aortic arch with aberrant right subclavian artery [3].

9. **What are the cyanotic heart lesions?**

The classic cyanotic heart lesions all start with the letter "T." Tetralogy of Fallot, truncus arteriosus, transposition of the great arteries, total anomalous pulmonary venous return and tricuspid valve atresia can all cause cyanosis.

10. **When and why can total anomalous pulmonary venous return (TAPVR) be a true congenital cardiac urgency?**

TAPVR describes anomalous drainage of the pulmonary veins into the systemic venous atrium. This can occur directly to the right atrium, via a remnant of the cardinal vein system (supra-cardiac), via a remnant of the umbilico-vitelline system (infra-cardiac) or as a mixture of these types. Due to drainage of all blood to the right atrium, an atrial level shunt must be present. If this shunt is restrictive to flow at the level of the accessory vein—profound respiratory distress and cardiogenic shock will result shortly after birth. This is considered obstructive TAPVR and is an indication for emergent repair or extra-corporeal support if the diagnosis is not clear [1].

11. **Why are ventricular septal defects (VSDs) approached with different treatment algorithms?**

A VSD is a defect in the interventricular septum that results in blood flow from the left ventricle to the right ventricle and can result in too much blood flow to the lungs (heart failure). Many VSDs, both muscular and peri-membranous, have potential to close on their own. Therefore, if a VSD is small enough (restrictive to flow) that a patient can be medically managed (diuretics) and grow, surgery can be deferred. Larger VSDs or those with associated defects often need to be closed in infancy.

12. **Where is the heart's conduction tissue and when is it in jeopardy?**

The sino-atrial node is located on the atrial side of the junction of the right atrium and superior vena cava on the epicardial surface of the heart. It should be considered with any right atrial or superior vena cava manipulation. The AV node lies within the triangle of Koch—bounded by the coronary sinus, the tendon of Tedaro and the anteroseptal commissure of the tricuspid valve. It is at risk with operations near the crux of the heart such as a VSD or atrioventricular septal defect (AVSD) closure.

13. **What is a "tet spell?"**

Tetralogy of Fallot (TOF) is a common cardiac diagnosis caused by anterior malalignment of the conal septum and resulting in 4 defects—VSD, overriding aorta, pulmonary stenosis and right ventricular hypertrophy (RVH). As the RVH worsens, more blood is forced away from the lungs and into the aorta—especially with a catecholamine surge – resulting in a cyanotic spell. Anything that increases systemic vascular resistance (alpha agonists) and decreases the catecholamine response (soothing, narcotic, beta blocker) will help mitigate the cyanosis [1].

14. **Which heart defect is most likely in a child born with trisomy 21 and how likely?**

Approximately 40% of patients with trisomy 21 have an AVSD. Conversely, approximately 75–80% of patients with AVSD have trisomy 21 [1].

15. **What does "unbalanced" AVSD mean?**

Some patients with an AVSD have a common atrioventricular valve that does not sit above 2 equally sized ventricles. Some have severe enough ventricular hypoplasia that the heart cannot be divided into 2 systems and a single ventricle pathway is necessary.

16. **When is a pulmonary artery band (PAB) needed and what are the pitfalls of placing one?**

Pulmonary artery banding is a palliative procedure used to limit excessive pulmonary blood flow from a large left-to-right shunt and ameliorate heart failure. In contemporary times, this is mostly limited to single ventricle patients with excessive pulmonary blood flow and occasional scenarios where complete repair of a 2 ventricle patient is deferred. Achieving appropriate band tightness can be difficult as there are numerous and dynamic factors affecting pulmonary blood flow and pulmonary vascular resistance. The band being placed too distally or migrating distally can cause right pulmonary artery impingement as well.

17. **What is a Blalock Taussig (BT) Shunt and when is one needed?**

The modern version of the BT shunt is anastomosing a polytetrafluoroethylene (PTFE) tube graft from the right subclavian artery to the right pulmonary artery. This is performed to augment pulmonary blood flow and is frequently used as the initial palliation or part of the initial palliation in cyanotic single ventricle patients, but is also occasionally used to palliate 2 ventricle patients needing additional pulmonary blood flow if a complete repair is deferred.

18. **What is the Norwood Procedure?**

The Norwood procedure is the complex operation performed for hypoplastic left heart syndrome. It consists of: anastomosing the aorta to the pulmonary artery (Damus-Kaye-Stansel), enlarging the aortic arch, atrial septectomy and either a systemic to pulmonary artery (BT) shunt or right ventricle to pulmonary artery (Sano) shunt.

19. **What are the 2nd and 3rd stages of the single ventricle pathway?**

As an infant's pulmonary vascular resistance falls after the first few months of life, their physiology gradually becomes better suited to tolerate the continuous single ventricle circuit of a Fontan. The 2nd stage (in some cases actually referred to as hemi-Fontan) is a step toward the Fontan and is typically done between 3 and 6 months of age. Most centers perform a bidirectional Glenn procedure, which is anastomosing the superior vena cava to the right pulmonary artery and removing the initial palliative shunt. The Fontan completion is performed at about 2–5 years of age. It consists of directing the inferior vena cava blood to the pulmonary artery via a tunnel or graft. Upon completion, all the blood returning from the body is passively directed to the lungs.

20. **What are some known long-term complications of Fontan circulation?**

Among other things, plastic bronchitis and protein-losing enteropathy, occurring in up to 14% and 13% respectively, are both long-term complications of Fontan that carry a poor prognosis [1].

References

1. Jonas R. Comprehensive Surgical management of congenital heart disease. 2nd ed. Taylor & Francis Group: CRC Press; 2014.
2. Selke FW, del Nido PJ, Swanson SJ. Sabiston and spencer, Surgery of the chest, 8th ed. Saunders Elsevier; 2010.
3. Mavroudis C, Backer CL. Pediatric cardiac surgery, 4th ed. Wiley-Blackwell; 2013.
4. Stark JF, de Leval MR, Tsang VT. Surgery for congenital heart defects, 3rd ed. Wiley; 2006.

Chapter 15
Hemangiomas and Vascular Malformations

Jo Cooke-Barber and Roshni Dasgupta

Abstract Vascular Anomalies are a broad term used to describe a wide array of complex vascular lesions. Their complex nature and nomenclature have added to their ambiguity over the past few decades. Recent advances in gene sequencing have created a genetic basis for classification which is becoming the standard of diagnosis. There are new medical and surgical techniques being developed to improve the quality of life of these complex patients.

Keywords Hemangioma · Vascular malformation · Surgery · Sirolimus

Questions

1. **How are vascular anomalies classified?**

In 1996 the International Society for the Study of Vascular Anomalies (ISSVA) adopted a classification system proposed in 1982 by Mulliken and Glowacki, and most recently expanded it at the General Assembly in Amsterdam, the Netherlands in 2018 [1]. The ISSVA classification system (Fig. 15.1) divides lesions into two categories—tumors and vascularmalformation malformations and then further categorizes them based on endothelial characteristics. Tumors are further divided, into benign, locally aggressive or borderline, and malignant categories. This classification system can be used to aid providers in predicting the disease course. Vascularmalformation malformations can be simple, combined, associated with major named blood vessels, or associated with other anomalies such as congenital syndromes.

J. Cooke-Barber · R. Dasgupta (✉)
Division of Pediatric General and Thoracic Surgery, Cincinnati Children's Hospital Medical Center, University of Cincinnati, 3333 Burnet Ave, Cincinnati, OH 45229, Unites States
e-mail: Roshni.Dasgupta@cchmc.org

J. Cooke-Barber
e-mail: Jo.Cooke-Barber@cchmc.org

M. Lacher et al. (eds.), *Pearls and Tricks in Pediatric Surgery*,
https://doi.org/10.1007/978-3-030-51067-1_15

ISSVA Classification for vascular anomalies

Vascular anomalies				
Vascular tumors	Vascular malformations			
	Simple	Combined°	of major named vessels	associated with other anomalies
Benign Locally aggressive or borderline Malignant	Capillary malformations Lymphatic malformations Venous malformations Arteriovenous malformations* Arteriovenous fistula*	CVM, CLM LVM, CLVM CAVM* CLAVM* others	See details	See list

° defined as two or more vascular malformations found in one lesion
* high-flow lesions

Fig. 15.1 ISSVA classification for vascular anomalies

2. **What causes vascular anomalies to develop?**

Vascular anomalies usually arise sporadically and are generally not due to germline mutations. The exceptionally inherited vascularmalformation malformation syndromes typically follow an autosomal dominant inheritance pattern.

3. **What is the standard for diagnosing vascular malformations?**

Thanks to advances in gene mapping abilities such as next generation sequencing (NGS), many different genes have been identified as the primary mutations that lead to the development of vascularmalformation malformations. A biopsy of the affected tissue should be sent for pathologic evaluation and gene testing, as many vascularmalformation malformations are due to somatic mutations and mosaicism and not germ line mutations. Many diagnoses are made with a combination of phenotype, radiology studies and clinical history and exam.

4. **What is the best imaging technique?**

MRI has been recently suggested to be the standard for diagnostic imaging of these complex lesions, especially involving the extremity. Advanced imaging should be performed prior to any invasive procedure such as biopsy, debulking, or sclerotherapy.

5. **What type of vascularmalformations are high-flow?**

Arteriovenous malformations are characteristically high-flow lesions, similar to flow dynamics seen in surgically created arteriovenous fistulas.

6. **What is Kasabach-Merritt syndrome?**

Kasabach-Merritt syndrome is a phenomenon associated primarily with KHE lesions which can create a consumptive coagulopathy and severe thrombocytopenia with platelet count of<30,000.

7. **Which vascular tumors are typically benign?**

Infantile, congenital hemangiomas, spindle-cell hemangiomas, epithelioid hemangiomas, pyogenic granulomas, and tufted angiomas are typically benign tumors. Some vascular tumors are locally aggressive and therefore borderline malignant, but classically do not have a risk of distant metastases. These include Kaposiform hemangioendothelioma (KHE), retiform hemangioendothelioma, Dabska tumor or papillary intralymphatic angioendothelioma, composite hemangioendothelioma, and Kaposiform sarcoma. Angiosarcoma and epithelioid type hemangioendotheliomas are considered malignant tumors.

8. **What are the stages of growth of infantile hemangiomas?**

Infantile hemangiomas classically present at birth or soon after birth as a flat or raised vascular stain that can even be mottled or bruise-like in appearance. The lesions can be deep or superficial. Soon after the appearance of the lesion, a rapid growth phase occurs with the lesion reaching 80% of its maximal size by 3 months of life. This is typically followed by a rapid involuting phase. Most lesions will involute gradually over a period of years and are usually completely involuted by 10 years old [2].

9. **What are treatment modalities for infantile hemangiomas (IH)?**

Multidisciplinary management is typically required for complex hemangiomas. Propranolol is a widely accepted oral medication to treat hemangiomas. It is generally well tolerated, even by infants, with few side effects. It is given in the proliferative phase of the lesions and may be continued for 1–2 years of life or more. Propranolol may be contraindicated in PHACE syndrome patients who have underlying cardiac or cerebral lesions. Local therapy includes timolol cream, laser treatment and surgical debulking or excision [2, 3].

10. **What are the complications of hemangiomas?**

Hemangiomas can ulcerate, become infected, and cause disfigurement due to dermal thickening and permanent skin changes. Lesions involving the periorbital area can lead to cortical blindness in infant if left untreated. Airway lesions can lead to airway obstruction or compromise. Liver hemangiomas can cause organ compromise, hypothyroidism, and high output cardiac failure (dependent on type and number of lesions) [2].

11. **What are the subtypes of congenital hemangiomas?**

Congenital hemangiomas are fully grown at birth (Fig. 15.2), and have recently been subdivided based on their involution characteristics. These include rapidly involuting congenital hemangiomas (RICH) which involute shortly after birth, and non-involuting congenital hemangiomas, called NICH. Additionally, congenital hemangiomas that have focal areas which display some involution and other areas in the same lesion which do not involute are called partially involuting congenital hemangiomas (PICH) [2].

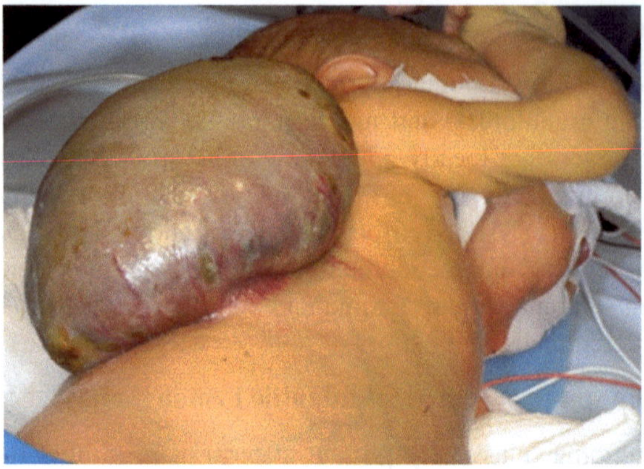

Fig. 15.2 Congenital hemangiomas are fully grown at birth

12. **What are capillary malformations and how do they present?**

Capillary malformations are composed of a large network of cutaneous capillary redundancies and have historically been referred to as "port-wine stains". Typically, these sporadic anomalies manifest as flat, red lesions on the head and neck with a characteristic blush on physical examination. They can be associated with underlying venous or lymphatic malformations, as well as overgrowth of a limb.

13. **What are venous malformations and where are they found?**

Venous malformations are lesions that display characteristic radial distribution with venous endothelium that has a markedly dilated channel (Fig. 15.3). Can be found throughout the body—within the subcutaneous fat, muscle and bone [4].

14. **What is the most common treatment for venous malformations?**

They are commonly treated with compression garments. Function threatening malformations can be treated with sclerotherapy or a combination of embolization and excision or surgical debulking alone [4].

15. **What are lymphatic malformations?**

Lymphatic malformation (Fig. 15.4) can occur anywhere in the body, but are most commonly (50% of lesions) seen in the head and neck as these areas are rich in lymphatic tissue. In general, these are divided into macrocystic and microcystic lesions based on their size. Lesions smaller than 2 cm are microcystic and larger than 2 cm are considered macrocystic [5].

16. **How are lymphatic malformations treated?**

Lymphatic malformations can be treated with multiple modalities either alone or in combination. Compression therapy is a mainstay of treatment with all patients

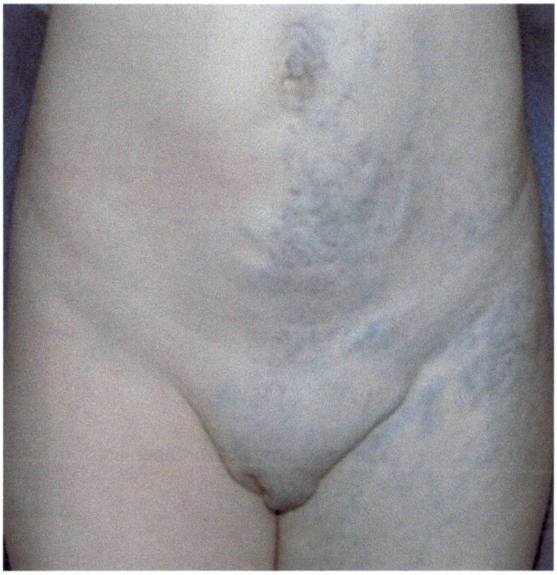

Fig. 15.3 Venous malformations demonstrating a characteristic radial distribution with dilated venous channels

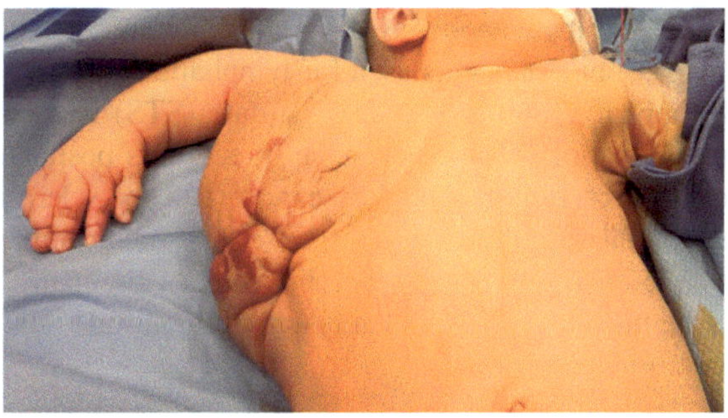

Fig. 15.4 Lymphatic malformation involving the chest wall

with significant malformations being prescribed a compression garment. If symptoms are ongoing, sclerotherapy is the next step in management. Surgical resection of lymphatic malformations can be done if form or function is threatened. Medical therapy with sirolimus should be also be used for significant lesions [5, 6].

17. **What is CLOVES syndrome?**

Congenital Lipomatous Overgrowth, Vascularmalformation malformations, and Epidermal Nevi Syndrome, or CLOVES Syndrome, is a genetic disorder caused by mutation of the gene PIK3CA on chromosome 3q26, which can be attributed to postzygotic, somatic mosaicism. The hallmark sign of this disorder is hemihypertrophy and overgrowth (Fig. 15.5). These vascular anomalies are generally low-flow, with the exception of peri-spinal vascularmalformation malformations which have been documented as high-flow in some individuals. There are also

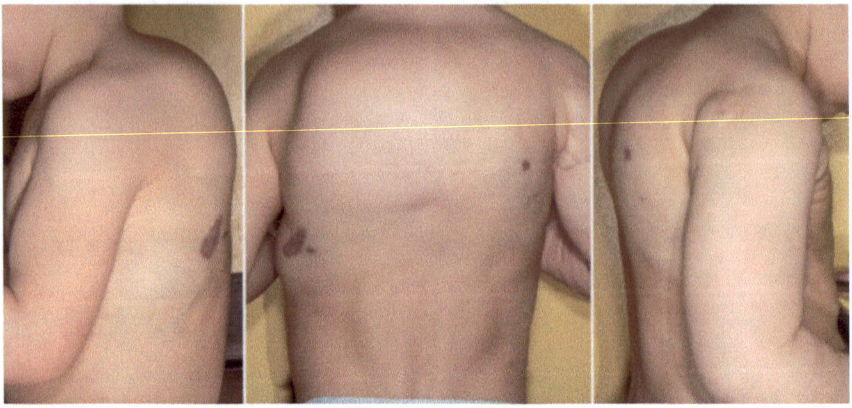

Fig. 15.5 CLOVES syndrome displaying lipomatous overgrowth involving the upper extremity and torso

several skeletal and spinal anomalies associated with this condition as well as extremity hamartomas and epidermal nevi.

18. **What is sclerotherapy and how is it used?**

Sclerotherapy can be used for symptomatic lymphatic and venous malformations. Common agents used for lymphatic malformations include doxycycline and bleomycin. Sodium tetradecyl sulfate (STS) is used most commonly for venous malformations. The mechanism of action is postulated by initiation of an inflammatory reaction mediated by exposure of the sclerosant to the endothelium of the abnormal vascular tissue, response to percutaneous sclerotherapy can be affected by the open or closed-cell architecture of the malformations. Sclerotherapy tends to be more efficacious with macrocystic lesions rather than microcystic lymphatic malformations [4, 5].

19. **What are compression garments and when do you use them?**

Compression garments allow for compression of vascularmalformation malformations—venous or lymphatic which are symptomatic. They decrease edema and venous distension associated with these anomalies. Custom garments can be fit for infants and children and should be remeasured every 6 months to adjust for growth of the child and wear of the garment. Garment compression should start at 20–30 mmHg and titrate upward to maximize therapeutic effect [5].

20. **What surgical therapies are used to treat vascular**malformation **malformations?**

Surgical therapy can be divided into a few classifications based on the goal of intervention: debulking procedures, resection, and sclerotherapy. Surgery should take into account the complex anatomy of these malformations, a judicious use of sealants and post-operative drains. Advances in interventional radiology have led to the development of minimally invasive techniques of obliterating flow through lesions through angioembolization techniques which can be an excellent adjunct to surgical procedures. Glue embolization of venous malformations prior to debulking procedures to reduce blood loss and allow for vascular control for resection of venous malformations.

21. **What are the indicated for use of sirolimus?**

Sirolimus is indicated in PIK3CA associated overgrowth syndromes and complicated vascularmalformation malformations which are limb, life, or function threatening, or disfiguring. Clinical trials have demonstrated sirolimus is effective particularly for lymphatic malformations and well tolerated. Side effects include headaches, mouth ulcers, hypertriglyceridemia, hyperglycemia, and bone marrow toxicity. Sirolimus levels, lipid levels, and liver function should be assessed with labs every 3 months [6].

22. **Are there any novel drugs to treat PIK3CA associated overgrowth syndromes?**

There are now multiple targeted drug therapies for patients with PIK3CA associated overgrowth syndromes such as CLOVES syndrome. Newer drugs specifically targeting the genetic mutations involved have been developed, a drug called BYL719 has been studied in a CLOVES mouse model and is now in clinical trials in patients with PIK3CA related overgrowth syndromes including CLOVES. The results have been promising. Other drugs inhibiting the AKT pathway are also being tested in clinical trials [7, 8].

References

1. www.issva.org.
2. Liang MG, Frieden IJ. Infantile and congenital hemangiomas. Semin Pediatr Surg. 2014;23:162–7.
3. Leaute-Labreze C, de la Roque EM, Hubiche T, Boralevi F. Propranolol for severe hemangiomas of infancy. N Engl J Med. 2008;358:2649–51. https://doi.org/10.1056/NEJMc0708819.
4. Dasgupta AR, Patel M. Venous malformations. Semin Pediatr Surg. 2014;23:198–202.
5. Elluru RG, Balakrishnan K, Padua HM. Lymphatic malformations: diagnosis and management. Semin Pediatr Surg. 2014;23:178–85.
6. Adams DM, et al. Efficacy and safety of sirolimus in the treatment of complicated vascular anomalies. Pediatrics. 2016; (137)2. https://doi.org/10.1542/peds.2015-3257.
7. Quitterie V, Blanc T, Smail HR, Bareloot L, et al. Targeted therapy in patients with PIK3CA-related overgrowth syndrome. Nature. 2018;28:540–6.
8. Fritsch C, et al. Characterization of the novel and specific PI3Ka inhibitor NVP-BYL719 and development of the patient stratification strategy for clinical trials. Mol Cancer Ther. 2014;(13)1117–1129.

Chapter 16
Umbilical Problems

Jeffrey J. Dehmer

Abstract Disorders of the umbilicus are a common cause for pediatric surgery referral. This chapter will briefly review the workup and management of several frequent umbilical problems.

Keywords Omphalitis · Urachus · Omphalomesenteric duct · Umbilical hernia

1. **What 5 structures are present in the umbilicus?**

The umbilical vein, 2 umbilical arteries, the omphalomesenteric (or vitelline duct), and the urachus (or allantois).

2. **How long does it take for the umbilical cord stump to fall off?**

On average, about 10–14 days but it can vary widely.

3. **What is omphalitis?**

A newborn infection of the umbilical tissues and surrounding skin.

4. **How is omphalitis managed?**

If severe, it requires parenteral antibiotics and possibly debridement. Most cases however, will respond to oral antibiotics and careful hygiene measures. Topical alcohol can be used to dry out the tissue.

5. **What is an umbilical granuloma?**

A small fleshy appearing nodule of granulation tissue in the umbilicus after the umbilical cord stump has fallen off.

J. J. Dehmer (✉)
New Hanover Regional Medical Center, Pediatric Surgery, 2131 S. 17th Street, PO Box 9000, Wilmington, NC 28402-9000, USA
e-mail: jeff.dehmer@nhrmc.org

M. Lacher et al. (eds.), *Pearls and Tricks in Pediatric Surgery*,
https://doi.org/10.1007/978-3-030-51067-1_16

6. **How are umbilical granulumas treated?**

Classically, they are treated with topical silver nitrate over the course of several applications. Care must be taken not to burn the surrounding skin. Silver nitrate can stain the skin and clothing. Topical steroids may also be an effective therapy [1].

7. **What if there is bilious drainage from the umbilicus?**

There would be concern for a patent omphalomesenteric duct or an omphalomesenteric cyst. Further workup is not typically necessary if the physical exam confirms the diagnosis. If it is unclear a contrast study or an ultrasound might be helpful.

8. **How is an omphalomesenteric duct remnant treated?**

These require operative exploration and excision. If there is a connection to the bowel, it should be closed in a fashion so as not to narrow the bowel lumen. Often, this can be done just through an umbilical incision without needing a larger laparotomy.

9. **What if the drainage is more consistent with urine?**

This is highly suspicious for a patent urachus. Similarly, a contrast study or an ultrasound could be helpful. Some advocate obtaining a voiding cystourethrogram to evaluate for a distal urinary obstruction prior to surgery, however this may not be necessary. The operation to remove the patent urachus can be done through an open umbilical incision or via a laparoscopic approach where excision and ligation are done down to the level of the dome of the bladder [2].

10. **Can urachal anomalies present later?**

There can be urachal sinuses or cysts that manifest later with infectious complications. If so, they can be treated with antibiotics and then excised electively. Although exceptionally rare, there can be malignant degeneration into urachal cancer [3].

11. **What causes an umbilical hernia and how common are they?**

After the umbilical cord stump falls off, the ring is supposed to close spontaneously. Umbilical hernias occur when the umbilical ring doesn't close. They are extremely common, affecting up to 23% of newborns in the US each year [4].

12. **Are umbilical hernias more common in certain types of patients?**

Premature infants have a very high incidence of umbilical hernia at birth. Also, African Americans have a higher incidence than other races.

13. **Do all umbilical hernias require urgent repair?**

No, many will close spontaneously. Unless there are symptoms of incarceration or strangulation, watchful waiting is appropriate. Furthermore, there is some data to suggest that early repair is associated with a higher rate of complications [5].

14. **What is the right time to repair an asymptomatic umbilical hernia?**

There is no consensus regarding optimal timing for repair of an asymptomatic umbilical hernia. However, the risk of complications such as incarceration or strangulation is quite low, so waiting until age 4–5 years is a reasonable approach and is not affected by the size of the hernia [4, 5].

15. **How do you repair an umbilical hernia?**

Classically, a curved infra-umbilical incision is used. The apex of the hernia sac is separated from the umbilical dermis and the sac excised down to healthy fascia. The fascia is closed with absorbable suture and then the umbilical dermis tacked down to the fascia. The skin is closed and a compressive dressing is applied.

References

1. Ogawa C, Sato Y, Suzuki C, et al. Treatment with silver nitrate versus topical steroid treatment for umbilical granuloma: a non-inferiority randomized control trial. PLoS One. 2018;13;13(2):e0192688.
2. Dethlefs CR, Abdessalam SF, Raynor SC, et al. Conservative management of urachal anomalies. J Pediatr Surg. 2019;54(5):1054–8.
3. Szarvas T, Módos O, Niedworok C, et al. Clinical, prognostic, and therapeutic aspects of urachal carcinoma: a comprehensive review with meta-analysis of 1,010 cases. Urol Oncol. 2016;34(9):388–98.
4. Zens T, Nichol PF, Cartmill R, et al. Management of asymptomatic pediatric umbilical hernias: a systematic review. J Pediatr Surg. 2017;52(11):1723–31.
5. Zens TJ, Rogers A, Cartmill R, et al. Age-dependent outcomes in asymptomatic umbilical hernia repair. Pediatr Surg Int. 2019;35(4):463–8.

Chapter 17
Hernias—Epigastric, Inguinal and Incisional

Jill Sutherland Quirt and Annie Fecteau

Abstract Hernias are a common pediatric surgical presentation. Hernias develop from an inherent weakness in the abdominal wall. With respect to inguinal hernias, they can be direct or indirect. Indirect hernias result from weakening of the fascia of the transversalis muscle fibers at the internal inguinal ring and the potential space from a persistent processus vaginalis. Direct hernias protrude through Hesslebach's triangle. Almost all pediatric inguinal hernias are indirect. All inguinal hernias require surgical repair. The timing of the repair is dependent on the presentation being acute or subacute. Pediatric patients who present with an incarcerated inguinal hernia require emergent surgical repair. Hernias can also develop in the epigastric region due to either a congenital or acquired anterior abdominal wall defect, or at the site of prior abdominal wall incision sites. These can also present with complications including incarceration. They should be repaired surgically if symptomatic. Overall, pediatric hernias are a common presentation warranting either emergent or elective surgical repair with either an open or laparoscopic approach depending on the patient characteristics, acute nature of presentation and the nature of the hernia itself.

Keywords Hernia · Inguinal · Epigastric · Incisional · Incarceration · Hernia repair · Laparoscopic

---

J. S. Quirt
Department of General Surgery, University of Toronto, Toronto, Canada
e-mail: jillquirt@gmail.com

A. Fecteau (✉)
Hospital for Sick Children, Department of Surgery,
University of Toronto, Toronto, Canada
e-mail: Annie.fecteau@sickkids.ca

M. Lacher et al. (eds.), *Pearls and Tricks in Pediatric Surgery*,
https://doi.org/10.1007/978-3-030-51067-1_17

17.1 Inguinal Hernia

1. **What are the anatomical landmarks of the inguinal canal?**

The inguinal region is between the anterior superior iliac spine and the pubic symphysis. The inguinal canal anatomical landmarks are: the inguinal ligament, the internal and external inguinal rings, the spermatic cord in males and the round ligament in females (Fig. 17.1) [1].

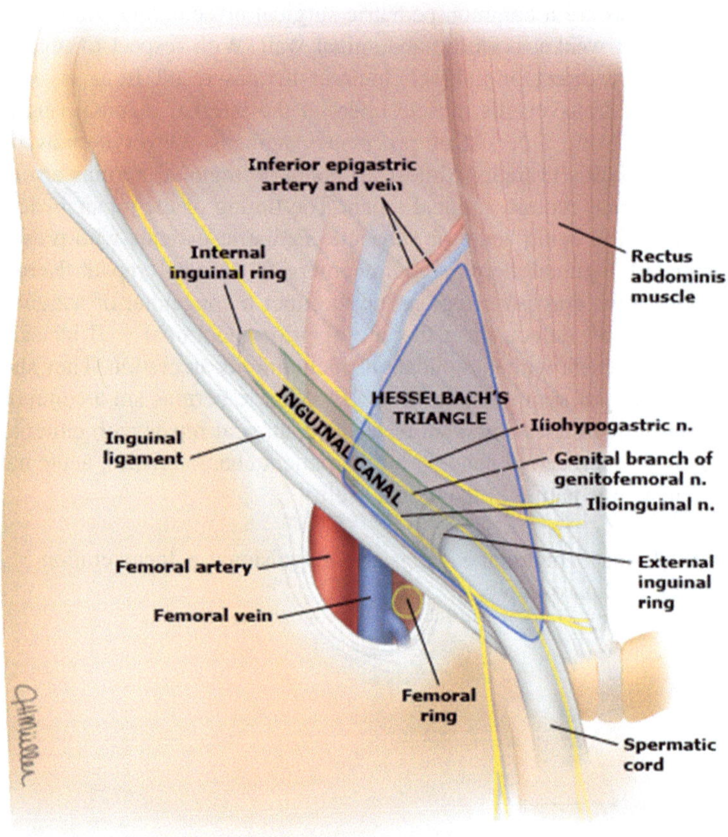

Fig. 17.1 The aponeurosis of the external oblique muscle forms the anterior aspect of the inguinal canal, the transversalis fascia and the transversus abdominus muscle form the posterior aspect. The external inguinal ring is formed by the external oblique muscle. The internal ring is within the transversalis fascia and composed of the transversus abdominus and internal oblique muscles. The femoral artery and vein leave the abdomen posterior to the inguinal canal. Indirect hernias develop at the internal inguinal ring, lateral to the inferior epigastric artery. Direct inguinal hernias occur through Hesselbach's triangle. Femoral hernias develop in the empty space at the medial aspect of the femoral canal, inferior to the inguinal ligament

Hesslebach's triangle is defined inferiorly by the inguinal ligament, laterally by the inferior epigastric artery, and medially by the lateral border of the rectus muscle. Hesselbach's triangle helps differentiate indirect from direct hernias. Direct hernia's protrude into this space, while indirect hernias pass outside the triangle through the inguinal canal.

Indirect hernias result from: weakening of the fascia of the transversalis muscle fibers at the internal inguinal ring and the potential space from a persistent processus vaginalis.

2. **What is the processus vaginalis?**

The processus vaginalis is a peritoneal diverticulum. It extends through the internal ring at 3 months gestation.

3. **What is the physiology of testicular descent and the pathophysiology of the development of inguinal hernias and hydroceles in infants and children?**

The testis descends through the processus vaginalis between the seventh and ninth months of gestation. A portion of the processus vaginalis attaches to the testes and is pulled with the descent of the testes into the scrotum. The portion of the processus vaginalis surrounding the testis becomes the tunica vaginalis. The remainder of the processus vaginalis obliterates, eliminating the communication between the peritoneal cavity and scrotum.

In males, the processus vaginalis obliterates during the first two years of life. However, up to 40% remain patent, of which 20% will later develop into inguinal hernias or hydroceles. The female counterpart of the processus vaginalis obliterates by eight months of gestation, although occasionally this will persist into childhood, which is then termed the canal of Nuck.

Indirect inguinal hernias occur more frequently on the right, as this is the side where the migration of the testicle or round ligament occurs last.

4. **What is a hydrocele vs a hernia?**

Both hydroceles and hernias result due to incomplete obliteration of the processus vaginalis. In a hydrocele, the processus vaginalis obliterates such that there is proximal and distal obliteration, but patency of the midportion. This results in a small peritoneal opening allowing fluid accumulation around the testicle or the cord structures. This fluid may or may not communicate with the peritoneal cavity.

A hernia in comparison, is a larger peritoneal opening resulting from distal obliteration of the processus vaginalis yet the proximal aspect remains patent or there is a complete failure of obliteration allowing fluid, bowel and rarely ovaries to be present within the sac.

5. **What type of inguinal hernia do infants and children get vs adults?**

Almost all inguinal hernias in infants and children are indirect hernias. However, with rising incidence of obesity in childhood, it is possible we will see a resulting rise in incidences of direct inguinal hernias.

6. **What is the incidence of inguinal hernias in infants and children?**

The incidence of inguinal hernias is approximately 1–5% in term infants and 9–11% in infants born less than 33 weeks of gestational age [2]. The incidence in boys is 3–4 times higher than in girls, with the right side being more commonly affected.

7. **What patient populations are at higher risk of inguinal hernias?**

Preterm infants and low-birth-weight infants are at a higher risk of inguinal hernias. Inguinal hernias are more common in children with abdominal wall defects, conditions resulting in an increased intraabdominal pressure such as VP shunts or peritoneal dialysis, connective tissue disease, genitourinary abnormalities, or family history of inguinal hernia.

8. **What is the risk of incarceration of groin hernias in premature infants?**

The reported incidence of incarcerated inguinal hernias is between 14–31% [2], usually in infants younger than 12 months. Incarceration is the presenting sign in as many as 65% of inguinal hernias. Due to the high incidence of incarceration, efforts are made to repair inguinal hernias shortly after diagnosis, and whenever possible prior to discharge for infants diagnosed during a NICU admission.

9. **What is the anatomic distribution of inguinal hernias?**

The right side is more commonly affected in both sexes. This is related to the later descent of the right testicle and obliteration of the processus vaginalis. Bilateral inguinal hernias are relatively common, with reported incidence of ~10% in full term infants, and 50% in premature and low-birth-weight infants [2].

10. **How do non-incarcerated inguinal hernias present?**

Most inguinal hernias present with an intermittent bulge in the groin. Often this is noticed by parents at times of increased intraabdominal pressure—straining, coughing, or crying; or commonly during bath time at the days end. Often the trigger to seek medical care is when the inguinal mass is not spontaneously reducing or the inguinal mass is significantly large.

11. **How do you differentiate an inguinal hernia vs a hydrocele?**

Communicating hydroceles are essentially hernias containing peritoneal fluid; they are differentiated through transillumination, irreducibility, nontender nature on examination and cystic in nature. A noncommunicating hydrocele will be nonreducible and unchanging with increased intraabdominal pressure. However, there should be normal spermatic cord felts superior to the hydrocele, often described as being able to "get above" the hydrocele. While a hernia should be reducible as long as it is not incarcerated. An acute hydrocele of the spermatic cord can be difficult to differentiate from an incarcerated inguinal hernia.

12. **What is the differential diagnosis of inguinal swelling in children?**

Males or Females
Inguinal hernia (indirect or direct) Inguinal lymphadenopathy Granuloma inguinale Femoral hernia Amyand hernia (appendicitis within the hernia sac) Benign or malignant tumor: lipoma, hematomas, mesothelioma, dermoid cyst, sarcoma
Males
Hydrocele Retractile testis Ectopic or undescended testis Traumatically dislocated testis Testicular tumour
Females
Herniation of the ovary or fallopian tube

13. **What are the symptoms and signs of an incarcerated inguinal hernia?**

Infants or children with incarcerated inguinal hernias are often irritable and crying. They may develop nausea, vomiting, abdominal distention and obstipation depending on presence of prolonged incarceration or obstructed bowel. A firm, discrete inguinal mass can be palpated which may extend into the scrotum or labia majora. This is often tender, edematous, with possible erythema of the overlying skin. In males, venous congestion can cause the testicle to appear dark blue.

14. **What structures can become incarcerated within an inguinal hernia?**

Small or large bowel, omentum, appendix, ovary or fallopian tube, and extremely rarely a benign or malignant tumour.

15. **What is the silk glove sign?**

A palpable smooth bandlike thickening of the cord that may sometimes be appreciated by placing a single finger parallel to the inguinal canal at the level of the pubic tubercle and rubbing it from side to side. The tissues are felt to be sliding, as if sliding a silk scarf over itself. This is thought to represent the sac sliding over the cord structures. This is can be a very reliable sign in experienced hands, but requires experience to appreciate confidently.

16. **Should you reduce an inguinal hernia, what are some of the considerations prior to attempting reduction?**

Manual reduction is successful in 95–100% of pediatric patients [3]. The duration of incarceration and the age of the child influence the success rates for manual reduction, with younger patients and longer durations of symptoms reducing the overall success rates of reduction.

Elective repair after successful manual reduction has a lower complication rate than emergent operative reduction [3].

If a patient presents extremely ill with evidence of peritonitits, prolonged intestinal obstruction or toxicity from gangrenous bowel, manual reduction is generally contraindicated. Often these hernias are non-reducible in nature. The risk is that you will reduce bowel that has or is at risk of perforation, which can then result in delayed recognition and patient deterioration. However, often in this setting, the hernia is non-reducible.

17. **How do you reduce an inguinal hernia?**

Place the patient in Trendelenburg position if possible. Align the sac using gentle traction on the scrotum to help align the hernia sac with the external ring. With gentle traction, you can then attempt to decompress the contents with gentle pressure on either side of the hernia neck from distal to proximal. Moving your distal hand to the apex of the mass, apply constant pressure on the inguinal canal with your other hand, pressure is applied to continue to reduce the contents, slowly walking up the groin towards the internal ring until the contents are fully reduced (Fig. 17.2) [2].

18. **How do you manage an inguinal hernia that is not palpable on physical examination?**

Observe the patient with frequent examinations, consider surgical exploration based on strong history and reliable guardians. Often, guardians will have photographs, which can be a good reference. Indications for imaging with US, CT or MRI are in the setting of chronic groin or pelvic pain with unclear cause for concern of an occult inguinal hernia.

19. **How do you repair an indirect inguinal hernia?**

High ligation and excision of the hernia sac using either a laparoscopic or open approach. Plication of the floor of the inguinal canal may be necessary when the inguinal ring has been enlarged with repetitive herniation. In the setting of complete break down of the transversalis fascia, a complete reconstruction of the floor of the inguinal canal using the conjoint tendon may be required. Males who have an associated undescended testis should have an orchidopexy at the time of the inguinal hernia repair. In females, often they will have closure of the external ring in addition to the high ligation of the hernia sac.

20. **What are the advantages and disadvantages of a laparoscopic or open approach for repair?**

Herniotomy (open surgery)	Laparoscopic inguinal hernia repair
Advantages:	Advantages:
– Teachable technique and replicable at all levels – Laparoscopic equipment is not required – Can be performed under local anesthesia if required	– Precise detection and simultaneous repair of contralateral patent processus vaginalis – Cosmesis

Herniotomy (open surgery)	Laparoscopic inguinal hernia repair
Disadvantages:	Disadvantages:
– Inability to evaluate contralateral side – Cosmesis (debated due to the ability to hide the small incisional scar in natural skin lines and below future pubic hair lines)	– Availability of experienced surgeons to perform laparoscopic approach – Prolonged operative time – Unclear long-term recurrence rates – Potential complications can be more severe in nature due to intra-abdominal approach. – Failure of laparoscopic approach can result in requirement of an open conversion

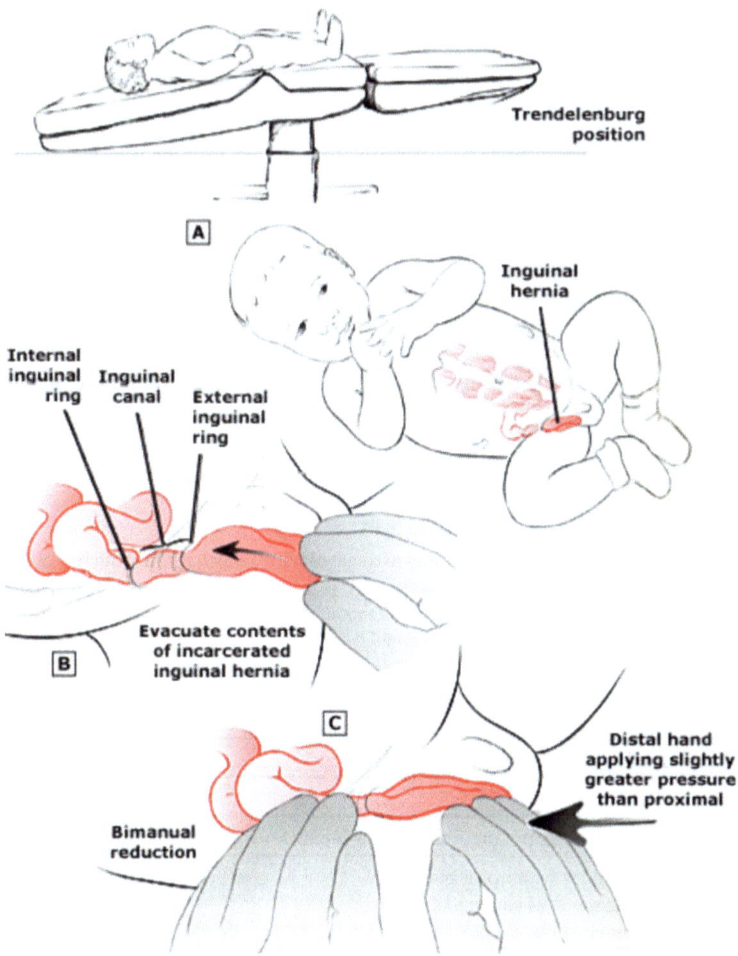

Fig. 17.2 Indirect hernia reduction

21. **Where is the hernia sac located within the hernia?**

The hernia sac should be located anterior and medial to the spermatic cord structures/round ligament.

22. **When is it appropriate to repair an inguinal hernia?**

With presenting incarcerated inguinal hernias, immediate surgical repair following inguinal hernia reduction eliminates the risk of recurrence. Risk of recurrent incarceration is 16–35%, with the recurrence occurring between 0.5–120 days following the initial incarceration [3]. However, this can be a technically difficult time to perform a repair. Tissue edema secondary to incarceration can cause distortion of the anatomical landmarks, placing cord structures at a higher risk of injury, and poor healing of the primary repair, increasing the risk of recurrence or developing a subsequent direct hernia.

A short delay in definitive operative management can allow the tissues to heal. A general recommendation is to perform a definitive hernia repair within five days (two days for premature infants) of manual reduction of incarcerated inguinal hernias to minimize the risk of recurrence, while allowing for some recovery from the initial incarceration [3].

For children with asymptomatic inguinal hernias, a longer wait time for elective surgery is associated with an increased risk of incarceration, particularly in children under one year of age [3]. Therefore, the recommendation is to perform definitive repair within 14 days of presentation.

Of course included in the decision regarding timing of the repair is the balance of risk of incarceration versus the risks associated with required anesthetic.

23. **What are the complications associated with inguinal hernia repair?**

Complications of both open and laparoscopic inguinal hernia repair
– Vascular injury – Post-operative seroma/hematoma (5–25%) – Wound infection (1–2%) – Neuralgias (0.5–4.6%)—more commonly associated with a mesh repair, which is not commonly used in pediatric patients. Nerves at risk are: lateral cutaneous nerve of the thigh, gentiofermoral nerve, intermediate cutaneous nerve of the thigh. Usually involved by mesh-induced fibrosis or entrapment by a tack – Recurrence (1%) – Vas Deferens injury (<1%) – Testicular atrophy
Complications of open inguinal hernia repair
– Wound infection rate is higher
Complications of laparoscopic inguinal hernia repair
– Bladder or bowel injury with trocar placement – Identification of anatomical landmarks – Pneumoperitoneum complications

24. **What are the relative indications for exploration of the contralateral side?**

Contralateral exploration was previously common practice, however this has declined in recent years based on large prospective studies that demonstrated children with unilateral inguinal hernias had an overall risk of metachronous hernia of 5–12% [4]. It was therefore concluded that the low incidence of contralateral hernia did not justify the routine exploration. Contralateral exploration therefore is only warranted for children at particular risk for metachronous inguinal hernias including those with increased intraabdominal pressure, connective tissue disease, ventriculoperitoneal shunts, or chronic pulmonary disease, or in patients with an underlying medical condition, which increases their risk of anesthetic complications.

In the setting of a laparoscopic repair, the contralateral side is always inspected for possible contralateral hernia. This is a highly sensitive and specific means of exploring the contralateral inguinal region.

17.2 Epigastric Hernia

1. **What is the pathogenesis of an epigastric hernia?**

Epigastric hernias can be congenital or acquired defects in the anterior abdominal wall. Congenital epigastric hernias arise from defects in the linea alba or in an abnormally wide orifice for a blood vessel. Other studies have suggested epigastric hernias are acquired defects from a unique pattern of aponeurotic decussation in the upper abdominal wall. Which may be related to traction from fibers originating from the diaphragm that insert on the linea alba between the umbilicus and xiphoid.

2. **How do epigastric hernias present?**

Epigastric hernias typically present with a circumscribed midline epigastric abdominal mass that may be painful or tender.

3. **What is the incidence of epigastric hernias in the pediatric population?**

Epigastric hernias represent about 4% of all abdominal hernias operated on in children [5].

4. **What are the indications for surgical intervention?**

All symptomatic or enlarging epigastric hernias should be surgically corrected. Smaller or asymptomatic epigastric hernias can be observed until they either present with complications secondary to their hernia, or for cosmetic reasons, the patient would like surgical correction. The timing of the non-symptomatic repairs is a decision made in balancing the risks associated with anesthesia if general anesthesia is required.

5. **What is the surgical approach to repair?**

Epigastric hernias have been traditionally repaired with an open surgical approach with incision over the fascial defect and primary closure. However, more recently, some are employing a laparoscopic technique.

17.3 Incisional Hernia

1. **What are the risk factors for development of an incisional hernia in the pediatric population?**

The risk factors for an incisional hernia in the pediatric population overlap somewhat with the adult population, but there are also specific pediatric incisional hernia risk factors. Risk factors for pediatric patients of developing an incisional hernia include: malnutrition, immunosuppression (due to medical conditions or immunosuppressive therapy), connective tissue disorders, obesity and operation in the neonatal period.

Procedures that carry a higher risk of incisional hernia post operatively in pediatric patients include: laparotomy for necrotizing enterocolitis, stoma closure, and pyloromyotomy.

2. **What is the incidence of incisional hernias in pediatric patients?**

The incidence of incisional hernia in adults has been reported as 10–50% following any type of abdominal wall incision, with the highest being following midline incisions. There is a paucity of data relating to the pediatric population, however recent single institution based studies have reported incidence as low as 1–3% [6]. This is likely secondary to pediatric patients having fewer patient risk factors including smoking and higher incidences of obesity.

3. **How do incisional hernias present?**

An incisional hernia should be suspected in a patient with a prior abdominal surgery who presents with abdominal pain or discomfort, skin changes overlying a prior incision, or symptoms of bowel obstruction or strangulation. This will often be associated with a palpable abdominal mass in the location of their prior incision sites.

4. **How are incisional hernias diagnosed?**

Generally a physical examination is all that is required to diagnose an incisional hernia. However, if there is no palpable mass appreciated, symptoms not entirely in keeping with an incisional hernia, or a complex surgical history and complex possible incisional hernia based on history or examination, an ultrasound or CT scan may be indicated to confirm diagnosis and delineate the abdominal anatomy.

5. **What are the indications for surgical intervention?**

Symptomatic incisional hernias, particularly in the setting of incarcerated or strangulated bowel, require immediate operative management. Discomfort and cosmetic complaints are also valid indications for surgical repair in the pediatric setting, but the timing and ultimate decision to operate is balanced with the patient's overall health and risks of anesthesia or recurrence.

6. **What is the surgical approach to repair?**

Incisional hernias are repaired with either an open or laparoscopic approach. In pediatrics, the repair is a primary repair unless the abdominal wall defect precludes this requiring a mesh repair, however this is much less common than in the adult patient population.

References

1. Mathison D. Evaluation of Inguinal Swelling in Children Waltham, Massacheusetts: Up to Date; 2019 [updated November 2018].
2. Ramsook C. Inguinal Hernia in Children Waltham, Massachusetts: Up to Date; 2019 [updated November 2018].
3. Gahukamble DB, Khamage AS. Early versus delayed repair of reduced incarcerated inguinal hernias in the pediatric population. J Pediatr Surg. 1996;31(9):1218–20.
4. Miltenburg DM, Nuchtern JG, Jaksic T, Kozinetz CA, Brandt ML. Meta-analysis of the risk of metachronous hernia in infants and children. Am J Surg. 1997;174(6):741–4.
5. Coats RD, Helikson MA, Burd RS. Presentation and management of epigastric hernias in children. J Pediatr Surg. 2000;35(12):1754–6.
6. Mullassery D, Pedersen A, Robb A, Smith N. Incisional hernia in pediatric surgery—experience at a single UK tertiary centre. J Pediatr Surg. 2016;51(11):1791–4.

What are the indications for surgical intervention?

[illegible]

References

[illegible]

Chapter 18
Abdominal Wall Defects, Gastroschisis and Omphalocele

Kevin Johnson and Saleem Islam

Abstract Abdominal Wall Defects comprise of two distinct entities, gastroschisis and omphalocele. While often considered together, these congenital anomalies are quite different and pose unique management issues. These issues will be discussed in this chapter.

Keywords Gastroschisis · Omphalocele · Atresia · Prenatal diagnosis · Congenital defect · Neonatal surgical emergency · Short bowel syndrome

1. **What is the incidence of gastroschisis and omphalocele?**

The incidence of gastroschisis is 1 in 4,000 live births, the incidence of omphalocele is 1 in 4–6,000 live births. The incidence of gastroschisis has been increasing in all maternal age groups over the last two decades without a known etiology. The incidence of omphalocele has remained stable over time [1].

2. **What are risk factors for gastroschisis and omphalocele?**

Known risk factors for gastroschisis include young maternal age, lower socioeconomic status, vasoactive recreational drug use, aspirin use, low body mass index, prematurity, gestational diabetes, use of antidepressants and cigarette smoking. Risk factors for omphalocele include numerous syndromes and chromosomal abnormalities that will be outlined below.

3. **What is the pathophysiology of gastroschisis and omphalocele?**

The exact etiology remains unknown for abdominal wall defects. The most widely accepted theory for the etiology of gastroschisis is the lateral ventral body folds theory, which suggests the condition stems from failure of migration of the lateral

K. Johnson · S. Islam (✉)
Division of Pediatric Surgery, University of Florida, Gainesville, FL, USA
e-mail: saleem.islam@surgery.ufl.edu

M. Lacher et al. (eds.), *Pearls and Tricks in Pediatric Surgery*,
https://doi.org/10.1007/978-3-030-51067-1_18

folds. Omphalocele is thought to arise from failure of the viscera to return to the abdomen during development due to a developmental arrest at that time. In both instances, there is an accompanying loss of abdominal domain which substantially impacts management [1].

4. **Presentation of gastroschisis and omphalocele?**

Gastroschisis presents as eviscerated bowel without a covering membrane, usually to the right of umbilicus [2]. Omphalocele presents as a membrane covered bowel and liver in the midline. Care must be taken not to mistake ruptured omphalocele for gastroschisis [3].

5. **What anomalies are associated with gastroschisis and omphalocele?**

Gastroschisis is associated with other intestinal atresia in 10–15% cases. Omphalocele is more frequently associated with other anomalies, including chromosomal (trisomy 13, 18, 21, and 45X), syndromic (Beckwith-Weideman, pentalogy of Cantrell) and non-syndromic organ system abnormalities (cardiac defects) [1–3].

6. **How are gastroschisis and omphalocele diagnosed prenatally?**

In most cases AWD are detected prenatally. They are both associated with elevated maternal serum alpha-fetoprotein levels and are diagnosed on ultrasonography. Gastroschisis has intestinal loops floating in amniotic fluid and growth retardation. Omphaloceles have a variable size and contents, with potential anomalies in other organ systems.

7. **How are patients with abdominal wall defects followed prenatally?**

For gastroschisis, factors to watch for on prenatal imaging include intra-abdominal bowel dilation, bowel wall thickening, gastric dilation, IUGR, polyhydramnios, liver or urinary bladder herniation, and changes in bowel dilation during the gestation. For omphalocele, karyotyping via amniocentesis and prenatal ultrasound, particularly looking for cardiac and central nervous system anomalies that may affect survival and whether termination of the pregnancy is considered [1–3].

8. **What timing/mode of delivery is optimal for gastroschisis and omphalocele?**

Vaginal delivery has been shown to be both safe and beneficial to the mother and baby. Cesarean should be reserved for specific obstetric or fetal indications. Term or close to term delivery is recommended for both.

9. **Initial management of a patient with gastroschisis**

The intestines need to be covered with a ‘bowel bag’, and intravenous fluid resuscitation should be started. Babies should be positioned laterally to reduce mesenteric kinking. The defect should be enlarged at the fascial level if it is too tight.

10. **Initial management of a patient with omphalocele**

Care should be taken to prevent damage to the sac, and cover with a moist gauze. Intravenous fluid resuscitation should be started at the same time that a cardiac evaluation is performed and examination for other syndromes and defects is carried out [3].

11. **How is the decision made to use a silo versus primary closure in gastroschisis?**

Regardless of which approach is used, maintaining adequate bowel perfusion by avoiding kinking of the mesenteric vessels and high intra-abdominal pressures is key to maintaining bowel viability. Overall, outcomes are equivalent for simple gastroschisis that is closed primarily versus being placed in a silo. Definitive closure can be obtained in a variety of ways, ranging from sutured closure of the skin and fascia, to sutureless closure using the umbilical stalk as a patch to close the skin defect and allowing the defect to close spontaneously.

12. **How should the fascial opening be enlarged in a patient with gastroschisis if the bowel appears to be ischemic in the silo?**

If the fascial defect appears to be causing bowel compromise the fascia can opened. The facial opening is generally extended to the patient's right (opposite the umbilical cord) to avoid injury to the umbilical vein medially. The skin does not need to be opened in most cases.

13. **What is closing or vanishing gastroschisis?**

Closing or vanishing gastroschisis refers to when the fascial defect decreases in size or closes completely prior to birth. This can result in bowel compromise with an atresia and potential for short bowel syndrome [2].

14. **What defines complex gastroschisis?**

Complex gastroschisis is defined as those patients with intestinal complications including atresia, ischemia, or perforation at birth. Development of NEC was considered to be complex, however that is not present at birth and has been excluded [1, 2].

15. **What is a ruptured omphalocele?**

The amniotic sac can rupture prenatally in patients with omphalocele. While the basic principles of the bowel requiring coverage to prevent dehydration and infection still apply, recognition of this is critical as it affects the workup that the patient requires and the comorbidities that will affect the patient's course. In general, these patients will not have adequate abdominal domain to be able to place a spring-loaded silo and will require a silo or mesh to be sewn to the fascia and skin for placement. These are difficult conditions to manage [3].

16. **What are the key points of postoperative care for patients with abdominal wall defects?**

Following abdominal closure, patients should be closely monitored for signs of abdominal compartment syndrome, including respiratory compromise, hypotension, and impaired renal function. Nutritional support with parenteral nutrition will be required until bowel function returns.

17. **Why do patients with gastroschisis have difficulties with feeding, even after reduction?**

Impaired bowel motility and ability to absorb nutrients both lead to feeding difficulties in neonates with gastroschisis. This bowel dysfunction is thought to be related to the inflammatory peel that occurs as a result of contact of the bowel with amniotic fluid, as well as to decreased numbers of interstitial cells of Cajal seen on pathologic analysis. Use of prokinetic agents has not been shown to improve time to goal feeds. It takes 2–4 weeks in cases of simple GS for the dysmotility to resolve [2].

18. **What are the surgical options for closure of omphaloceles?**

A variety of options exist that are used based on the size of defect and the ability of the patient to undergo surgical interventions. Primary repair can be performed in some patients with small defects (with those <1.5 cm commonly called hernias of the cord) when the patient has adequate abdominal domain and the associated anomalies do not preclude surgical intervention. Other methods include staged closure, in which the amniotic sac is inverted to serially reduce the abdominal content until the abdomen can be closed primarily or with mesh. Delayed closure involves excising the amniotic sac and sewing a mesh to the abdominal wall fascia or skin that can be used for reduction prior to closure. Scarification involves the use of topical agents to promote formation of an eschar over the amniotic sac that will gradually epithelialize over time. If closure of the abdomen does not involve closure of fascia, the resulting ventral hernia is generally closed primarily or in stages when the child is several years old [1, 3].

19. **What are the long-term outcomes for patients with abdominal wall defects?**

Overall outcomes for patients with gastroschisis are largely based on whether it is a simple or complex defect. Those with complex GS have longer length of stay and are far more likely to develop intestinal failure and liver disease. Gastroschisis remains the leading cause of intestinal failure requiring intestinal transplant. It is also associated with cryptorchidism, which is generally addressed at one year of age. Malrotation is part of the defect, but rarely leads to volvulus. Intestinal obstruction may occur and present with bilious emesis and should be promptly assessed [1, 2].

For patients with omphalocele, outcomes are likely related to several factors, most notably associated cardiac and neurologic anomalies. Additionally, pulmonary hypoplasia is common in omphalocele patients with large defects and can lead to long term respiratory failure requiring tracheostomy. Several risk stratification categories have been created, but none is commonly used [1, 3].

20. **What are the neurodevelopmental outcomes for patients with abdominal wall defects?**

Neurodevelopmental outcomes among patients with gastroschisis have not been well studied and are largely unknown to date. Patients with omphalocele overall have decreased motor and language score for age, with 35% having severe neurodevelopmental delay, which may reflect the multiple congenital issues. Simple gastroschisis patients are not considered to have any long-term neurodevelopmental issues [1–3].

References

1. Islam S. Abdominal wall defects. In: Holcomb, Murphy, St. Peter, editors. Ashcraft's pediatric surgery, 7th ed. New York, NY, USA: Elsevier; 2020.
2. Islam S, Gollin G, Koehler S, Wagner AJ. Gastroschisis. In: Powel, Hirschl, Waldhausen, editors. Pediatric surgery NaT. Unbound Medicine. https://www.pedsurglibrary.com/apsa/view/Pediatric-Surgery-NaT/829060/all/Gastroschisis.
3. Islam S, Ledbetter DJ, Olutoye OO. Omphalocele. In: Powel, Hirschl, Waldhausen, editors. Pediatric surgery NaT. Unbound Medicine. https://www.pedsurglibrary.com/apsa/view/Pediatric-Surgery-NaT/829059/all/Omphalocele.

Chapter 19
Exstrophy-Epispadias Complex

Abdulrahman E. Alshafei and Raimondo Maximilian Cervellione

Abstract The bladder exstrophy complex represents a spectrum of severe congenital malformations which range from epispadias, an isolated penile abnormality, to classic cloacal exstrophy, one of the most severe abnormalities compatible with life. In this chapter the authors have provided an extract of the expertise developed in the treatment of this conditions at Royal Manchester Children's Hospital following the centralisation of the treatment of exstrophy in the UK in 1999.

Keywords Bladder exstrophy · Cloacal exstrophy · Epispadias · Osteotomy

1. **What anomalies make up the spectrum of the Exstrophy-Epispadias complex?**
    - Epispadias: The urethra is a partial or complete open plate on the dorsal penis. There is always severe dorsal chordee and it can be associated with vesico-ureteric reflux (VUR) and urinary incontinence.
    - Classic bladder exstrophy (CBE): There is pubic diastasis with subsequent diastasis of the anterior abdominal wall. The bladder is an open plate often associated with congenital pseudo-polyps and it is incarcerated within the abdominal defect in an extraperitoneal position. The umbilical cord is usually lower in the abdomen compared to normal children. It is always associated with epispadias and the length of the urethral plate represents a critical factor in the reconstruction.
    - Cloacal exstrophy (CE): It is one of the most severe congenital malformations compatible with life. Over 70% of the patients have severe associated

A. E. Alshafei · R. M. Cervellione (✉)
Department of Paediatric Urology, Royal Manchester Children's Hospital,
Oxford Rd., Manchester M13 9WL, UK
e-mail: raimondo.cervellione@mft.nhs.uk

M. Lacher et al. (eds.), *Pearls and Tricks in Pediatric Surgery*,
https://doi.org/10.1007/978-3-030-51067-1_19

anomalies including spinal dysmorphism and limbs abnormalities [1]. There is extreme pubic diastasis and an omphalocele which both contribute to a large anterior abdominal wall defect. Two hemi-bladders are incarcerated in the abdominal defect and between them there is the cecum which is opened, and the ileum prolapses through the defect like an elephant trunk.

- Exstrophy variants: Partial manifestations of the above anomalies, which may lack symmetry in the sagittal plane [2]. There is significant variability of clinical manifestations and it is imperative to rule out associated anomalies.

2. **Which embryological structure is commonly implicated in the pathogenesis of exstrophic anomalies?**

- The cloacal membrane.

By the 4th week of gestation, the cloacal membrane forms the ventral wall of the urogenital sinus [1]. With further development, mesoderm fuses in the midline to form the lower abdominal wall with simultaneous caudal progression of the urorectal septum to separate the cloaca into the urogenital canal and rectum [1]. The *Marshall and Muecke's theory* states that rupture of the cloacal membrane after complete separation of the GU and GI tracts results in CBE and prior to descent of the urorectal septum results in CE [3].

Epispadias occurs when there is failure of midline mesodermal fusion of the most distal part of the anterior cloacal membrane.

Normally the bladder forms around the 4th–8th week of gestation and represents the most anterior lower abdominal organ [4]. The two hemi-bony-pelvises form laterally to the sacrum and subsequently start to internally rotate which completes around the 10th week of gestation with the formation of the pubic symphysis [4]. The Cervellione's theory speculates that the bladder remains trapped between the two pubic bones during their migration to the midline and the detrusor fuses to the pubic bones and the lower abdominal wall leading to perforation of the bladder. The positive intra-abdominal pressure inverts the bladder 'inside-out'. The corpora cavernosa remain attached to the pubic bones and cannot externally rotate as normally happens with the consequent dorsal chordee.

3. **What is the risk of recurrence of exstrophy in the family of a known index case?**

Current counselling recommendations [2]:

- 1% sibling recurrence
- 1:70 chance of transmission from parent to child.

4. **What is the prevalence of CBE, CE, and epispadias?**

The following figures are according to a recent European prospective trial [5]:

- Male epispadias ~1 in 101,000
- Female epispadias ~1 in 1,300,000
- CBE ~1 in 46,000. M:F 3:1
- CE ~1 in 317,000. M:F 6:1.

5. **What is the rate of associated anomalies in CBE, CE, and epispadias?**

- Epispadias ~3%: renal, chromosomal [5]
- CBE ~5%: renal, chromosomal, cardiac, anorectal malformation[5]
- CE ~71%: Gastrointestinal 65% (malrotation, short gut, duodenal atresia), Sacral agenesis 60%, spinal dysraphism 50%, orthopaedic 40% (club foot, hip dysplasia), cardiovascular <10%, and renal anomalies 7% (ectopic kidney, agenesis) [1].

6. **What antenatal ultrasound findings suggest a diagnosis of an exstrophy-epispadias complex?**

- Failure to visualize the bladder (usually visible at ~14 weeks gestation)
- Lower abdominal wall mass
- Low-set umbilical cord
- Abnormal genitalia
- Widening of the iliac crests.

Data suggests that approximately 25% of bladder and cloacal exstrophy patients are detected antenatally [5].

7. **What are the key external characteristics of CBE in male and female patients?**

The bladder is open on the lower abdominal wall and the urothelium fully exposed. In males, the penis is short and wide with a short urethral plate and a dorsal chordee. In females, the clitoris is bifid with the labia displaced laterally. The vagina is displaced anteriorly and the mons pubis is absent. In both sexes, the pubic symphysis is widely separated with divergent recti muscles.

8. **What is the rate of inguinal hernias in patients with bladder exstrophy?**

>80% males
>10% females.

Indirect inguinal hernias are commonly associated with bladder exstrophy [1, 2]. The wide pubic diastasis and external rotation of the anterior pelvis means that the internal and external rings lie in an anterior-posterior plane rather than the usual oblique plane seen in non-exstrophy children.

9. **In addition to ligation of the patent processus vaginalis (PPV), what additional step must be undertaken during inguinal hernia repair in exstrophy patients?**

- Narrowing of the internal ring.

This operative step, incorporating simple absorbable sutures, reduces the hernia recurrence rate. Care must be taken to not strangulate the spermatic cord.

10. **A term baby is born with CBE and is awaiting operative repair. What pre-operative measures must be taken during this period?**

A hydrated gel dressing or plastic wrap is secured over the bladder and changed daily with normal saline irrigation. Parents must be warned about the possibility for the baby to develop an inguinal hernia and occasionally rectal prolapse. Patients with CBE often have no life-threatening anomalies and should be encouraged to remain with their recovering mothers until surgical repair is planned. Feeding need not be restricted and breast-feeding encouraged. Antibiotic prophylaxis is usually not required.

Pre-operative renal ultrasound is necessary to rule out upper tract dilatation and as a baseline for future ultrasound studies. Spinal ultrasounds are necessary to rule out spinal cord anomalies. In CE, an echocardiogram is always needed due to the higher rate of cyanotic heart disease (<10%) [1]. Antibiotics are also needed peri-operatively.

11. **What are the pathological hallmarks of exstrophic bladders?**

Exstrophic bladders demonstrate a similar amount of type 1 collagen but a 3-fold increase in type 3 collagen compared to controls [6]. Patients with adequate bladder capacity post closure demonstrate a significant decrease in the ratio of collagen to smooth muscle, provided the bladder remained infection free [6]. Based on experimental studies, exstrophy patients have similar cholinergic receptor density and binding affinity, but a significant decrease of myelinated nerves per field [6].

12. **What are the key external characteristics of CE?**

There is a central hind-gut plate with two separated bladder halves. The ileum intussuscepts through the ileocaecal valve and into the hindgut creating an elephant trunk appearance. One or two appendices may be seen on either side of the ileum.

Pubic diastasis is almost twice that seen in children with classic exstrophy and the two phallic halves may be completely separated and asymmetrical with a dominant hemiphallus or hemiscrotum. Patients with CE almost always required pelvic osteotomies for proper pelvic closure.

The anus is imperforate, sacrum short, and spinal dysraphism may be evident. There is usually an associated omphalocele (>88%) [1].

13. **What are the main operative approaches to anatomic reconstruction?**

a. Primary versus staged
b. Early versus delayed.

The author's surgical preference is the Manchester delayed exstrophy closure technique. This staged approach involves initial bladder closure with ureteric re-implantation at 3–9 months followed by epispadias repair at 12–18 months. In this approach, further bladder neck surgery or bladder augmentation may or may not be necessary at 5–6 years depending on continence outcomes and only after vigorous biofeedback training.

The complete primary repair (Mitchell technique) includes bladder closure, urethroplasty, and genital reconstruction. Due to penile ischaemic complications, this technique should be considered obsolete. However, a modification of the technique with a less aggressive penile dissection is still adopted in some centres in North America.

14. **What are the main components of the staged closure technique?**

   a. Bladder closure with ureteric re-implantation and tubularisation of the proximal urethra at 3–9 months of age with pelvic osteotomies and insertion of a pelvic external fixator
   b. Epispadias repair (12–18 months)
   c. Potty training and biofeedback between the age of 3 and 5 years
   d. ± Bladder neck reconstruction (~6 years) if continence not attained after biofeedback training
   e. ± Bladder augmentation if small non-compliant high pressure bladder.

15. **What is the sequence of reconstruction in CE patients?**

1. Initial management of the associated anomalies and prematurity when appropriate. Severe lung hypoplasia may require prolonged ventilation after birth and occasionally can be fatal.
2. If a large omphalocele is present, gradual reduction of the omphalocele is performed in the NICU suspending the umbilical cord to the roof of the incubator to facilitate the descend of the liver into the abdominal wall.
3. First stage of reconstruction is performed when the baby is stable, usually in the first few weeks of life:
   a. Insertion of central line for parenteral nutrition (PN)
   b. Laparotomy with Ladd's procedure if required
   c. Separation of the cecum from the hemi-bladders, tubularisation of the cecum after washout of the atretic colon and formation of an ileostomy
   d. The two hemi-bladders are sutured together
   e. The omphalocele is reduced when possible.
4. Bladder closure with para-exstrophy skin flaps to reconstruct the absent urethra with pelvic osteotomies is performed when the patients is about 6–7 kg.

16. **What are the advantages of performing pelvic osteotomies at the time of initial bladder closure?**

   - Facilitates closure of the pubic symphysis
   - Decreased abdominal wall tension and reduced risk of wound dehiscence
   - Placement of bladder and urethra deep within the pelvis
   - Increased pelvic floor support around the bladder neck which may improve future continence.

Studies have shown that exstrophy patients tend to have shorter pubic bones than controls [7]. Although this was originally been thought to be a congenital phenomenon, recent evidence shows that this is an acquired condition resulting from the lack of tension across epiphyseal plates in an incomplete pelvic ring and epiphyseal plate damage following osteotomy [7]. Tension across epiphyseal plates has been shown to increase bone growth [7].

17. **Incision of what anatomic structure is essential to move the bladder and urethra posteriorly in the pelvis?**

- The intersymphyseal bands: This structure represents part of the anterior detrusor abnormally attached to the medial portion of the pubic bones.

Failure to divide the intersympheseal bands does not allow positioning of the bladder deep in the pelvis and appropriate securement of the pubic bones in the midline.

18. **What is the most common complication following exstrophy closure?**

The most commonly reported complication is a urethrocutaneous fistula (5–40%), commonly in the peno-pubic angle in males [2]. Since they may close spontaneously, they can initially be managed conservatively via catheter drainage. If the fistula does not close, cystoscopy must be performed to evaluate for possible bladder neck obstruction.

Wound dehiscence is associated with increased tension on the wound and may be reduced with pelvic osteotomies. Complete breakdown of the repair is rare and usually associated with severe infection or technical errors.

19. **What is the incidence of vesico-ureteric reflux (VUR) following exstrophy closure?**

Small bladder size, increased detrusor pressures, and increased outlet resistance following closure results in VUR in almost all patients. Moreover, the ureters often enter the bladder with a short submucosal tunnel predisposing to reflux. For this reason, the authors prefer to perform ureteric re-implantations in all patients at the time of primary bladder closure.

Following closure, patients must be followed closely with 3–6 monthly ultrasound scans to look for any signs of upper tract deterioration. Progressive dilatation, especially when associated with urinary tract infections, may require a period of anticholinergics, intermittent catheterization and eventual bladder augmentation to reduce bladder pressures and protect the upper tracts.

20. **A 35-year old woman born with classic bladder exstrophy underwent a ureterosigmoidostomy in childhood for urinary diversion. What are the long-term complications of this procedure?**

Continent and incontinent urinary diversion techniques (i.e. Indiana pouch, ureterosigmoidostomy, ileal conduit) have largely been abandoned in favour of anatomic reconstruction. However, these procedures may be useful to achieve dryness in patients who have failed multiple attempts at anatomic reconstruction.

Long-term complications associated with ureterosigmoidostomy [2]:

- Hyperchloremic metabolic acidosis
- Chronic pyelonephritis
- Bladder calculi
- 250–300-fold increased risk of adenocarcinoma at the anastomosis.

Any attempt at reversal of a ureterosigmoidostomy must include excision of a cuff of normal colonic tissue at the site of the implanted ureters to prevent future malignancy [2].

21. **A concerned mother asks you about her daughter's fertility potential after undergoing a successful staged exstrophy closure. How do you respond?**

In contrast to males, most females have normal fertility [8]. Women must have an elective caesarean section to avoid injury to the reconstructed urinary tract. In addition, females often have normal sexual desire, are adequately sexually active, and have normal menstruations [8]. However, the vagina is often short and vertically lying, which may require an introitoplasty or vaginoplasty in adulthood to allow normal sexual intercourse. Uterine prolapse is a common occurrence (30–60%) and may be precipitated by pregnancy [8]. In cases of refractory prolapse, complex uro-gyne reconstruction may be required.

In males, fertility potential is significantly reduced and normal sperm counts are reported in 16–63% of patients [8]. The volume of ejaculate of often low and up to 50% experience retrograde ejaculation [8]. The effect on fertility potential is likely attributed to previous bladder neck surgery. Although the penile length is short, most male patients have normal libido and erections adequate for sexual function [8].

22. **What are the psychosocial outcomes following exstrophy closure?**

Both males and females suffer from psychosocial disturbances due to body image and genital perception. Exstrophy patients have higher rates of anxiety, depression, and suicidal ideation than controls [8]. Therefore, early psychiatric assessment and parental education is warranted.

References

1. Thomas DFM, Duffy PG, Rickwood AMK. Essentials of paediatric urology. CRC Press; 2008.
2. Holcomb GW, Ashcraft KW. Ashcraft's pediatric surgery. Saunders Elsevier; 2014.
3. Marshall VF, Muecke EC. Variations in exstrophy of the bladder. J Urol. 1962;88(6):766–96.
4. Liaw A, Cunha GR, Shen J, Cao M, Liu G, Sinclair A, et al. Development of the human bladder and ureterovesical junction. (1432-0436 (Electronic)).
5. Cervellione RM, Mantovani A, Gearhart J, Bogaert G, Gobet R, Caione P, et al. Prospective study on the incidence of bladder/cloacal exstrophy and epispadias in Europe. J Pediatr Urol. 2015;11(6):337.e1–6.
6. Puri A, Mishra K, Sikdar S, Unni KE, Jain AK. Vesical preservation in patients with late bladder exstrophy referral: histological insights into functional outcome. (1527-3792 (Electronic)).
7. Stephens L, Mantovani A, Keene DJ, Dickson AP, Khan T, Shabani A, et al. Shortened pubic bones in bladder exstrophy: a congenital or acquired phenomenon? J Pediatr Urol. 2014;10(2):325–8.
8. Ansari MS, Cervellione RM, Gearhart JP. Sexual function and fertility issues in cases of exstrophy epispadias complex. Indian J Urol. 2010;26(4):595–7.

A concerned mother asks you about her daughter's fertility po[illegible] tial after undergoing a successful staged exstrophy closure. How do you [illegible]

Chapter 20
Prune Belly Syndrome

A. J. Pomajzl and Gwen M. Grimsby

Abstract Prune belly syndrome is characterized by three cardinal features: bilateral undescended testicles, dilated urinary tract, and deficient abdominal wall musculature. These manifestations place patients with prune belly syndrome at risk for testicular malignancy, infertility, urinary tract infections, and renal failure. In addition, extra-genitourinary manifestations may also affect the gastrointestinal, orthopedic, and cardiopulmonary organ systems. The syndrome affects males in 95% of cases with up to 29% of patients dying during the peri-natal period, the majority from complications of pulmonary hypoplasia. The complexity of these patients requires a thorough understanding of their pathophysiology by pediatric surgeons and pediatric urologists alike.

Keywords Prune belly syndrome · Eagle-Barrett syndrome · Cryptorchidism · Hydronephrosis · Vesicoureteral reflux

1. **By what other names is prune-belly syndrome (PBS) known?**
   - Eagle-Barrett syndrome
   - Abdominal musculation syndrome
   - Triad syndrome
2. **What is the incidence of PBS?**
   - PBS has a contemporary incidence of 3.6–3.8 per 100,000 live male births [1].
   - It is a predominantly male diagnosis as <5% of those diagnosed are female [1].

A. J. Pomajzl
Department of Urology, Creighton University School of Medicine, Omaha, NE, USA

G. M. Grimsby (✉)
Division of Urology, Phoenix Children's Hospital, Phoenix, AZ, USA
e-mail: ggrimsby@phoenixchildrens.com

M. Lacher et al. (eds.), *Pearls and Tricks in Pediatric Surgery*,
https://doi.org/10.1007/978-3-030-51067-1_20

3. **What are theories regarding the embryology of the development of PBS?**

    - No single embryological explanation has universal acceptance and many theories overlap.
    - Some theories emphasize that a severely dilated urinary tract—either from early in utero posterior urethral obstruction or an intrinsic defect in the urinary tract—leads to redundancy in the abdominal wall.
    - Another theory ascribes the syndrome to a yolk sac defect.
    - A final theory points to a possible defect in the lateral plate mesoderm which gives rise to the ureters, bladder, prostate, urethra and gubernaculum.

4. **What are the major manifestations of PBS, giving rise to its alternative name of the triad syndrome?**

    - A deficiency of abdominal musculature leading to a wrinkled "prune-like" appearance of the abdominal wall.
    - Bilateral intra-abdominal testes.
    - Urinary tract dysmorphism. The urinary tract anomalies are characterized by differing degrees of renal dysplasia, hydronephrosis, dilated tortuous ureters, an enlarged bladder and a dilated prostatic urethra.

5. **What percentage of patients with PBS are female? What major manifestations of PBS does a female with the diagnosis exhibit?**

    - Only 5% of PBS diagnoses are female.
    - Females exhibit only deficiency of abdominal wall musculature and the anomalous urinary tract without any gonadal abnormality [2].

6. **Besides the triad, what are other manifestations of PBS and how common are they?**

    - 75% of children with PBS have non–urinary tract abnormalities [3].
    - These abnormalities include respiratory (58%, e.g. pulmonary hypoplasia), cardiac (25%, e.g. patent ductus arteriosus, atrial septal defect, ventricular septal defect, tetralogy of Fallot), gastrointestinal (63%, e.g. constipation, incomplete rotation of the midgut) and musculoskeletal anomalies (65%, e.g. talipes equinovarus, scoliosis, hip dysplasia) [2, 4].

7. **How common is prematurity in those born with PBS?**

    - The incidence of prematurity in the PBS population is nearly 50% [3].

8. **What is the perinatal mortality of those born with PBS? Which factor most limits survival?**
   - Perinatal mortality ranges between 10–29% in contemporary studies [1].
   - Perinatal mortality is directly connected to the level of prematurity and severity of pulmonary hypoplasia [2].
9. **What is the most common urinary tract dysmorphism found in PBS?**
   - Hydroureteronephrosis is almost always present and most commonly bilateral [2].
   - The distal ureter is usually where massive dilation occurs, however the presentation is variable.
   - Hydroureteronephrosis is almost never due to obstruction within the ureter, rather, culprits include lower urinary tract obstruction (posterior urethral valves), vesicoureteral reflux, and a histologic deficiency of smooth muscle and preponderance of fibrous tissue in the ureters leading to ineffective peristalsis [3].
10. **How common is vesicoureteral reflux in PBS?**
    - 75% of patients have vesicoureteral reflux with most cases being bilateral [2].
11. **What percentage of patients with PBS have renal dysplasia?**
    - 50% of patients will have dysplasia in varying degrees and laterality [3].
12. **How common is it for PBS patients to require renal replacement therapy? What are two clinical predictors for satisfactory long-term renal function in a newborn with PBS?**
    - 40–50% of patients will require renal replacement therapy at some point in time.
    - Positive prognostic indicators include at least one normal-appearing kidney on ultrasound and a nadir serum creatinine of less than 0.7 mg/dL over their first year of life [2].
13. **What characteristic appearance of the bladder one would expect in PBS?**
    - On imaging, the bladder is commonly enlarged with a volume 2 to 4 times that of expected capacity [5].
    - These large bladders often demonstrate a smooth wall without trabeculation.
    - The dome of the bladder is often diverticular-shaped and a patent urachus is found in 25–30% of patients [3].

- The bladder neck is commonly wide with a dilated prostatic urethra due to prostatic hypoplasia.

14. **What type of bladder dynamics would you expect to find in a patient with PBS?**

    - PBS bladders are large-capacity, hypotonic bladders. Because of this, patients are often unable to adequately empty their bladder [2].

15. **How common are urinary tract infections (UTI) in this patient population?**

    - Nearly 80% of patients will have at least one documented UTI. One third of these patients will develop pyelonephritis [2].
    - The high likelihood of infection owes largely to the common co-morbidities of vesicoureteral reflux, ureteral urinary stasis due to ineffective peristalsis, and poor bladder emptying.
    - Prophylactic antibiotics and circumcision are commonly recommended by urologists to reduce the risk of UTI.

16. **Where are the testes usually located in patients with PBS?**

    - The testes typically lie intra-abdominally, bordering the dilated ureters at the level of the iliac arteries.

17. **Histologically, is there any difference between testes in patients with PBS and those of normal, age-matched controls?**

    - A lower concentration of Leydig cells have been found in testicles in patients with prune belly syndrome. The number and size of seminiferous tubules are equivalent to patients without PBS [6].
    - Germ cell counts, spermatogonia, and Leydig cells are essentially identical in intraabdominal testes of boys with and without PBS [3, 7].

18. **What is the future reproductive potential in children born with PBS?**

    - Infertility is considered multi-factorial, largely due to cryptorchidism, retrograde ejaculation from an incompetent bladder neck, and prostatic hypoplasia.
    - Prior to 1992, men with PBS were considered infertile as there had been no reported cases of paternity [8]. Since that time however, there have been several cases of men with PBS fathering children via sperm retrieval techniques and intra-cytoplasmic sperm injection.
    - There have been reports of a normal pregnancy with vaginal birth in a woman with PBS [9].

19. **What is the likelihood that patients with PBS will pass the syndrome to future offspring?**

  - Given the propensity of the syndrome to exist in males, occasional reported diagnosis in male siblings or cousins and the increased incidence in twins, it has been suggested that PBS has an underling genetic etiology [10].
  - An exact inheritance pattern has yet to be described, and most cases are considered sporadic with patients having normal karyotypes.
  - Of the few reported cases of patients with PBS fathering or mothering children reported in the literature, there have been no offspring diagnosed with PBS.
  - Given what little is known at this point about the genetic basis of the syndrome, patients should be counseled about the potential, yet still unknown, risk of transmission to their future children [8].

20. **Are patients with PBS at an increased risk of testicular malignancy?**

  - There have been three cases of testis tumor reported in the literature [3].
  - The risk of malignancy appears to be increased in PBS, but it is no higher than that of non-PBS patients with cryptorchidism.
  - This emphasizes the importance of placement of the testes into the scrotum in a timely manner is necessary to both reduce the risk of developing malignancy as well as enhancing detection of potential tumors.

21. **What area of the abdominal wall is most commonly deficient in patients with PBS?**

  - While rare cases have reported completely absent abdominal wall musculature, the usual deficiency lies in the lower portion of the abdominal wall [11].
  - The rectus muscles and internal and external obliques are less well developed than in the upper abdomen and in severe cases, skin subcutaneous fat and a single fibrous layer may be all that is overlying the peritoneum [12].

22. **Do children born with PBS commonly carry their characteristic wrinkled appearance of the abdomen into adolescence?**

  - As PBS children grow, adipose tissue deposits in the subcutaneous layer of the abdominal wall. This tends to diminish the wrinkled appearance of the abdominal wall over the first year of life when their abdomen begins to take on more of a pot-bellied appearance owing to the deficiency of musculature [3].

23. **Is there a characteristic gait associated with PBS? Are PBS children able to sit up normally?**
    - Walking style usually is not affected; however achievement of the walking milestone may be delayed [3].
    - Since the usual musculature responsible for sitting up is commonly deficient in PBS, patients tend to sit up by rolling to their sides and using their arms to push themselves up [3].
24. **Why does the deficiency of abdominal wall musculature place patients with PBS at greater anesthetic risk?**
    - The deficiency in abdominal wall musculature compromises the cough effectiveness, potentially leading to retention of pulmonary secretions and subsequent pneumonia [13, 14].
25. **What radiologic studies should be obtained in newborns with PBS?**
    - A chest radiograph should be obtained to rule out early pulmonary problems, especially in cases of oligohydramnios.
    - Once the patient is stable, renal bladder ultrasound will give information of nature and severity of the urinary tract dysmorphism.
    - Voiding cystourethrogram (VCUG) is indicated to assess for presence of vesicoureteral reflux and to study the bladder outlet and bladder emptying ability.
    - Ultrasound studies of the heart and the abdomen will help identify cardiac and gastrointestinal anomalies common in the syndrome.
26. **Broadly speaking, what are the three types of surgeries a PBS patient may require?**
    - Orchiopexy is almost always indicated in patients with PBS for surveillance for testicular malignancy and facilitation of fertility [2].
    - Urinary tract reconstruction may be indicated in patients with recurrent febrile urinary tract infections or progressive renal deterioration.
    - Abdominal wall reconstruction is indicated in children with moderate to severe abdominal wall deficiencies.
27. **By what age should orchiopexy be performed? Abdominoplasty?**
    - The current recommendation for bilateral orchiopexy is at 6 months corrected gestational age. Elective orchiopexy any sooner brings with it higher anesthetic risk, and elective orchiopexy any later makes it less likely the adequate mobilization can be achieved for single-stage scrotal placement [15].
    - Abdominoplasty may be performed at any time, but is usually performed in coordination with any other indicated surgeries, including orchiopexy, vesicostomy or urinary tract reconstruction [16].

References

1. Routh JC, Huang L, Retik AB, Nelson CP. Contemporary epidemiology and characterization of newborn males with prune belly syndrome. Urology. 2010;76(1):44–8.
2. Seidel NE, Arlen AM, Smith EA, Kirsch AJ. Clinical manifestations and management of prune-belly syndrome in a large contemporary pediatric population. Urology. 2015;85(1):211–5.
3. Wein A, Kavoussi LR, Partin AW, Peters CA. Campbell-Walsh Urology; 2016.
4. Grimsby GM, Harrison SM, Granberg CF, Bernstein IH, Baker LA. Impact and frequency of extra-genitourinary manifestations of prune belly syndrome. J Pediatr Urol. 2015;11(5):280 e1–6.
5. Zugor V, Schott GE, Labanaris AP. The prune belly syndrome: urological aspects and long-term outcomes of a rare disease. Pediatr Rep. 2012;4(2):e20.
6. Favorito LA, Costa SF, Costa WS, Vieiralves R, Bernardo FO, Sampaio FJB. Study of testicular structure in fetuses with prune belly syndrome. Adv Urol. 2017;2017:3254980.
7. Nunn IN, Stephens FD. The triad syndrome: a composite anomaly of the abdominal wall, urinary system and testes. J Urol. 1961;86:782–94.
8. Kolettis PN, Ross JH, Kay R, Thomas AJ Jr. Sperm retrieval and intracytoplasmic sperm injection in patients with prune-belly syndrome. Fertil Steril. 1999;72(5):948–9.
9. Hillman RT, Garabedian MJ, Wallerstein RJ. Pregnancy outcome in a woman with prune belly syndrome. BMJ Case Rep. 2012;2012.
10. Iqbal NS, Jascur TA, Harrison S, Chen C, Arevalo MK, Wong D, et al. Copy number variations in a population with prune belly syndrome. Am J Med Genet Part A. 2018;176(11):2276–83.
11. Randolph J, Cavett C, Eng G. Abdominal wall reconstruction in the prune belly syndrome. J Pediatr Surg. 1981;16(6):960–4.
12. Mininberg DT, Montoya F, Okada K, Galioto F, Presutti R. Subcellular muscle studies in the prune belly syndrome. J Urol. 1973;109(3):524–6.
13. Smith CA, Smith EA, Parrott TS, Broecker BH, Woodard JR. Voiding function in patients with the prune-belly syndrome after Monfort abdominoplasty. J Urol. 1998;159(5):1675–9.
14. Woodard JR. Lessons learned in 3 decades of managing the prune-belly syndrome. J Urol. 1998;159(5):1680.
15. Fallat ME, Skoog SJ, Belman AB, Eng G, Randolph JG. The prune belly syndrome: a comprehensive approach to management. J Urol. 1989;142(3):802–5.
16. Denes FT, Park R, Lopes RI, Moscardi PR, Srougi M. Abdominoplasty in prune belly syndrome. J Pediatr Urol. 2015;11(5):291–2.

Chapter 21
Normal Embryology, Anatomy, and Physiology of the Gastrointestinal Tract

Faten Al Rubian and Richard Keijzer

Abstract Understanding the developmental embryology, anatomy and the unique physiologic properties of the Gastrointestinal Tract is essential for the surgeon to provide proficient surgical treatment for the pediatric patient. This chapter aims to equip the surgeon with the foundational knowledge needed to manage the broad spectrum of congenital and acquired pathology that can affect the gastrointestinal tract.

Keywords Embryology · Omphalomesenteric duct · Cloaca · Gastrointestinal tract · Auerbach plexus · Meissner plexus

1. **What are the three germ layers in embryological development?**

The gastrointestinal (GI) system involves three germ layers: mesoderm, endoderm, ectoderm

– The mesoderm gives rise to the connective tissue, including the wall of the gut and the smooth muscle.

– The endoderm is the source of the epithelial lining of the gastrointestinal tract, liver, gallbladder, and pancreas.

– The ectoderm divides into the surface ectoderm, neural tube, and neural crest [1].

F. Al Rubian · R. Keijzer (✉)
Health Sciences Centre-Children's Hospital, Children's Hospital Research Institute of Manitoba and University of Manitoba, Winnipeg, MB, Canada
e-mail: richard.keijzer@umanitoba.ca

F. Al Rubian
e-mail: Faten.alrubian@gmail.com

F. Al Rubian
King Abdulla Specialist Children Hospital, Riyadh, Saudi Arabia

M. Lacher et al. (eds.), *Pearls and Tricks in Pediatric Surgery*,
https://doi.org/10.1007/978-3-030-51067-1_21

2. **How can the gastrointestinal tract be divided embryologically?**

The gastrointestinal system has three divisions: the foregut, midgut, and hindgut.

- The foregut starts with the oral cavity and ends at the first part of the duodenum, blood supply is from the celiac artery.
- The midgut covers the mid-duodenum to the proximal two-thirds of the transverse colon, blood supply is from the superior mesenteric artery.
- The hindgut extends from the latter one-third of the transverse colon to the upper portion of the anus, blood supply is from the inferior mesenteric artery [1].

3. **When does midgut herniation occur?**

At week 6–10 of gestation the midgut herniates through the umbilical ring. The midgut then develops almost entirely outside of the peritoneal cavity, then rotates and returns back into the abdominal cavity around week 10 of gestation [1].

4. **What is the omphalomesenteric duct?**

The omphalomesenteric duct or vitelline duct forms a connecting tract between the embryonic yolk sac and primitive midgut. It usually obliterates during week 8 of gestation.

Failure of complete obliteration of the omphalomesenteric duct produces several malformations including a Meckel's diverticulum, patent omphalomesenteric duct and omphalomesenteric sinus [3].

5. **What is the definition of a cloaca?**

A cloaca is the common channel found at 4–6 weeks gestation in the terminal portion of the fetal hindgut. This common channel will be separated by a septum into a dorsal gastrointestinal component and ventral renal/genital component (urogenital sinus). Failure of the urorectal septum to partition the cloaca results in a persisting cloacal malformation [1].

6. **What is the blood supply of the esophagus?**

The arterial blood supply of the esophagus is segmental. The cervical esophagus is supplied by the inferior thyroid artery and drains into the corresponding vein. Esophageal arteries paired from the aorta supply the thoracic esophagus with blood. The most distal segment of the esophagus receives its blood supply from the left gastric artery and a branch of the left phrenic artery and drains into the left gastric vein which drains into the portal vein system [2].

7. **What are the narrow anatomical areas of the esophagus?**

- Cricopharyngeus muscle (C5, C6)
- Aortic arch (T4, T5)
- At the level of the diaphragm (T10) [2].

8. **Define the lower esophageal sphincter (LES)?**

LES is a high-pressure zone in the lower part of the esophagus at the level of the diaphragm. It serves as a functional sphincter [2]. Its action is reinforced by the right crus of the diaphragm, intra-abdominal length of the esophagus, and the angle of His.

9. **Describe the different parts of the stomach in Fig.** 21.1**?**

10. **How is the blood supply to the stomach?**

The stomach has a rich blood supply. The gastric arteries arise from all three branches of the celiac trunk:

- The left gastric artery is one of the three direct branches coming of the celiac trunk.
- The right gastric artery is a branch of the hepatic artery.
- The right gastroepiploic artery originates from the gastro-duodenal branch.
- The left gastroepiploic artery and the short gastric arteries arise from the splenic artery.

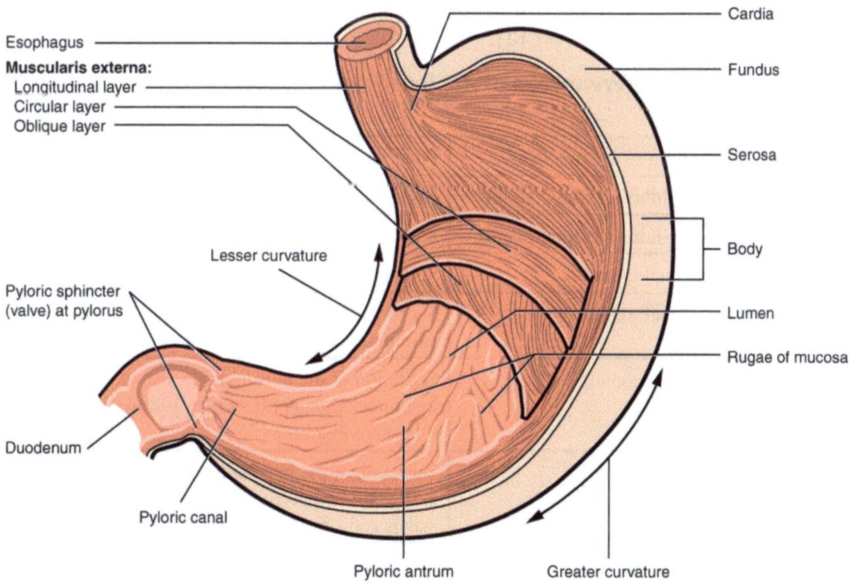

Fig. 21.1 Adapted from Wikimedia Commons contributors. File:2414 Stomach.jpg [Internet]. Wikimedia Commons, the free media repository; 2017 Nov 25, 23:25 UTC [cited 2019 Aug 1]. Available from: https://commons.wikimedia.org/w/index.php?title=File:2414_Stomach.jpg&oldid=269243795

The corresponding veins, running alongside the arteries, drain into the portal vein system, mostly either into the splenic or superior mesenteric vein, although some pass directly into the portal vein [4].

11. **What are the four major secretory cells of the stomach?**

- Parietal cells: secrete hydrochloric acid.
- Chief cells: secrete pepsin, a proteolytic enzyme.
- G cells: secrete the hormone gastrin.
- Mucous cells: secrete a mucus which has a high Ph that protects the epithelium against stress and acid [4].

12. **What are the landmarks of the duodenum?**

Its C-shaped curve begins at the pyloric and ends at the ligament of Treitz, at the level of L2. The duodenum consists of 4 parts. The papilla of Vater is located in the second part [5].

13. **What is the blood supply to the small intestine?**

The small intestine is supplied with blood from the superior mesenteric artery (a branch of the abdominal aorta) and the superior pancreaticoduodenal artery (a branch of the hepatic artery). The venous return from the small intestine consists of the superior mesenteric vein, which, with the splenic vein, forms the portal vein, which drains into the liver [5].

14. **What are the different cells of the intestinal mucosa?**

Cell type	Location in the mucosa	Function
Absorptive	Epithelium/intestinal glands	Digestion and absorption of nutrients and chyme
Goblet	Epithelium/intestinal glands	Secretion of mucus
G cells	Intestinal glands	Secretion of hormone intestinal gastrin
I cells	Intestinal glands	Secretion of the hormone cholecystokinin which stimulates release of pancreatic juice and bile
K cells	Intestinal glands	Secretion of the hormone glucose–dependent insulinotropic peptide which stimulates the release of insulin
M cells	Intestinal glands	Secretion of the hormone motilin, which accelerates gastric emptying, stimulates intestinal peristalsis and stimulates the production of pepsin
S cells	Intestinal glands	Secretion of the hormone secretin

15. **What are the Auerbach and Meissner plexi?**

The Auerbach plexus is located between the circular muscle layer and the longitudinal muscle layer in the lower esophagus, stomach, and intestines. The Meissner plexus is located in the submucosal tissue, which connects the surface mucous membrane lining to the deeper muscle layers in the stomach and intestines [5].

16. **In which part of the alimentary tract does absorption occur?**

Absorption of most of the nutrients occurs in the jejunum.

17. **Where do the following nutrients absorb?**

- Iron—The absorption of iron nutrients occurs in the duodenum.
- Lipids and water—The absorption of lipids and water occurs through passive diffusion within the small intestine.
- Bile salts—These are absorbed within the terminal ileum.
- Vitamin B12—In the terminal ileum after binding to the intrinsic factor which is secreted from the stomach.
- The Fat-Soluble Vitamins: A, D, E, and K—Need lipids and bile salts to be absorbed in the ileum [5].

18. **What is the blood supply of the large colon?**

The superior mesenteric artery supplies the cecum, ascending, and proximal two-thirds of the transverse colon from blood. The inferior mesenteric artery supplies the splenic flexure, descending colon and sigmoid. The venous drainage of the colon is similar to the arterial supply, the superior mesenteric and inferior mesenteric veins ultimately empty into the hepatic portal vein [6].

19. **What is the blood supply of the rectum and anal canal?**

- **Superior rectal artery** originates from the inferior mesenteric artery
- **Middle rectal arteries**, which are branches of the internal iliac arteries
- **Inferior rectal arteries** from the internal pudendal arteries
- The submucosal venous plexus above the pectinate line drains into the superior rectal veins (portal circulation)
- The submucosal plexus below the pectinate line drains into the inferior rectal veins (systemic circulation) [6].

20. **What are the porto-systemic anastomoses?**

- It is the connection between the veins of the systemic venous system and the portal vein system.
- The major anastomoses sites are:

Lower esophagus	Left gastric veins (portal system) and the oesophageal tributaries to the azygous system
Rectal	Superior rectal veins (portal) and inferior and middle rectal veins (systemic)
Paraumbilical	Paraumbilical veins (portal) and epigastric veins (systemic)
Retroperitoneal	The portal tributaries of the mesenteric veins and the retroperitoneal veins

21. **What is the role of the ileocecal sphincter?**

The ileocecal sphincter creates a mechanical barrier to prevent the entry of bacteria into the small intestine. It assists in controlling the movement of nutrients and fluids into the colon.

The loss of an ileocecal sphincter can also cause a condition known as small bowel bacterial overgrowth. The illness causes poor absorption of vitamin B12 and fat, as well as diarrhea. Other effects of the condition include bile salts' de-conjugation, liver damage, abdominal pains, and loss of fluid [5].

22. **Which characteristic features differentiate the large intestine from the small intestine?**

- The large intestine has fat-filled, peritoneal bags attached to its surface called epiploic appendices.
- The large intestine contains the teniae coli that move vertically along the large intestine's surface, which diverges at the recto-sigmoid junction to form an extensive coating in the rectum.
- The teniae coli's contraction reduces the wall of the large intestine, thereby leading to haustration.
- The ascending and descending part of the colon are fixed to the retroperitoneum [6].

23. **What is a watershed area?**

A watershed area refers to any region within the body that receives a dual supply of blood from the two large arteries' most distal branches and has the least vascular collaterals. The watershed areas in the body are highly susceptible to ischemia. It includes the splenic flexure of the colon and the rectosigmoid area [6].

References

1. Bhatia A, Bordoni B. Embryology, gastrointestinal [Internet]. Treasure Island (FL): StatPearls Publishing; 2019 [cited 1 August 2019]. https://www.ncbi.nlm.nih.gov/books/NBK537172/.
2. Oezcelik A, DeMeester SR. General anatomy of the esophagus. Thorac Surg Clin. 2011;21(2):289–97.

3. Wyllie R, Hyams JS. Pediatric gastrointestinal and liver disease E-Book. Elsevier Health Sciences; 2010.
4. Wilson R, Stevenson C. Anatomy and physiology of the stomach. In: CJ Yeo, editor. Shackelford's surgery of the alimentary tract, 2 Volume Set. 8th ed. Philadelphia, PA: Elsevier; 2019, p. 634–6.
5. Campbell J, Berry J, Liang Y. Anatomy and physiology of the small intestine. In: Charles JY, editor. Shackelford's surgery of the alimentary tract. 8th ed. Philadelphia, PA: Elsevier; 2019. p. 817–41.
6. Kelley M, Efron J, Fang S, Safar B, Gearhart S. Operative anatomy of the colon, rectum, and anus. In: C Yeo, editor. Shackelford's surgery of the alimentary tract. 8th ed. Philadelphia, PA: Elsevier; 2019. p. 1662–75.

Chapter 22
Small Intestinal Obstruction

Justin L. Hunter and Hanna Alemayehu

Abstract Small intestinal obstruction in children can have a wide range of etiologies. Neonatal intestinal obstructions are often related to specific gastrointestinal pathology such as intestinal atresias, meconium ileus, meconium plug syndrome, small left colon syndrome, Hirschsprung disease, anorectal malformation, necrotizing enterocolitis, malrotation with midgut volvulus, incarcerated inguinal hernia, anterior abdominal wall defects and more. In older children, intestinal obstruction are also seen in the setting of intussusception, vitelline duct remnants, perforated appendicitis, malrotation with or without midgut volvulus, foreign bodies, tumors and more. This chapter will focus on post-operative adhesive small bowel obstruction (ASBO) in children including incidence, epidemiology, management and outcomes.

Keywords Small bowel obstruction · Adhesive small bowel obstruction · Intestinal obstruction · Non-operative management · Recurrent bowel obstruction

J. L. Hunter
Department of Surgery, University of South Alabama, 1601 Center Street, Strada Patient Care Center, Suite 1E, Mobile, AL 36604, USA
e-mail: jlhunter@health.southalabama.edu

H. Alemayehu (✉)
Department of Surgery, Division of Pediatric Surgery, University of South Alabama, Children and Womens Hospital, 1601 Center Street, Strada Patient Care Center, Suite 1E, Mobile, AL 36604, USA
e-mail: halemayehu@health.southalabama.edu

M. Lacher et al. (eds.), *Pearls and Tricks in Pediatric Surgery*,
https://doi.org/10.1007/978-3-030-51067-1_22

1. **How common is adhesive small bowel obstruction (ASBO) in the pediatric population?**

Overall, ASBO occurs in 1–6% of children following abdominal surgery [1].

2. **Which patients are at the highest risk for developing ASBO?**

High rates of ASBO have been reported after the following index operations: ileostomy formation and closure (25%), Ladd procedure for malrotation (24%), and nephrectomy for Wilm's tumor (8.9%) [1, 2]. Younger patients who have undergone index operation during infancy are also at higher risk (13%), particularly within two years of the initial operation [3].

3. **Which patients are at lowest risk for developing ASBO?**

The rate of ASBO is <1% in patients who have undergone appendectomy but may be more common in patients with perforated appendicitis [1].

4. **How do patients with ASBO present?**

Patients commonly present with anorexia, crampy abdominal pain, emesis, and obstipation. Lethargy, significant abdominal distension and constant abdominal pain are late findings.

5. **What are the clinical signs and symptoms of bowel ischemia?**

The signs and symptoms of bowel ischemia can be difficult to determine in the pediatric population. Peritonitis is an obvious sign. Other indicators are fever, tachycardia and an elevated white blood cell count and lactic acidosis on laboratory work-up.

6. **What are radiologic findings of small bowel obstruction on abdominal plain films?**

Two-view plain radiographs should be obtained in all patients with suspected ASBO. Dilated loops of small bowel, presence of air-fluid levels, bowel wall thickening and lack of colonic or rectal air may be seen on X-ray. Paucity of bowel gas can also be seen and may be a more worrisome finding.

7. **What are the radiologic signs and symptoms of bowel ischemia?**

On plain film pneumoperitoneum is a clear indication of perforation likely secondary to bowel ischemia. Other concerning findings include bowel wall thickening, pneumatosis intestinalis and portal venous gas. On computed tomography (CT) scan, free peritoneal fluid is also concerning for bowel ischemia [1].

8. **What other imaging modalities aid in the diagnosis of ASBO?**

The diagnosis of small bowel obstruction (SBO) can often be made by history, physical examination, and abdominal plain films only. CT scan has a sensitivity of 87–92% in diagnosing SBO and can be useful in determining the site and cause of obstruction in children. However, risks of ionizing radiation and possible need for sedation preclude routine use of CT in children [1]. Administration of oral water-soluble contrast can be used as a diagnostic tool and as a way to predict potential failure of non-operative management. It may have therapeutic effects in non-operative resolution of ASBO in children [4].

9. **When is CT indicated in pediatric patients suspected of having an ASBO?**

CT scan can be useful in identifying high grade obstruction with signs of bowel ischemia; however, it is most useful for clinical decision-making when used to differentiate benign from worrisome pneumatosis intestinalis beyond infancy. Additionally, CT can help differentiate ileus versus SBO in children with concern for concomitant intra-abdominal abscess (for example in the post-appendectomy patient). CT images can then be used to aid in the drainage of these abscesses [1].

10. **Can CT scan be used to predict failure of non-operative management in children?**

CT findings associated with the need for an operation have been describe in adults, including lack of fecalization of the small bowel, free intraperitoneal fluid, mesenteric edema and the presence of a transition point [1]. However, this has not been specifically studied in children, and CT scan should be used judiciously in children.

11. **When should water soluble contrast studies be used?**

Children undergoing trial of non-operative management may benefit from upper gastrointestinal series with water-soluble contrast. Delayed plain films are performed at 10 and 24 hours. These studies should be performed on initial presentation, if they are to be used, in order to limit delay in surgical intervention. Failure of contrast to reach the colon within 24 hours predicts failure of non-operative management and surgical exploration should then be considered. Oral administration of water-soluble contrast may improve success rate of non-operative management of ASBO in children [4].

12. **Which patients with ASBO should undergo trial of non-operative management?**

Children presenting with clinical signs and symptoms of small bowel obstruction who have undergone previous abdominal operation and do not have any of the following: signs of bowel ischemia, hemodynamic compromise or evidence of end-organ distress. Those with bowel ischemia, perforation, sepsis, and severe physiologic disruption should undergo prompt surgical exploration after appropriate resuscitative measures.

13. **What does non-operative management of ASBO consist of?**

Initial fluid resuscitation is imperative in all children with SBO. Standard non-operative treatment of ASBO includes bowel rest, nasogastric tube decompression with a large diameter sump tube, intravenous fluid replacement and correction of electrolyte abnormalities. An abdominal plain film is the initial imaging modality of choice when SBO is suspected in children. Serial abdominal examinations should be performed, ideally by the same examiner. Analgesics should be administered as needed.

14. **When treating pediatric patients with ASBO non-operatively, how is their progress monitored?**

Strict monitoring of patient fluid status, urine output and daily nasogastric tube output is imperative. Serial abdominal exams should be performed. Water-soluble contrast administration can be used to determine progress of contrast to the colon, predicting successful non-operative management with 96% sensitivity and 98% specificity [4]. If nasogastric tube output does not significantly decrease within 24–48 hours, the abdominal exam worsens, or there are aberrant changes in vital signs, prompt surgical exploration is warranted.

15. **What are the clinical indicators that an ASBO has resolved?**

Nasogastric tube output will decrease significantly and appear less bilious. The movement of swallowed air through the GI tract will be evident by the passing of flatus, and resolution of obstipation with a bowel movement.

16. **How can nasogastric tube output be falsely elevated?**

If the distal tip of the nasogastric tube is post-pyloric and within the duodenum, the output will be falsely elevated and frankly bilious.

17. **How long should a patient with ASBO be managed non-operatively without improvement?**

Observation periods greater than 48 hours carry a higher risk of small bowel resection at the time of surgical exploration [1]. Additionally, in patients who have undergone water soluble contrast administration, the failure of contrast to reach the colon within 24 hours is predictive of failure of non-operative management and surgical exploration should be considered [4].

18. **What are clinical factors associated with failure of non-operative management?**

Children less than 1 year of age are more likely to require an operation than older children. Obstipation, previous ASBO, number of prior abdominal operations, history of a hernia, and history of malignancy are associated with the need for an operation in adults, however this has not been validated in children [1].

19. **When should surgical exploration be the initial management choice for ASBO?**

All children who present with peritonitis, pneumoperitoneum, hemodynamic instability, or findings concerning for bowel ischemia should undergo surgical exploration after resuscitation has been initiated.

20. **What role does laparoscopy have in the surgical treatment of ASBO?**

Laparoscopic surgery has been shown to be a safe and viable option for the surgical management of ASBO, despite initial concerns regarding difficulty with dilated bowel and potential for increased iatrogenic injuries. Literature suggests that laparoscopy for ASBO reduces morbidity and length of hospital stay compared to laparotomy [5].

21. **What are the long-term effects of ASBO?**

Recurrent SBO is a significant cause of readmission and re-operation in children with previous ASBO. Infertility in women and chronic abdominal pain in both men and women (24%) who underwent childhood operations account for significant distress, hospital admissions and resource utilization in people with previous ASBO.

22. **What is the rate of recurrence of ASBO?**

ASBO recurs in 9–36% in children as reported in several series [1, 6]. Younger children and those within their first post-operative year may have higher rates of recurrence [4].

23. **Is there a difference in recurrence rate of ASBO managed operatively versus non-operatively?**

Children managed non-operatively have a higher recurrence rate (14–35%) than those managed with an operation (9–19%) [6]. The cumulative rate of recurrence increases over time in adults (18% after ten years and 29% after thirty years), and the risk of ASBO recurrence increases with each successive episode of ASBO [1].

24. **Is a small bowel obstruction in the immediate post-operative period managed differently?**

The mainstay of non-operative management, bowel rest and nasogastric tube decompression, are similar. Studies in adults suggest that SBO in the immediate postoperative period may be observed for 10–14 days, however in children this has not been specifically supported. Intussusception is a specific cause of early post-operative bowel obstruction in children, and the majority require surgical exploration. Therefore, intussusception should be excluded in children prior to attempting prolonged non-operative management in the early post-operative period [1]. Additional consideration should be given to the possibility of incomplete lysis of adhesions as a technical cause of persistent post-operative obstruction.

25. **Are there any surgical techniques that can be utilized to decrease the risk of ASBO post-operatively?**

Neonatal operations have a 13% incidence of ASBO; stoma formation, duration of surgery >1 hour and post-operative complications were risk factors for development of ASBO, and so should be avoided if possible [3]. Gentle surgical technique and minimization of bowel manipulation are standard techniques to prevent ASBO. Additionally, literature suggest that ASBO rates lower with laparoscopy compared to open surgery [1, 5]. The use of adjuncts such as a bioresorbable membrane composed of sodium hyaluronate and carboxymethylcellulose has been shown to decrease ASBO in adults, and recently in children as well. Newer products including sprays, gels and liquids have been formulated but not assessed in the pediatric population [7].

References

1. Lautz TB, Barsness KA. Adhesive small bowel obstruction-Acute management and treatment in children. Semin Pediatr Surg. 2014;23(6):349–52.
2. Grant HW, Parker MC, Wilson MC. Adhesions after abdominal surgery in children. J Pediatr Surg. 2008;43(1):152–7.
3. Fredriksson F, Christofferson RH, Lilja HE. Adhesive small bowel obstruction after laparotomy during infancy. BJS. 2016;103:284–9.
4. Linden AF, Raiji MT, Kohler JE, et al. Evaluation of a water-soluble contrast protocol for non-operative management of pediatric adhesive small bowel obstruction. J Pediatr Surg. 2019;54:184–8.
5. Miyake H, Shogo S, Pierro A. Laparoscopy or laparotomy for adhesive bowel obstruction in children: a systematic review and meta-analysis. Pediatr Surg Int. 2018;34:177–82.
6. Akgur FM, Tanyel FC, Buyukpamukcu N, et al. Adhesive small bowel obstruction in children: the place and predictors of success for conservative treatment. J Pediatr Surg. 1991;26(1):37–41.
7. Mikihiro I, Keiichi U, Kohei O, et al. Efficacy of Seprafilm for preventing adhesive bowel obstruction and cost–benefit analysis in pediatric patients undergoing laparotomy. J Pediatr Surg. 2013;48:1528–34.

Chapter 23
Intestinal Atresia and Webs

Raphael H. Parrado and Daniel J. Ostlie

Abstract Congenital intestinal obstruction occurs in approximately 1 in 2000 live births and is one of the most common causes for admission to a neonatal care unit. Morphologically they are divided into either atresia and stenosis depending the continuity of the intestine. Furthermore, they are divided by the region of the gastrointestinal tract involved: duodenal, jejunoileal and colonic. Prenatally they present as polyhydramnios and dilation of the intestine on ultrasound. Neonatally infants present with obstructive symptoms. Usually a radiograph is enough to make the diagnosis of any of these conditions, depending the point of obstruction there might be a "double-bubble" sign or more diffuse intestinal dilation with or without pneumoperitoneum. For more distal obstruction a contrast enema might be needed. Treatment is surgical with a thorough exploration and repair through a single anastomosis or resection with or without anastomosis depending the portion of the gastrointestinal tract involved, other abnormalities and if perforation had occurred.

Keywords Intestinal atresia · Duodenal atresia · Jejunal atresia · Colonic atresia · Duodenoduodenostomy

R. H. Parrado · D. J. Ostlie (✉)
Phoenix Children's Hospital, Phoenix, USA
e-mail: dostlie@phoenixchildrens.com

R. H. Parrado
e-mail: parrado@musc.edu

D. J. Ostlie
Mayo Clinic School of Medicine, Rochester, USA

D. J. Ostlie
University of Arizona College of Medicine, Tucson, USA

M. Lacher et al. (eds.), *Pearls and Tricks in Pediatric Surgery*,
https://doi.org/10.1007/978-3-030-51067-1_23

1. **What is the incidence of congenital intestinal obstruction?** [1]

The incidence of congenital intestinal obstruction is about 1 in 200 live births. The incidence of both duodenal and jejunal atresia (the most common) is 1 per 5,000 live births, and the incidence of colonic atresia is 1 in 20,000 live births.

2. **What is the cause of congenital duodenal obstruction?**

Congenital duodenal obstruction occurs secondary to intrinsic or extrinsic lesions. The most common intrinsic lesion is duodenal atresia. As of today, the mechanism is unclear, however some theories aim towards defects in the epithelial plugging of the duodenum in early development related with fibroblast growth receptor. Other intrinsic causes include duodenal webs and diaphragm. Extrinsic causes include annular pancreas, or abnormalities in the biliary tree such as biliary atresia, gallbladder agenesis, common bile duct stenosis or choledochal cysts.

3. **How is congenital duodenal obstruction classified?**

Duodenal obstructions are classified as three types of stenosis or atresia. Type I is depicted below (Fig. 23.1a). In type I there is either a membrane (Fig. 23.1b) or a web (Fig. 23.1c) leading to the obstruction. In type I the duodenum remains in continuity. Type II duodenal atresia is characterized by complete obliteration of the duodenal lumen, replaced by a fibrous cord. Type III is the result of compete separation of the proximal and distal duodenal segments.

4. **How often are other abnormalities associated with duodenal atresia?** [2]

Associated abnormalities have been encountered in about 45–65% of the cases. Trisomy 21 and cardiac defects have been encountered in up to 30% of the cases followed by other gastrointestinal abnormalities (such as malrotation) in 25% of the cases. Other abnormalities are renal, esophageal atresia, imperforate anus or skeletal abnormalities.

5. **Where is the obstruction most commonly located in congenital duodenal obstruction?**

It is estimated that 85% of the obstructions occur distal to the ampulla.

6. **How is duodenal obstruction diagnosed?**

Polyhydramnios should raise a concern as 32–81% of congenital duodenal obstruction presents with this finding. Sonographic evaluation can identify the two

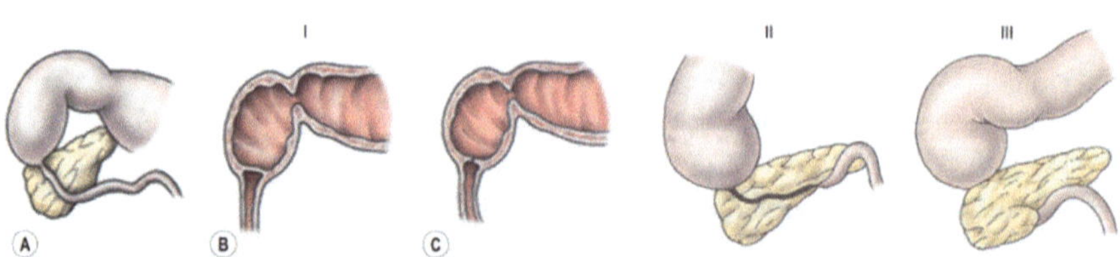

Fig. 23.1 Duodenal Atresias. From Ref. [1]

fluid filled strictures (double-bubble sign) in about 44% of the cases, this is mostly accomplished by week 28–32 due to lower gastric pressure in early development phases. Neonatally, a plain radiograph is usually enough.

7. **What is the double bubble sign and how can it be reproduced?**

The double bubble sign is commonly related to duodenal obstruction. The proximal bubble represents the air-fluid stomach whereas the second bubble represents the dilated distal duodenum. In cases of duodenal atresia is often encountered with a concomitant gasless distal abdomen. However, presence of air does not exclude the diagnosis of congenital duodenal obstruction as there might be abnormalities in the biliary tree that could let the air bypass the obstruction. This sign can often be reproduced by instilling 40–60 ml of air into the stomach. Is important to note that this sign is often not present in stenosis as the obstruction is not complete.

8. **What is the treatment of duodenal atresia?**

The treatment that is now preferred is an open or laparoscopic proximal transverse and distal longitudinal (diamond-shaped) duodenoduodenostomy. If a web is the cause a vertical duodenotomy with a web excision and transverse closure is enough.

9. **Should the duodenoduodenostomy be performed laparoscopic or open?** [3]

Since its first description by Rothenberg in 2002, multiple studies have compared laparoscopic vs open duodenal duodenoduodenostomy. Literature shows that the laparoscopic repair is safe, allows better visibility and offers the advantage of early feeding and shorter hospitalization time.

10. **During a duodenal atresia repair should the intestine be evaluated for malrotation or other atresia?**

Abdomen should be inspected for malrotation is it has been related to up to 30% of the cases of duodenal atresia. Historically it was recommended to evaluate the intestine for other atresia, however recent literature shows that the rate of other intestinal atresia is less than 1% for which extensive inspection does not appear necessary.

11. **What are the issues related to long side to side duodenoduodenostomies and duodenojejunostomies?** [3]

The use of a long side to side duodenostomy has been related to a high incidence of anastomotic dysfunction and prolonged obstruction (12%). Duodenojejunostomies have been related to an increased risk of blind loop syndrome.

12. **What is the cause of jejunoileal atresia**

Several hypotheses and clinical data point towards a vascular disruption that results in mesenteric disruption and interference with the segmental blood supply of the small bowel resulting in atresia and stenosis. It usually occurs latter in the small bowel development as an intrauterine insult. However there has been reports of hereditary forms that occur way early in development that are related with multiple atresia and poor survival.

13. **Is jejunoileal atresia related to other abnormalities?** [4]

As the mechanism is different from other abnormalities and is often secondary to a vascular insult, jejunoileal atresia is related to other abnormalities in less than 1% of the cases. There have been reports relating it with patients with Hirschsprung's Disease, cystic fibrosis (10%), malrotation, Down syndrome, congenital heart disease and other atresias (6%).

14. **How is jejunoileal atresia classified?** [1]

The Louw's classification system (and then modified by Grosfield) is shown below and divides them in four groups. This classification depends on the most proximal segment and has both diagnostic and prognostic value (Fig. 23.2).

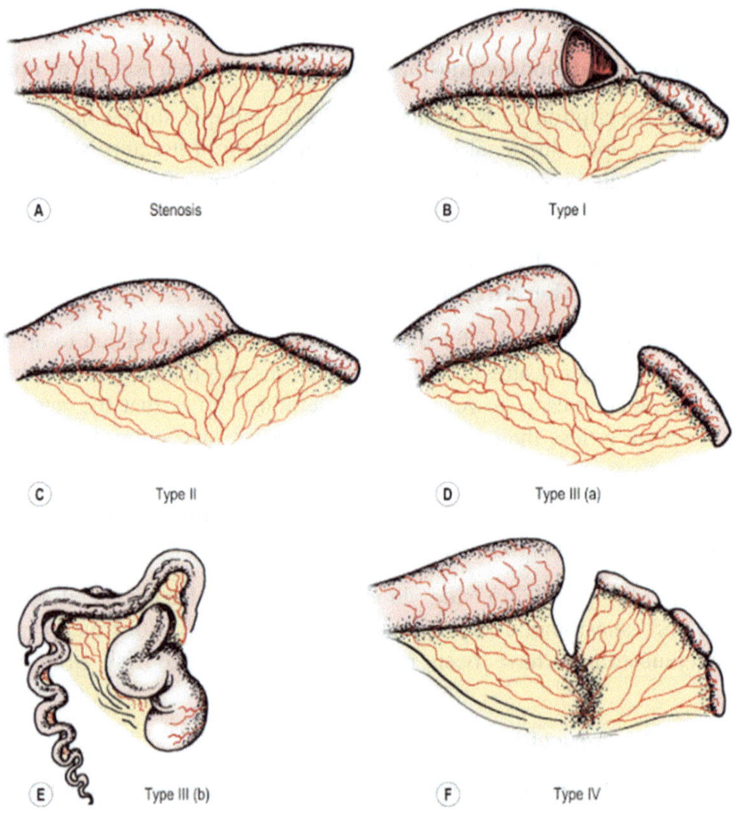

Fig. 23.2 Classification system for Jejunoileal Atresias. From Ref. [1]

15. **How is the clinical presentation of jejunoileal atresia?**

Prenatal ultrasound might show dilated loops of bowel and polyhydramnios, however the majority of this atresias are not diagnosed prenatally. In the neonatal period, symptoms are of bowel obstruction (bilious emesis and abdominal distension). Meconium can appear to be normal but often there can be gray plugs or blood (in type II(b)).

16. **What are the radiological findings of jejunoileal atresia?**

Usually a plan radiograph with swallowed air is enough to make diagnosis. In cases of proximal atresia there are some gas-filled and fluid filled loops with the remainder of the abdomen being gasless. Distal atresias are harder to differentiate from colonic atresias due to absence of haustral markings so contrast enema can be used to aid the diagnoses. About 10% of the patients can present with meconium peritonitis with radiologic findings of a large pseudocyst with a large-air-fluid level.

17. **What are some important operative considerations when performing an abdominal exploration for a neonate with suspected jejunoileal atresia?**

   - A usual transverse abdominal incision can be used, however a circumbilical incision has been found to be as effective with best cosmetic results. We usually perform a vertical umbilical incision due to the ease of small bowel exteriorization.
   - Careful examination must be performed to avoid missing segments or other atresias. Intraoperative contrast enema or cannulation with a red rubber catheter can be used.
   - Resection of the dilated and hypertrophied proximal segments with primary end-to-end anastomosis is the most common technique.
   - The proximal bowel can also be tapered or imbricated to maintain mucosal surface.
   - Mesenteric repair must be done carefully to avoid damage to the blood supply due to rotating or kinking movements.
   - In cases of concomitant gastroschisis we recommend facial closure, gastric decompression, total parenteral nutrition (TPN) and repair of the atresia 4–6 weeks later.
   - Special care has to be taken for type III(b) atresia, restricting bands should be released and mesentery should be placed in a way to prevent torsing of the single marginal artery that irrigates the segment.
   - No intestinal lengthening procedures should be attempted in the first intervention.
   - Remaining bowel length should be carefully measured as it is a vital prognostic factor.

18. **What are the most important prognostic factors after management of a jejunoileal atresia?** [5]

Bowel length and presence/absence of the ileocecal valve are the most important factors. Usually neonates with <25 cm of bowel will require long-term TPN and intestinal lengthening procedures, whereas <100 cm will require at least short-term TPN. Other factors include the location of the atresia (ileum adapts better) and the maturity of the intestine (premature infant might have more time for growth).

19. **What are the types of colonic atresia?**

   – Type I mucosal atresia with intact bowel wall and mesentery

   – Type II Atretic ends are separated by a fibrous cord

   – Type III atretic ends are separated by a V-shaped mesentery.

20. **What is the cause of colonic atresia?**

Studies nowadays point towards a vascular insult to the colon as in jejunoileal atresia.

21. **What are the abnormalities related to colonic atresia?** [6]

The rate of other abnormalities is low. Colonic atresia can be found in 2.5% of the children with gastroschisis. There have been some reports in patients with Hirschsprung's Disease (HD), complex urological abnormalities, multiple jejunoileal atresias and skeletal abnormalities.

22. **How is colonic atresia diagnosed?**

Initial evaluation with abdominal X-ray might show large and dilated intestinal loops difficult to difference from other atresias or pneumoperitoneum. Diagnosis is made by a contrast enema showing an abrupt halt where the obstruction is.

23. **How is colonic atresia treated?**

Operative exploration is warranted as this type of atresia has higher risk of perforation. Is important to exclude other atresias and stenoses. Is recommended to perform a frozen biopsy for HD as it may lead to anastomotic leak or obstruction. For right sided colonic atresia resection and primary anastomosis is possible: for left sided a staged approach with a colostomy with a mucous fistula with resection of both proximal and distal edges is recommended. Closure is then performed months later.

References

1. Ogle S, Nichol P, Ostlie DJ. Duodenal and Intestinal Atresia and Stenosis. In: Holcomb and Ashcraft's pediatric surgery, 7th ed. Philadelphia: Saunders/Elsevier; 2020.
2. Escobar M et al. Duodenal atresia and stenosis: long-term follow-up over 30 years. J Pediatr Surg. 39(6):867–71.
3. Kay S, Yoder S, Rothenberg S. Laparoscopic duodenostomy in the neonate. J Pediatr Surg. 44(5):906–8.
4. Dalla Vecchia LK, Grosfeld JL, West KW, Rescorla FJ, Scherer LR, Engum SA. Intestinal Atresia and Stenosis: a 25-year experience with 277 cases. Arch Surg. 1998;133(5):490–7. https://doi.org/10.1001/archsurg.133.5.490.
5. Adams SD, Stanton MP. Malrotation and intestinal atresias. Early Hum Dev. 2014. https://doi.org/10.1016/j.earlhumdev.2014.09.017.
6. El-Asmar KM, Abdel-Latif M, El-Kassaby AA, Soliman MH, El-Behery MM. Colonic Atresia: association with other anomalies. J Neonatal Surg. 2016;5(4):47. https://doi.org/10.21699/jns.v5i4.422.

References

Chapter 24
Malrotation and Midgut Volvulus

R. Ellen Jones, Jordan S. Taylor, and Matias Bruzoni

Abstract Disorders of intestinal rotation arise during gestation and represent the failure of normal 270-degree counterclockwise rotation of the intestines around the superior mesenteric artery (SMA). Malrotation is associated with a narrow mesenteric base and intestines what are not fixed to the abdominal sidewall or retroperitoneum. This anatomy predisposes the gastrointestinal (GI) tract to volvulus, in which the bowel twists around the SMA, forming a closed loop obstruction of the entire small bowel with interruption of arterial inflow and venous drainage. Bilious emesis in an infant is the clinical finding that signals this life-threatening complication, and must be addressed with expedient operative exploration if the patient is in extremis versus rapid upper GI contrast study. The definitive surgical management of malrotation with midgut volvulus is Ladd's procedure, which includes reduction of volvulus, lysis of adhesive bands, and placement of the small bowel in the right abdomen and large bowel in the left abdomen. This chapter discusses the embryology, presenting features, acute clinical management, and the role of laparoscopy and prophylactic Ladd's procedure for children with malrotation.

Keywords Malrotation · Midgut volvulus · Bilious emesis · Ladd's procedure

R. Ellen Jones · J. S. Taylor · M. Bruzoni (✉)
Division of Pediatric Surgery, Department of Surgery, Stanford University Medical Center, 300 Pasteur Dr Rm M116, Alway Bldg MC 5733, Stanford, CA 94305, USA
e-mail: Mbruzoni@Stanford.edu

R. Ellen Jones
e-mail: Rejones7@Stanford.edu

J. S. Taylor
e-mail: Jtaylor4@Stanford.edu

M. Lacher et al. (eds.), *Pearls and Tricks in Pediatric Surgery*,
https://doi.org/10.1007/978-3-030-51067-1_24

1. **What defines normal intestinal rotation and fixation?**

Normal rotation is defined as a 270-degree counterclockwise rotation of the intestines around the superior mesenteric artery (SMA) axis. The stomach resides above and anterior to the SMA. Progressing along the intestinal tract, the second part of the duodenum lies to the right of the SMA, while the third part of the duodenum is posterior to the SMA. The duodenum again crosses the midline, with the fourth portion to the left of the SMA. Finally, the cecum and ascending colon lie to the right of the SMA. Peritoneal attachments hold the duodenojejunal flexure in fixation at the ligament of Treitz, and the ascending and descending colon are likewise fixed to the retroperitoneum. The normal axis of the mesentery thus lies between the ligament of Treitz and ileocecal fold; this wide fixation prevents twisting of the intestines.

2. **What is the normal embryologic process of intestinal rotation?**

Intestinal development begins in the fourth to eighth week of gestation, in which the intestinal tract is a straight tube [1]. The jejunum, ileum, cecum, right colon and part of the transverse colon enter into the umbilical cord, while the stomach remains in its position. The duodenojejunal loop begins to curve downward and to the right of the super mesenteric artery (SMA) forming a 90-degree arc, then continues to rotate below the SMA to complete a 180-degree movement. Finally, the duodenojejunal loop continues to the left of the SMA to achieve a full 270-degree rotation, which coincides with return of the rest of the intestines from the cord during the tenth week of gestation. The return of the small bowel to the abdominal cavity pushes the fourth portion of the duodenum and the jejunum to the left of the SMA. Finally, the cecum and right colon return to the abdomen and are fixed on the right side of the abdomen.

3. **What is the incidence of intestinal malrotation and midgut volvulus?**

Autopsy series suggest that 1:200–500 live births harbor some variant of intestinal malrotation [2]. The incidence of midgut volvulus is significantly lower, estimated to occur in 1:6,000 live births. The majority of patients (58%) who develop symptoms from rotational abnormalities present during the first year of life, with 30% presenting in the first month of life [3].

4. **What conditions are associated with intestinal malrotation?**

Malrotation is most commonly associated with congenital diaphragmatic hernia, congenital heart disease, and omphalocele [4]. Up to 62% of patients present with some associated anomaly, including intestinal atresia, intussusception, anorectal malformations and Hirschsprung's disease [1]. Gastroschisis patients all have malrotation.

5. **What are the classifications of various disorders of intestinal rotation and fixation?**

While any rotation less than 270 degrees is considered malrotation, there are several distinct categories of malrotation. Complications and risks associated with each category of malrotation vary [5].

a. **Incomplete rotation** is any degree of counterclockwise rotation less than 270 degrees about the SMA axis. Because of the broad definition, the position of the bowel and its attachments are highly variable.
b. **Nonrotation** occurs when the bowel returns to the abdominal cavity without any additional rotation and the cecum resides in the left upper quadrant of the abdomen. It occurs in 0.5–2% of patients and is not typically pathologic.
c. **Reverse rotation** is an abnormal clockwise rotation of the midgut, resulting in an anterior duodenum to the right of midline. The underlying transverse colon is often obstructed.
d. **Paraduodenal (mesocolic) hernias** are a result of incomplete fixation of either the ascending or descending colon in the retroperitoneum. Small bowel can herniate into that paraduodenal space and cause obstructive symptoms.
e. **Mobile cecum** describes a proximal colon that is not appropriately fixed in the right lower quadrant; however, the more proximal midgut (jejunum) is fixed in the left upper quadrant. These patients are still at a risk for volvulus.

6. **How does malrotation lead to midgut volvulus?**

Midgut volvulus is the most common and potentially devastating complication of malrotation, defined as a twisting of the bowel around its mesenteric base (Fig. 24.1). Risk of midgut volvulus is related to length of the mesenteric base; a narrower based malrotation has a higher risk of volvulus. Malrotation has a higher risk of volvulus than any of the variants [5].

7. **What are the presenting features of midgut volvulus?**

Bilious emesis in an infant is assumed to represent malrotation with midgut volvulus until proven otherwise. This symptom alone should prompt surgical consultation with high index of suspicion for midgut volvulus. Midgut volvulus can rapidly progress to severe systemic illness and hemodynamic compromise. Other presenting features may include scaphoid abdomen. This results from initial proximal intestinal obstruction followed by proximal and distal intestinal emptying. Crampy abdominal pain and blood per rectum may be encountered, though these can be late features of the disease process. Because the obstruction is proximal, there may be no abdominal distension.

8. **What is the worst-case scenario for patients with midgut volvulus and how can this be prevented?**

The midgut volvulus can compromise blood supply to large portions of the small and large intestines. The bowel can quickly become necrotic and cause severe metabolic derangements. Mortality from a midgut volvulus ranges from 2–24%, with worse prognosis in patients with necrotic bowel, younger age, or associated anomalies. Preventing bowel necrosis is best achieved by rapid diagnosis with an upper GI, aggressive resuscitation and broad-spectrum antibiotics, and early operative intervention to reduce the volvulus.

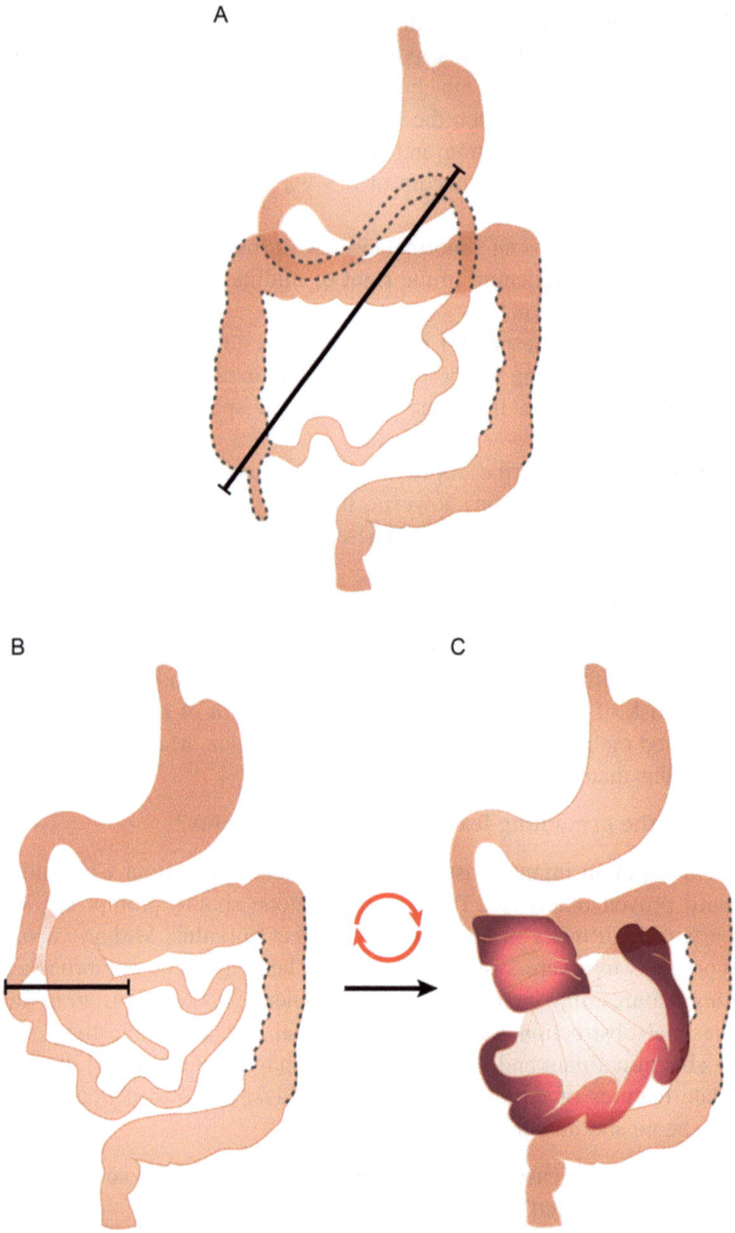

Fig. 24.1 Normal rotation and attachment versus malrotation and midgut volvulus. a Schematic of normal intestinal fixation (small bowel is truncated for ease of viewing). The solid black line indicates the wide-based mesenteric axis that prevents twisting of the small intestine around its vascular pedicle. The dotted lines signify portions of bowel which are normally fixed into position by peritoneal attachments. **b** Malrotation is illustrated with a narrow small bowel mesenteric base, as indicated by the solid black line. The right colon is not fixed to the retroperitoneum, as indicated by absence of the black dotted lines. Ladd's bands (adhesions) are noted between the duodenum and the right colon. **c** The narrow mesenteric base of malrotation predisposes the intestine to twisting around its vascular pedicle in a clockwise direction (red arrow). This leads to vascular compromise and ischemia of the small intestine

9. **What is the differential diagnosis of infants who present with bilious vomiting?**

Bilious emesis in a newborn infant is malrotation until proven otherwise by an upper GI study that shows normal rotation. The differential for bilious emesis in a newborn includes duodenal atresia beyond the Ampulla of Vater. Bilious emesis can also be caused by a functional or mechanical obstruction such as Hirschsprung's disease, intussusception, or intestinal atresia. Other etiologies like gastroenteritis or neonatal sepsis can also cause bilious emesis but have additional clinical features (profuse diarrhea, fever, etc.) that distinguish them from midgut volvulus.

10. **How is midgut volvulus diagnosed?**

A thorough history and physical exam should be performed on all patients suspected of a midgut volvulus secondary to malrotation. Most infants (93%) present with bilious emesis that is otherwise unexplained [6]. If a plain film radiograph has been obtained, it may show gastric outlet obstruction, a large stomach bubble, duodenal obstruction ("double bubble"), or may be without any focal abnormalities. A normal plain film radiograph cannot rule out malrotation or a midgut volvulus, again because of a proximal obstruction there aren't distended loops. Most pediatric surgeons prefer an upper GI to diagnose malrotation, though contrast may not pass beyond the point of obstruction. For a patient in extremis, rapid resuscitation and operative exploration without contrast studies may be indicated. Abdominal ultrasound can diagnose midgut volvulus based on abnormal positioning of the superior mesenteric artery (SMA) and vein (SMV). CT scans are generally not recommended for the diagnosis of malrotation or midgut volvulus.

11. **What radiologic findings define normal rotation and rule out malrotation?**

Contrast leaves the stomach and crosses the patient's midline from left to right on anteroposterior view. The patient is turned to the accommodate a lateral view, and contrast will flow posterior to the stomach through the retroperitoneal second portion of the duodenum. The patient is transitioned back to an anteroposterior view, where contrast will then cross the midline from right to left of the spine while ascending towards the ligament of Treitz. Finally, the duodenojejunal junction should be located at the same level as the gastric pylorus. If all of these features are present, malrotation is ruled out. On ultrasound with doppler, normal rotation is defined by location of the SMV on the right and SMA on the left.

12. **What radiologic findings are associated with malrotation and/or midgut volvulus?**

On upper GI contrast study, the duodenojejunal junction will fail to cross midline to the left, and will lie inferior to the duodenal bulb. Additionally, the second and third portion of the jejunum will not be located in the normal retroperitoneal location (Fig. 24.2a). On ultrasound with doppler, reversal of the normal orientation of the mesenteric vessels is diagnostic of malrotation. With abnormal rotation, the

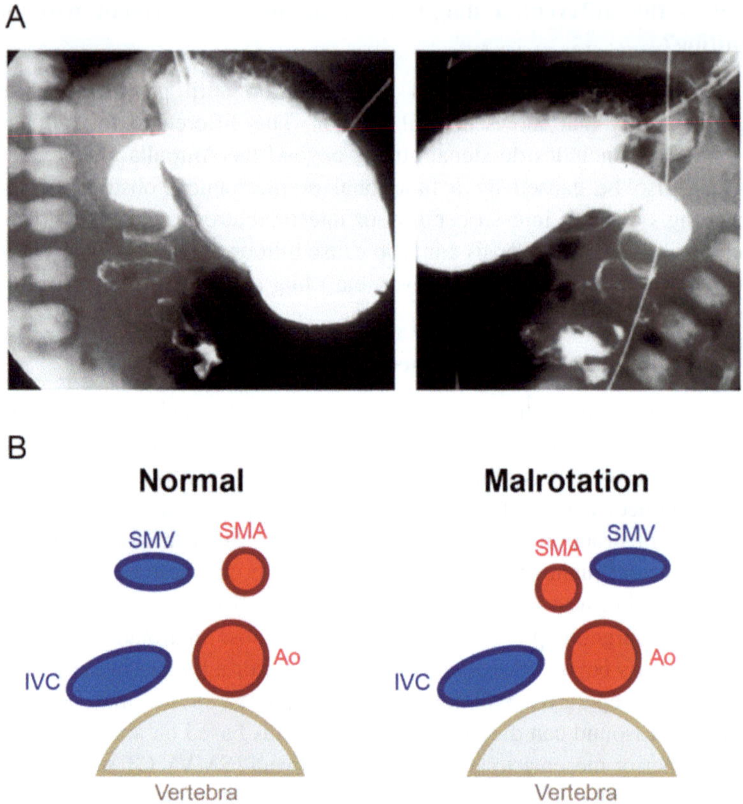

Fig. 24.2 Imaging for malrotation and midgut volvuolus. a Upper GI contrast study showing malrotation with midgut volvulus. The left panel shows an anteroposterior view, and the right panel shows a lateral view. The duodenojejunal junction is abnormally positioned and remains on the right side of the patient and does not cross over the midline (spine). The duodenum fills with a corkscrew sign. **b** Schematic illustration of Doppler ultrasound findings associated with normal rotation and malrotation. The left panel shows normal findings with the SMV on the right and SMA on the left. The right panel indicates malrotation since this relationship is reversed. SMV: superior mesenteric vein. SMA: superior mesenteric artery. IVC: inferior vena cava. Ao: aorta. Upper GI images provided courtesy of the PEIR database and used with permission. Available at: http://peir.path.uab.edu/library/

SMA will appear on the right, and the SMV will appear on the left. Specific radiologic findings associated with midgut volvulus include a corkscrew appearance of the duodenum and proximal jejunum (Fig. 24.2b). Additionally, "whirlpool" appearance of the SMV and mesentery around the SMA may be seen on ultrasound in association with midgut volvulus.

13. **What is the initial management of midgut volvulus?**

Midgut volvulus should be managed with rapid diagnosis (upper GI), resuscitation and expedited operative exploration, with the goal of restoring blood flow to the bowel. Resuscitation is best achieved with two large-bore IVs and 20 cc/kg bolus of normal saline or lactated ringer's solution. A nasogastric tube should be placed on suction to decompress the obstructed bowel proximally. Broad spectrum antibiotic should be administered to cover translocation of enteric bacteria and possible perforation.

14. **What is the surgical management of midgut volvulus?**

Midgut volvulus is managed by the Ladd procedure, which begins with detorsion of the bowel in a counterclockwise fashion (as the volvulus is always in a clockwise direction). "Turn back the hands of time" is a useful device to remember the counterclockwise direction of small bowel detorsion (Fig. 24.3). Additionally, the abnormal peritoneal attachments (Ladd's bands) between the duodenum and the right colon must be divided and the bowel should be repositioned a non-rotated position (see below).

15. **How is a Ladd procedure performed?**

The traditional Ladd procedure is performed through an upper transverse incision, though midline and laparoscopic approaches are commonly used. After entering the abdomen, the bowel must be rotated in a counterclockwise direction, typically 720 degrees. The degree of detorsion can vary from one to multiple 360 degree turns. As the bowel can appear initially dusky, purple, or black, sufficient time must be given for the reperfusion and recovery of the bowel. The procedure then

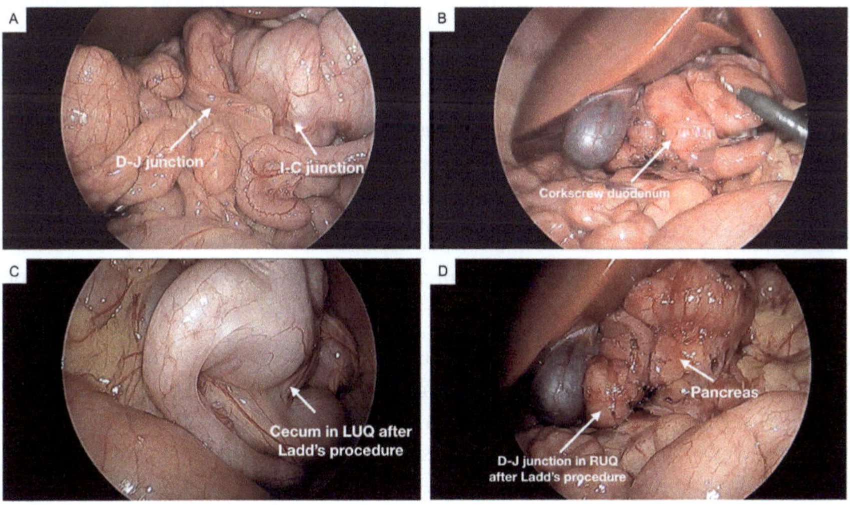

Fig. 24.3 Intraoperative photographs from laparoscopic surgery for malrotation and midgut volvulus. **a** Evidence of malrotation with the duodenojejunal junction right next to the ileocecal junction. **b** Midgut volvulus as noted by the duodenum's corkscrew configuration. During Ladd's procedure, **c** the cecum is placed in the left upper quadrant, **d** and the duodenojejunal junction is placed in the right upper quadrant

begins by identifying and dividing the abnormal peritoneal attachments to the duodenum, right colon and cecum (Ladd's bands). Division of these bands allows for the bowel to be placed in a position that maximizes the distance between the duodenum and the cecum. The bowel is then returned to the abdomen with the small bowel on the right side of the abdomen and the large bowel on the left, with the cecum situated in the left upper quadrant. The procedure is completed with an appendectomy, as the abnormal position of the appendix will obscure a possible acute appendicitis diagnosis in the future. Bowel resection and diversion may have to be performed if there is frankly necrotic bowel or perforated bowel identified after untwisting the bowel *and* after sufficient time has passed to allow for bowel recovery intraoperatively.

16. **What is the role of laparoscopic surgery in the surgical management of midgut volvulus?**

Laparoscopic surgery can be useful in diagnosing malrotation when imaging findings are equivocal [7]. Laparoscopic Ladd's procedure for malrotation is widely accepted. Some centers also advocate for a laparoscopic Ladd procedure in symptomatic patients without suspected volvulus, with conversion rates to open between 8 and 30% [8, 9]. Laparoscopy should not be used in a decompensated patient; patients with suspected midgut volvulus typically undergo an open Ladd procedure [10].

17. **What is the postoperative care of a patient with midgut volvulus?**

Broad spectrum antibiotics should be started preoperatively in patients with midgut volvulus and continued until the child appears well. Antibiotics are targeted against bacterial translocation from compromised bowel. Postoperative antibiotics for an uncomplicated Ladd procedure without midgut volvulus are not indicated.

Feeding postoperatively is dependent upon the degree and length of compromised bowel, as well as the return of bowel function. Most surgeons opt to leave a decompressive nasogastric tube and await resolution of bilious output as an indication to begin to advance the diet. Alternative means for providing nutrition parenterally should be considered in patients who may have delayed enteral intake.

18. **What is are the potential complications of surgery for midgut volvulus and how are they managed?**

Complications following a Ladd procedure are relatively rare if no bowel resection is performed. A ten-year follow up study determined an overall complication rate of 9%, with the most common complications being bowel obstruction, incisional hernias and recurrent volvulus [11]. If compromised bowel does need to be resected, patients are at risk for short bowel syndrome. While laparoscopic procedures may reduce the risk for adhesive small bowel obstructions, they may increase the risk for recurrent volvulus. Overall, risk of recurrent volvulus is around 2% [12]. Additionally, patients who have undergone a Ladd procedure have risks for intussusception and prolonged postoperative ileus.

19. **What is chronic midgut volvulus and how is it managed?**

Though the majority of infants are diagnosed within hours of developing symptoms, older children and adults may have chronic symptoms of intermittent midgut volvulus that fail to be recognized. Patients with undiagnosed malrotation may experience intermittent abdominal pain with or without emesis. Most surgeons recommend a Ladd procedure in symptomatic patients, particularly in younger patients.

20. **What is the treatment of asymptomatic or subclinical intestinal malrotation?**

Treatment of asymptomatic malrotation or malrotation identified incidentally is somewhat controversial. While most individuals present early in life, the risk of midgut volvulus does not completely disappear with age. Determining the risk of volvulus by imaging is also limited, as no study can reliably identify a narrow-based mesentery. Most surgeons advocate for elective surgery when malrotation is encountered incidentally in children [1, 13]. However, the benefit of prophylactic Ladd's surgery dwindles after childhood, so adults over the age of 20 may defer surgery if truly asymptomatic [14] (Fig. 24.4). Laparoscopy can also be used to evaluate the mesentery width and mobility of the bowel. It is important to note that upper GIs carry a false-positive rate that can be as high as 15% [15].

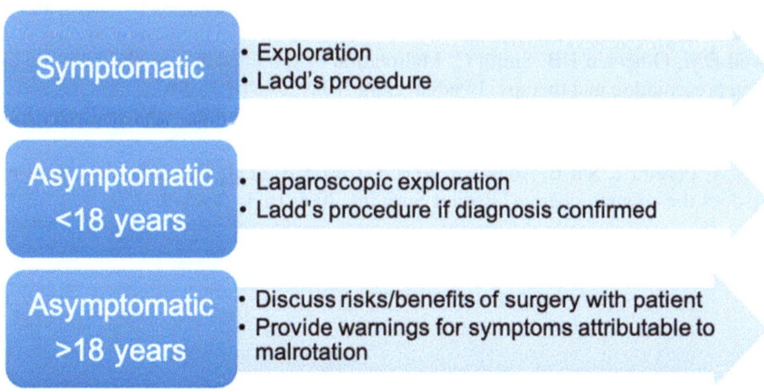

Fig. 24.4 Algorithm for suggested management of malrotation with and without symptoms. Permissions Upper GI images provided courtesy of the PEIR database and used with permission. Available at: http://peir.path.uab.edu/library/

References

1. Filston HC, Kirks DR. Malrotation—the ubiquitous anomaly. J Pediatr Surg. 1981;16(4):614–20.
2. Torres AM, Ziegler MM. Malrotation of the intestine. World J Surg. 1993;17(3):326–31.
3. Aboagye J, Goldstein SD, Salazar JH, Papandria D, Okoye MT, Al-Omar K, et al. Age at presentation of common pediatric surgical conditions: reexamining dogma. J Pediatr Surg. 2014;49(6):995–9.
4. Graziano K, Islam S, Dasgupta R, Lopez ME, Austin M, Chen LE, et al. Asymptomatic malrotation: diagnosis and surgical management: an American Pediatric Surgical Association outcomes and evidence based practice committee systematic review. J Pediatr Surg. 2015;50(10):1783–90.
5. Dassinger MS, Smith SD. Disorders of intestinal rotation and fixation. In: Coran AG, Adzick S, Krummel TM, Laberge J-M, Shamberger RC, Caldamone AA, editors. Pediatric surgery, 7th ed. Elsevier; 2012.
6. Nehra D, Goldstein AM. Intestinal malrotation: varied clinical presentation from infancy through adulthood. Surgery. 2011;149(3):386–93.
7. Hsiao M, Langer JC. Value of laparoscopy in children with a suspected rotation abnormality on imaging. J Pediatr Surg. 2011;46(7):1347–52.
8. Fraser JD, Aguayo P, Sharp SW, Ostlie DJ, Peter SDS. The role of laparoscopy in the management of malrotation. J Surg Res. 2009;156(1):80–2.
9. Stanfill AB, Pearl RH, Kalvakuri K, Wallace LJ, Vegunta RK. Laparoscopic Ladd's procedure: treatment of choice for midgut malrotation in infants and children. J Laparoendosc Adv Surg Tech. 2010;20(4):369–72.
10. Hsiao M, Langer JC. Surgery for suspected rotation abnormality: selection of open vs laparoscopic surgery using a rational approach. J Pediatr Surg. 2012;47(5):904–10.
11. El-Gohary Y, Alagtal M, Gillick J. Long-term complications following operative intervention for intestinal malrotation: a 10-year review. Pediatr Surg Int. 2010;26(2):203–6.
12. Stehr W. Intestinal Rotational Abnormalities. Pediatric Surgery NaT: American Pediatric Surgical Association; 2018.
13. Powell DM, Othersen HB, Smith C. Malrotation of the intestines in children: the effect of age on presentation and therapy. J Pediatr Surg. 1989;24(8):777–80.
14. Malek MM, Burd RS. The optimal management of malrotation diagnosed after infancy: a decision analysis. Am J Surg. 2006;191(1):45–51.
15. Dilley A, Pereira J, Shi E, Adams S, Kern I, Currie B, et al. The radiologist says malrotation: does the surgeon operate? Pediatr Surg Int. 2000;16(1–2):45–9.

Chapter 25
Gastrointestinal Surgical Aspects of Cystic Fibrosis

Ross M. Beckman and Samuel M. Alaish

Abstract Cystic fibrosis is an autosomal recessive disorder caused by mutations to the CFTR chloride channel protein that results in increased viscosity of epithelial secretions throughout multiple organ systems. While the effects on the lung are most detrimental, there are a multitude of manifestations throughout the gastrointestinal tract of particular interest to the pediatric surgeon, including meconium ileus, distal intestinal obstruction, biliary disease, pancreatic insufficiency and rectal prolapse. Although there is currently no cure for cystic fibrosis, there are many effective medical and surgical treatments for combating the complications of the disease.

Keywords Cystic fibrosis · Meconium ileus · Distal intestinal obstruction syndrome · Gastroesophageal reflux disease · Nissen fundoplication · Pancreatic insufficiency · Rectal prolapse

1. **What is cystic fibrosis?**

Cystic Fibrosis (CF) is an autosomal recessive disorder caused by mutations in the cystic fibrosis transmembrane conductance regulator (CFTR) gene resulting in an abnormal cell membrane chloride channel. This manifests as an inability to properly regulate electrolyte content with thickening of secretions along secretory epithelium. Poor clearance of desiccated secretions is the primary cause of morbidity across multiple organ systems.

R. M. Beckman
Johns Hopkins University School of Medicine, Baltimore, MD, USA

S. M. Alaish (✉)
Division of Pediatric Surgery, Johns Hopkins University School of Medicine, Baltimore, MD, USA
e-mail: salaish1@jhmi.edu

M. Lacher et al. (eds.), *Pearls and Tricks in Pediatric Surgery*,
https://doi.org/10.1007/978-3-030-51067-1_25

2. **How is CF diagnosed?**

The two most common newborn screening tests are the serum immunoreactive trypsinogen (IRT), which is elevated in the first weeks of life, and DNA analysis for CFTR mutations. In patients with a positive screen, sweat chloride testing should subsequently be performed as the gold standard diagnostic test. A value of >60 mmol/L on two occasions is diagnostic [1, 2].

3. **What organ systems are affected?**

The most affected organ systems include the respiratory tract with chronic obstruction and infection, the gastrointestinal tract with obstruction and dysfunction of the biliary tract, pancreas, and alimentary canal, the sinus tracts with obstruction, infection and nasal polyposis, as well as the testes with defective sperm transport mechanisms resulting in infertility in males.

4. **What is the earliest clinical manifestation of CF?**

Meconium ileus is caused by obstruction of the small intestine by inspisssated meconium usually at the level of the terminal ileum. It presents as abdominal distention and inability to pass meconium in the first few days of life. It occurs in approximately 10–20% of neonates with CF, and 80–90% of all meconium ileus cases occur in infants with CF [2].

5. **What causes meconium ileus?**

Abnormally functioning CFTR ion channels within the pancreas and small intestine cause intraluminal dehydration and hyperviscous meconium that obstructs the mid to distal ileum.

6. **What prenatal findings may be seen?**

Meconium ileus may be identified on prenatal ultrasound by visualization of dilated small intestine associated with hyperechoic intraluminal masses, representing the inspissated meconium. Non-visualization of the gallbladder on prenatal ultrasound is another non-specific finding.

7. **How does meconium ileus appear on plain film radiography?**

The classic radiographic appearance includes dilated loops of small bowel without air-fluid levels and a soap bubble appearance as air mixes with inspissated meconium.

8. **How is meconium ileus classified?**

Meconium ileus is termed complicated if intestinal atresia, volvulus, bowel necrosis, perforation or meconium peritonitis are present. Meconium peritonitis may be seen on prenatal ultrasound or plain radiographs as scattered calcifications. Approximately 40% of patients will present with complicated disease. Simple meconium ileus includes obstruction without any of the complications listed above [2].

9. **How is simple meconium ileus diagnosed?**

The gold standard diagnostic test is a hyperosmotic contrast enema with gastrografin, which will typically reveal a small caliber colon, meconium pellets in the distal ileum, and dilated, proximal small intestine.

10. **What is the initial treatment for simple meconium ileus?**

Following a confirmatory diagnostic enema, therapeutic gastrografin enemas are performed under close fluoroscopic guidance. The hyperosmotic solution draws water into the lumen to soften and clear the obstructing meconium. Complications of this procedure can include massive fluid shifts and subsequent hypovolemic shock, as well as bowel perforation. IV access should be obtained prior to the procedure to allow adequate fluid resuscitation. N-acetylcysteine solution may also be added to the enema to aid in breaking up the obstructing meconium. If necessary, repeated gastrografin enemas may be performed [2].

11. **When is surgery indicated for meconium ileus?**

Surgery is the mainstay of treatment for all cases of complicated meconium ileus, but it is also indicated in patients with simple disease who have failed non-operative management.

12. **What are the surgical options for meconium ileus?**

For uncomplicated disease, an enterotomy is performed to allow intraoperative irrigation of the bowel to flush out the obstructing meconium, with either primary closure or creation of an enterostomy for continued irrigation post-operatively. For complicated disease, the necrotic bowel is resected. Primary anastomosis is generally not recommended, because it does not allow for postoperative irrigation and carries a risk of anastomotic leak. Temporary diverting stomas (ileostomy and mucous fistula) have the benefits of not requiring complete evacuation of meconium at the time of operation resulting in a shorter operative time and elimination of the risk of anastomotic leak. Ostomy-in-continuity operations, such as the Bishop-Koop or Santulli enterostomies, allow access for irrigation and maintenance of intestinal continuity via an end-to-side anastomosis of the proximal and distal ends (or vice versa, respectively). These procedures reduce fluid losses, preserve the distal bowel as a site of nutrient absorption and protect the anastomosis with adequate decompression via the "chimney" limb which is brought up as a stoma [2].

13. **What is distal intestinal obstruction syndrome (DIOS)?**

DIOS can occur at any age outside the newborn period and results from inspissation of thickened intestinal contents causing impaction and obstruction typically at the terminal ileum or ileocecal valve. The mechanism isn't fully understood, but it is likely multifactorial, including pancreatic insufficiency, resulting in increased intraluminal fat content and increased intestinal transit time, as well as altered water and electrolyte content of ileal mucus, and global dehydration [3].

14. **How is DIOS diagnosed?**

A careful history typically reveals colicky abdominal pain, abdominal distention, constipation, nausea, and emesis when it progresses to full obstruction. A mass in the right lower quadrant can sometimes be palpated. Plain radiographs may show a stool bulk in the right lower quadrant with a "bubbly" appearance, along with dilated loops of proximal bowel with air fluid levels. Computed tomography (CT) may be useful to delineate the location of the obstruction and exclude other pathology. A water-soluble contrast enema may reveal non-filling of the terminal ileum [3].

15. **How is DIOS treated?**

These patients may often be successfully treated with osmotic agents, such as hyperosmolar contrast during a diagnostic enema or an osmotic laxative bowel preparation, as well as oral hydration to loosen up and remove the inspissated stool. Patients who are fully obstructed require decompression with a nasogastric tube. The few patients that do not respond to contrast enema and oral laxative treatments may require operative intervention via a laparoscopic or open approach. Postoperatively, optimization of pancreatic enzymes, long-term laxative initiation, such as daily polyethylene glycol, and maintaining oral hydration are important to prevent recurrence [3].

16. **How does GERD affect pulmonary function in CF?**

While GERD is hypothesized to contribute to pulmonary disease through micro-aspiration, increased airway reactivity, and airway inflammation, there is limited evidence to support this relationship. As there is no clear link between GERD and poor respiratory outcomes, invasive testing in patients who do not exhibit reflux symptoms is unwarranted.

17. **What is the role of acid suppression in CF?**

Proton pump inhibitors (PPI) and histamine blockers are frequently used to manage GERD symptoms in CF patients; however, there is limited evidence to support their use for secondary improvement of pulmonary disease. The benefit of acid suppression may be offset by the increased risk of pneumonia attributed to increased colonization of pathogens in the upper GI tract in the setting of a higher pH. Acid suppression is also commonly used in the CF population to enhance the efficacy of pancreatic enzyme replacement therapy; however, supportive data is lacking.

18. **What is the role of anti-reflux surgery in CF?**

Anti-reflux procedures may be beneficial for GERD that is refractory to medical management. Improved outcomes may be partially attributed to the better nutritional status provided by gastrostomy tube placement that often accompanies these procedures. Anti-reflux procedures should not be performed to improve pulmonary function alone in the absence of refractory reflux symptoms [4, 5].

19. **Why are CF patients prone to gallstone formation?**

Pancreatic insufficiency without adequate enzyme replacement results in the loss of bile acids through the GI tract with subsequent fat malabsorption. The enterohepatic reuptake of bile acids becomes disrupted, and cholesterol becomes supersaturated within the gallbladder, leading to stone and sludge formation. Pancreatic enzyme replacement is the best way to prevent gallstones.

20. **How is pancreatic insufficiency treated?**

The mainstay of treatment of pancreatic insufficiency is supplementation with enteral pancreatic enzymes that are titrated based on weight gain and presence of steatorrhea.

21. **What causes rectal prolapse in patients with CF?**

Rectal prolapse is most commonly associated with chronic constipation, but it may be associated with diarrhea, as well as other causes of increased intra-abdominal pressure, including chronic cough. It is more common in children whose pancreatic insufficiency is poorly managed or whose pulmonary disease is not well-controlled [6].

References

1. Boyle MP, De Boeck K. A new era in the treatment of cystic fibrosis: correction of the underlying CFTR defect. Lancet Respir Med. 2013;1(2):158–63.
2. Waldhausen JHT, Richards M. Meconium Ileus. Clin Colon Rectal Surg. 2018;31(2):121–6.
3. Hort A, Hameed A, Middleton PG, Pleass HC. Distal intestinal obstruction syndrome: an important differential diagnosis for abdominal pain in patients with cystic fibrosis. ANZ J Surg. 2019. https://doi.org/10.1111/ans.15357.
4. Boesch RP, Acton JD. Outcomes of fundoplication in children with cystic fibrosis. J Pediatr Surg. 2007;42(8):1341–4.
5. Sheikh SI, Ryan-Wenger NA, McCoy KS. Outcomes of surgical management of severe GERD in patients with cystic fibrosis. Pediatr Pulmonol. 2013;48:556–62.
6. El-Chammas KI, Rumman N, Goh VL, Quintero D, Goday PS. Rectal prolapse and cystic fibrosis. J Pediatr Gastroenterol Nutr. 2015;60(1):110–2.

Chapter 26
Necrotizing Enterocolitis (NEC)

Xiaoyan Feng and Martin Lacher

Abstract Necrotizing enterocolitis (NEC) is the most common lethal gastrointestinal (GI) disease in preterm infants worldwide. It is characterized by severe inflammatory response and intestinal necrosis, and may have a different pathogenesis with than intestinal perforation (FIP). The symptoms of NEC range from feeding intolerance to lethal courses characterized by perforation, peritonitis, sepsis and shock. An abdominal X-ray is helpful to identify dilated or fixed bowel loops, pneumatosis, portal venous gas or free air. Exploratory laparotomy with enterostomy is the most frequently performed surgical treatment. Alternatives include primary anastomosis or the placement of a primary peritoneal drain. In case of panintestinal NEC (<25% viable bowel), the options range from aggressive surgical management to comfort measures only. Long-term sequelae include strictures, short-bowel syndrome, growth retardation and neurodevelopmental delay.

Keywords Necrotizing enterocolitis · Pathology · Prevention

1. **Which infants develop NEC? [1]**

Children with low birth weight, small for gestational age, low gestational age, assisted ventilation, premature rupture of membranes, black ethnicity, sepsis, and hypotension.

2. **How does the incidence of NEC correlate with birth weight (BW)?**

The incidence of NEC in children with LBW (<1500 g) varies worldwide (USA/Canada 7%, Netherlands 3.9–6.8%, Germany 2.9%). It accounts for 1–5% of all NICU admissions in the USA and depends on the birth weight. From stage II

X. Feng · M. Lacher (✉)
Department of Pediatric Surgery, University of Leipzig, Leipzig, Germany
e-mail: martin.lacher@medizin.uni-leipzig.de

M. Lacher et al. (eds.), *Pearls and Tricks in Pediatric Surgery*,
https://doi.org/10.1007/978-3-030-51067-1_26

onwards (pneumatosis but no surgery; Bell classification, see below) it is reported as follows: 11% with BW 401–750 g, 9% with 751–1000 g, 6% with 1001–1250 g, and 4% with 1251–1500 g.

3. **What is the typical gestational week (GW) and age of life?**

Neonates <28 GW and especially 28–31 GW. The typical age for NEC is 14–21 days of life.

4. **Which is the associated mortality rate of NEC?**

Mortality is as high as 30–50% in those infants requiring surgical management.

5. **Which are the predominant sites of intestinal involvement in NEC?**

Isolated small intestinal involvement is noted in 30% of cases. NEC is limited to the colon in 25% of cases, and the splenic flexure is the most common site of colonic involvement. In ~10%, nearly the entire intestine can be involved (panintestinal NEC).

6. **What are the characteristic pathologic changes of the intestine seen in NEC?**

On abdominal X-ray the bowel loops are distended. The intestines may be encased in a fibrinous exudate. Subserosal gas collections called pneumatosis intestinalis may be seen. The extent of the pathologic changes may be classified as focal, multifocal, or pan-intestinal (<25% viable bowel).

7. **What does histologic sectioning of NEC lesions show?**

In early stages histopathologic changes in NEC include pneumatosis intestinalis in the submucosa. In advanced disease transmural necrosis and loss of villus and crypt architecture is seen.

8. **What are the key factors involved in NEC pathogenesis? [2]**

Epidemiologic studies demonstrate that NEC incidence is inversely proportional to gestational age at birth. Therefore, immature intestinal host defenses are thought to play a major role in its pathogenesis. These key immature defenses include intestinal barrier function, intestinal regulation of microbial colonization, regulation of intestinal circulation, and intestinal innate and adaptive immunity.

9. **Which to other phenotypes of neonatal bowel perforation or "pretenders of NEC" are frequently seen? [3]**

Focal intestinal perforation (FIP; syn: spontaneous/segmental intestinal perforation): with no demonstrable cause a bowel perforation is typically found in the terminal ileum. Compared to NEC children are younger, typically <1500 g and most often present in the first week of life. The definite diagnosis is made at the time of laparotomy. Prognosis of FIP is better compared to NEC.

Neonatal bowel perforation on the basis of congenital heart defects: A bowel perforation may happen prior or after cardiac surgery most likely due to circulatory disturbances (bowel ischemia). The typical anatomic location of the perforation is the left colonic flexure.

10. **What are the clinical signs of NEC at presentation?**

The clinical findings are often nonspecific: physiologic instability including lethargy, temperature instability, recurrent apnea, bradycardia, hypoglycemia, and shock. As the disease progresses, abdominal distention/tenderness, blood per rectum, high gastric residuals after feeding or vomiting may occur. At a later stage palpable bowel loops, a fixed or mobile mass, or edema and erythema of the abdominal wall or scrotum may be seen.

11. **What alterations in the complete blood count and arterial blood gas analysis are typically associated with NEC?**

A frequent combination is neutropenia, thrombocytopenia, and metabolic acidosis.

12. **What are the radiologic findings of NEC on a plain-film?**

Early signs: multiple gas-filled loops of intestine with thickened bowel walls. Pneumatosis intestinalis (presence of gas in the bowel wall with a sensitivity and specificity for NEC of 44% and 100% respectively). It is caused by hydrogen, a by-product of the metabolism of translocated intramural bacteria.

13. **In which layer does pneumatosis start?**

In the submucosa, progressing to the muscularis and subserosal layers.

14. **Portal venous gas—how does it get there? Does it affect prognosis?**

It is hypothesized that the genesis of portal venous gas, seen in ~33% of cases, may involve accumulation of gas in the bowel wall as a result of bacterial invasion up the venous system from the intestinal wall into the portal veins. It is associated with worse prognosis (Mortality as high as 54%; 25% panintestinal NEC).

15. **Are contrast studies useful in NEC?**

Not in making the diagnosis of NEC, even in case of bowel perforation. However, contrast enemas or antegrade studies with water soluble contrast media have a value in the evaluation of bowel strictures after NEC prior to closure of the enterostomy.

16. **Who is "Bell", what is the role of his classification for NEC?**

Martin J Bell is a pediatric surgeon from St. Louis, USA who did his fellowship at Cincinnati Children's Hospital Medical Center. In 1978 Bell defined three stages of NEC [4]. According to this classification the severity of NEC is sub grouped into "suggestive of NEC" (Stage I), "definitive NEC" (Stage II) and "evidence of bowel necrosis and clinical deterioration" (Stage III) based on the patient's history, gastrointestinal or systemic symptoms and radiologic findings.

17. **What are the components of conservative management of NEC?**

Nasogastric decompression, total parenteral nutrition, and broad-spectrum antibiotics. In case of fungal sepsis empirical antifungal therapy should be considered.

18. **How many children with NEC need surgery?**

Approximately 50% of VLBW children.

19. **What are the indications for surgical intervention?**

Free air on X-ray (pneumoperitoneum). Relative indications include a positive paracentesis, palpable abdominal mass, abdominal wall erythema, portal venous gas, fixed intestinal loop, and clinical deterioration despite maximal medical therapy.

20. **How does one determine the extent of bowel to resect?**

The goal is to remove only gangrenous bowel and preserve intestinal length. All other bowel loops with potential for recovery should be left in place and may be reevaluated by multiple-look laparotomies to allow for adequate resuscitation and abdominal decompression.

21. **What do you do in case of multisegmental disease (>50% viable bowel)?**

Depending on the case the options include resection with enterostomy, resection with anastomosis, proximal enterostomy, the "clip-and-drop" technique, and the "patch, drain, and wait" technique.

22. **In case of focal NEC, is it safe to perform a primary anastomosis?**

Yes, in selected cases, but the classic approach is to create an enterostomy proximal to the resected segment and bring out the distal intestine as a mucous fistula leading to immediate decompression of the bowel in the postoperative period.

23. **What are your options in case of Pan involvement (NEC totalis, <25% viable bowel)?**

Some surgeons take the decision to forego any treatment as the mortality rate is 42 to 100%. Another option is diverting the intestinal stream by high proximal jejunostomy (without bowel resection) in the hope that the injured bowel heals through distal intestinal decompression.

24. **Does the placement of a primary peritoneal drain (PPD) have better outcome than laparotomy? [5]**

PPD versus laparotomy was evaluated in two multicenter RCT. The US-American NECSTEPS trial (117 children, GA < 34 weeks, BW < 1500 g) had a comparable outcome after 90 days. The European NET trial (69 children, BW <1000 g) showed similar results. The mortality rate of the two treatment groups was the same in both trials. However, in the NET-trial secondary laparotomy was necessary in 74% of cases after 2.5 days. Other studies show that the highest mortality is seen in children treated by PPD only.

25. **Which intraoperative event during exploratory laparotomy is life threatening?**

Spontaneous intraoperative liver hemorrhage caused by retractors or finger dissection. Therefore liver retraction must be gentle at all times.

26. **Does the location of the stoma and mucous fistula in the same incision cause more wound infection?**

No, there is no increase in wound infection rates.

27. **Which are the associated long-term problems of children with NEC?**

Strictures, short-bowel syndrome, growth retardation and neurodevelopmental delay.

28. **Which probiotics are given for prevention of NEC, what is the evidence for this treatment? [6]**

The most common strains are Lactobacillus and Bifidobacterium. Multiple RCT and several meta-analyses show that probiotics can lower the risk of late-onset-sepsis and NEC. However, in children < 1500 g the evidence for the benefit of routine probiotic supplementation for NEC prevention is less clear. Also unanswered questions include dosage, type of microorganism and duration of treatment.

References

1 Samuels N, van de Graaf RA, de Jonge RCJ, Reiss IKM, Vermeulen MJ. Risk factors for necrotizing enterocolitis in neonates: a systematic review of prognostic studies. BMC Pediatr. 2017 Apr 14;17(1):105
2 Eaton S, Rees CM, Hall NJ. Current research on the epidemiology, pathogenesis, and management of necrotizing enterocolitis. Neonatology. 2017;111(4):423–30.
3. Vongbhavit K, Underwood MA. Intestinal perforation in the premature infant. J Neonatal Perinatal Med. 2017;10(3):281–9.
4. Bell MJ. Neonatal necrotizing enterocolitis. N Engl J Med. 1978 Feb 2;298(5):281-2
5. Rees CM, Eaton S, Khoo AK, Kiely EM. Members of NET Trial Group, Pierro A. Peritoneal drainage does not stabilize extremely low birth weight infants with perforated bowel: data from the NET Trial. J Pediatr Surg. 2010 Feb;45(2):324–8
6. Thomas JP, Raine T, Reddy S, Belteki G. Probiotics for the prevention of necrotising enterocolitis in very low-birth-weight infants: a meta-analysis and systematic review. Acta Paediatr. 2017 Nov;106(11):1729-1741

Chapter 27
Meckel's Diverticulum & Vitelline Duct Remnants

R. Cartland Burns and Matthew P. Landman

Abstract The vitelline, or omphalomesenteric, duct usually regresses during the first trimester of fetal development. Several structures can remain if the duct fails to regress. The clinical presentation can be variable. The most common vitelline duct remnant is the Meckel's diverticulum. Imaging selection to evaluate for vitelline duct remnants is dictated by the patient's symptoms at presentation. In all symptomatic cases, surgical resection is recommended.

Keywords Vitelline duct · Omphalomesenteric duct · Meckel's diverticulum · Meckel's scan

1. **What is the vitelline duct?**

The vitelline duct, also known as the omphalomesenteric duct, is the embryonic structure that connects the extracoelomic yolk sac with the developing midgut [1].

2. **When does the vitelline/omphalomesenteric duct regress?**

The regression of this embryonic duct occurs between weeks 5 and 9 of fetal development [2].

3. **What are the potential remnants of the vitelline/omphalomesenteric duct if complete regression does not occur?**

If complete regression of the vitelline duct does not occur, several different remnants are possible. These remnants include Meckel's diverticulum, omphalomesenteric cyst, congenital band, umbilical sinus and omphalomesenteric duct fistula. If present, they usually occur in isolation; however, case reports of more than one anomaly have been described. The most common remnant is Meckel's diverticulum [3].

R. C. Burns · M. P. Landman (✉)
Division of Pediatric Surgery, Indiana University, Indianapolis, IN 46202, USA
e-mail: landman@iu.edu

M. Lacher et al. (eds.), *Pearls and Tricks in Pediatric Surgery*,
https://doi.org/10.1007/978-3-030-51067-1_27

4. **How do these remnants present in pediatric patients?**

Most of these remnants are asymptomatic and remain that way for a lifetime. If symptoms present, they are directly related to the portion of the vitelline duct that remains.Meckel's diverticulum can present with painless bloody stools, abdominal pain mimicking appendicitis, or symptoms of intestinal obstruction. Omphalomesenteric duct cysts can present with abdominal pain, abdominal wall cellulitis or umbilical drainage. A congenital band usually presents with symptoms of intestinal obstruction. Umbilical sinus presents with umbilical drainage or umbilical cellulitis. In the case of an omphalomesenteric duct fistula, intestinal contents can be noted at the umbilicus in the newborn.

5. **How does intestinal obstruction occur in patients with Meckel's diverticulum?**

There are several different underlying etiologies for intestinal obstruction in Meckel's diverticula. In pediatric patients, a congenital band may attach to the Meckel's which serves as a fixed point around which intestinal volvulus can occur. An internal hernia may be formed from bands between the Meckel's and surrounding mesentery. The Meckel's can serve as a lead point for intussusception. More uncommonly, chronic inflammation secondary to diverticulitis may cause an intestinal stricture. Perforation with adjacent abscesses may also cause obstruction or ileus [4]. A foreign body may be lodged in the Meckel's or it may become incarcerated in a hernia defect, called a Littre hernia.

6. **What are the "rule of 2′s" as they relate to Meckel's diverticulum?**

In general, Meckel's diverticula occur in 2% of the population, 2% are symptomatic, they are 2 feet from the ileocecal valve, most are approximately 2 inches in length, they can contain 2 types of heterotopic mucosa (gastric and pancreatic) and most are symptomatic before the age of 2. Meckel's diverticula occur 2:1 in males versus females.

7. **What imaging modalities are recommended to diagnose Meckel's diverticula or other vitelline/omphalomesenteric duct remnants?**

In addition to a quality physical examination, imaging can be utilized to assist in making the diagnosis of these remnants. In cases of intestinal obstruction, abdominal flat and decubitus plain films may be the only imaging obtained preoperatively. CT scan or MRI may assist in diagnosing a vitelline duct remnant as the source of symptoms, but many cases of obstruction are not fully delineated until the operating room. A Meckel's scan can assist in diagnosing a Meckel's diverticulum. Abdominal ultrasonography can diagnose omphalomesenteric duct cysts [4].

8. **What is a Meckel's scan?**

The Meckel's scan is a technetium-99 m (Tc99m)-pertechnetate scintigraphy study. Tc99m accumulates in the parietal cells of ectopic gastric mucosa within the diverticulum. The sensitivity is 85% and specificity is 95% [4].

9. **What pharmacologic adjuncts can be used to improve the sensitivity of the Meckel's nuclear medicine scan?**

Diagnostic accuracy of the Meckel's scan has been improved with pentagastrin, histamine-2-blockers and glucagon [4].

10. **What is the treatment recommendation for symptomatic Meckel's diverticula?**

Symptomatic Meckel's diverticula are treated with surgical resection in all cases. This involves open or minimally-invasive approaches to diverticulectomy versus segmental small intestinal resection.

11. **What is the appropriate operation for a symptomatic Meckel's?**

As mentioned above, symptomatic Meckel's diverticula require surgical resection. This resection can be performed in an open or laparoscopic fashion. In the absence of significant inflammation or intestinal wall thickening, an isolated diverticulectomy stapled or handsewn is sufficient. It is important to note that in a minority of patients, ectopic tissue may be present in the base of the diverticulum and this area may not feel abnormal. Segmental small intestine resection may be required if the diverticulum has resulted in significant surrounding inflammation, intestinal thickening at the diverticulum's base or if there is concern for bleeding ulcerations in the remaining small intestine.

12. **What should be done with an asymptomatic Meckel's diverticulum discovered incidentally at the time of surgery for a different indication?**

Incidental removal of an asymptomatic Meckel's diverticulum is controversial. Zani and colleagues noted a low lifetime mortality risk in patients. Additionally, they noted a higher postoperative complication rate than morbidity rate of Meckel's diverticulum left in situ. By their calculations, nearly 800 Meckel's would need to be removed to prevent one mortality. Park and colleagues reviewed a large, retrospective series of patients of all ages at the Mayo Clinic with Meckel's diverticula of which 16% were symptomatic. They recommend considering selective excision of asymptomatic Meckel's in patients less than 50 years of age, male patients, diverticula with a length greater than 2 cm or those containing abnormal/ectopic tissue [5, 6].

References

1. Hegazy AA. Anatomy and embryology of umbilicus in newborns: a review and clinical correlations. Front Med. 2016;10(3):271–7.
2. Kadian YS, et al. Vitellointestinal duct anomalies in infancy. J Neonatal Surg. 2016;5(3):30.
3. Francis A, et al. Pediatric Meckel's Diverticulum: Report of 208 Cases and Review of the Literature. Fetal Pediatr Pathol. 2016;35(3):199–206.
4. Bagade S, Khanna G. Imaging of omphalomesenteric duct remnants and related pathologies in children. Curr Probl Diagn Radiol. 2015;44(3):246–55.

5. Zani A, et al. Incidentally detected Meckel diverticulum: to resect or not to resect? Ann Surg. 2008;247(2):276–81.
6. Park JJ, et al. Meckel diverticulum: the Mayo Clinic experience with 1476 patients (1950–2002). Ann Surg. 2005;241(3):529–33.

Chapter 28
Appendicitis

Tomas Wester and Jan F. Svensson

Abstract Acute appendicitis is the most common surgical emergency in children. Standard treatment for both non-perforated and perforated appendicitis is laparoscopic appendectomy. In recent years there has been great interest in treatment of non-perforated appendicitis with antibiotics. Treatment with antibiotics is also the first-line management for appendiceal mass or abscess. This chapter includes questions related to clinical presentation, diagnostic investigations, imaging, treatment and outcomes.

Keyword Appendicitis · Non-perforated · Perforated · Abscess · Appendectomy · Laparoscopic

1. **Is knowledge of appendicitis important in the surgical care of children**?

Acute appendicitis is the most common surgical emergency in children. The life-time risk of developing appendicitis is 7–8%, with a peak incidence during the second decade of life. Appendectomy remains the standard treatment for acute appendicitis. Although appendectomy is generally a simple procedure, it requires general anesthesia and it is an abdominal operation with potential complications.

2. **What is the cause of appendicitis?**

The cause of acute appendicitis remains poorly understood. Traditionally, luminal obstruction was considered the most important factor. It has been shown that other factors contribute to the etiology. Both genetic and environmental factors as well as infections are important [1].

T. Wester (✉) · J. F. Svensson
Department of Pediatric Surgery, Karolinska University Hospital, Stockholm, Sweden
e-mail: tomas.wester@sll.se

M. Lacher et al. (eds.), *Pearls and Tricks in Pediatric Surgery*,
https://doi.org/10.1007/978-3-030-51067-1_28

3. **Does acute appendicitis always progress to perforation?**

The definition of perforated appendicitis varies from perforation verified by the histopathologist to a visible hole in the appendix or a free fecalith in the abdomen seen by the surgeon. Approximately 25% of children with acute appendicitis have perforated appendicitis. The perforation rate is even higher in young children. The traditional understanding has been that acute appendicitis always progresses to perforation. However, it has been convincingly shown that the inflammation resolves without treatment in a subset of patients. The increasing proportion of perforations over time is explained by selection due to resolution of inflammation in patients with non-perforated appendicitis [2].

4. **How do children with appendicitis present?**

Typical presentation begins with vague periumbilical pain. Older children describe that the pain migrates to the right lower quadrant. Fever is common and usually low-grade in acute appendicitis. Nausea and vomiting often follows the onset of pain. Diarrhea is common in perforated appendicitis. Atypical symptoms are common in children with appendicitis.

5. **How is appendicitis diagnosed and what is the role of "appendicitis scores"?**

Appendicitis risk scores are designed to estimate the risk for appendicitis. The most commonly used scores, Alvarado score and Pediatric Appendicitis Score (PAS), were initially shown to have high sensitivity, specificity, negative predictive value and positive predictive value. However, validation studies have shown less favourable outcomes. The more recently described Appendicitis Inflammatory Response (AIR) score appears preferable in young children. Scores should not be used as the only diagnostic modality and for the decision-making it is important to take into account both history, clinical findings, laboratory tests, as well as imaging results. In many centers acute appendicitis is confirmed by imaging, primarily ultrasound, in more or less all children.

6. **What are the clinical findings of acute appendicitis?**

Tenderness in the right lower quadrant is the main finding in children with acute appendicitis. Particularly rebound tenderness increases the likelihood of appendicitis.

7. **Are laboratory tests important?**

A moderately elevated white blood cell count, particularly elevated neutrophils, increases the risk for appendicitis. In non-perforated appendicitis CRP is usually slightly elevated. On the other hand, normal white blood cell count and CRP do not exclude appendicitis. Recent findings indicate that hyponatremia increases the risk for perforation in patients with appendicitis.

8. **Is imaging useful?**

One important advantage with imaging is that the negative appendectomy rate can be significantly reduced. Although ultrasound is depending on the experience of the examiner it generally has a high sensitivity and specificity to diagnose appendicitis in children. Ultrasound should be the first option to limit exposure to radiation. In approximately 10% of children a computed tomography is needed in addition to ultrasound. Magnetic resonance imaging may be useful to diagnose appendicitis but its availability is limited in most centres.

9. **What other diagnoses can be confused with appendicitis?**

The workup to diagnose suspected appendicitis in children should always include the possibility of differential diagnoses. The differential diagnoses include gastrointestinal disorders (mesenteric lymphadenitis, Crohn's disease, Meckel diverticulitis, viral gastroenteritis, pancreatitis, cholecystitis), genitourinary tract disorders (urinary tract infection, hydronephrosis, ovarian torsion, ruptured ovarian cyst, salpingitis, testicular torsion), and other conditions (pneumonia, Henoch-Schönlein purpura, sickle cell disease, porphyria).

10. **How is uncomplicated, non-perforated acute appendicitis treated?**

Laparoscopic appendectomy is the standard approach for non-perforated acute appendicitis. Three-port appendectomy is the most common approach, although single-incision laparoscopy has similar outcomes.

11. **Is laparoscopic appendectomy better than open appendectomy?**

Laparoscopic appendectomy is currently the treatment of choice for acute appendicitis in children. The risk for wound infections as well as adhesive small bowel obstruction is lower compared to open appendectomy.

12. **How common are negative appendectomies?**

The incidence of negative appendectomy has dropped below 5% in many major centres. This is explained by the introduction of both active expectancy and imaging. Also introduction of appendicitis scores may have contributed.

13. **Is there a role for non-operative treatment of non-perforated appendicitis with antibiotics?**

Recent data suggest that non-perforated appendicitis can be treated with antibiotics, with a success rate of about 90%. After the initial success some patients will have a relapse in acute appendicitis. Antibiotics can very well be used as an alternative in cases where surgery or general anaesthesia is associated with an increased risk. When more long-term follow-up data becomes available, antibiotic treatment of non-perforated appendicitis will be included as an alternative treatment option for patients and parents to choose [3].

14. **How often does appendicitis recur after treatment with antibiotics?**

After initial successful treatment with antibiotics about 10% may recur during the first year and another 10–20% during the following five years. The data on this outcome in children are very limited.

15. **How is perforated appendicitis treated?**

Perforated appendicitis in children should be treated with surgery. But, the most important initial treatment is fluid resuscitation and intravenous antibiotics, and surgery should be performed after stabilisation.

16. **For how long should the patient remain on antibiotics after perforated appendicitis?**

Traditionally, perforated appendicitis has been treated with seven to ten days of broad-spectrum antibiotics. More recently, it has been shown that, when the patient tolerates a light diet, it is safe to change intravenous to per oral antibiotics and discharge the patient. Also, when the patient tolerates a light diet and has no leukocytosis, it is safe to discharge the patient home without any antibiotics at all [4].

17. **How should an appendiceal mass or abscess be treated?**

An appendiceal mass should be treated with antibiotics, with or without a drain, to minimize the risk of complicated surgery, bowel injury and/or generalized peritonitis during early surgery.

18. **When should an abscess be drained?**

Most appendiceal masses or abscesses can be treated with antibiotics only. In focal abscesses larger than approximately five centimetres is it likely that the evacuation of pus will shorten the course of the disease. This has to be weighed against the increased morbidity associated with the drain itself.

19. **Is it wrong to do an appendectomy in patients with an appendiceal mass or abscess?**

In a setting where you perform an interval appendectomy the total complications and hospital stay is similar if you perform an early appendectomy or initial non-operative treatment followed by an interval appendectomy. If you do not include the interval appendectomy, the non-operative approach would be preferable.

20. **Is there a role for interval appendectomy after conservative treatment?**

Traditionally, an interval appendectomy has been performed after initial non-operative treatment of an appendiceal mass or abscess, mainly to prevent the risk of recurrence. This regimen has been questioned and stopped in many centres since decades. A recent randomized controlled trial showed that the risk of recurrence was low and that interval appendectomy should be restricted to patients who develop recurrent symptoms. Less than a quarter of the patients had to undergo a late appendectomy using this wait-and-see approach [5].

21. **What are the short term complications of appendectomy?**

Laparoscopic appendectomy is a safe procedure with a low risk of complications. 1–2% of patients develop a wound infection and 3–5% of patients develop a post-operative abscess. In children with perforated appendicitis this risk may be as high as 10%.

22. **Is there a risk for future mechanical small bowel obstruction?**

The risk of small bowel obstruction is small, but present. Hospitalization for small bowel obstruction after appendectomy is 0.5–1.0% with about half the patients undergoing adhesiolysis. The risk is greater after open appendectomy than after laparoscopic appendectomy and greater after perforated than after non-perforated appendicitis. The risk may also be greater after surgery when no appendicitis were found.

23. **Is there a risk for impaired fertility in girls with appendicitis?**

There is no impaired risk for impaired fertility in girls after appendicitis. One meta-analysis described a slight increased risk of ectopic pregnancy. The question has been raised due to the risk of adhesion after appendectomy and that the adhesions may cause infertility. As there is an increased risk of adhesions after open compared to laparoscopic appendectomy it may very well be the surgical intervention rather than the inflamed, sometimes perforated, appendix that causes these adhesions.

24. **How common are appendiceal tumors in children?**

The incidence of carcinoid tumors in histopathology specimens after appendectomy is about 1 in 300. Other appendiceal tumours such as appendiceal adenocarcinoma and lymphoma are even rarer. Most appendiceal tumors are found in histopathological specimens without clinical suspicion of a tumor and most of them are most likely asymptomatic.

References

1. Bhangu A, Soreide K, Di Saveria S, et al. Acute appendicitis; modern understanding of pathogenesis, diagnosis, and management. Lancet. 2015;386:1278–87.
2. Andersson RE. The natural history and traditional management of appendicitis revisited: spontaneous resolution and predominance of prehospital perforations imply that a correct diagnosis is more important than early diagnosis. World J Surg. 2007;31:86–92.
3. Svensson JF, Patkova B, Almström M, et al. Nonoperative treatment of antibiotics versus surgery for acute nonperforated appendicitis in children: a pilot randomized controlled trial. Ann Surg. 2015;261:67–71.
4. Desai AA, Alemayehu H, Holcomd GW 3rd, et al. Safety of a new protocol decreasing antibiotic utilization after laparoscopic appendectomy for perforated appendicitis in children: a prospective observational study. J Pediatr Surg. 2015;50:912–4.
5. Hall NJ, Eaton S, Stanton MP, et al. Active observation versus interval appendicectomy after successful non-operative treatment of an appendix mass in children (CHINA study): an open-label, randomised controlled trial. Lancet Gastroenterol Hepatol. 2017;2:253–60.

Chapter 29
Intussusception

Alexander T. Gibbons, Alejandra M. Casar Berazaluce, Rachel E. Hanke, and Todd A. Ponsky

Abstract Intussusception is a "telescoping" of the intestine, resulting in obstruction and bowel wall edema that can cause ischemia. It is most frequently seen in children under the age of three years. The most common type is ileocolic. Usual presentation includes vomiting and colicky abdominal pain. Patients are evaluated with ultrasound, which frequently shows a target sign. However, the gold standard for diagnosis is a contrast enema, which is also usually therapeutic. In stable patients with ileocolic intussusception, reduction can be attempted with an air contrast enema (up to 120 mmHg) or with an ultrasound-guided saline enema (up to 88 mmHg). If reduction is successful, the patient can be observed for several hours and then sent home. If reduction is unsuccessful, it can be repeated for a total of three times. If all three attempts are unsuccessful, or if the patient is unstable, surgery with manual reduction is necessary. Surgery can be attempted laparoscopically, but there should be a low threshold to convert to a laparotomy. The key to successful reduction is milking the intussusceptum out from its distal extent, rather than pulling proximally. Bowel resection is not needed unless there is perforation or necrosis, or if reduction is not possible.

Keywords Intussusception · Enema reduction · Ileocolic · Small bowel · Hydrostatic reduction · Pneumatic reduction · Ultrasound

A. T. Gibbons
Akron Children's Hospital, Akron, OH, USA
e-mail: agibbons68@gmail.com

A. M. Casar Berazaluce · R. E. Hanke · T. A. Ponsky (✉)
Cincinnati Children's Hospital, Cincinnati, OH, USA
e-mail: tponsy@gmail.com

R. E. Hanke
e-mail: rachel.hanke@cchmc.org

M. Lacher et al. (eds.), *Pearls and Tricks in Pediatric Surgery*,
https://doi.org/10.1007/978-3-030-51067-1_29

1. **What is intussusception?**

Intussusception is a full-thickness telescoping of the bowel where a proximal segment invaginates and is propelled forward by peristalsis into a distal segment. This telescoping results in obstruction and bowel wall edema that can eventually cause ischemia.

2. **What is an intussusceptum?**

An intussusceptum is the proximal segment of bowel that constitutes the internal component of an intussusception.

3. **What is an intussuscipiens?**

An intussuscipiens is the distal segment of bowel that constitutes the outer layer in an intussusception. Quick tip: Remember it as the *recipient.*

4. **What is the most common site for intussusception?**

Due to the abrupt change in lumen size between the terminal ileum and the cecum, the most common site of intussusception is at the ileocecal valve.

5. **What are features of small bowel intussusception?**

Small bowel intussusception, in which both the intussusceptum and intussuscipiens are segments of the small intestine, occurs in up to 25% of cases [1]. It typically occurs in the central abdomen, involves a short length of bowel, and is usually self-resolving [2].

6. **What is the most common cause of ileocolic intussusception?**

In most cases (90%), the etiology is *idiopathic*. It is thought that *lymphoid hyperplasia* of Peyer's patches, which occurs after a viral illness, acts as a lead point that is then propelled forward by peristalsis [3]. In the remaining 10% of cases, a *pathologic lead point* causes the intussusception.

7. **What is a pathologic lead point?**

This is any recognizable intraperitoneal condition that tethers or obstructs the bowel, initiating the process of intussusception. Examples include Meckel's diverticulum, intestinal polyps, intestinal lymphoma, and hemangiomas [4]. Indwelling tubes, like a gastrojejunal feeding tube, can also act as lead points for cases of small bowel-small bowel intussusception.

8. **What patient population is most commonly affected by ileocolic intussusception?**

Children under the age of three years are most commonly affected, representing 90% of cases [5].

9. **What risk factors suggest a pathologic lead point?**

Intussusception in a patient over 3 years old is suspicious for pathology. These patients are more likely to have a Meckel's' diverticulum act as a lead point (14% vs. 2%), but not more likely to have a tumor act as a lead point (6% vs. 5%) [5].

10. **What is the usual presentation?**

Symptoms include vomiting (78%), colicky abdominal pain (69%), and lethsargy/irritability (67%). A sausage-shaped mass identified by palpation may be associated with intussusception, but is often hard to appreciate in a distressed child and is only found in 50% of patients [4].

11. **What are currant jelly stools?**

Edema, lymphatic obstruction, local venous hypertension, and vascular stasis cause mucosal sloughing. These tissue fragments, combined with blood and intraluminal fluid, create the currant jelly appearance. "Currant jelly stools," classically taught as being pathognomonic in intussusception, occur late in the disease process and are only found in 35% of patients.

12. **How is the diagnosis confirmed?**

Ultrasound is most frequently used and first line to evaluate for intussusception.

13. **What findings on ultrasound are consistent with ileocolic intussusception?**

Ultrasound showing a target sign is pathognomonic for intussusception (see Fig. 29.1). Ultrasound can also show the intussuscipiens and intussusceptum in the longitudinal view and can reveal a pathologic lead point if one is present.

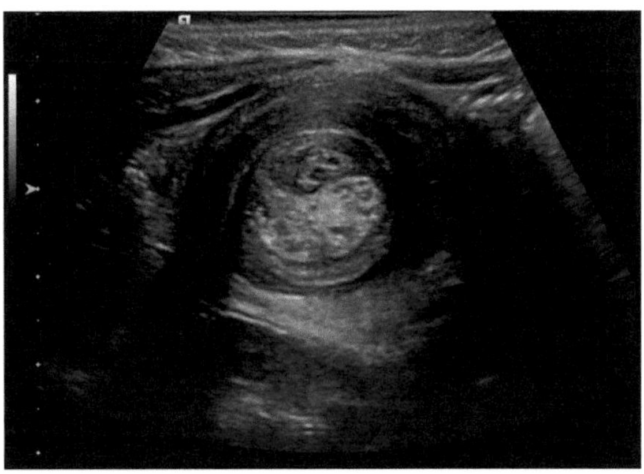

Fig. 29.1 Target sign seen on ultrasound (transverse view)

14. **What are the most common findings on abdominal plain film?**

Common findings include intestinal obstruction (54%), presence of an intracolonic mass or target sign (29%), and paucity of air in the right lower quadrant (10%). Plain films are normal in 24% of patients [6].

15. **How should ileocolic intussusception be managed initially?**

If a patient is hemodynamically unstable or has peritonitis or pneumoperitoneum, they should be managed surgically. Otherwise, initial management should involve fluid resuscitation, attempts at enema reduction, and a surgical consult.

16. **How should small bowel intussusception be managed?**

Since small bowel intussusception self-reduces in the vast majority of cases, most of these patients will not require any intervention. However, if the length of intussusception seen on imaging is greater than 3.5 cm, the patient will likely require an operation [7]. Additionally, if symptoms do not resolve and radiographic evidence of small bowel intussusception persists, operative intervention is necessary.

17. **Which enema reduction method is most effective for ileocolic intussusception?**

The two most commonly used methods of reduction are pneumatic (air-contrast enema) or hydrostatic (ultrasound-guided saline enema). A randomized controlled trial showed that saline enema is the more successful of the two (97% vs. 84%), while also utilizing lower intraluminal pressure (74–88 mmHg vs. 80–120 mmHg) [8].

18. **How frequently does intussusception recur after enema reduction?**

Intussusception recurs in approximately 7.5% of patients reduced hydrostatically and 8.5% of patients reduced pneumatically [9].

19. **How many times can a successful enema reduction be completed for recurrence?**

As long as the intussusception is successfully reduced, enema reduction can be repeated indefinitely. Clinical practice varies by clinician and health system.

20. **How should a patient with successful reduction be managed?**

Historically, practice often involved observing the patient post-reduction for at least 24 hours. Most recent evidence supports safely discharging the patient after four hours of observation in the Emergency Department. While under observation, they are given clear liquids after 3 hours. If they have no recurrence of symptoms, they can be discharged home. If symptoms return, a repeat ultrasound is recommended, with repeat reduction if intussusception is seen [10].

21. **How many *unsuccessful* attempts should be made at enema reduction before proceeding with an operation?**

If initial reduction is not successful, attempts can be repeated twice. If, after three times, reduction is still not successful, that patient should be taken to the operating room for manual reduction [10].

22. **How should operative reduction of intussusception be performed?**

Operative reduction can be performed laparoscopically. The key principle of reduction is milking the intussusceptum out from its most distal point (similar to squeezing out toothpaste), rather than pulling on the proximal bowel. Due to technical limitations of laparoscopy, the reduction is usually completed with controlled tension from the proximal edge. Bowel resection is only needed in cases of perforation or necrosis, or if the reduction is not possible. Patients must be evaluated for a pathologic lead point, which should be resected if present.

23. **Should the appendix be removed at the time of reduction?**

Some surgeons advocate for performing an appendectomy if the patient requires an operative reduction of intussusception, as it removes appendicitis as a differential diagnosis for future episodes of abdominal pain and prevents the appendix from acting as a potential pathologic lead point for recurrence. However, this upstages the wound classification in cases where no bowel resection is needed. A database study showed that performing an appendectomy slightly increased the length of stay and total cost, with no difference in the risk for recurrence, suggesting that routine appendectomy is not beneficial [11].

References

1. Lioubashevsky N, Hiller N, Rozovsky K, Segev L, Simanovsky N. Ileocolic versus small-bowel intussusception in children: can US enable reliable differentiation? Radiology. 2013;269(1):266–71.
2. Navarro O, Daneman A. Intussusception. Pediatr Radiol. 2004;34(4):305–12.
3. Xie X, Wu Y, Wang Q, Zhao Y, Xiang B. Risk factors for recurrence of intussusception in pediatric patients: a retrospective study. J Pediatr Surg. 2018;53(11):2307–11.
4. Blanch AJ, Perel SB, Acworth JP. Paediatric intussusception: epidemiology and outcome. Emerg Med Australas. 2007;19(1):45–50.
5. Savoie KB, Thomas F, Nouer SS, Langham MR, Huang EY. Age at presentation and management of pediatric intussusception: a Pediatric Health Information System database study. Surgery. 2017;161(4):995–1003.
6. Hernandez JA, Swischuk LE, Angel CA. Validity of plain films in intussusception. Emerg Radiol. 2004;10(6):323–6.
7. Munden MM, Bruzzi JF, Coley BD, Munden RF. Sonography of pediatric small-bowel intussusception: differentiating surgical from nonsurgical cases. AJR Am J Roentgenol. 2007;188(1):275–9.

8. Xie X, Wu Y, Wang Q, Zhao Y, Chen G, Xiang B. A randomized trial of pneumatic reduction versus hydrostatic reduction for intussusception in pediatric patients. J Pediatr Surg. 2018;53(8):1464–8.
9. Gray MP, Li S-H, Hoffmann RG, Gorelick MH. Recurrence rates after intussusception enema reduction: a meta-analysis. Pediatrics. 2014;134(1):110–9.
10. Sujka JA, Dalton B, Gonzalez K, Tarantino C, Schroeder L, Giovanni J, et al. Emergency department discharge following successful radiologic reduction of ileocolic intussusception in children: a protocol based prospective observational study. J Pediatr Surg [Internet] (2018). https://linkinghub.elsevier.com/retrieve/pii/S0022346818305499. Accessed 17 July 2019.
11. Wang A, Prieto JM, Ward E, Bickler S, Henry M, Kling K, et al. Operative treatment for intussusception: should an incidental appendectomy be performed? J Pediatr Surg. 2019;54(3):495–9.

Chapter 30
Small Left Colon Syndrome (SLCS)

Colleen M. Fitzpatrick

Abstract SLCS was originally described by Davis, et al., in 1974. It is a rare clinical entity in which newborns present with symptoms of distal intestinal obstruction. Infants of insulin dependent diabetic mothers are at increased risk for developing SLCS. Contrast enema demonstrates a small caliber colon up to the level of the splenic flexure with dilated proximal bowel. This is a functional obstruction, which typically resolves after a diagnostic and therapeutic contrast enema. If normal, spontaneous bowel movements follow the contrast enema, no further intervention is warranted. Surgical intervention is indicated in cases of complicated SLCS. Additional diagnostic evaluation is appropriate in patients who do not resume a normal, spontaneous stooling pattern. There are no sequelae of SLCS at long-term follow-up.

Keywords Distal obstruction · Maternal diabetes · Contrast enema

1. **What is the typical clinical presentation of SLCS?**

Term or near-term infants typically present within the first 24–48 h of life with abdominal distention, failure to pass meconium, and bilious emesis[1]. These infants may also manifest sequelae of a diabetic gestation including hypoglycemic cardiomyopathy, cyanosis and persistent fetal circulation. Plain radiographs demonstrate dilated loops of bowel. Occasionally, pneumoperitoneum may be present on initial plain radiographs [2].

C. M. Fitzpatrick (✉)
Division of Pediatric Surgery, St. Louis University, St. Louis, MO, USA
e-mail: colleen.fitzpatrick@health.slu.edu

Division of Pediatric Surgery, SSM Health Cardinal Glennon Children's Hospital, 1465 S. Grand Blvd, St. Louis, MO 63104, USA

M. Lacher et al. (eds.), *Pearls and Tricks in Pediatric Surgery*,
https://doi.org/10.1007/978-3-030-51067-1_30

2. **What patients are at risk for developing SLCS?**

Patients born to diabetic mothers are at increased risk for developing SLCS. In the original series described by Davis, 40% of patients of patients with SLCS were born to insulin-dependent diabetic mothers [1]. Subsequent series have demonstrated this rate to be as high as 50% [3, 4].

In a study of asymptomatic patients born to diabetic mothers, six of twelve infants were found to have features of small left colon on contrast enema [5].

As most efforts to identify an etiology for SLCS have focused on diabetes, no other specific risk factors have been identified.

3. **What is the cause of SLCS?**

The cause of SLCS has not been clearly defined. In the original series by Davis, et al., histology samples in four patients demonstrated an increased ratio of small cells to multipolar ganglion cells in the myenteric plexus. This was felt to reflect immaturity of the myenteric plexus, though these changes were found in both the normal caliber and contracted bowel thus making it difficult to ascribe the presence of SLCS to these changes.

A subsequent series by Philippart et al. demonstrated normal ganglion cells in all cases where biopsy was performed. They concluded SLCS, in the setting of maternal diabetes, is due to a hypoglycemia-induced alteration in intestinal motility that is a composite neurohumoral response. Increased glucagon levels decrease motility in the descending colon while increased vagal output stimulates the midgut leading to the typical abrupt splenic flexure transition. They further postulated a similar mechanism may account for SLCS seen in infants of non-diabetic mothers who may have elevated glucagon levels due to neonatal stress response.

No recent studies have further evaluated the etiology of SLCS.

4. **How is SLCS diagnosed?**

SLCS is diagnosed with contrast enema. From the anus to the splenic flexure, the colon has a decreased caliber. At the splenic flexure, there is an acute transition to dilated proximal bowel. The descending colon may be foreshortened and lack normal tortuosity. Contrast is promptly evacuated [1].

Meconium plugs may be found on contrast enema in the setting of SLCS and are thought to be secondary to impaired colonic motility rather than to the intrinsic composition of the meconium.

5. **Are there other conditions that mimic SLCS?**

Patients with Hirschsprung's disease and SLCS present with similar patterns. However, there are features on contrast enema that can be used to distinguish the two entities. In SLCS, the descending colon has a significantly decreased caliber consistent with microcolon, the transition between proximal dilation and distal microcolon is located at the splenic flexure, and the transition is relatively abrupt. Patients with Hirschsprung's disease differ in that the aganglionic segment is normal in caliber (not a microcolon), most patients with Hirschsprung's disease will have a rectosigmoid transition zone, and the transition zone is typically gradual and cone-shaped. If an abnormal stooling pattern persists in a patient diagnosed with SLCS, further evaluation for the presence of ganglion cells should be undertaken.

Furthermore SLCS may be difficult to distinguish from meconium plug syndrome (originally described by Clatworthy in 1956) and colonic inertia (originally described by Berdon in 1968), and there is likely overlap in the clinical spectrum, diagnostic criteria and nomenclature of these entities [6]. Reports have associated meconium plug syndrome with both Hirschsprung's disease and cystic fibrosis. Given the overlap between meconium plug syndrome and SLCS, it is important to note that a recent review of meconium plug syndrome found no association with cystic fibrosis and a 13% incidence of Hirschsprung's disease in meconium plug syndrome [4].

6. **How is SLCS treated?**

The contrast enema in SLCS is often diagnostic and therapeutic. There is typically prompt evacuation of contrast and meconium with subsequent normal stooling. Repeat enemas may be necessary if abdominal distention persists.

7. **Is operative intervention required in patients with SLCS?**

In cases of complicated SLCS where pneumoperitoneum is identified, surgical exploration is necessary and temporary intestinal diversion is usually performed. Perforation may occur at the time of initial presentation or may be delayed. Persistent abdominal distention following contrast enema has been reported in patients presenting with delayed perforation. The cecum is the most common site of perforation.

8. **Is rectal biopsy necessary in SLCS?**

The diagnosis of SLCS does not mandate rectal biopsy. Rectal biopsy is indicated only if abnormal stooling follows attempted therapeutic enemas.

9. **What are the long-term consequences of SLCS?**

No long-term sequelae of SLCS have been reported. Most series report follow-up duration of 1–2 years and all report normal stooling patterns.

In the original series by Davis et al. repeat enemas were performed on three separate patients at different intervals of follow-up in each patient. These intervals were 1, 2, and 11 months of age. In each patient, the left colon remained small despite a normal stooling pattern. One patient had a repeat enema at 6 years of age and the colon appeared normal [1].

References

1. Davis WE, Allen RP, Favara BE, Slovis TL. Neonatal small left colon syndrome. Am J Roentgenol Radium Ther Nucl Med. 1974 Feb;120(2):322–9.

2. Stewart DR, Nixon G, Johnson DG, Condon VR. Neonatal small left colon syndrome. Ann Surg. 1977 Dec;186(6):741–5.
3. Philippart AI, Reed JO, Georgeson KE. Neonatal small left colon syndrome: intramural not intraluminal obstruction. J Pediatr Surg. 1975 Oct;10(5):733–40.
4. Keckler SJ, St. Peter SD, Spilde TL, Tsao KJ, Ostlie DJ, Holcomb III GW, Snyder CL. Current significance of meconium plug syndrome. J Pediatr Surg. 2008 May;43(5):896–898.
5. Davis WS, Campbell JB. Neonatal small left colon syndrome, occurrence in asymptomatic infants of diabetic mothers. Am J Dis Child. 1975 Sept;129(9):1024–7.
6. Berdon WE, Slovis TL, Campbell JB, Baker DH, Haller JO. Neonatal small left colon syndrome: its relationship to aganglionosis and meconium plug syndrome. Radiology. 1977 Nov;125:457–62.

Chapter 31
Disorders of Colonic Motility/Hirschsprung Disease

Rebecca M. Rentea and Marc A. Levitt

Abstract Hirschsprung disease (HD) is characterized by a variable amount of aganlionosis of the bowel. Enterocolitis both pre-and postoperative requires irrigation and treatment. Following an operation for HD, children should thrive. Recurrent episodes of obstruction require workup. Functional constipation is a common problem seen by pediatric surgeons following failure of medical management. Following workup, motility testing may help determine medical and surgical management.

Keywords Hirschsprung disease · Soave cuff · Aganlionosis · Enterocolitis · Colonic motility · Failed medical management · Functional constipation · Malone · Appendicostomy · Encopresis

1. **Describe Hirschsprung disease.**

Hirschsprung disease (HD), characterized by the absence of enteric ganglia along a variable length of intestine, is the main genetic cause of functional intestinal obstruction. The enteric ganglia are derived from the vagal neural crest cells.

2. **Describe the incidence and the most common sites of aganlionosis.**

The prevalence of HD is approximately 1 in 5000 live births with a male to female ratio of 1. Presentation of HD is influenced by the length of colon (or in rare cases

R. M. Rentea (✉)
Comprehensive Colorectal Center, Children's Mercy Hospital, 2401 Gillham Road, Kansas City, MO 64108, USA
e-mail: rrentea@cmh.edu

M. A. Levitt
Division of Colorectal and Pelvic Reconstructive Surgery, Children's National Hospital, 111 Michigan Ave NW, Washington, DC 20010, USA
e-mail: mlevitt@childrensnational.org

M. Lacher et al. (eds.), *Pearls and Tricks in Pediatric Surgery*,
https://doi.org/10.1007/978-3-030-51067-1_31

small bowel too) that is affected. HD can occur in the rectum and various lengths of proximal intestine. The length correlates with illness severity and diagnostic difficulty. The length of colon affected is variable; including the rectosigmoid colon (75% of patients), a longer segment above the sigmoid (17%), or the entire colon and variable lengths of the small intestine (8%).

3. **Is Hirschsprung disease genetically inherited?**

Between 15 and 25% of children born with HD have other congenital anomalies.

4. **What percent of patients with Hirschsprung's disease have other congenital anomalies?**

HD occurs as an isolated trait in 70% of patients. Familial cases of HD account for approximately 10–20% of total cases. A newborn with an affected sibling has a 1 in 200 chance of having HD. The most common chromosome abnormality associated with HD is Trisomy 21 which occurs in conjunction in 2–10% of HD cases.

5. **Which diseases are associated with Hirschsprung disease?**

Neural crest abnormalities, Trisomy 21, Smith-Lemili-Opitz syndrome, Waardenberg's syndrome, Ondine's curse Congenital Central hypoventilation syndrome, Mowat-Wilson, MEN-2A/Familial Medullary Thyroid Cancer, MEN-2B [1].

6. **In what layer of the bowel are ganglion cells missing with Hirschsprung disease?**

There is an absence of ganglion cells in the intramuscular plexus and the submucosal plexsus. The internal sphincter is also dysfunctional; there is an absence of the rectoanal inhibitory reflex (RAIR).

7. **What is the differential diagnosis of Hirschsprung disease?**

Malrotation with volvulous, intestinal atresias or stenoses, duodenal obstruction, meconium ileus, meconium plug syndrome, hypothyroidism, anorectal malformation, constipation, milk protein allergy, opoid affect transmitted from the mother, angnesium sulfate toxicity from maternal labor.

8. **What is the presentation of HD and how is it diagnosed?**

Most infants present in the first 24-hours after birth with delayed passage of meconium and associated abdominal distension, constipation, and bilious emesis. Digital examination of the anus may result in explosive passage of meconium/stool and gas.

The diagnosis is suspected with plain abdominal films demonstrating a colon distended with gas and an nondilated rectum. A contrast enema usually identifies a transition zone. Contrast retained in the colon great than 24 hours and on a post evacuation film are typical. The rectosigmoid ratio is utilized by radiologists and is calculated from the contrast enema. It divides the widest diameter of the rectum by the widest diameter of the sigmoid loop when the colon is fully distended by contrast media. The normal rectosigmoid index is >1, and in HD it is <1. A suction rectal biopsy or full thickness rectal biopsy for permanent pathology confirms the diagnosis, and both the absence of ganglion cells and the presence of hypertrophic nerves (greater than 40 microns) must be observed.

9. **In Hirschprung Disease, which should be used as first line therapy in the treatment of Hirschsprung associated enterocolitis (HAEC)?**

Irrigations and metronidazole. The reported incidence of HAEC varies widely (due largely to a broad definition) ranging from 6 to 60% prior to definitive pull-through surgery and from 25–37% following surgery [2]. The principles of treatment are to decompress the colon/intestine, perform rectal irrigations, initiate broad-spectrum antibiotics, and correct dehydration and electrolyte imbalances. Prompt rectal irrigations should be initiated immediately in the emergency department, neonatal intensive care unit, or clinic. A rectal irrigation is performed with a large bore soft silicone catheter, 20-French for children less than 1 year of age, or a 24-French for children greater than 1 year of age. Using room temperature or warm saline, 10–20 mL of saline should be instilled into the colon via the catheter to allow gas and stool to empty through the catheter. This process should be repeated with aliquots of 10–20 mL of saline until the effluent runs clear.

10. **What is the best, most reliable intervention to perform for a sick child with enterocolitis if irrigations are not working?**

Leveling colostomy or an ileostomy. Both are correct answers depending on the clinical circumstances.

11. **In obtaining a suction rectal biopsy in a neonatal infant, what are important technical components of the biopsy for the diagnosis of Hirschsprung disease?**

A diagnostic biopsy should be performed 1 cm above the dentate line. The biopsy should be performed at this level and not distal to it as the epithelium is different than that visualized in the large intestine- squamous epithelial cells vs. columnar epithelial cells. Mucosa and submucosa should be included in the tissue sampled.

12. **At the time of the surgical procedure, when you do a biopsy to determine the colonic level at which to do the pull-through, you should:**

Take a full thickness biopsy (which includes submucosa) either laparoscopic, transumbilical, or open in the part of the colon above the visualized transition zone. The reason for this biopsy technique is to avoid the potential pitfall of sampling only the seromuscular layer which could have ganglion cells while submucosal layer could have hypertrophic nerves.

13. **What size nerve is considered hypertrophic?**

Greater than 40 microns.

14. **During the pull-through, where is the ideal location to begin the transanal dissection?**

0.5–1.0 cm above the dentate line. Starting the trans-anal dissection too low in the anal canal (too distal) results in loss of the dentate line and will negatively impact future continence.

15. **Describe the operative differences in the three most common types of pull-through operations performed for Hirschsprung disease**.

Swenson: Full thickness rectosigmoid dissection with end-to-end anastomosis (A).

Soave: originally performed as a way to avoid the risks of injury to pelvic structures inherent in the Swenson dissection plane (which occurred when the surgeon was in the incorrect surgical plane). Consists of removing the mucosa and submucosa of the rectum and placing the pull-through bowel within a "cuff" of aganglionic muscle (B).

Duhamel: The aganglionic colon is resected to the rectum and the normal proximal bowel is brought retrorectally. The ganglionated colon and rectum are brought together in a side-to side anastomosis (C).

16. **Laparoscopy as part of a pull-through for Hirschsprung disease is helpful for:**

Mobilization of the splenic flexure, ligation of the inferior mesenteric and sigmoidal arcades, mobilization of the left colon off the retroperitoneum, and distal dissection of rectum into the pelvis.

17. **In the Soave procedure, what complication can result by having too long of a cuff or an incised cuff that has fused back together or rolled up?**

An obstructing cuff, which surrounds the pull-through, and physiologically causes external compression.

18. **What goals should be achieved prior to the performance of a pull-through on a child with total colonic Hirschsprung Disease to reduce the incidence of perineal excoriation?**

HD may extend to the small intestine (total colonic type)and males and females are equally affected. Imaging may demonstrate a normal or small caliber colon. Prior to ileo-anal or ileo-Duhamel pull-through the patient must demonstrate the ability to have thickened ileostomy output as liquid stools are difficult to control, good nutrition and growth (check urinary sodium—should be >30 mmol/L), and the availability of products to treat perineal rash. Timing for these milestones is between 6–12 months of age.

19. **What are early complications of a pull-through for Hirschsprung disease?**

Anastomotic leak, stricture, intestinal obstruction, wound infection, and enterocolitis.

20. **In a post pull-through Hirschsprung patient with recurrent enterocolitis, what potential problems with the pull-through can cause obstructive symptoms?**

A stricture at the anastomosis, obstructing Soave cuff, twist of the pull-through, Duhamel spur, or dilated pouch, persistently dilated segment of bowel, retained transition zone, or aganglionic pull-through. In Hirschsprung Disease, the most likely cause of postoperative fecal incontinence is:

Iatrogenic, related to the loss of the dentate line, overstretching of the sphincters, or both [3].

21. **A Hirschsprung patient at the age of 12 is soiling. Work-up for this patient should include:**

Contrast enema, digital and visual exam of the anal canal and dentate line under anesthesia, and anorectal manometry.

22. **Anal manometry (AMAN) is performed for fecal soiling demonstrating no recto anal inhibitory reflex (RAIR) and low resting pressures. Given these findings on AMAN, what likely findings will be visualized on operative visualization of anal canal and dentate line under anesthesia?**

Injured sphincters without tone or complete loss of the dentate line.

23. **What finding on anorectal manometry suggests a diagnosis of Hirschsprung Disease?**

Absence of the recto anal inhibitory reflex (RAIR). The physiology of voluntary bowel evacuation relies on the RAIR. The normal internal sphincter relaxation in response to distention of the rectum is absent in Hirschsprung disease. When a bolus of fecal material is delivered to the rectum, increased rectal pressure and distension causes transient relaxation of the internal anal sphincter, allowing a small sample of the rectal contents to come in contact with the sensory afferent somatic nerves innervating the anorectum. Then the individual can choose if and when to tighten the external (voluntary) sphincters.

24. **What are some different histologic stains utilized to assist in diagnosing Hirschsprung disease?**

H+E or hematoxylin and eosin—one of the principal stains in histology.

Acetylcholinesterase (AChE)—only good for the distal colon.

Calretinin—stains thin nerve fibrils (neurites) and can add diagnostic value to specimens with inadequate submucosa or rarely seen ganglion cells.

25. **Is the content of acetylcholinesterase increased or decreased in the nerve fibers of the lamina propria and muscularis mucosa in patients with Hirschsprung disease?**

It is significantly increased, and is one of the essential points of diagnosis in some institutions when assessing a rectal biopsy for HD. However, it is useful only in rectal biopsies and in biopsies of the left colon because there usually is no acetylcholinesterase activity proximal to the splenic flexure.

26. **Should the evaluation for ganglion cells in the appendix be utilized for pathologic diagnosis of Hirschsprung's disease?**

The appendix should not be utilized to determine whether there is Hirschsprung disease as many normal appendices have no ganglion cells [4].

27. **Define functional constipation? What is the most current indication for surgical management in children with constipation?**

Constipation is defined as infrequent bowel movements (2 or fewer per week) that are painful, or large in caliber stools that require excessive straining. The *Rome III criteria* for constipation are utilized in infants and children up to 4 years of age. This includes one month of at least 2 of the following: 2 or fewer defecations per week, at least 1 episode per week of incontinence after acquiring toileting skills, history of excessive stool retention, history of painful or hard bowel movements, presence of a large fecal mass in the rectum, history of large diameter stools that may obstruct the toilet. Accompanying symptoms include irritability with decreased appetite and/or early satiety. The accompanying symptoms disappear immediately following passage of a large stool.

28. **What imaging and workup aids in understanding functional constipation and potentially rules out other causes of constipation?**

A thorough understanding of which laxatives or enemas have been utilized and to what effect, as well as anorectal examination, contrast enema, anorectal manometry, and colonic motility testing. Colonic motility testing (sitzmarkers, radionuclides, or colonic manometry) is reserved only for those patients who have failed medical management (laxative or enema therapy).

29. **What is the most common indication for surgical management in children with constipation?**

The most common indication for surgical intervention in a child with functional constipation is for one who has failed medical management; high dose laxatives do not work or cause intolerable cramping and enemas do not empty the colon or are not tolerated. For these patients, anal manometry (AMAN) is performed to see if Botox or pelvic floor biofeedback is indicated and colonic manometry (CMAN) is performed to determine whether motility is normal, diffusely abnormal or segmentally (usually the sigmoid) abnormal. Based on the motility testing an antegrade option can be offered which is usually successful, but if flushes do not work a colonic resection may be required.

30. **How is functional constipation treated?**

Through a combined multidisciplinary approach with the implementation of laxatives, dietary modifications, defecation trials, psychosocial support and appropriate testing. Psychosocial counseling often benefits the patient and family as part of a multimodality management.

31. **What are some surgical options for children with medically refractory functional constipation?**

A number of surgical procedures have been proposed that include anal and pelvic floor procedures (such as Botox and biofeedback training), antegrade continence enema procedures (Malone antegrade continence enemas or cecostomy), colonic resections and sacral nerve stimulation (SNS) [5].

32. **What colonic manometry/colonic motility test finding is consistent with poor colonic motility?**

The absence of high amplitude propagating contractions (HAPC) in response to a stimulant medication.

33. **Which patients are most likely to have a good response to antegrade enema flushes?**

Children with poor motility that is limited to the sigmoid as well as children with normal colon motility.

34. **What percentage of neurologically normal children with fecal incontinence have functional constipation as an underlying disorder?**

>95% of children.

References

1. Amiel J, Sproat-Emison E, Garcia-Barcelo M, Lantieri F, Burzynski G, Borrego S, et al. Hirschsprung disease, associated syndromes and genetics: a review. J Med Genet. 2007;45(1):1–14.
2. Gosain A, Frykman PK, Cowles RA, Horton J, Levitt M, Rothstein DH, et al. Guidelines for the diagnosis and management of Hirschsprung-associated enterocolitis. Pediatr Surg Int. 2017;33(5):517–21.
3. Levitt MA, Dickie B, Pena A. Evaluation and treatment of the patient with Hirschsprung disease who is not doing well after a pull-through procedure. Semin Pediatr Surg. 2010;19(2):146–53.
4. Lane VA, Levitt MA, Baker P, Minneci P, Deans K. The appendix and aganglionosis. A note of caution-how the histology can mislead the surgeon in total colonic Hirschsprung disease. Eur J Pediatric Surg Rep. 2015;3(1):3–6.
5. Wood RJ, Yacob D, Levitt MA. Surgical options for the management of severe functional constipation in children. Curr Opin Pediatr. 2016;28(3):370–9.

Chapter 32
Inflammatory Bowel Disease

Sebastian King

Abstract Inflammatory bowel disease is an increasingly important condition in the practice of pediatric surgeons. In the last three decades, there has been an exponential increase in the diagnosis of both Crohn's disease and ulcerative colitis in children worldwide. The conditions continue to be more prevalent in Western countries, though many countries in Asia are also seeing increases in pediatric diagnoses. The introduction of biological agents has transformed the medical management of both Crohn's disease and ulcerative colitis, with a resultant change in the requirements for operative intervention.

Keywords Inflammatory bowel disease · Crohn's disease · Ulcerative colitis · Biological agents · Magnetic resonance enterography

1. **What are the common types of inflammatory bowel disease (IBD) in children?**

Classic IBD consists of Crohn's disease (CD) and ulcerative colitis (UC).

Unclassified IBD (IBD-U) is of increasing importance, and must be diagnosed accurately to reduce the risk of inappropriate surgical interventions for the incorrect type of IBD. Approximately 10–15% of pediatric patients will be diagnosed with IBD-U, as they cannot be definitively categorized with CD or UC. A diagnosis of indeterminate colitis (IC) may only be used in the situation in which a colectomy has been performed, and the distinction between CD and UC still remains uncertain.

2. **What are the predisposing risk factors for Crohn's disease?**

Crohn's disease is most likely the result of an interplay between genetic susceptibility, exposure to environmental factors, and intestinal microflora. The result is

S. King (✉)
Department of Paediatric Surgery, The Royal Children's Hospital, Melbourne, Australia
e-mail: sebastian.king@rch.org.au

M. Lacher et al. (eds.), *Pearls and Tricks in Pediatric Surgery*,
https://doi.org/10.1007/978-3-030-51067-1_32

an abnormal mucosal immune response, leading to compromised epithelial barrier function and adaptive immune dysregulation [1].

A family history of CD is seen in up to 12% of patients at diagnosis, though this rate may change during the patient's life. Ashkenazi Jews exhibit a 3–4 times increased risk of developing the disease. There is an increasing number of alleles that have been associated with pediatric CD.

Commonly detected variants in the risk loci for both CD and UC are able to explain only a small fraction of the expected heritability. Causative genes include NOD2, IL23R, CARD9 and RNF186.

3. **What are the predisposing risk factors for ulcerative colitis?**

Similar to CD, UC is most likely the result of an interplay between genetic susceptibility, exposure to environmental factors, and intestinal microflora [1]. The estimated prevalence of IBD among family members with UC is 8–12%.

The advent of Genome Wide Association Study (GWAS) has led to greater understanding of the links between HLA loci and UC. Strong associations have been shown with HLA DRB1, HLA DQA1 and HLA-DRB*01:03 [2].

4. **hen does inflammatory bowel disease most commonly affect children?**

Approximately 25% of IBD patients will present before the age of 20 years. The peak onset in children is during adolescence, with a pediatric incidence of 10 per 100,000 children in USA and Canada [1]. Pediatric UC has a tendency to have more extensive disease than adult-onset UC at the time of diagnosis. However, the gene expression in adult and pediatric patients is shared.

5. **How does inflammatory bowel disease typically present in children and adolescents?**

Presenting symptom	Crohn's disease (% patients)	Ulcerative colitis (% patients)
General		
- Weight loss	55–80	31–38
- Fever	38	Not applicable
- Anorexia	2–25	6
- Growth retardation	3–4	0
- Lethargy	13–27	2–12
Gastrointestinal tract		
- Abdominal pain	67–86	43–62
- Diarrhea	30–78	74–98
- Rectal bleeding	22–49	83–84
- Nausea/vomiting	6	<1
- Constipation	1	0

Presenting symptom	Crohn's disease (% patients)	Ulcerative colitis (% patients)
- Perianal disease	6–15	0
- Mouth ulcers	5–28	13

6. **What are the extra-intestinal symptoms of inflammatory bowel disease?**

Dermatological	Erythema nodosum, pyoderma gangrenosum
Musculoskeletal	Arthritis, growth failure, osteopenia, osteoporosis, ankylosing spondylitis
Hepatic	Primary sclerosing cholangitis, autoimmune hepatitis
Ocular	Episcleritis, uveitis, iritis
Renal	Nephrolithiasis
Pancreatic	Pancreatitis
Hematological	Anemia, venous thromboembolism

7. **What is very early onset inflammatory bowel disease (VEO-IBD)?**

The age at onset of IBD is intimately linked with the clinical presentations and progression of the disease. Pediatric-onset IBD (<17 years), early-onset IBD (<10 years), VEO-IBD (<6 years), infantile-onset IBD (<2 years), and neonatal-onset IBD (<28 days) may all present in different ways with regards to disease location and severity. Children with onset during the neonatal or infantile periods suffer from a more severe disease course, are known to have higher rates of affected first-degree relatives, and are more resistant to immunosuppressive therapies. In addition, it has been demonstrated that patients with VEO-IBD have an increased gene-variant burden, compared with patients that are older at diagnosis. It is important to consider a potential immunodeficiency syndrome in children with VEO-IBD, due to the high prevalence of gastrointestinal symptoms in children with an immunodeficiency.

8. **Describe the common laboratory findings in patients with inflammatory bowel disease.**

According to the European Society of Pediatric Gastroenterology, Hepatology and Nutrition (ESPGHAN), initial blood tests should include a complete blood count, at least two inflammatory markers, albumin, transaminases and γGT. It has been established that fecal calprotectin is superior for the detection of intestinal inflammation to any blood investigation. The sensitivity for fecal calprotectin in the diagnosis of IBD has been shown to be as high as 0.97.

9. **How has the radiological investigation of patients with inflammatory bowel disease changed in the last decade?**

The radiological investigation of pediatric IBD has been significantly altered in the last decade by the increasing utilization of magnetic resonance imaging (MRI). The main advantage of MRI, particularly in the pediatric population, is the avoidance of ionizing radiation. Pelvic MRI is particularly useful in the assessment of perianal disease, which is a common presenting feature in pediatric CD.

Whilst upper gastrointestinal contrast studies (small bowel follow-through) were previously the mainstay of small bowel imaging, magnetic resonance enterography (MRE) is now considered the modality of choice for evaluation of the small bowel. This is particularly useful when assessing children prior to colectomy, as the presence and extent of small bowel disease is critical to operative planning.

10. **How do the endoscopic findings differ between Crohn's disease and ulcerative colitis?**

Endoscopic findings	Crohn's disease	Ulcerative colitis
Anus	Fistulae often present	Rare to have anal lesions
Rectum	Usually spared	Present in the majority
Colon	Skip lesions Cobble-stone appearance	Contiguous Circumferential
Small bowel	Involvement common (>25%)	Backwash ileitis (10%)
Oesophagus	Ulceration	Spared

11. **What are the standardized scoring systems for pediatric inflammatory bowel disease?**

The pediatric Crohn's disease activity index (PCDAI) was developed in 1991 by Hyams and colleagues to provide a reproducible stratification system for disease severity [3]. The components of the PCDAI include: (1) subjective recall of symptoms (abdominal pain, stool frequency and character, general well-being); (2) objective measures (gender, age, hematocrit, ESR, albumin); and; (3) examination findings (weight, height, abdomen, perianal disease, extra-intestinal manifestations). The combined score may then be used to determine the severity of disease (<10 = remission, 11–30 = mild disease, >30 = moderate/severe). The PCDAI has been shown to closely correlate with the global assessment performed by physicians, and may be used to assess the effect of treatments.

The pediatric ulcerative colitis activity index (PUCAI) was developed in 2007 by Turner and colleagues. [4] The authors sought to create a non-invasive activity index of UC that was reproducible, and accurately assessed response to treatment. The components of the PUCAI include: (1) abdominal pain; (2) rectal bleeding; (3) stool consistency; (4) stool frequency; (5) nocturnal stools; and; (6) activity level. The combined score may then be used to determine the severity of disease (<10 = remission, 11–34 = mild disease, 35–64 = moderate; 65–85 = severe). In addition, a change in the PUCAI score ≥20 was defined as significant.

12. **Describe the medical management of a pediatric patient with inflammatory bowel disease.**

The introduction of biologic therapies, with a greater focus upon targeting of the immune system, has radically altered the management of pediatric IBD. These therapies, including anti-TNF agents and monoclonal antibodies to lymphocytes and interleukins, now augment the more traditional treatments in pediatric patients.

The predominant goals of medical therapy are control of symptoms, induction and maintenance of remission, and avoidance of complications (stricture, fistula, abscess, malignancy). The mainstays of therapy include: (1) corticosteroids (largely used for induction therapy); (2) 5-aminosalicylates (exert a topical immunomodulatory and anti-inflammatory effect); (3) thiopurines (immunosuppressive agents effective in maintaining remission); (4) methotrexate (immunomodulator effective at inducing and maintaining remission); (5) exclusive enteral nutrition (useful in induction, but rarely tolerated for prolonged periods); and; (6) biologics (used in both induction and maintenance).

13. **Is the use of Infliximab associated with an increased risk of long-term malignancy?**

Biologic agents have transformed the management of pediatric IBD, with particular efficacy in children with perianal and fistulizing disease [4]. However, there have been concerns regarding the potential increased risk of malignancy associated with prolonged administration. Hyams and colleagues demonstrated, in a large prospective study of 5766 pediatric IBD patients, that there was no increased risk of malignancy, nor development of hemophagocytic lymphohistiocytosis, with infliximab [5].

14 **What are the nutritional implications for children with inflammatory bowel disease?**

A detailed and purposeful approach to nutrition in children with IBD is essential to reduce the long-term risks of the disease, and should be an integral part of the follow-up of pediatric IBD patients. Children with IBD exhibit greater risks for malnutrition and impaired linear growth, as well as self-imposed food elimination diets. In addition, steroid therapies are well known to exert a direct effect on patient growth. During periods of active disease, it may be required to further supplement macronutrients, including proteins, carbohydrates and fats.

15 **Which children with Crohn's disease require operative intervention?**

The requirement for operative intervention in pediatric CD has decreased significantly due to the marked improvements in medical management of the disease.

However, one-third of children with CD will still require an operation within 5 years of diagnosis for variable indications, including fistula formation, stricturing and/or bowel obstruction [6]. Unlike UC, operative interventions in CD are palliative, and preservation of bowel length is critical.

Children with CD may require elective or emergency operative interventions. Elective indications include stricture formation, enteric fistula formation, failure to comply with medical therapy, complications related to medical therapy, growth retardation, and delayed puberty. Emergency indications include perforation, complete small bowel obstruction, hemorrhage, abscess formation and/or generalized peritonitis. Proximal diversion, with the formation of a temporary ileostomy within unaffected ileum, may be useful to reduce the inflammatory load in children with significant colonic disease.

16. **Which children with ulcerative colitis require operative intervention?**

Unlike CD, UC is a mucosal disease confined to the colon and rectum and is, therefore, able to be cured with resection. In addition, UC carries a greater risk of developing cancer related to colitis, with 5% of patients affected. Children with UC may require elective or emergency operative intervention, with up to 45% of all patients requiring surgery at some stage.

Elective indications include children with active or steroid-dependent UC, failure of maximal medical therapy, and/or colonic dysplasia. These patients require a procto-colectomy, J-pouch formation and ileal pouch-anal anastomosis, with sparing of the dentate line. The majority of surgeons will employ a two-stage procedure, with covering ileostomy formation, dependent upon the age of the patient and the duration of disease.

Emergency indications include colonic perforation, severe rectal bleeding, and/or toxic megacolon. In these settings, an abdominal colectomy with ileostomy formation and retention of a Hartmann pouch, will reduce the long-term risks for the patient.

17. **What are the psychological impacts of pediatric inflammatory bowel disease?**

The psychological impact of IBD in children and adolescents should not be underestimated. Potential risk factors for increased psychological morbidity include an older age at diagnosis, a lower socioeconomic status, female gender in adolescent patients, increased severity of disease, and use of corticosteroids. Increased psychological morbidity may lead to poorer medication compliance, increased episodes of abdominal pain, and increased utilization of antidepressant medications.

References

1. Torres J, et al. Crohn's disease. Lancet. 2017;389:1741–55.
2. Goyette P, et al. High-density mapping of the MHC identifies a shared role for HLA-DRB*01:03 in inflammatory bowel disease and heterozygous advantage in ulcerative colitis. Nat Genet. 2015;47(2):172–9.

3. Hyams J, et al. Development and validation of a pediatric Crohn's disease activity index. J Pediatr Gastroenterol Nutr. 1991;12(4):439–47.
4. Turner D, et al. Development, validation, and evaluation of a pediatric ulcerative colitis activity index: a prospective multicentre study. Gastroenterology. 2007;133(2):423–32.
5. Hyams J, et al. Infliximab is not associated with increased risk of malignancy or hemophagocytic lymphohistiocytosis in pediatric patients with inflammatory bowel disease. Gastroenterology. 2017;152(8):1901–14.
6. Stewart D. Surgical care of the pediatric Crohn's disease patient. Semin Pediatr Surg. 2017;26(6):373–8.

Chapter 33
Gastrointestinal Bleeding

Aaron T. Scott and Julia Shelton

Abstract Gastrointestinal bleeding (GIB) in children is a relatively common condition, affecting patients of all ages in both the inpatient and outpatient settings. Presentation is varied and depends on the anatomic location and severity of bleeding. In patients who present with GIB, a broad differential diagnosis must be considered based on patient age and symptomatology. Endoscopic evaluation is the procedure of choice for the management of pediatric GIB, and the majority of cases will be localized and successfully treated using this modality. Depending on the etiology, a number of other diagnostic tests and therapeutic interventions may be required. Although brisk bleeding can lead to hemodynamic instability requiring urgent surgery, angiography, or endoscopic intervention, children with GIB generally have an excellent prognosis. This chapter concisely summarizes the presentation, etiology, diagnosis and treatment of GIB in pediatric patients.

Keywords Gastrointestinal bleeding · GI bleed · Pediatrics · Surgery · Hematemesis · Melena · Hematochezia · Anemia · Gastritis · Ulcer · Colitis

1. **How is gastrointestinal bleeding classified?**

Gastrointestinal bleeding (GIB) is broadly divided into upper and lower GIB. Upper GIB arises from the esophagus, stomach or duodenum, proximal to the ligament of Treitz, while lower GIB arises distally in the small bowel, colon and rectum [1, 2]. Though there are many commonalities, it is useful to consider

A. T. Scott · J. Shelton (✉)
Department of Surgery, Division of Pediatric Surgery, University of Iowa Stead Family Children's Hospital, 200 Hawkins Drive 2966-Z JPP, Iowa City, IA 52242, USA
e-mail: julia-shelton@uiowa.edu

M. Lacher et al. (eds.), *Pearls and Tricks in Pediatric Surgery*,
https://doi.org/10.1007/978-3-030-51067-1_33

the etiology, presentation, diagnosis and treatment of upper and lower GIB separately.

2. **What are the signs and symptoms of gastrointestinal bleeding?**

Gastrointestinal bleeding may present in a variety of ways depending on the location, underlying cause, and pace of the bleeding. Common terminology used to describe GIB includes hematemesis, vomitus containing frank blood; coffee ground emesis, vomitus containing black or dark brown material representing digested blood; melena, dark, tarry stools containing blood from a proximal source; and hematochezia, the passage of frank blood from the rectum [1, 3]. Depending on the underlying etiology, other symptoms such as abdominal pain, nausea and vomiting may accompany bleeding and help to guide the diagnostic workup [2]. Obscure GIB refers to bleeding without an identifiable source despite thorough workup [1]. Slow bleeding from any location in the GI tract may present as anemia without overt signs of bleeding, and is termed occult.

3. **How does upper gastrointestinal bleeding present?**

Upper GIB most commonly presents with hematemesis, followed by melena and finally coffee ground emesis [2, 4]. Uncommonly, brisk upper GIB may present with hematochezia [2, 3].

4. **How does lower gastrointestinal bleeding present?**

Lower GIB characteristically presents with hematochezia, but slower, more proximal sources of lower GIB may also present with melena [2, 3].

5. **How common is gastrointestinal bleeding in children?**

Data describing the incidence of GIB in children are sparse. In a review of emergency department admissions from a nationally representative sample of US-based pediatric hospitals from 2006 to 2011, GIB accounted for approximately 1.5% of all ED visits. Upper GIB accounted for 20% of these visits, lower GIB for 30%, and the location of bleeding was not specified in the remaining 50%. Over the time period studied, the rate of GIB-associated ED visits increased from 82.2 to 93.9 per 100,000 children per year [5].

6. **What are the most common causes of upper gastrointestinal bleeding?**

The differential diagnosis in children presenting with upper GIB is broad and depends on age, as shown in Table 1. The most common etiologies include gastritis, peptic ulcers (often *H.pylori* related), and vomiting induced hematemesis, which includes Mallory-Weiss tears and prolapse gastropathy syndrome [1, 2, 4].

7. **What are the most common causes of lower gastrointestinal bleeding?**

As with upper GIB, the differential diagnosis for children presenting with lower GIB depends on age and is shown in Table 2. The most common etiologies include colorectal polyps, inflammatory bowel disease (IBD) and both infectious and non-infectious colitis [1–3].

8. **What are the initial priorities in children with gastrointestinal bleeding?**

Prior to embarking on an extensive diagnostic workup, patients should be rapidly assessed for hemodynamic stability. Hemodynamically unstable patients may present with tachycardia, tachypnea, orthostatic hypotension, or altered mental status. In these patients, prompt resuscitation with isotonic fluid and/or blood products is the first priority. Initial laboratory studies should include a complete blood count, electrolytes, liver function panel, and coagulation tests to help quantify the severity of blood loss, clarify comorbid conditions and identify bleeding diathesis. Severe ongoing blood loss or persistent hypotension necessitates urgent surgical, angiographic, or endoscopic intervention to control the bleeding [1–3].

9. **Does acid suppression benefit children with gastrointestinal bleeding?**

Medical therapy for pediatric GIB should be directed by the suspected etiology of the bleeding. For patients with upper GIB, treatment with proton pump inhibitors (PPIs) has been shown to reduce the rate of re-bleeding, transfusion requirement, and need for surgery [1]. In addition, administration of a PPI in the first 48 h is associated with lower mortality [6].

10. **What is the medical treatment for patients with portal hypertension and gastrointestinal bleeding?**

In patients with portal hypertension and GIB, treatment with somatostatin or the somatostatin analog octreotide, vasopressin, or non-selective beta-blockers reduces portal venous pressure, decreasing variceal bleeding [1]. Endoscopy can be used prophylactically to prevent progression to variceal bleeding.

11. **What is the role of endoscopy in the diagnosis of gastrointestinal bleeding?**

Endoscopy, including esophagogastroduodenoscopy (EGD) and colonoscopy is the diagnostic test of choice in children with GIB, with the patient's presentation determining the initial test [2–4]. Those presenting with hematochezia, suggesting a lower GIB should undergo colonoscopy first, while those presenting with melena or hematemesis, suggesting a proximal source, should undergo EGD [2].

12. **What are the next steps in patients with a negative EGD and colonoscopy?**

The diagnostic yield of repeat colonoscopy or EGD is low in these patients, and there is no established algorithm which can be applied to all patients [2, 3]. In patients with painless lower GIB, technetium-99 pertechnetate disodium scintigraphy (Meckel scan) can be used to diagnose Meckel's diverticulum with a sensitivity of 89.7% and specificity of 97.1% [7]. Cross sectional imaging, including CT and MRI, can also be used to located a Meckel's diverticulum or bleeding tumor, and double-balloon enteroscopy or video capsule enteroscopy can identify luminal bleeding inaccessible by EGD or colonoscopy [3]. Due to the risk of capsule retention, the latter technique should not be used when there is suspicion for an stricture or tumor. A technetium labeled red blood cell scan, or angiography may also be used to localize GIB, but both of these techniques require relatively brisk bleeding [3]. Ultimately, the source of GIB will not be identified in 10–20% of patients who present with GIB [2, 4].

13. **What is the role of endoscopy in the treatment of gastrointestinal bleeding?**

Endoscopy is employed both diagnostically and therapeutically in pediatric GIB. Hemostasis can be achieved endoscopically using injection of epinephrine or sclerosants, electrocautery, argon beam coagulation, or application of clips [1, 3].

14. **What is the role of interventional radiology in gastrointestinal bleeding?**

For patients who present with brisk, arterial GIB, mesenteric angiography can be used both to identify the site, and to embolize the offending vessel [1, 3].

15. **When is surgery indicated for pediatric gastrointestinal bleeding?**

Surgical intervention is generally reserved for patients with significant ongoing bleeding refractory to endoscopic treatment, hemodynamic instability, signs of peritonitis, bleeding tumor, or Meckel's diverticulum [2, 7].

16. **What is a Meckel's diverticulum?**

A Meckel's diverticulum is a remnant of the vitelline duct which manifests as an outpouching of the distal small bowel. According to the approximately correct and easily remembered "rule of 2's" which states that they occur in 2% of the population, within 2 feet of the ileocecal valve, are 2 inches in length, with 2 possible types of heterotopic tissue (gastric and pancreatic), and present before the age of 2 [7].

17. **How often does a Meckel's diverticulum present with bleeding?**

Meckel's diverticula most commonly present with painless lower GIB, intestinal obstruction, or local inflammation which may mimic appendicitis. Roughly 25% of symptomatic Meckel's diverticula in children will present with GIB [7].

18. **How is a bleeding Meckel's diverticulum managed?**

A Meckel scan will reveal the diverticulum due to uptake of the radiotracer in heterotopic gastric mucosa, though false positives and negatives are possible, and other modalities including cross sectional imaging or angiography identifying the vitelline artery as the source of GIB can be used to make the diagnosis. The treatment of a bleeding Meckel's diverticula is surgical resection, either via a laparoscopic or open approach [7].

19. **What is the prognosis for children with gastrointestinal bleeding?**

The prognosis for pediatric patients with GIB is generally excellent. Roughly 80% of pediatric ED visits for GIB are discharged from the ED, suggesting that the majority of children with GIB have a relatively benign course [5]. In a nationally representative database study of children with GIB, the overall mortality was 2.07%. However among patients whose principal diagnosis was GIB, the mortality was only 0.37%, demonstrating the favorable prognosis of isolated GIB compared to GIB in the setting of other significant illness [6].

References

1. Romano C, Oliva S, Martellossi S, Miele E, Arrigo S, Graziani MG, et al. Pediatric gastrointestinal bleeding: Perspectives from the Italian Society of Pediatric Gastroenterology. World J Gastroenterol. 2017;23:1328–37.
2. Franke M, Geiss A, Greiner P, Wellner U, Richter-Schrag HJ, Bausch D, et al. The role of endoscopy in pediatric gastrointestinal bleeding. Endosc Int Open. 2016;4:E1011–6.
3. Sahn B, Bitton S. Lower gastrointestinal bleeding in children. Gastrointest Endosc Clin N Am. 2016;26:75–98.
4. Cleveland K, Ahmad N, Bishop P, Nowicki M. Upper gastrointestinal bleeding in children: an 11-year retrospective endoscopic investigation. World J Pediatr. 2012;8:123–8.
5. Pant C, Olyaee M, Sferra TJ, Gilroy R, Almadhoun O, Deshpande A. Emergency department visits for gastrointestinal bleeding in children: Results from the nationwide emergency department sample 2006–2011. Curr Med Res Opin. 2015;31:347–51.
6. Attard TM, Miller M, Pant C, Kumar A, Thomson M. Mortality associated with gastrointestinal bleeding in children: A retrospective cohort study. World J Gastroenterol. 2017;23:1608–17.
7. Hansen CC, Soreide K. Systematic review of epidemiology, presentation, and management of Meckel's diverticulum in the 21st century. Medicine (Baltimore). 2018;97:e12154.

Chapter 34
Anorectal Malformations

Hira Ahmad and Marc A. Levitt

Abstract Anorectal malformations (ARM) malformation are complex, heterogeneous disorders ranging from perineal fistulas to more complex malformations such as cloaca. Rectourethral fistula is the most common malformation in males and imperforate anus with a rectovestibular fistula is the most common anomaly in females. Patients with ARM require long term follow up for bowel management.

Keywords Anorectal malformation · Rectourethral fistula · Rectovesticbular fistula · Cloaca · Cloacal exstrophy · Bowel management · Krickenbeck classification · Hydrocolpos

1. **What is an anorectal malformation (ARM)?**

ARM is an abnormal termination of the anorectum, which presents across a wide spectrum of anatomic manifestations ranging from a fistula to the perineum, vaginal and urethral structures to a blind-ending rectum without a fistula.

2. **What is the incidence of ARM?**

1 in 5,000 live births and is slightly more common in males.

H. Ahmad (✉)
Center for Colorectal and Pelvic Reconstruction, Nationwide Children's Hospital, Faculty Office Building, 611 E. Livingston Ave. Columbus, 6th Floor, Columbus, OH 43205, USA
e-mail: Hira.Ahmad@nationwidechildrens.org

M. A. Levitt
Division of Colorectal and Pelvic Reconstructive Surgery, Children's National Hospital, 111 Michigan Ave NW, Washington, DC 20010, USA
e-mail: mlevitt@childrensnational.org

M. Lacher et al. (eds.), *Pearls and Tricks in Pediatric Surgery*,
https://doi.org/10.1007/978-3-030-51067-1_34

3. **How are anorectal malformations classified?**

In the past, ARMs were classified according to gender and as low, intermediate, or high, depending on the termination of the rectum relative to the puborectalis muscle complex based on Wingspread classification. Currently, ARMs are classified by the precise anatomical abnormality of the distal rectum and the location of the fistula in relationship to the perineum and urogenital system. The Krickenbeck classification is utilized as it helps predict the type of surgery required (Table 34.1).

4. **What are the most common variants of anorectal malformation in males? In females?**

The most common anorectal malformation in males is imperforate anus with rectourethral fistula. The most common ARM in females is imperforate anus with rectovestibular fistula (Fig. 34.1).

5. **What are the most common associated anomalies?**

A child with an anorectal malformation can have anomalies in multiple systems including vertebral, anal, cardiac, trachea-esophageal, renal, and limb (VACTERL). 8% of infants have esophagealatresia atresia, 3% have duodenalatresia atresia, 30% have a cardiovascular condition, but only one third of these infants have hemodynamic lesions that require medical or surgical management. Tethered spinal cord occurs in 25% of children. Approximately 50% of children with anorectal malformations are born with an associated urologic condition (Table 34.2).

6. **A patient with an anorectal malformation without a fistula defect (blind ending rectum) on high pressure distal colostogram, is most commonly associated with which syndrome?**

Trisomy 21.

Table 34.1 Krickenbeck classification for ARM [6]. Reprinted with permission from Holschneider A, Hutson J, Peña A, Beket E, Chatterjee S, Coran A, et al. Preliminary report on the International Conference for the Development of Standards for the Treatment of Anorectal Malformation. Journal of Pediatric Surgery. 2005;40(10):1521–6

Major clinical groups	Rare/regional variants
Perineal (cutaneous) fistula	Pouch colon
Rectourethral fistula	Rectal atresia/stenosis
Bulbar	Rectovaginal fistula
Prostatic	H-Type fistula
Rectovesical fistula	Others
Vestibular fistula	
No fistula	
Anal stenosis	

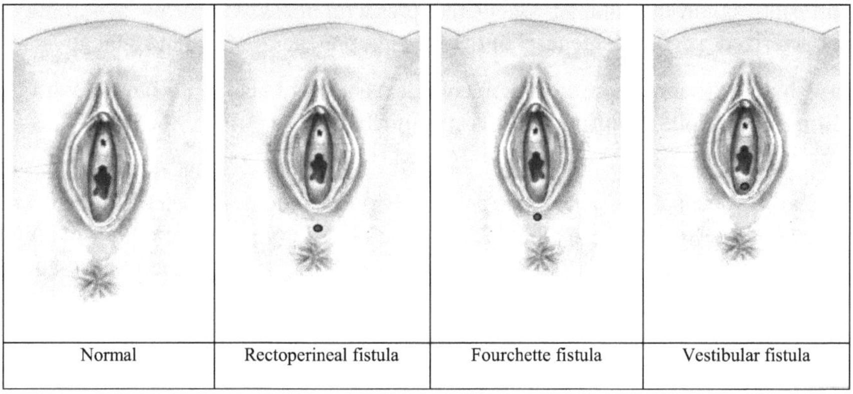

Fig. 34.1 Various ARM anomalies in a female patient (author's personal picture)

Table 34.2 Associated anomalies in ARM. Table 2: Created from information in Stoll C, Alembik Y, Dott B, Roth MP. Associated malformations in patients with anorectal anomalies. European Journal of Medical Genetics. 2007;50(4):281–90. And Stoll C, Dott B, Alembik Y, Roth MP. Associated anomalies in cases with anorectal anomalies. American journal of medical genetics Part A. 2018;176(12):2646–60

System	Type of anomaly	Frequency (%)
Urinary	Vesicoureteric reflux	50
	Hydronephrosis	
	Renal agenesis	
	Renal dysplasia	
Genital	Vaginal septum	50
	Uterine didelphys/Bicornuate uterus	35
	Cryptorchidism	3–19
	Vaginal duplication, vaginal agenesis, absent ovary	
Vertebral	Lumbosacral anomalies	30–35
	Tethered cord	
	Cord lipomas	
	Syringohydromyelia	
Cardiovascular	VSD	25–30
	Tetralogy of fallot	
	Transposition of great vessels	
	Hypoplastic left heart syndrome	
Gastrointestinal	Tracheo-esophageal fistula	10
	Duodenal obstruction	
	Malrotation	

7. **A child with a rectal atresia and anal stenosis requires which workup?**

With a normal appearance of the anal canal and dentate line, the typical appearance of this rare type of malformation, a workup should specifically evaluate for

Currarino syndrome and an associated presacral mass. Currarino syndrome is characterized by partial agenesis of the sacrum, pre-sacral mass, and anal atresia.

8. **What is the most common gynecologic associated issue in a female with an anorectal malformation- rectovestibular fistula?**

Vaginal septum. Vaginal anomalies such as vaginal septum (longitudinal or transverse) occur in 5% of females with ARM. Usually a vaginal septum can be resected at the same time as the PSARP. The clinician must have a high index of suspicion for other gynecological anomalies, albeit rare, such as distal vaginal atresia. Thus, careful examination under anesthesia of the vagina at the same time as PSARP is prudent.

9. **A female patient with a normal anus, urogenital sinus and hypertrophy of the clitoris requires evaluation for:**

Congenital adrenal hyperplasia (CAH).

10. **A male infant is born via spontaneous vaginal delivery at 35-weeks' gestation. Physical examination reveals no anus, but a well-defined buttock crease and a bucket-handle deformity on the perineum. Crosstable lateral film performed at 20 h of life shows the rectal air column to be within 1 cm of the perineal skin marker. What is the next best step in management?**

It is important to observe this infant for 24 h for passage of meconium, looking for drainage of meconium through a fistula to the perineum or the urinary tract because this significantly alters treatment. The cross table lateral film shows the rectum to be within 1 cm of the perineal skin marker making it amenable to a primary posterior sagittal anorectoplasty. The bucket handle was a key to this type of malformation (rectoperineal fistula).

The absence of passage of meconium in the first 24 to 48 h increases the likelihood of a malformation to the urinary tract or a blind ending rectum and requires a diverting colostomy and subsequent high pressure colostogram via the distal stoma at a few months of age to define the distal rectal anatomy (Fig. 34.2).

11. **Why is it important to wait for up to 24 h prior to creating a colostomy?**

A newborn infant with an anorectal malformation requires up to 20 to 24 h for enough distal colonic pressure to build up in order to delineate a fistula. A cross table x-ray can be done to see the distal aspect of the rectum or a perineal ultrasound which can guide the decision as to whether a primary repair or a colostomy should be performed (Fig. 34.3).

12. **Name the key steps in managing an infant with imperforate anus?**

Infants require a complete physical examination, with focus on evaluation of the perineum, and workup to evaluate for comorbidities and associated anomalies. This includes imaging of the spine (spinal ultrasound), urinary system (renal

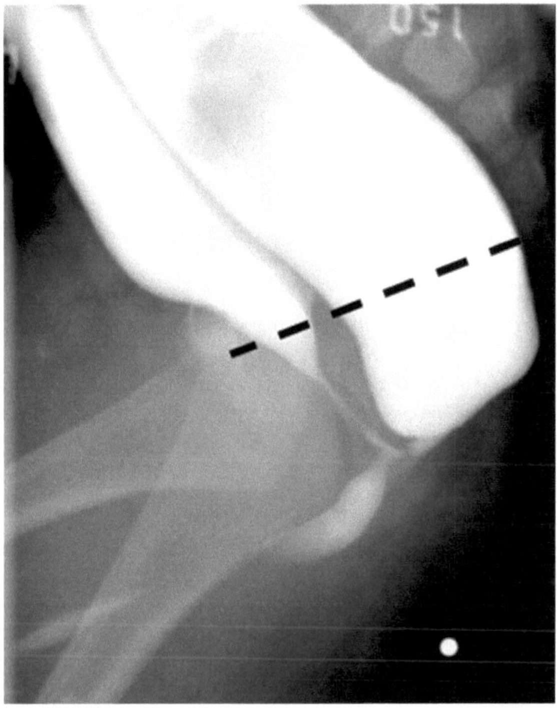

Fig. 34.2 Distal colostogram of a male patient born with an ARM. The pubococcygeal line (dotted line) may be useful in predicting the need for laparoscopy or laparotomy at the time of PSARP. If the rectum is the first structure encountered from a posterior sagittal approach, then the case can more likely be performed using only a posterior sagittal approach. If the urinary tract is the first structure that would be encountered via a posterior sagittal incision, then it is more likely that laparoscopy or laparotomy will be needed [5]

ultrasound) and heart (echocardiogram). If no fistula is delineated within 24-48 h, the infant will require a divided colostomy.

13. **Describe the ideal colostomy to create in a child with an anorectal malformation?**

Divided descending colostomy with mucous fistula. The colostomy should be performed at the junction of the descending colon and sigmoid colon to ensure that adequate distal length remains to perform the posterior sagittal anorectoplasty (PSARP) without having to take the mucus fistula down. Attention should also be paid to the peritoneal reflection attachments which will prevent future stoma prolapse. Another advantage of a divided stoma versus a loop colostomy is to limit fecal contamination of the urinary tract if a fistula is suspected. A well-constructed loop which avoids this is also acceptable.

14. **What are the potential disadvantages to a loop or a transverse colostomy?**

With a loop stoma, the likelihood of a prolapse increases and spillage into the distal limb can potentially result in urinary tract infections, and a fecaloma. For a transverse colostomy, it may be challenging to establish enough pressure to perform an adequate distal colostogram. The possibility of absorption of urine into the colon via a rectourethral fistula may lead to acidosis.

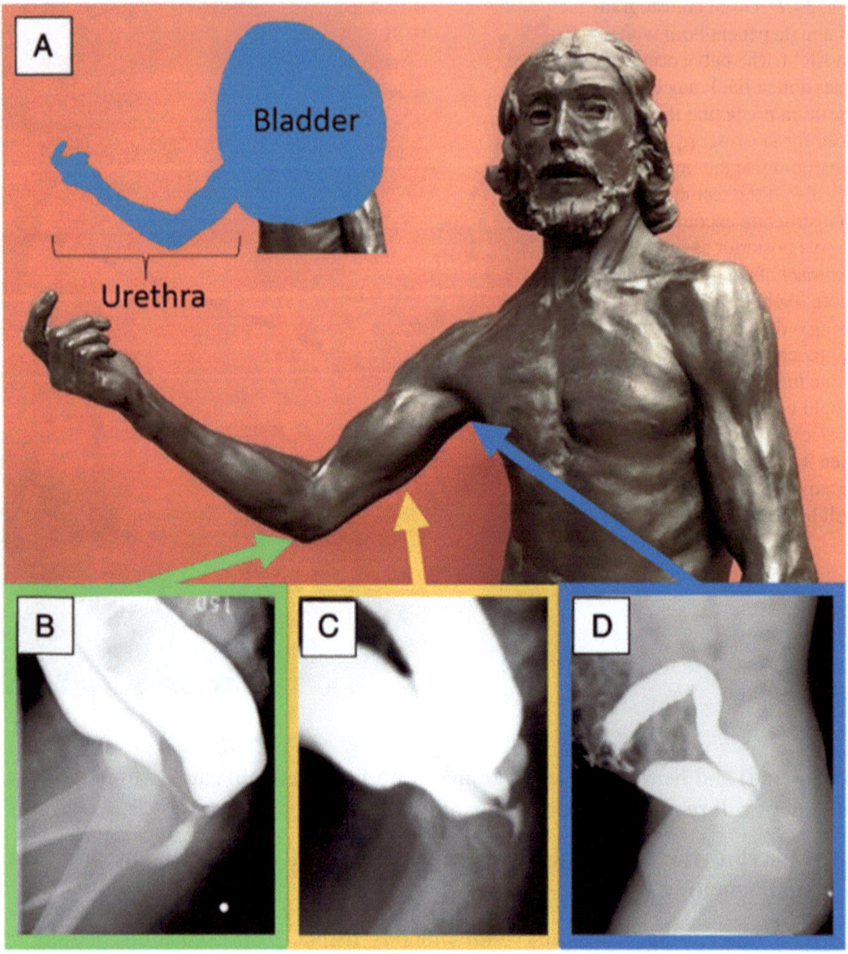

Fig. 34.3 Auguste Rodin's Saint John the Baptist sculpture (1880) in the Musée d'Orsay, Paris, France. The right arm is used to represent the course of the male urethra (**a**). The elbow represents the bulbar urethra (**b**), the humerus represents the prostatic urethra (**c**), and the axilla represents the bladder neck (**d**) [5]. Figures 34.2 and 34.3: Reprinted with permission from Halleran DR, Ahmad H, Bates DG, Vilanova-Sanchez A, Wood RJ, Levitt MA. A call to ARMs: Accurate identification of the anatomy of the rectourethral fistula in anorectal malformations. J Pediatr Surg. 2019

15. **What is a high pressure distal colostogram?**

A high pressure distal colostogram is performed through the mucous fistula at several months of life in order to delineate the length of the rectum, rectum to perineal distance, and the location of the fistula. Without a properly performed distal colostogram, the surgeon will not know the precise location of the distal rectum. There are risks of injuring adjacent structures including the vas deferens, urethra, seminal vesicles and bladder neck. Recent work with water injection and visualization using ultrasound could replace the use of ionizing radiation used during fluoroscopy [1].

16. **A 4-year old male presents with a history of an international adoption and prior anorectal malformation repair, (original malformation unknown). He voids incompletely and dribbles urine after voiding. How would you evaluate this child?**

Children who have undergone surgery for an anorectal malformation who present with fecal and/or urinary incontinence always require a complete workup for associated anomalies especially in the setting where their surgical record is unknown. In this case the child could have a remnant of the original fistula (ROOF) leading to urinary dribbling [2]. This can be evaluated by pelvic MRI and cystoscopy. The possibility of a neurogenic bladder must also be investigated. A voiding cystourethrogram (VCUG) and video urodynamics (UDS) should be included in the work up as well.

17. **In a male with ARM, distal colostogram shows a high rectum with no fistula. On the contrast study the distal end of the rectum appears flat. What should be the next step in management?**

Request a repeat distal colostomy with higher pressure.

18. **In a male ARM patient with a rectobladderneck fistula, mobilization of a very high rectum requires:**

Dissection of the distal IMA branches thus preserving the intramural rectal blood supply to the distal rectum.

19. **In a male ARM patient, unilateral hydronephrosis is likely related to:**

Vesicoureteral reflux.

20. **In a male ARM patient, the "no fistula" defect is almost always located at the level of:**

Bulbar urethra.

21. **A previously repaired ARM patient is found to have mislocated anus with rectal prolapse. MRI of the pelvis reveals a mass behind the urethra. Reoperation is considered. The posterior urethral mass most likely represents:**

R.O.O.F. Remnant Of Original Fistula.

22. **What are appropriate ways to manage an infant with imperforate anus and a rectovestibular or rectoperineal fistula?**

This infant has several options depending on the comfort and expertise of the surgeon and parental preferences. (1) A colostomy can be performed in the newborn period followed by repair at 3–10 months of age and eventually colostomy closure. (2) Dilations of the fistulous tract to Hegar # 10 with delayed repair at 3 to 6 months of age. (3) Primary PSARP in the newborn period with or without a protecting colostomy (Fig. 34.4).

23. **What are the indications for the treatment of a rectoperineal fistula in a female?**

First, it is crucial to delineate the location of the fistula in relation to the sphincter complex. The definitive diagnosis is with an examination under anesthesia with electrical stimulation of the sphincter complex. The goals of the operation are then to relocate the anus within the sphincter mechanism, make the anal opening an appropriate size for patient's age, and create an adequate length of perineal body. If, however, the anal opening is circumferentially surrounded by the sphincter muscle complex, then a short or inadequate perineal body alone is not an indication for operation.

24. **What are the key steps of a posterior sagittal anorectoplasty (PSARP)?**

- Place a Foley catheter (Coude tip preferred)
- Position the patient prone, elevate the pelvis, prep and drape
- Identify the center of the sphincter complex with an electrical stimulator and mark the site
- Make a posterior sagittal incision
- Separate the fistula/rectum from the urethra
- Divide and close the fistula
- Stimulate the sphincter muscle complex again while the muscle complex is open to confirm the site of the anoplasty
- Reapproximate the levators and midline structures incorporating the rectum with at least 3–4 sutures to prevent prolapse.
- Place the rectum in the center of the sphincter complex
- Perform the anoplasty and size the neoanus with a Hegar dilator.

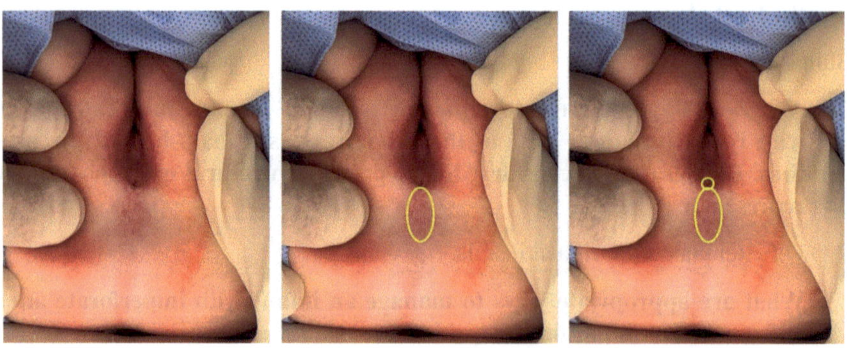

Fig. 34.4 ARM: rectovestibular fistula in a female (arrow), circle demonstrates the location where the sphincter mechanism is located. Finally, fistula and location of sphincter mechanism where the anal opening belongs are both circled (author's personal picture)

25. **A female newborn is found to have only two perineal openings, what are the defects that could be responsible?**

Rectovaginal fistula, urogenital sinus, a blind ending rectal fistula, vestibular fistula with vaginal atresia.

26. **Describe the anorectal malformation in which a female infant with imperforate anus, has only a single perineal opening?**

Cloaca. In this malformation, rectum, vagina and urinary tract empty into a single common channel.

27. **You are asked to perform a fetal consultation for a pregnant woman with a 24-week female fetus who on prenatal ultrasound has a cystic pelvic mass, an absent radial bone, and a single kidney with hydronephrosis. What is the most likely diagnosis?**

Cloaca. A single perineal orifice in a female that forms a common channel consisting of the urinary tract, reproductive tract and rectum. The cystic mass is likely a vagina filled with mucous and urine (hydrocolpos), and the radial and renal anomalies are part of the VACTERL complex.

28. **What is the incidence of cloaca?**

1 in 50,000 females.

29. **What is hydrocolpos?**

Hydrocolpos is the distension of the vagina caused by accumulation of fluid in the vagina (mucous and urine). It may be problematic when it obstructs the distal ureters by compressing the bladder trigone and resulting in hydronephrosis. In these cases, hydrocolpos needs to be drained.

30. **In the management of a newborn with a cloaca, how do you determine whether a hydrocolpos requires drainage?**

If there is hydronephrosis associated with the pelvic mass, the hydrocolpos will need to be drained.

31. **How can a hydrocolpos be drained?**

There are two options for the drainage of hydrocolpos. (1) Intermittent catheterization of the common channel, with confirmation of decompression and resolution of hydronephrosis by ultrasound (2) A transabdominal vaginostomy tube either by interventional radiology or at the time of colostomy creation.

32. **Which anatomic details are vital to surgical planning in cloaca?**

Length of the common channel (<3 cm short common channel vs. >3 cm long common channel) and urethral length (measurement based on a cloaca up to one year of age). These are vital in deciding whether a total urogenital mobilization or a urogenital separation with preservation of the common channel as urethra should be performed [6] (Fig. 34.5).

33. **Identify key steps in the newborn management of cloacal malformations.**

- Identify the single perineal opening and confirm the diagnosis.
- Divert the fecal stream via a divided descending colostomy
- Determine whether a hydrocolpos causing hydronephrosis is present, and if so drain it via perineal catheterizations or vaginostomy.
- Evaluate for associated anomalies (VACTERL)
- Perform a cystoscopy, vaginoscopy, and a contrast study to visualize the anatomy (3D reconstructed fluoroscopy) at 5 to 6 months of age
- Perform a definitive cloacal repair between 6 months to 1 year of age.

34. **A 13 years old previously repaired cloacal patient, presents with cyclical, monthly left lower quadrant abdominal pain. What is the most likely diagnosis?**

Hematometrocolpos associated with an obstructed Mullerian structure.

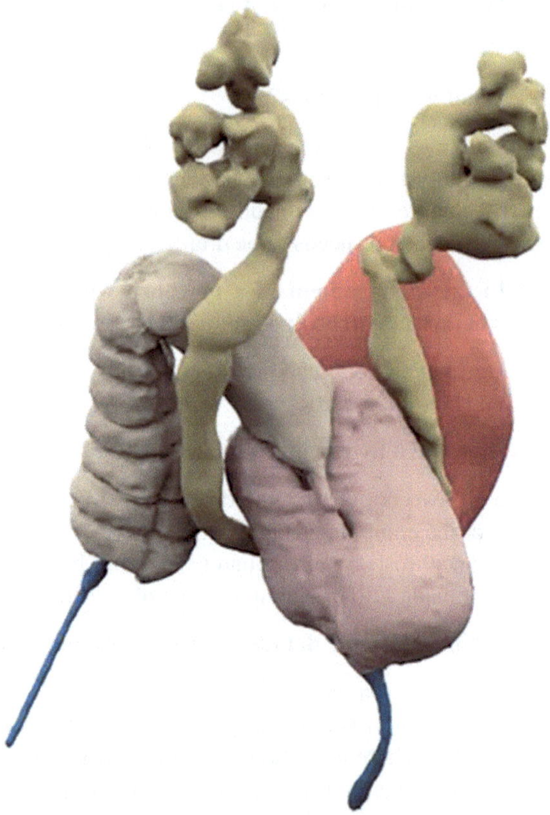

Fig. 34.5 3D reconstructed cloacagram with bladder marked in magenta, vaginas in pink, bowel in tan and common channel in blue [3]. Reprinted with permission from Wood RJ, Reck-Burneo CA, Dajusta D, Ching C, Jayanthi R, Bates DG, et al. Cloaca reconstruction: a new algorithm which considers the role of urethral length in determining surgical planning. J Pediatr Surg. 2017

35. **What is the most common indication for a reoperation in patients with previously repaired cloaca?**

Persistent urogenital sinus, i.e. only the rectal component was previously repaired.

36. **In a patient with previously repaired ARM patient, what is the most important predictor of continence? Type of malformation? Status of the spine? Quality of the Sacrum?**

All three are important variables to consider when counseling patients on their continence potential. We use Fig. 34.6 to counsel families. A recent study has shown that the type of ARM was the only factor that predicted fecal continence in children with ARM.

37. **An ARM patient has successful bowel management program with enemas and requests an antegrade enema route. For his urine, he does intermittent catheterization but leaks at 2 h. What is the next step in management? What are his options for antegrade route?**

For patients on intermittent catheterization leaking at 2 h, strong consideration should be given to urology referral. The patient should undergo urology evaluation

			NUMBER
ARM TYPE	Perineal Fistula	1	
	Anal Stenosis	1	
	Rectal Atresia	1	
	Rectovestibular Fistula	1	
	Rectobulbar Fistula	1	
	ARM without Fistula	1	
	Cloaca < 3 cm Common Channel	2	
	Rectoprostatic Fistula	2	
	Rectovaginal Fistula	2	
	Rectobladderneck Fistula	3	
	Cloaca > 3 cm Common Channel	3	
	Cloacal Exstrophy	3	

SPINE	Normal termination of the conus (L1-L2)	1	
	Normal filum appearance	1	
	Abnormally low termination of the conus (below L3)	2	
	Abnormal fatty thickening of filum	2	
	Myelomeningocele	3	

SACRUM	Sacral Ratio equal to or greater than 0.7	1	
	Sacral Ratio less than 0.69 or greater than 0.4	2	
	Hemisacrum	2	
	Sacral hemivertebrae	2	
	Presacral mass	2	
	Sacral Ratio less than 0.4	3	

TOTAL NUMBER

3-4 = Good Potential for Continence

5-6 = Fair Potential for Continence

7-9 = Poor Potential for Continence

Fig. 34.6 Anorectal malformation (ARM) continence predictor index. An educational handout developed at Nationwide Children's Hospital for counseling patients on their continence potential

with urodynamics, VCUG, and renal ultrasound. If patient needs a Mitrofanoff, then consideration should be given to split appendix Malone/Mitrofanoff. If the length of the appendix is not adequate then appendix should be used for Mitrofanoff and neomalone should be constructed. If the cecum is not amenable to neomalone due to vascular supply, then a cecostomy should be considered (Fig. 34.7).

38. **What is cloacal exstrophy?**

It is a severe form of anorectal malformation with ventral abdominal wall defects. The classic features of cloacal exstrophy include anorectal malformation, omphalocele, blind ending micro-colon, exstrophic hemibladders, and an everted cecum with prolapse between them. Boys often have a rudimentary hemiphallic structures on each side. Females may have many gynecologic anomalies. The incidence of cloacal exstrophy is 1 in every 400,000 births with a male predominance [4].

39. **Name the key steps in the management of a newborn with cloacal exstrophy**.

- Careful preoperative investigation
- Omphalocele closure
- Separation of the gastrointestinal tract from the hemibladders with tubularization of the cecum and construction of an end colostomy (gastrointestinal stoma)
- Closure of hemibladders, if possible, or if not, joining them together and keeping them inverted
- Pelvic osteotomies of the time of bladder closure
- Delayed additional urogenital reconstruction, depending on gender assignment
- Colonic pull through plus malone if end stoma is capable of forming solid stool.

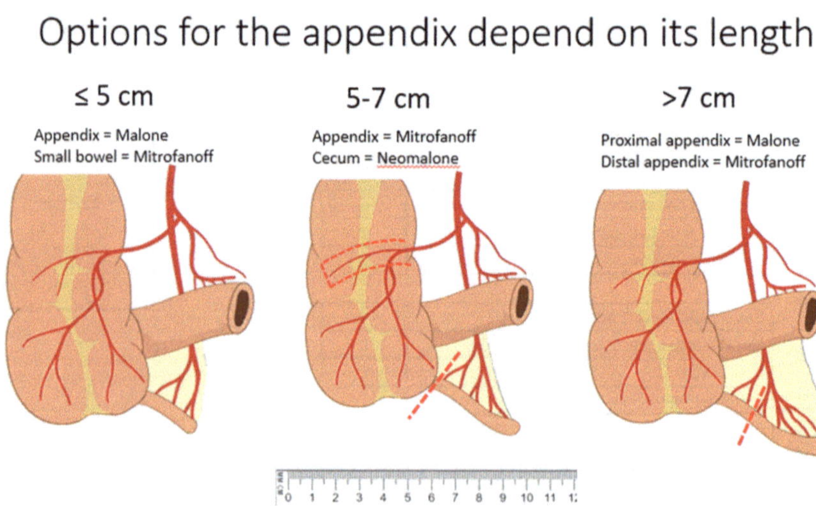

Fig. 34.7 Options for the appendix depend on its length. Developed and used at Nationwide Children's Hospital

References

1. Chow JS, Paltiel HJ, Padua HM, McNamara E, Dickie BH. Contrast-Enhanced Colosonography for the Evaluation of Children With an Imperforate Anus. Journal of ultrasound in medicine: official journal of the American Institute of Ultrasound in Medicine. 2019.
2. Rentea RM, Halleran DR, Vilanova-Sanchez A, Lane VA, Reck CA, Weaver L, et al. Diagnosis and management of a remnant of the original fistula (ROOF) in males following surgery for anorectal malformations. Journal of pediatric surgery. 2019.
3. Wood RJ, Reck-Burneo CA, Dajusta D, Ching C, Jayanthi R, Bates DG, et al. Cloaca reconstruction: a new algorithm which considers the role of urethral length in determining surgical planning. J Pediatr Surg. 2017.
4. Woo LL, Thomas JC, Brock JW. Cloacal exstrophy: A comprehensive review of an uncommon problem. Journal of Pediatric Urology. 2010;6(2):102–11.
5. Halleran DR, Ahmad H, Bates DG, Vilanova-Sanchez A, Wood RJ, Levitt MA. A call to ARMs: Accurate identification of the anatomy of the rectourethral fistula in anorectal malformations. J Pediatr Surg. 2019.
6. Holschneider A, Hutson J, Peña A, Beket E, Chatterjee S, Coran A, et al. Preliminary report on the International Conference for the Development of Standards for the Treatment of Anorectal Malformation. Journal of Pediatric Surgery. 2005;40(10):1521–6.

References

Chapter 35
Anorectal Complaints (Proctology): Hemorrhoids, Fissures, Abscesses, Fistulae

Brian C. Gulack, Justyna M. Wolinska, and Sharifa Himidan

Abstract Anorectal diseases occur commonly in pediatric patients but are often benign and self-limiting. These conditions include haemorrhoids, anal fissures, perianal abscesses and fistulae-in-ano. The pediatric surgeon and those who work with the pediatric population should be familiar with the presentations of these diseases, along with associated issues, management, and complications. The vast majority will improve with time or medical management, but failure of conservative management will often necessitate operative intervention. In this chapter, we discuss some basic questions related to these conditions and their management.

Keywords Anorectal disease · Haemorrhoid · Anal fissure · Perirectal abscess · Fistulae-in-ano

35.1 Hemorrhoids

1. **What is a hemorrhoid?**

Hemorrhoidal veins are arteriovenous connections which lie in the submucosal space above the dentate line. There are three hemorrhoidal venous plexi. They are located in the left lateral, right anterior, and right posterior positions. During periods of high venous pressure, these veins can become engorged.

B. C. Gulack · J. M. Wolinska · S. Himidan (✉)
Division of General and Thoracic Surgery, The Hospital for Sick Children, Toronto, ON M5G1X8, Canada
e-mail: sharifa.himidan@sickkids.ca

B. C. Gulack · J. M. Wolinska · S. Himidan
Department of Medicine, University of Toronto, Toronto, ON M5S3H2, Canada

M. Lacher et al. (eds.), *Pearls and Tricks in Pediatric Surgery*,
https://doi.org/10.1007/978-3-030-51067-1_35

2. **How do patients with hemorrhoids present?**

Hemorrhoids are an extremely uncommon finding in healthy young children. About a third of children with portal hypertension are affected by anorectal varices, but these are often asymptomatic. Parents may report a "protrusion" from the anus, but it is important to differentiate hemorrhoids from other similarly presenting pathology such as rectal prolapse and rectal polyps. If hemorrhoids are symptomatic, painless hematochezia is a typical presenting symptom. Adolescents may develop hemorrhoids which present more classically like those seen in adults, including painful thrombosed external hemorrhoids or prolapsing internal hemorrhoids.

3. **How are hemorrhoids classified?**

Hemorrhoids are classified as internal or external, depending on their relation to the dentate line. Internal hemorrhoids arise from the superior hemorrhoidal plexus above the dentate line, and are insensate, while external hemorrhoids arise from the inferior hemorrhoidal plexus and have associated pain. Internal hemorrhoids can be further classified by the extent of their prolapse (Table 35.1).

4. **What are the initial treatment options for hemorrhoids?**

Hemorrhoid management depends on the etiology. In children with anorectal varices secondary to portal hypertension, treatment of the underlying hepatic pathology is necessary. In older children, hemorrhoids are likely due to prolonged constipation. Management of this should focus on increasing dietary fiber and water. Stool softeners can be used as adjuncts, but overly loose stools can aggravate symptoms. Behavioral changes such as promotion of healthy toilet habits (reduction of prolonged toilet time and avoidance of reading or using electronic devices while stooling) are encouraged. Sitz baths may help relieve symptoms.

5. **If medical management fails, what are the other options for hemorrhoid treatment?**

Internal Grade II or III hemorrhoids recalcitrant to medical management can be treated with rubber band ligation. In this procedure, a hemorrhoid banding ligator is used to launch a rubber band around the base of the hemorrhoid and results in hemorrhoidal ischemia and necrosis. It is important to avoid banding external hemorrhoids. Their location below the dentate line renders them highly sensitive

Table 35.1 Classification of internal hemorrhoids

Grade of internal hemorrhoid	Extent of prolapse
I	No prolapse outside of anal canal
II	Prolapse outside of anal canal but reduces spontaneously
III	Prolapse outside of anal canal but requires manual reduction to reduce
IV	Prolapsed outside of anal canal and cannot be reduced

and banding will cause extreme pain from the ischemia. Other techniques including injection sclerotherapy and infrared coagulation have been employed, but are less common.

Should medical management and non-operative procedures fail, surgery can be considered. The majority of hemorrhoidectomies are performed by resecting the hemorrhoidal column free from the internal anal sphincter up to its vascular pedicle, which is then ligated. Some practitioners recommend avoiding resection of more than two hemorrhoidal columns at once as this may increase the risk of anal stenosis. Stapled hemorrhoidopexy is another option, which may be less painful as the incision is kept above the dentate line; however, this approach is less popular as it is associated with a higher stricture risk.

6. **Are there any concerns practitioners should keep in mind when working up children with hemorrhoids?**

Rectal prolapse is often confused with hemorrhoids and vice versa. Rectal polyps can also mimic prolapsed internal hemorrhoids. Other rare diagnoses such as rectal hemangioma, rectal duplication and venous malformation of the anal canal can also occur. A thorough physical examination is pertinent to ensure an accurate diagnosis.

7. **Are there any long-term complications from hemorrhoid management?**

Described complications are limited to the postoperative period. Rectal stenosis from overly aggressive hemorrhoid resection, pelvic sepsis from infection, and fecal incontinence from sphincter complex injury are among these.

35.2 Anal Fissures

1. **What is an anal fissure?**

An anal fissure is a tear in the anoderm, or the squamous epithelial mucosa distal to the dentate line. Anal fissures can be painful and associated with the passage of bloody stools.

2. **At what age do anal fissures occur?**

Anal fissures most commonly occur in children at the time of introduction to solid foods. The stool consistency subsequently changes from loose and seedy, to formed. The passage of harder stools leads to the tear, subsequent pain and possible stool retention. This may result in harder and bulkier stools which worsen the tear and may prevent healing.

3. **What are the symptoms associated with anal fissures?**

Anal fissures tend to be painful, resulting in crying during defecation. Often, they are identified after finding bright red blood in the stool in small volume.

4. **How do I diagnose an anal fissure?**

Anal fissures can be diagnosed clinically. The buttocks and anoderm should be spread apart and the anus inspected. The vast majority of anal fissures are in the posterior midline.

5. **Are there medical conditions I should be concerned about when identifying an anal fissure?**

Anal fissures occurring in older children and those that are not in the midline should raise concern for inflammatory bowel disease. Anal malignancy is extremely rare in children, but should be considered in non-healing fissures in older children. Additionally, the presence of concomitant bruising or other trauma should raise concern for the possibility of non-accidental trauma.

6. **What is the medical management for anal fissures?**

The vast majority of anal fissures heal without any surgical management. The mainstay of medical management for anal fissures is relief of constipation and loosening of the stools (Fig. 35.1). Increasing water consumption and fiber intake are central to this management. Stool softeners can be helpful, but should be used cautiously since overly loose stools can aggravate the fissure. Regular sitz baths can also be helpful.

7. **If dietary changes fail, are there any non-surgical procedures that should be trialed prior to more invasive methods?**

Numerous methods have been reported to accelerate fissure healing. Topical anesthetic creams (ex EMLA), topical nitroglycerin ointments, and topical calcium channel blockers have been utilized to assist with fissure healing, however high recurrence rates have been reported.

8. **Are there surgical procedures available for anal fissures?**

If the above therapies fail, surgical options may be considered. It is important to consider alternative diagnoses among these recalcitrant fissures. Numerous

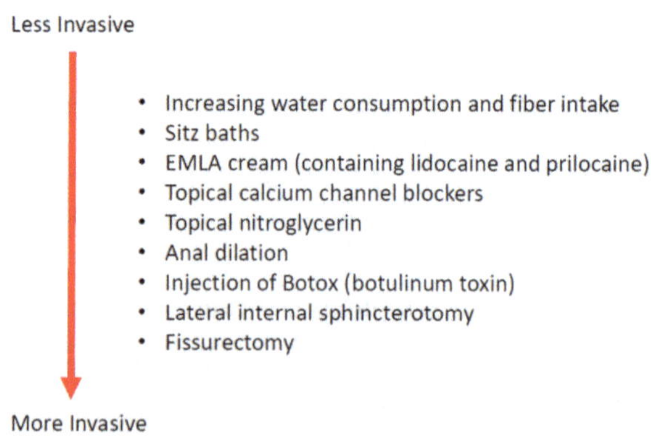

Fig. 35.1 Treatment options for anal fissure

procedures have been reported for the management of anal fissures. Anal dilation, the injection of botulinum toxin (Botox), and lateral internal sphincterotomy have all been described, but with mixed results. Botulinum toxin injections have temporary effects, with reduced risk of long-term incontinence, however lateral internal sphincterotomy has been shown to have the lowest long-term rate of recurrence. Fissurectomy, or the removal of the fissure with primary closure, has been reported with reasonable outcomes when combined with Botox to prevent recurrence.

9. **What are the complications of associated with surgical management anal fissures?**

Long-term complications are rare, mainly due to the rarity of surgical management of this disease process. Anal dilations and Botox injections can lead to temporary fecal incontinence, while lateral internal sphincterotomies can lead to long term incontinence if an aggressive sphincterotomy is performed.

35.3 Abscesses

1. **What children get perirectal abscesses?**

Abscesses are a very common benign condition in infants. Roughly 90% occur in males. Abscesses can also develop in older children, especially in those immunocompromised or with inflammatory bowel disease.

2. **How do perirectal abscesses present?**

The majority of perirectal abscesses in children occur in males under one year of age. These children tend to present with an inflamed perianal mass, which may or may not be spontaneously draining. There are usually no systemic signs of infection. However, older children and those who are immunocompromised, may present with apparent signs of systemic infection including fever and lethargy along with perirectal pain.

3. **How are perirectal abscesses classified?**

Traditionally, perirectal abscesses are grouped in four distinct categories based on location. Perianal abscesses are located near the anus and tend to be superficial. These are the most common abscesses presenting in infants. Ischiorectal abscesses occur lateral to the external sphincter complex, but superficial to the pelvic floor. Intersphincteric abscesses can be found between the internal and external sphincter and are often not visible on the skin. Lastly, supralevator abscesses extend above the levator ani.

4. **Are there any disease processes associated with perirectal abscesses?**

Perirectal abscesses are most commonly benign and not associated with other disease processes, but certain children are at higher risk for recurrent abscesses.

Children with perirectal Crohn's disease can present with chronic abscesses and fistulae. It is important to note that these children are managed uniquely and practitioners should always consider this diagnosis in children with recurrent, intractable disease. Additionally, children with immunocompromised states (e.g. diabetes, treatment with steroids, chemotherapy) have a higher incidence of perirectal abscesses.

5. **Do perirectal abscesses need to be aspirated or drained?**

Management of perirectal abscesses has changed over the past few years. Traditionally, drainage of the abscess was common, but recent literature has shown that abscess incision and drainage may be associated with a higher rate of fistula formation. Therefore, in children who are not systemically ill, treatment with antibiotics, warm compresses/sitz baths, and observation is recommended. If large, abscess aspiration can also be entertained. Caution is urged when considering incision and drainage among children with inflammatory bowel disease as these children are also at high risk for fistula formation; however this should not be a contraindication in children who are systemically ill.

6. **If I elect to perform an incision and drainage, should I investigate for concomitant fistula-in-ano?**

Attempts to probe for a fistula in an inflamed field may lead to inadvertent "false tracking" or sphincter injury and therefore should be avoided. Furthermore, many fistulae will heal spontaneously and further intervention may not be necessary.

7. **If I perform an incision and drainage on a perirectal abscess, does the child require antibiotics? Should I pack the wound?**

Antibiotics may not be necessary after incision and drainage unless the child has systemic signs of infection, or is immunosuppressed. However, recent data have demonstrated that empiric antibiotic coverage may reduce the incidence of persistent fistula-in-ano after healing. Following incision and drainage, many practitioners leave packing in the wound to be removed between 24 and 72 h afterwards. This can help with hemostasis but is not necessary and can make postoperative care more complicated and uncomfortable. Children may return with recurrent abscesses due to retained packing. An alternative option is to make two counter-incisions in the abscess and pass a vessel loop or surgical tie through the incisions to allow drainage, with removal at a later date.

8. **What is the appropriate follow-up for patients treated for peri-rectal abscesses?**

Infants with simple perianal abscesses likely do not need surgical follow-up, but should be seen by their pediatricians within a short interval of time. Children who present with recurrent abscesses, or have other concerning signs or symptoms should undergo a more thorough work-up for underlying causes (e.g. immunosuppressed state or inflammatory bowel disease).

35.4 Fistulae

1. **What is fistula-in-ano?**

Fistula-in-ano is an abnormal connection from the anal crypt to the peripheral skin. In children, these often arise from crypts proximal to the dentate line, and travel in a straight line subcutaneously. They may involve the sphincter complex.

2. **What is Goodsall's rule?**

Goodsall's rule describes the expected route of a fistula-in-ano from the skin to the anal canal depending on the location of the fistula on the skin. Anterior fistulae tend to travel in a straight linc and have an internal opening in a similar radial location, while posterior fistulae can travel in a curvilinear manner, having an internal opening in the posterior midline (Fig. 35.2). Longer fistulae, and fistulae associated with inflammatory bowel disease may not conform to this generalization.

3. **How are fistulae categorized?**

Fistulae are traditionally described by Park's classification, which classifies the fistula based on its location with the sphincter muscle complex. Fistulae involving only a portion of the inferior sphincter complex are termed transphincteric, and are among the most common. Intersphincteric fistulae travel through the internal sphincter, and then travel to the skin through the intersphincteric space. Suprasphincteric fistula travel above the sphincter complex, and extrasphincteric fistula travel from higher in the rectum and are usually the result of trauma, however these are much rarer.

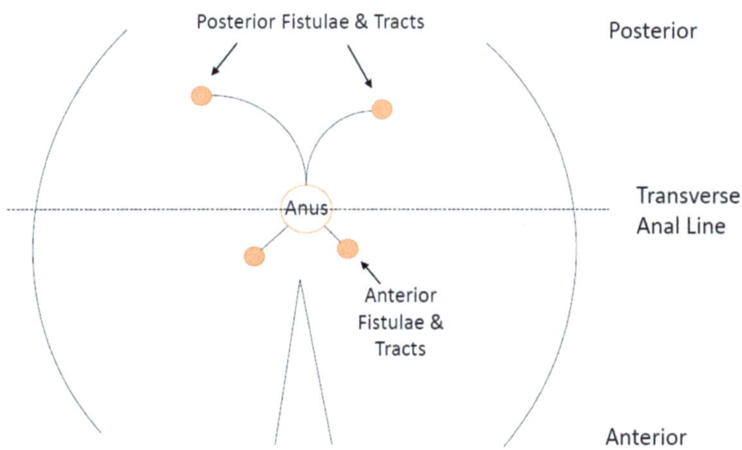

Fig. 35.2 Figure depicting Goodsall's rule

4. **Are fistulae benign or associated with other diseases?**

As with perirectal abscesses, fistulae in children tend to be a benign, self-healing processes. Weight loss, recurrence, multiple fistulae, and those that do not follow Goodsall's rule should raise concern for inflammatory bowel disease or other disease processes.

5. **Which fistulae require intervention?**

The vast majority of fistulae in children, especially in infants, will close spontaneously. Fistulae that fail to close spontaneously should be considered for operative intervention. Fistulae secondary to inflammatory bowel disease should have an attempt at medical management primarily.

6. **Is there any work-up that should be performed prior to intervention?**

Children with straightforward fistulae and no warning signs for other disease processes do not need other work-up prior to undergoing operative intervention. Children with signs or symptoms concerning for inflammatory bowel disease or immunosuppression should have further work-up. Magnetic resonance elastography (MRE) of the pelvis can be very useful in helping to define the location and type of fistulae.

7. **What are the options for surgical intervention for fistulae and how do I decide which to use?**

There are multiple options available for management of a fistula, depending on the depth of the fistula and its involvement with the sphincter. Superficial fistulas which do not involve a substantial amount of the sphincter complex can be managed with fistulotomy alone. This involves identification of the fistula and opening of the fistula along its entire tract. This procedure should not be performed in patients with Crohn's disease due to poor healing. If a substantial portion of the sphincter complex is involved, most surgeons opt for placement of a seton in order to spare the sphincter. The loose seton helps drainage and granulation and can be removed at a later date if it does not fall out spontaneously.

There are additional procedures available, but these are rarely used in the pediatric population, with a few reports in teenagers. They include endorectal and dermal advancement flaps, fibrin sealant, fistula plugs, and ligation of the intersphincteric fistula (LIFT) procedure. Fibrin sealants and fistula plugs are traditionally utilized after a seton has been used for a short time period, and after curetting and debriding the fistula. The LIFT procedure is a more modern procedure for management of transphincteric fistulae and involves dissection of the intersphincteric space and ligation of the fistula tract within this space.

8. **If I place a seton in a fistula, when and how should this be followed?**

Most surgeons perform a follow-up exam under anesthesia around 6-12 weeks after the initial procedure to evaluate the fistula tract and consider seton removal.

References

1. Afşarlar CE, Karaman A, Tanır G, et al. Perianal abscess and fistula-in-ano in children: clinical characteristic, management and outcome. Pediatr Surg Int. 2011;27(10):1063–8.
2. Charalampopoulos A, Zavras N, Kapetanakis EL, et al. surgical treatment of perianal abscess and fistula-in-ano in childhood, with emphasis in children older than 2 years. J Pediatr Surg. 2012;47(11):2096–100.
3. Jamshidi R. Anorectal complaints, hemorrhoids, fissures, abscesses. Fistulae. Clin Colon Rectal Surg. 2018;31(2):117–20.
4. Joda AE, Al-Mayoof AF. Efficacy of nitroglycerine ointment in the treatment of pediatric anal fissure. J Pediatr Surg. 2017;52(11):1782–6.
5. Piazza DJ, Radhakrishnan J. Perianal abscess and fistula-in-ano in children. Dis Colon Rectum. 1990;33(12):1014–6.
6. Stties T, Lund DP. Common anorectal problems. Semın Pediatr Surg. 2007;16(1):71–8.

Chapter 36
Biliary Atresia

Federico Scottoni and Mark Davenport

Abstract Biliary Atresia (BA) is the most common surgical cause of conjugated jaundice in infancy, and consists of a progressive inflammatory destruction and obliteration of variable lengths of the biliary tract. If left untreated it leads to liver failure and death within few months. It is best treated by an attempt at restoration of bile flow from the native liver by excision of the extrahepatic bile ducts and reconstruction using a jejunal Roux loop (Kasai portoenterostomy). With this clearance of jaundice of 50–60% can be achieved in large centres with appropriate adjuvant therapy. Failure to clear jaundice or onset of complications such as recurrent cholangitis, ascites and recurrent bleeding from variceal formation are indications for liver transplantation.

Keywords Biliary atresia · Liver transplantation · Kasai portoenterostomy

36.1 Introduction

1. **What is biliary atresia?**

Biliary atresia (BA) is unique to the neonatal period and first described by the Scottish paediatrician John Thomson in 1892. It is the most common surgical cause of conjugated jaundice in infancy, and consists of a progressive inflammatory destruction and obliteration of variable lengths of the biliary tract. If left untreated it leads to liver failure and death within few months. A comprehensive aetiology for BA has not been exhaustively formulated yet. Nevertheless, it is clear that the pathogenesis of the disease includes both a mechanical obliteration and in some a destructive inflammatory process of the bile ducts [1].

F. Scottoni · M. Davenport (✉)
Department of Pediatric Surgery, Kings College Hospital, Denmark Hill,
London SE5 9RS, UK
e-mail: markdav2@ntlworld.com

M. Lacher et al. (eds.), *Pearls and Tricks in Pediatric Surgery*,
https://doi.org/10.1007/978-3-030-51067-1_36

2. **What is the incidence of BA?**

It varies across the globe with relatively high incidence in Taiwan, mainland China and Japan of 1 in 5–10,000 live births to 1 in 15–20,000 in North America and Europe.

3. **What classifications are in use for BA?**
Phenotypic classification

This classification is based on objective features and represents a useful tool for the clinical assessment and management of the patients. It is possible to recognise four main groups [2].

1. **Syndromic BA (10% of European and North America, much rarer in China)**
   a. **BA splenic malformation (BASM) syndrome**—Association of BA, splenic anomalies (i.e. polysplenia or asplenia), vascular anomalies (e.g. preduodenal portal vein and absence of vena cava), situs inversus and cardiac anomalies. Related to maternal diabetes. Some have *PKD1L1* mutations.
   b. **Cat eye syndrome**—BA and coloboma (defect of iris), anorectal malformations and cardiac anomalies. Due to chromosome 22 aneuploidy.
   c. Other more common congenital anomalies such as esophageal atresia, jejunal atresia and cardiac malformations can be associated with BA without a defined syndromic picture.
2. **Cystic BA (5–10%)**
   a. Characterized by an extrahepatic cyst formation in an otherwise obliterated biliary tract. Larger examples can be detected antenatally with ultrasonography.
   b. This type may be easily confused with an obstructed choledochal malformation, the differential is intraoperative and demonstrable on cholangiography. If mucus is obtained puncturing the cyst, that is a confirmation of BA. Cholangiogram may show dilating intrahepatic ducts characteristic of a choledochal malformation.
3. **Cytomegalovirus associated BA (10–20%—marked worldwide variation)**

This is defined by serology (IgM+ve). These infants are often associated with a later presentation and more deranged biochemical markers and a greater degrees of liver inflammation and fibrosis. Effectiveness of Kasai portoenterostomy (KPE) and overall survival are also poor in these patients. This has been negated by specific adjuvant anti-viral therapy (e.g. ganciclovir) in some studies.

4. **Isolated BA**

This is the largest group of patients, with heterogeneous features in terms of response to surgical management and prognosis.

Anatomical Classification

The most common anatomical classification, based on the Japanese Association of Pediatric Surgeons, divides BA in 3 categories based on the level of biliary obstruction (Fig. 36.1).

- Type 1: obstruction at the level of CBD (5–10%), often associated with cyst.
- Type 2: at the level of the CHD (rare)
- Type 3: at level of porta hepatis.

1. **How do children with BA present?**

The invariable triad of symptoms in infants with BA consists of jaundice, dark urine and pale, acholic stool. These signs are usually present from birth, while hepatosplenomegaly and ascites secondary to portal hypertension are usually later developments. Some may also have a coagulopathy secondary to vitamin K malabsorption and present with bleeding.

2. **How do you diagnose BA in infants with jaundice?**

The key biochemical differentiation is to determine whether there is an elevated conjugated (aka direct) bilirubin. All surgical causes have this. Most medical causes including "physiological jaundice" are predominantly unconjugated.

The differential diagnoses of "surgical jaundice" are: BA, choledocal malformations, inspissated bile syndrome and spontaneous perforation of the bile duct.

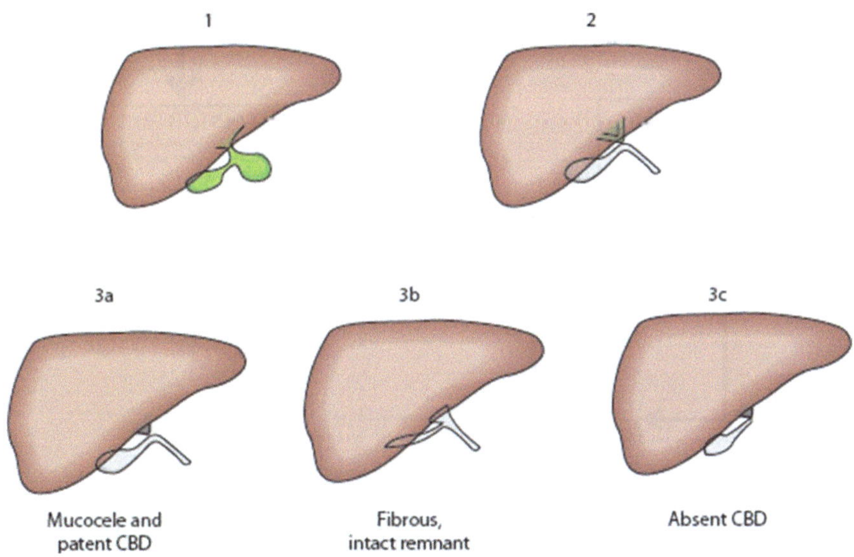

Fig. 36.1 Anatomical classification of BA. [Taken from Davenport M (2017) Biliary atresia. In: Davenport M, Heaton N and Superina R Surgery of the liver, bile ducts and pancreas in children, 3rd edn. CRC Press, London, pp. 71–86, with permission]

Ultrasonography should enable a more precise diagnosis showing intrahepatic duct dilation in all of these except for BA. An algorithm (Fig. 36.2) is suggested to lead to definitive pre-laparotomy diagnosis of BA. Although percutaneous liver biopsy is widespread, others simply opt for on-table laparoscopy or cholangiography. ERCP is certainly possible in infancy albeit uncommonly performed.

3. **What is the current treatment for BA?**

Most infants with BA should have an attempt at restoring bile flow and abbreviating the liver damage. The standard operation is termed Kasai portoenterostomy (KPE), but actually details of technique vary from surgeon to surgeon.

Age at KPE is important and delay is detrimental, but formerly held cut-offs values were simply naïve. Nevertheless, beyond 100 days of age outcome suffers. Late-presenting infants in this category may be considered for primary liver transplant certainly if cirrhotic features are obvious.

4. **What is a Kasai portoenterostomy?**

This was developed in the 1950s and 60 s in Japan by Morio Kasai and consists of excision of all apparently solid proximal bile duct remnants and Roux loop reconstruction to the denuded porta hepatis. The length of the Roux limb is typically 40 cm. Variations in the form of the creation of stomas in the loop are no longer done. Frozen section of the resected part is also redundant as the principle idea of

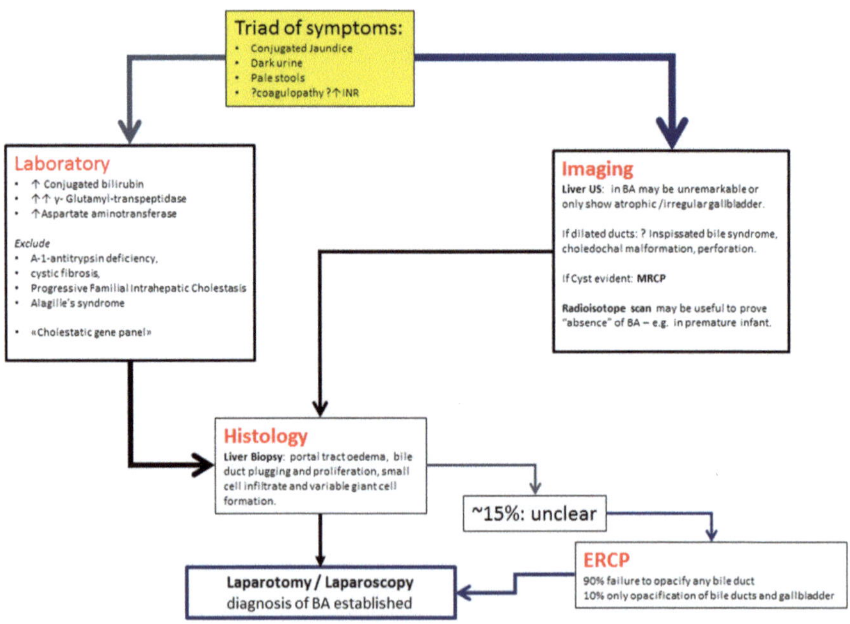

Fig. 36.2 Suitable diagnosis algorithm in infants with conjugated jaundice—as used at Kings College Hospital

a radical resection is to excise every visible part of the biliary tract, leaving nothing behind.

Beyond using the laparoscope for diagnosis, it is possible to perform a laparoscopic approximation of a KPE [3]. Nonetheless, the only large series have been from China and Japan and caution is advised. There is certainly no advantage, unless it is to the transplant surgeon later on!

Technical tips

- An on-table diagnosis should be clear as mostly the gallbladder is either full of clear mucus or so atrophic that a lumen can't be found to do a cholangiogram. Bile in an intact gallbladder implies it is not BA or if it is, it is Type 1 and then a cyst should be visible.
- In case of situs inversus the operator should be on the left side.
- In case of malrotation, extra-care has to be placed in forming the Roux loop to avoid mesenteric defects which might predispose to an internal hernia. Obviously, it can no longer be retrocolic, if a Ladd's procedure is also contemplated.
- The presence of portal hypertension can be challenging. Bipolar diathermy is the main hemostatic tool; however, this should not be applied to the transected portal plate in order to avoid bile ductule damage. Pressure or hemostatic material should suffice. Furthermore, full-thickness sutures or staples may be recommended for the jejuno-jejunal anastomosis.

1. **How are infants managed in the post-operative period?**

Prophylactic post-operative intravenous antibiotics should reflect the local microbiological policy. Some centers continue oral antibiotics for months after though the evidence in prevention of cholangitis is weak.

The use of more specific therapy is controversial [4]. High-dose steroids (≈4–5 mg/kg/day prednisolone) are widely prescribed, certainly outside of North America. The START randomized placebo controlled trial was equivocal, but underpowered to show a "significant" difference (though there was one of 15%) [5]. Ursodeoxycholic acid is less controversial, but has no evidence base. Anti-viral adjuvant therapy should be considered for those infants who are CMV IgM+ve.

2. **What complication can occur after KPE?**

KPE may be completely futile and not change the level of jaundice or pigment in their stool. Primary non-responders will need transplant consideration before 1–2 years of age. Other more specific complications may occur after KPE, including:

Cholangitis

Ascending bacterial cholangitis is described in up to 50% of the patients, usually within 2 years after KPE, then the risk diminishes. Gram negative bacteria are usually responsible and should be the target for appropriate antibiotics (e.g. meropenem, gentamicin, piperacillin-tazobactam). Clinically it presents with worsening jaundice, fever, rising inflammatory markers and altered biochemical liver function.

Portal Hypertension

Portal venous pressure is raised in >70% of infants at the time of KPE. Nevertheless, initial values correlate poorly with outcome, even development of varices. This implies that the formation of varices depends on the evolution of the fibrotic liver process following KPE rather than the condition of the liver at the time of the surgery. Endoscopic surveillance suggests endoscopically evident varices are present in 60% of patients, of which maybe half will bleed.

Acute bleeding should be treated medically at first with vasopressin or somatostatin analogues. In severe bleeding, a Sengstaken tube may have to be inserted as an emergency procedure. Endoscopic management includes banding in older children and adults while sclerotherapy is still the treatment of choice in infants.

Patients where gastrointestinal bleeding is associated with worsening liver function need evaluation for transplant.

Ascites

Ascites is often a consequence of portal hypertension but other features related to liver failure maybe involved (i.e. hypoalbuminemia and hyponatremia). Low salt diet and fluid balance management, including diuretics, are the first-line treatment. Persistent ascites may simply reflect end-stage liver failure and consideration of transplant.

Inguinal hernias

There is a higher incidence of these than the normal population possibly caused by ascites and increased abdominal pressure.

1. **What factors affect outcome?**

   - The state of the native liver is a key but not invariable prognostic factor. However, only cirrhosis is really detrimental and we lack real histological precision in defining this.
   - Increasing age is certainly detrimental but realistically only if >80 days or the BA is clearly developmental (BASM and cystic BA).
   - BA with associated anomalies has a worse outcome though whether this is because of the association with cardiac anomalies or it has an intrinsically worse outcome is not known.
   - Type 1 BA and Cystic BA have the best outcome.
   - Who does the operation. This is a rare disease and the porta hepatis is unfamiliar territory to most pediatric surgeons. Centralization of resources for this disease has been adopted in many countries outside North America (e.g. UK, Finland, Netherlands).

2. **What are the key outcome measures?**

- Median age at KPE—this reflects how quickly infants are referred in and delays in diagnosis—it should be 50–60 days;
- Proportion to clear jaundice after KPE (to normal levels <20 μmol/L or <1.5 mg/dL)—it should be >50% and values of >60–70% are possible;
- Native liver and true survival at 5 and 10 years. The former should be 45–50% with little change by 10 years, the second reflects the ease of access to safe transplantation [6].

References

1. Davenport M. Biliary Atresia: clinical aspect. Semin Pediatr Surg. 2012;21:175–84.
2. Davenport M. Biliary atresia. Davenport M, Heaton N and Superina R Surgery of the liver, bile ducts and pancreas in children. 3rd ed. London: CRC Press; 2017. p. 71–86.
3. Lishuang M, Zhen C, Guoliang Q, et al. Laparoscopic portoenterostomy versus open portoenterostomy for the treatment of biliary atresia: a systematic review and meta-analysis of comparative studies. Pediatr Surg Int. 2015;31:261–9.
4. Davenport M. Adjuvant therapy in biliary atresia: hopelessly optimistic or potential for change? Pediatr Surg Int. 2017;33:1263–73.
5. Bezerra JA, Spino C, Magee JC, et al. Use of corticosteroids after hepatoportoenterostomy for bile drainage in infants with biliary atresia: the START randomized clinical trial. JAMA. 2014;311:1750–9.
6. Davenport M, Ong E, Sharif K, et al. Biliary atresia in England and Wales: results of centralization and new benchmark. J Pediatr Surg. 2011;46:1689–94.

Chapter 37
Choledochal Cyst

Omid Madadi-Sanjani and Claus Petersen

Abstract Choledochal cysts are congenital, cystic dilatations of the biliary tree that can occur with an incidence of approximately 1:100,000–1:150,000 in the Western hemisphere and a reported incidence of 1:1,000 in the Asian population. The majority of patients with choledochal cysts remain asymptomatic and diagnosis is made due to an incidental finding. Only a minority presents with clinical signs of jaundice/obstruction, cholangitis/pancreatitis, or an acute abdomen due to secondary complications. Diagnostics include abdominal ultrasound and blood tests, an MRCP can further specify the anatomy if necessary and in cases of acute obstruction an ERCP with stenting is required. Choledochal cysts are premalignant conditions; therefore, the therapy consists of a complete choledochal cyst excision, early after diagnosis. This can be performed using "open" or "laparoscopic" surgery. The reconstruction afterwards includes a biliodigestive anastomosis, which can be either a hepatico-jejunostomy with a Roux-en-Y loop, or a hepatico-duodenostomy. Currently, there is no evidence for the superiority of any of these techniques. After choledochal cyst excision the lifetime risk for malignancies is reduced, but recent data suggest a lifelong elevated risk of up to 11% of cancer development even following operation. Therefore, lifelong follow-ups are necessary.

Keywords Choledochal cyst · Malformation · Pancreatobiliary maljunction · Premalignant condition · Cyst excision · Hepatico-jejunostomy · Hepatico-duodenostomy

O. Madadi-Sanjani (✉) · C. Petersen
Center of Pediatric Surgery, Hannover Medical School, Carl-Neuberg-Street 1, 30625 Hannover, Germany
e-mail: madadi-sanjani.omid@mh-hannover.de

M. Lacher et al. (eds.), *Pearls and Tricks in Pediatric Surgery*,
https://doi.org/10.1007/978-3-030-51067-1_37

1. **What are choledochal cysts?**

Choledochal cysts are rare congenital, cystic dilatations of the biliary tree that can occur anywhere between the duodenum and the intrahepatic bile ducts [1]. The etiology of this condition is still unknown. The first anatomical description was made in 1723 by the German anatomist and botanist Abraham Vater (1684–1751), who is also known for the ampulla of Vater and Lamellar corpuscles. Golder Lewis McWhorter (1888–1938) was the first surgeon to report on the surgical "cure" of a 49-year-old lady with choledochal cyst at the Presbyterian Hospital in Chicago/USA in 1924.

2. **What is the common classification for choledochal cysts?**

Todani classification. It was introduced in 1977 by Takuji Todani at the Department of Surgery/University Medical School in Okayama, Japan. Since then it has been modified, including information on the location and appearance of the choledochal dilatation (e.g. isolated or disseminated cysts) [Lee et al., Korean J Radiol. 2009 Jan-Feb;10(1):71–80)].

Type I: saccular/diffuse fusiform dilatation of common bile duct, typically inferior to the confluence of the left and right hepatic ducts (the most common type)
Type II: diverticulum of the common bile duct
Type III: intraduodenal dilatation of the common bile duct
Type IV: multiple cysts of the intra- or extrahepatic bile ducts (or both)
Type V: single or multiple intrahepatic cysts

3. **What is the common channel?**

The common channel describes the unification of the common bile duct and the pancreatic duct. In the majority of choledochal cysts, this unification already appears outside the duodenal wall, called pancreatobiliary maljunction and leading to a "long" common channel [Kamisawa T et al. (2017), J Gastroenterol., Feb;52(2):158–163].

4. **What are "forme fruste choledochal cysts"?**

The term "forme fruste" was introduced by John R Lilly of the Children's Hospital Denver in 1985, describing a stenosis of the distal common bile duct of unknown origin, with a "long common channel" and classical histopathological features of choledochal cysts (in the common bile duct wall). In the majority of cases the minimal (or nonexistent) dilatation of the extrahepatic bile duct and the pancreaticobiliary maljunction are present at first admission, without signs of stones, tumor, or inflammation.

5. **How common are choledochal cysts?**

The incidence of choledochal cysts is approximately 1:100,000–1:150,000 in the Western hemisphere, with high geographical variations and a reported incidence of 1:1,000 in the Asian population. While the majority is diagnosed during childhood, in some patients the diagnosis is delayed until adulthood. Higher numbers are expected, due to the fact that many patients remain undiagnosed during their lifetime.

6. **How do patients with choledochal cysts usually present?**

The majority of patients with choledochal cysts remain asymptomatic and diagnosis is made due to an incidental finding. Only a minority presents with clinical signs of jaundice/obstruction, cholangitis/pancreatitis, or an acute abdomen due to secondary complications. Recently, prenatal ultrasound diagnosis was reported.

7. **What are the possible complications of choledochal cysts?**

Choledocholithiasis and hepatolithiasis, leading to bile duct obstruction, jaundice, cholangitis, cholecystitis, pancreatic reflux and pancreatitis, and sepsis. Ascending cholangitis is a suspected carcinogen for malignant transformation of the cyst. Cyst rupture and peritonitis are rare complications of choledochal cysts.

8. **How does the diagnostic workup for suspected choledochal cyst look like?**

The diagnostic workup includes serologic markers for inflammation, cholestasis as well as imaging by sonography, CT scan, hepatobiliary scintigraphy with Technetium 99 (HIDA), MRCP, or ERCP (Figs. 37.1 and 37.2). Apart from an abdominal ultrasound, imaging in the typical age group of the patients has the disadvantage of a general anesthesia or sedation. In large centers an abdominal ultrasound is the only preoperative imaging needed. An MRCP can be added in unclear cases. ERCP and potential stenting are mainly reserved for patients with acute biliary obstruction.

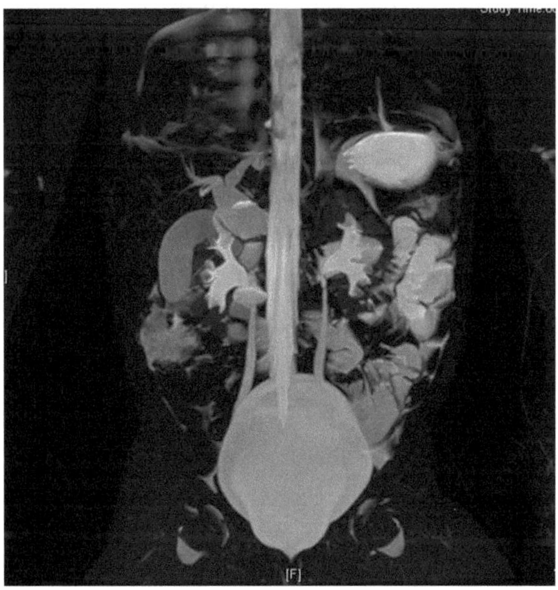

Fig. 37.1 MRCP demonstrating saccular dilatation of the common bile duct

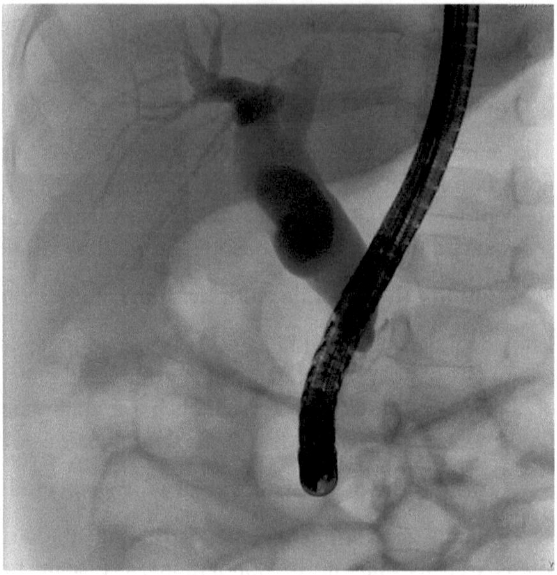

Fig. 37.2 ERCP demonstrating saccular dilatation of the common bile duct

9. **What is the most common complication following ERCPs?**

Acute pancreatitis, which occurs in approximately 5% of cases after ERCP. Less common complications include bleeding after sphincterotomy, duodenal perforation, and retroperitoneal abscesses.

10. **What is the treatment of choledochal cysts?**

Surgery with complete cyst excision. Based on preoperative imaging and classification, this may include cyst excision and hepatic resections. In rare cases with involvement of the pancreatic duct, a Whipple procedure needs to be considered.

11. **What is the best timing of surgery?**

Shortly after diagnosis, from three months of age onwards. If diagnosed during an inflammatory episode, broad-spectrum antibiotics should be given first followed by surgery after an inflammatory-free interval of 6–8 weeks.

12. **What is the major risk if a child with choledochal cyst is left untreated?**

Patients with untreated choledochal cysts have an increased risk of cholangiocarcinoma and gallbladder carcinoma. While cases of malignant transformation during childhood are extremely rare, the lifetime carcinoma risk in adults with untreated choledochal cysts is 6–30%, increasing with age. Furthermore, patients have a high risk of hepatolithiasis, recurrent cholangitis, and pancreatitis.

13. **What is Caroli's disease and how is it treated?**

Caroli's disease is a rare congenital condition with non-obstructive dilatation of the intrahepatic ducts, which can be localized in one hepatic lobe or disseminated all over the intrahepatic bile ducts. Based on the localization an (extended) hepatectomy in unilateral appearance and liver transplantation in bilateral, disseminated cases have been described [Lee HK, et al. (2009), Korean J Radiol., Jan–Feb; 10(1):71–80].

14. **What are surgical approaches to choledochal cyst excision?**

Choledochal cyst excisions can be performed by laparotomy or laparoscopy [2]. Based on the current literature, none of the approaches is superior. However, recent studies suggest that children undergoing laparoscopic cyst excision have longer operating times, less intraoperative bleeding (and blood transfusions), shorter hospital stay, and faster recovery.

15. **Is complete cyst excision always feasible?**

Any operation should always aim to excise the cyst completely. However, in some cases the cyst can expand into the porta hepatis, the head of the pancreas, or the duodenum. The extent of the resection then needs to be determined by the surgeon as remnants of the cyst predispose to malignancies.

Furthermore, in patients with recurrent inflammation prior to surgery, the cyst can be adherent the fragile tissues surrounding it. In these cases, the risk of vascular injury is increased. Whenever the decision for incomplete cyst excision is made, the surgeon should resect as much of the biliary epithelium as possible.

16. **Which anatomic reconstructions are performed following cyst excision?**

Hepatico-jejunostomy with a Roux-en-Y loop or hepatico-duodenostomy. Based on the lack of comparative studies in the current literature, none of the techniques is superior [3, 4]. However, recent studies suggest that while the frequency of postoperative bile leaks and anastomotic strictures are equivalent using both techniques, the rates of cholangitis and biliary reflux are higher following hepatico-duodenostomy. Cholecystectomy is always part of the operation.

17. **Is there any indication for cysto-enteric drainage?**

No. While cysto-enteric drainage was performed in the past, a complete cyst excision needs to be achieved according to the current consensus.

18. **What are the intraoperative complications of choledochal cyst excisions?**

Major intraoperative complications include bleeding, intraoperative cyst perforation, and narrowing of the pancreatic duct. Furthermore, all surrounding tissue/organs—especially the hepatoduodenal ligament should be handled with great caution.

19. **What are postoperative complications following choledochal cyst excisions?**

The most important postoperative complication is a bile leak or stricture of the biliodigestive anastomosis with recurrent episodes of cholangitis. In addition, postoperative anastomotic leaks of enteric anastomosis, fluid collections (hematoma, biloma, abscess), peritonitis, sepsis, bleedings, hepatolithiasis, biliary reflux, and pancreatitis can occur [5].

20. **Is there a potential postoperative risk of malignancies?**

After choledochal cyst excision the lifetime risk for malignancies is reduced significantly. However, recent data suggest a lifelong elevated risk of up to 11% of a local malignancy even following operation [6].

21. **Are postoperative follow-ups necessary?**

Due to the persistent risk of malignancies, even following cyst excision, lifelong follow-ups are necessary including transition to adult gastroenterology. For adults, a yearly abdominal ultrasound including measurement of CA19-9 are recommended.

References

1. Soares KC, Goldstein SD, Ghaseb MA, Kamel I, Hackam DJ, Pawlik TM. Pediatric choledochal cysts: diagnosis and current management. Pediatr Surg Int. 2017;33(6):637–50.
2. Shen H-J, Xu M, Zhu H-Y, Yang C, Li F, Li K, et al. Laparoscopic versus open surgery in children with choledochal cysts: a meta-analysis. Pediatr Surg Int. 2015;31(6):529–34.
3. Narayanan SK, Chen Y, Narasimhan KL, Cohen RC. Hepaticoduodenostomy versus hepaticojejunostomy after resection of choledochal cyst: a systematic review and meta-analysis. J Pediatr Surg. 2013;48(11):2336–42.
4. Santore MT, Behar BJ, Blinman TA, Doolin EJ, Hedrick HL, Mattei P, et al. Hepaticoduodenostomy vs hepaticojejunostomy for reconstruction after resection of choledochal cyst. J Pediatr Surg. 2011;46(1):209–13.
5. Grisotti G, Cowles RA. Complications in pediatric hepatobiliary surgery. Semin Pediatr Surg. 2016;25(6):388–94.
6. Ohashi T, Wakai T, Kubota M, Matsuda Y, Arai Y, Ohyama T, et al. Risk of subsequent biliary malignancy in patients undergoing cyst excision for congenital choledochal cysts. J Gastroenterol Hepatol. 2013;28(2):243–7.

Chapter 38
Pediatric Gallbladder Disease

Anna Elizabeth West and Matthew SClifton

Abstract Pediatric gallstone disease is on the rise in the United States, for two main reasons. First, improved diagnostic tools including high-resolution ultrasound have made the detection of small stones more readily apparent. Secondly, dietary changes have led to an increased incidence of cholesterol stones. Additionally, improved survival in the neonatal population, many of whom are maintained on parenteral nutrition for an extended period of time, has led to pathophysiology previously seen in very limited instances. Laparoscopic cholecystectomy remains the standard operation of choice for patients requiring surgical extirpation of the gallbladder alone. Regional variation in expertise dictates the management of choledocholithiasis using either laparoscopic common bile duct exploration or endoscopic retrograde cholangiopancreatography.

Keywords Gallbladder · Cholelithiasis · Cholecystitis · Choledocholithiasis · Cholangitis · Cholangiogram · Dyskinesia

1. **Describe the typical history and physical exam of a child presenting with acute cholecystitis.**

The classic history and physical exam of a patient with acute cholecystitis includes right upper quadrant pain associated with nausea and possibly fever. Older children and adolescents may provide additional details such as pain following ingestion of a fatty meal. However, younger children may manifest simply with decreased oral intake and dehydration. In infants, the development of jaundice following an illness or TPN use may be the first clues to gallbladder disease. Co-morbid conditions (described below) can increase the clinical suspicion for acute cholecystitis [1].

A. E. West · M. SClifton (✉)
Department of Surgery, Emory University/Children's Healthcare of Atlanta, 3rd Floor, Surgical Services, 1405 Clifton Road NE, Atlanta, GA 30322, USA
e-mail: mclifto@emory.edu

M. Lacher et al. (eds.), *Pearls and Tricks in Pediatric Surgery*,
https://doi.org/10.1007/978-3-030-51067-1_38

2. **What laboratory tests and imaging would you order to evaluate a child with right upper quadrant pain?**

CBC to evaluate for evidence of infection/inflammation. Chemistry to assess hydration status and electrolyte imbalances. Transaminases and bilirubin to determine if there is an obstructive component. Elevated direct bilirubin raises the concern for choledocholithiasis. Right upper quadrant ultrasound to evaluate for the presence of gallstones, sludge, peri-cholecystic fluid, gallbladder wall thickening, or biliary ductal dilatation.

3. **What are the causes of acute cholecystitis?**

   a. Acalculous: often occurs in the setting of severe illness/sepsis, lack of enteral feeding, and utilization of TPN. Since the gallbladder is not subjected to the hormonal impulses stimulating contraction, biliary stasis ensues. This, when combined with gallbladder distension and a low flow state, are a set up for infection.
   b. Calculous

      i. Hemolytic: This was previously the most common cause of cholelithiasis in the pediatric population, producing pigmented stones due to increased serum levels of unconjugated bilirubin. Pediatric patients with sickle cell disease and concurrent gallbladder sludge or cholelithiasis should be considered for elective cholecystectomy with appropriate pre-operative hydration to prevent peri-operative sickle cell crisis [1].
      ii. Non-hemolytic: The pathophysiology of non-hemolytic cholelithiasis in the pediatric population resembles that in adults, with cholesterol stone formation in association with obesity and estrogen exposure. Other lithogenic factors include conditions predisposing to gallbladder stasis, decreased enterohepatic circulation of bile (ileal resection, prolonged lack of enteral nutrition, TPN) or systemic illness. The incidence of non-hemolytic cholelithiasis has increased in incidence over time in children [3].

4. **Which pediatric patients are at increased risk of developing acute cholecystitis?**

Those with short gut/intestinal failure, history of severely prematurity, hemolytic diseases (sickle cell, hereditary spherocytosis, cystic fibrosis, obesity, and metabolic syndrome [1–3].

5. **What is the treatment for cholelithiasis and acute cholecystitis?**

The standard surgical treatment for both symptomatic cholelithiasis and acute cholecystitis is laparoscopic cholecystectomy. In acute cholecystitis, the patient should first be fluid resuscitated and given intravenous antibiotics [1–3].

6. **What are the important anatomical structures to identify during a laparoscopic cholecystectomy?**

The gallbladder is first grasped at the fundus and retracted cephalad. It is important to establish the “critical view of safety,” by retracting the infundibulum laterally. This allows the surgeon to visualize the infundibulum joining with the cystic duct and deflects these structures away from the common bile duct, which is located more posteriorly. This view allows easy access to the cystic artery. Important anatomic considerations in this area include the Triangle of Calot, which is bordered by the cystic duct, the common bile duct and the inferior edge of the liver; however, the common bile duct is often not exposed during the operation [4].

7. **What are the most common complications of the surgical treatment for acute cholecystitis? How are they managed?**

   a. Bile duct injury: if recognized during the time of operation, bile duct reconstruction with roux-en-Y hepaticojejunostomy is typically the operation of choice. If recognized post-operatively, percutaneous drainage of the biloma, decompression of the biliary tree, and delineation of the anatomy should be performed in order to determine the next step for operative reconstruction.
   b. Bleeding: The most commonly injured artery during the operation is the right hepatic artery. If recognized at the time of operation this should be addressed by either repair or ligation (if repair proves impossible). Post-operative hemorrhage is most often from the cystic artery. This, or the right hepatic artery, can be embolized with interventional radiology if necessary.
   c. Bile leak: Usually from a displaced clip off of the cystic duct stump. This is treated with ERCP with sphincterotomy and/or stent placement to provide a path of least resistance for bile to flow allowing the stump to heal [3].

8. **Describe the symptoms, physical exam and laboratory findings for a child with a stone is in their common bile duct.**

If a stone escapes the gallbladder and becomes lodged in the common bile duct, this is referred to as choledocholithiasis. If this is associated with obstruction that leads to infection it is referred to as ascending cholangitis. The presentation is similar to that for acute cholecystitis, however the child frequently has associated jaundice. Laboratory findings are notable for elevation of the transaminases, total and direct bilirubin due to obstruction of the common bile duct.

9. **What is the treatment for choledocholithiasis and cholangitis?**

Choledocholithiasis alone can be managed with either laparoscopic cholecystectomy and common bile duct exploration or ERCP followed by laparoscopic cholecystectomy in the same hospitalization. There are pros and cons of each treatment approach, but ultimately the decision relies on the regional expertise of the surgeon and the interventional gastroenterology team [3].

Ascending cholangitis should be treated with fluid resuscitation, IV antibiotics, and once stabilized, ERCP with sphincterotomy and/or stone retrieval. Laparoscopic cholecystectomy should be performed during the same hospital admission, after the patient has recovered from their acute illness but prior to discharge.

10. **What are the indications for performing intra-operative cholangiogram?**

Most commonly to evaluate for retained stones in the common bile duct, based on preoperative direct hyperbilirubinemia. It is also helpful with unclear anatomy and concern for intra-operative bile duct injury [1, 2].

11. **What is biliary dyskinesia and what are the elements from the history and physical that would heighten the clinical suspicion for this problem?**

Biliary dykinesia is usually defined as decreased/ineffective gallbladder contractility with an ejection fraction <20–35% on a cholecystokinin (CCK) HIDA scan [1–3].

Patients with biliary dyskinesia often have typical biliary symptoms including nausea, vomiting, & right upper quadrant pain however usually lack signs of systemic infection. Their pain may be more chronic in nature as opposed to intermittent episodes of acute pain.

12. **What are the typical laboratory and imaging findings of a patient with biliary dyskinesia?**

The laboratory data for a patient with biliary dyskinesia are often normal. Typically, gallbladder ultrasounds on these patients fail to demonstrate evidence of gallstones. The diagnosis is made by measuring the biliary ejection fraction using CCK-stimulated biliary scintigraphy (HIDA scan).

13. **What is the treatment for biliary dyskinesia?**

Laparoscopic cholecystectomy is offered for the treatment for biliary dyskinesia. Oftentimes this diagnosis is one of exclusion, and unfortunately this does not always provide symptomatic relief. As a generalization, patients with very low biliary ejection fraction are more likely to have symptomatic relief from cholecystectomy [2]. Persistent pain despite cholecystectomy will require further work-up.

References

1. Coran AG, Adzick NS, Krummel TM, Laberge JM, Shamberger R, Caldamone A. Pediatric Surgery. 7th ed. Philadelphia, PA: Elsevier Saunders; 2012.
2. Holcomb GW III, Murphy PJ, Ostlie DJ. Ashcraft's Pediatric Surgery. 6th ed. New York, NY: Elsevier Saunders; 2014.
3. Spitz L, Coran AG. Operative Pediatric Surgery. 7th ed. Boca Raton, FL: CRC Press, Taylor & Francis Group, LLC; 2013.
4. Brunt LM. "SAGES Safe Cholecystectomy Program." Retrieved from https://www.sages.org/safe-cholecystectomy-program/.

Chapter 39
Portal Hypertension

Alexander Dzakovic and Riccardo Superina

Abstract Portal hypertension in children has many causes, and the treatment depends very much on the underlying condition. The treatment may be quite observational in cases caused by mild intrinsic liver disease, to operative hepatic revascularization, or possible liver transplant in those children who have decompensated cirrhosis or severe manifestations of portosystemic shunting.

Keywords Portal hypertension · Meso-Rex-Bypass · Rex-Shunt

1. **What causes portal hypertension in infants and children?**

Intrinsic liver disease with subsequent fibrosis and cirrhosis caused by biliary atresia, metabolic and autoimmune diseases, vascular causes including extrahepatic portal vein occlusion, and rarely, post-hepatic Budd-Chiari syndrome and hepatic vein stenosis as well as high-flow intra-and extrahepatic arteriovenous communication.

2. **How is portal hypertension defined?**

Portal venous pressures exceeding 8–10 mmHg or a portal vein to hepatic pressure gradient greater than 5 mmHg. Direct portal pressure measurement is difficult in children. In children, indirect evidence of portal hypertension includes physical signs such as an enlarged spleen, caput medusa and thrombocytopenia. Esophageal varices are also indirect evidence of portal hypertension.

3. **What are the most common causes of portal hypertension in children?**

Biliary atresia (BA) and extrahepatic portal vein obstruction (EPVO).

A. Dzakovic (✉) · R. Superina
Loyola University Medical Center, Ann and Robert H. Lurie Children's Hospital of Chicago, Chicago, IL, USA
e-mail: adzakovic@luriechildrens.org

M. Lacher et al. (eds.), *Pearls and Tricks in Pediatric Surgery*,
https://doi.org/10.1007/978-3-030-51067-1_39

4. **How do patients typically present?**

Spontaneous hemorrhage from gastrointestinal sites, epistaxis, hematuria, menorrhagia, hypersplenism, thrombocytopenia, ascites.

5. **What are key treatment goals for an acute gastrointestinal bleeding episode?**

Volume resuscitation to restore hemodynamic stability with a target hemoglobin level of 8 mg/dl, platelet levels above 20,000, replacement of fresh frozen plasma, initiation of vasoactive intravenous medication such as octreotide or other somatostatin analogues, endoscopy with variceal banding (EVL) or sclerotherapy are the mainstays of initial therapy. ICU admission is generally recommended. Antibiotic prophylaxis is recommended in children with cirrhosis.

6. **Is transjugular intrahepatic portosystemic shunts (TIPS) a treatment option?**

Creation of a portosystemic shunt between portal and hepatic veins via inserted stent has limited use in children and is generally reserved for refractory treatment of variceal hemorrhage in patients with intrinsic liver disease as a bridge to transplantation.

7. **What are surgical management options of portal hypertension?**

Surgical treatment options are done to redirect portal hypertensive blood flow into the low pressure systemic venous circulation and need to consider underlying pathophysiology and severity of symptoms. Shunt procedures can be divided into non-selective and selective shunts. Mesocaval, proximal splenorenal and side-to-side porta-caval shunts essentially redirect the entire portal blood flow and are considered non-selective. Selective shunts such as the distal splenorenal shunt divert only the splenic and gastroesophageal portion of portal blood flow. The meso Rex shunt restores mesenteric venous circulation back to the intrahepatic portal circulation and as such, is more of a bypass than a shunt (MSB). Non shunt options include extensive gastric devascularization with distal esophageal transection and reanastomosis (Sugiura procedure), splenic artery ligation as well as liver transplantation but are reserved for high risk patients that are not candidates for shunt surgery. Splenectomy is NOT a surgical treatment option as it significantly reduces the chance of successful selective shunt surgery.

8. **What diagnostic imaging should be considered in the workup?**

Imaging objectives include confirming extrahepatic portal vein thrombosis and assessing size and patency of left portal vein and superior mesenteric vein for MRB feasibility. Furthermore, evaluation of large collaterals as alternative conduits for MRB as well as inferior vena cava, renal and splenic veins for alternative porto-systemic shunt (PSS) are considered. Abdominal ultrasonography with doppler can provide and assessment of the portal vein as well as liver parenchyma. Both triphasic computed tomography (CT) or magnetic resonance (MR) angiography provide an excellent road map. Transjugular wedged hepatic vein portography is the authors modality of choice to assess not only the patency of the left intrahepatic branch of the portal vein but also communication between left and right intrahepatic portal veins.

9. **What are the indications for surgical treatment of extrahepatic portal vein thrombosis?**

Failure of medical and endoscopic management of variceal hemorrhage, severe hypersplenism with thrombocytopenia below 50,000 and recurrent non-variceal bleeding, hepato-pulmonary syndrome and porto-pulmonary hypertension are considered absolute indications for shunt surgery. Neurocognitive testing suggestive of encephalopathy, increased serum ammonium levels and growth retardation are relative indications.

10. **How do treatment considerations differ for children with EHPVO as compared to those with Biliary Atresia?**

Portal hypertension develops early in the disease course of EHPVO while in BA portal hypertension may rarely develop when liver function is generally well compensated and overall mortality is less than 1%. However, unlike BA where the transplantation intervention prevents the disease progression, the natural course of PHT from EHPVO subjects children to a long variety of complications including splenomegaly, hypersplenism, spontaneous portosystemic shunting, encephalopathy, growth failure, coagulopathy and less commonly portal bilopathy and hepato-pulmonary syndrome. Rather than serial symptomatic treatment, definite surgical correction should be considered.

11. **When should MRB be considered preemptively?**

There is expert consensus on the use of MRB as primary prophylaxis of PHT complications in EHPVO [1]. Favorable anatomy confirmed on wedge portography, patent superior mesenteric, splenic and bilateral internal jugular veins, negative coagulopathy work up, body weight greater than 8 kg, normal echocardiogram and a multidisciplinary team with MRB experience are prerequisite for a greater than 90% success rate.

12. **What is the advantage of a MRB**

Both meso rex bypass and portosystemic shunt effectively relieve symptoms of portal hypertensive bleeding. However meso rex bypass improves somatic growth, liver synthetic function, coagulopathy, neurocognitive function, prealbumin and insulin like growth factor as well as platelets to levels higher than portosystemic shunts [2, 3].

13. **How did the Rex shunt get its name?**

Hugo Rex, an Austrian anatomist, described the anatomic correlation of the intrahepatic left portal vein branch with the base of the falciform ligament and ductus venosus in 1888, later referred to as the Rex recessus. Jean de Ville de Goyet first described direct bypassing of an obstructed extrahepatic portal vein into the Rex recessus in 1998 which became known as the Rex shunt or the meso Rex bypass [4].

14. **What does the preoperative workup include?**

In addition to preoperative imaging, liver function tests and biopsy must evaluate for intrinsic liver disease. Echocardiogram and possibly cardiac catheterization is performed to assess operative risk particularly pulmonary hypertension and hepato-pulmonary syndrome as both are contraindications for portosystemic shunts and relative indication for meso rex bypass. Hematological workup should rule out a hypercoagulable state.

15. **What are key technical components of a MRB?**

The recessus of Rex is dissected following the round ligament maintaining vascular control of segmental feeding branches and assuring adequate lumen and backbleeding of the left portal vein. Partial resection of liver segments III and IV allows wider exposure and passage of the subsequent vein graft. Then, the superior mesenteric vein is exposed and controlled at the base of the small bowel mesentery and the jugular vein is harvested. The narrower cephalic end is anastomosed to the exposed left portal vein and the wider thoracic end tunneled through the lesser sac over the pancreas posterior to the stomach and transverse mesocolon before anastomosing the distal wider end to the infrapancreatic superior mesenteric vein.

16. **How are Rex shunt patients managed post operatively?**

Systemic low level heparinization and transition to long-term antiplatelet therapy for 6 months. If in the preoperative work-up a hypercoagulable condition has been identified, long term anticoagulation may be necessary.

17. **How should patients be followed up?**

Outpatient follow up includes doppler US every 3 months for the first year and then every 6 months for the second year and yearly after that.

18. **What are complications of shunt surgery? How can they be managed?**

Shunt thrombosis in the immediate postoperative period requires urgent thrombectomy, shunt revision and systemic anticoagulation. If not salvageable alternative portosystemic shunts need to be considered. Shunt stenosis can successfully be managed by percutaneous endovascular interventions in the majority of cases with excellent long term patency rates and resolution of clinical symptoms [5]. Failure of percutaneous therapy requires operative shunt revision. Ascites from extensive dissection of retroperitoneal lymphatics resolves spontaneously in most cases but may require oral diuretics or reduced-fat diet.

19. **What are the long-term outcomes of MRB?**

Over 80% of patients with EHPVO can successfully be treated with MRB. A patent MRB obviates the need for esophageal endoscopy, banding or use of non-selective beta blockade. Age at the time of surgery does not appear to affect outcome but younger children tend to have shunt flows that are closer to normal portal flow when expressed per body surface area.

References

1. Primary prophylaxis of variceal bleeding in children and the role of MesoRex Bypass: Summary of the Baveno VI Pediatric Satellite Symposium. Shneider BL, de Ville de Goyet J, Leung DH, Srivastava A, Ling SC, Duché M, McKiernan P, Superina R, Squires RH, Bosch J, Groszmann R, Sarin SK, de Franchis R, Mazariegos GV. Hepatology. 2016 Apr;63(4):1368–80.
2. Advantages of the meso-Rex bypass compared with portosystemic shunts in the management of extrahepatic portal vein obstruction in children. Lautz TB, Keys LA, Melvin JC, Ito J, Superina RA. J Am Coll Surg. 2013 Jan;216(1):83–9.
3. Metabolic profile of children with extrahepatic portal vein obstruction undergoing meso-Rex bypass.Lautz TB, Eaton S, Keys L, Ito J, Polo M, Wells JCK, Pierro A, Superina RA.J Surg Res. 2018 Mar;223:109–114.
4. Direct bypassing of extrahepatic portal venous obstruction in children: a new technique for combined hepatic portal revascularization and treatment of extrahepatic portal hypertension. de Ville de Goyet J, Alberti D, Clapuyt P, Falchetti D, Rigamonti V, Bax NM, Otte JB, Sokal EM. J Pediatr Surg. 1998 Apr;33(4):597–601.
5. Outcomes of percutaneous interventions for managing stenosis after meso-Rex bypass for extrahepatic portal vein obstruction. Lautz TB, Kim ST, Donaldson JS, Superina RA.J Vasc Interv Radiol. 2012 Mar;23(3):377–83.

Chapter 40
Disorders of the Spleen

Jacob C. Langer

Abstract Splenectomy is indicated for a number of different conditions in children, including trauma, immune thrombocytosis purpura, cysts, and a variety of hemolytic anemias. The operation can usually be done laparoscopically, and in some cases partial splenectomy may be appropriate. Perioperative considerations are determined by the underlying disease. Because of the long-term risk of post-splenectomy sepsis, children undergoing splenectomy should be immunized against encapsulated organisms and should receive prophylactic antibiotics pos-operatively.

Keywords Splenectomy · Hemolytic anemia · Splenic injury · Immune thrombocytopenia purpura · Spherocytosis · Sickle cell disease · Post-splenectomy sepsis

1. **What are the functions of the spleen?**

The spleen is primarily a filter, which removes old and damaged red blood cells and platelets. It also contains immunological cells, including T- and B-cells and reticuloendothelial cells, which remove opsonized bacteria and other particles from the blood.

2. **What is the surgical anatomy of the spleen?**

The spleen is roughly divided into three sections: the upper pole, the body and the lower pole. The arterial supply and venous drainage of the upper pole is from the short gastric vessels, the body is supplied by the main hilar vessels, and the lower pole is supplied by gastroepiploic and omental vessels. The main splenic artery

J. C. Langer (✉)
Pediatric General and Thoracic Surgery, University of Toronto, Rm 1524, Hospital for Sick Children, 555 University Ave, Toronto, ON M5G 1X8, Canada
e-mail: jacob.langer@sickkids.ca

M. Lacher et al. (eds.), *Pearls and Tricks in Pediatric Surgery*,
https://doi.org/10.1007/978-3-030-51067-1_40

is a branch of the celiac artery, and the main splenic vein joins the superior mesenteric vein to form the portal vein which then drains into the liver. The spleen is fixed to the diaphragm and to the lateral abdominal wall by peritoneal attachments which prevent torsion or volvulus of the spleen.

3. **What are the steps of a splenectomy?**

The steps of a splenectomy are 1. Division of the attachments to the diaphragm and retroperitoneum, 2. Division of the lower pole vessels, 3. Division of the hilar vessels, 4. Division of the short gastric vessels, 5. Removal of the spleen, and 6. Identification and excision of accessory spleens. In most cases, the operation can be done laparoscopically, in which case division of the lateral attachments are often done at the end of the procedure after division of the vessels, and the spleen is placed into a bag inside the abdomen so the neck of the bag can be brought out through a port site and the spleen can be morcellated within the bag and removed in pieces.

4. **What is the technique of partial splenectomy?**

The goal of a partial splenectomy is to leave a sufficient amount of spleen behind to retain splenic function (although it is not known exactly how much residual spleen is necessary for that purpose). For spherocytosis, the preferred approach is to divide the lower pole vessels and the main hilar vessels, leaving the upper pole based on the short gastric vessels and stabilized with the phrenosplenic connections. For a splenic cyst or mass, the surgeon must assess the blood supply to the affected segment and make a decision which part of the spleen to leave behind with an intact blood supply. Because the spleen is very hard in patients with spherocytosis, the spleen must be divided with a sealing device; in patients with a splenic cyst or mass the residual normal spleen can usually be divided with a stapler.

5. **What is the best management for splenic trauma?** [1]

Most children with splenic injury can be managed non-operatively with activity restriction and fluid resuscitation. The indications for transfusion include unstable vital signs after receiving 20 cc/kg of isotonic fluid, a hemoglobin level of less than 7.0 gm/dl, or signs of active bleeding. The indication for emergency splenectomy is persistent hemodynamic instability despite blood transfusion. If laparotomy is necessary, the surgeon should attempt to salvage some or all of the spleen if possible. For those managed non-operatively, discharge can be done when the child is stable and eating, and activity limitation should be maintained for injury grade + two weeks.

6. **What are the indications for splenectomy in children with immune thrombocytopenia purpura (ITP)?**

ITP is an immunological condition in which the child makes antibodies to his own platelets, which are then destroyed by the spleen. Most children have the acute form that resolves on its own. Many children with the chronic form can be successfully treated medically with steroids or intravenous immunoglobulin (IVIG). Splenectomy is recommended for those who have persistent recurring thrombocytopenia despite medical therapy, or for those who have complications from the medical therapy itself.

7. **What are the perioperative considerations when doing a splenectomy for a child with ITP?**

Ideally, the platelet count should be at least 50,000 at the time of splenectomy. This can usually be accomplished by treating with IVIG within a week of the planned surgery. For those who cannot achieve an adequate platelet count, platelets should be infused just prior to surgery and continued until after the arterial supply to the spleen has been taken. Key technical points during the surgery include ensuring that the spleen is completely excised without spilling any splenic tissue, and ensuring that any accessory spleens are identified and excised.

8. **What should be done with a child who has persistent or recurrent thrombocytopenia after a splenectomy for ITP?**

The two main reasons for thrombocytopenia after a splenectomy are retained accessory splenic tissue, or breakdown of platelets by reticuloendothelial cells in the liver or bone marrow. A nuclear spleen scan should be done to identify any residual splenic tissue, and if found this tissue should be removed at a second operation.

9. **What are the indications for splenectomy in children with sickle cell disease (SCD)?**

Most children with SCD undergo auto-amputation of the spleen by the age of 10 or so and are therefore not candidates for splenectomy. However, a small minority will develop a sequestration crisis before that time, which can result in extremely low hemoglobin levels and can be fatal. Therefore, any child with SCD who has had even one sequestration crisis should have a splenectomy.

10. **What are the perioperative considerations when doing a splenectomy for a child with sickle cell disease?** [2]

Children with SCD are susceptible to acute chest syndrome after a general anesthetic and surgical procedure, which can be severe and even fatal. There is general agreement that these children should be well-hydrated and should have an adequate hemoglobin level prior to surgery, but there is continuing controversy about what that level should be, and whether routine preoperative transfusion is beneficial. Postoperatively it is important to maintain hydration and hemoglobin level, and to adequately prevent postoperative pain.

11. **What are the indications for splenectomy in children with spherocytosis?**

Children with moderate or severe forms of spherocytosis may be considered for splenectomy because of ongoing transfusion requirements, lethargy, jaundice, or discomfort from a massively enlarged spleen.

12. **What are the advantages and disadvantages of partial splenectomy for children with spherocytosis?** [3]

Partial splenectomy, removing approximately 80% of the spleen, has been shown to be very effective in treating the anemia, jaundice and symptoms in children with spherocytosis, while theoretically decreasing the long-term risks of post-splenectomy sepsis and thrombosis. The operation can be done laparoscopically, but is associated with a higher perioperative transfusion requirement, more pain, and a longer hospital stay than laparoscopic total splenectomy. There is also a 10–15% risk of regrowth of the splenic remnant with recurrent symptoms and need for a completion splenectomy in the future.

13. **What are the perioperative considerations when doing a splenectomy for a child with spherocytosis?**

Most children with spherocytosis are otherwise healthy and can tolerate splenectomy well. Almost half of patients with spherocytosis will develop gallstones; if they are symptomatic the gallbladder should be removed at the time of splenectomy. There is controversy about whether asymptomatic gallstones should be removed at the time of splenectomy.

14. **How should splenic cysts be managed?**

Splenic cysts are usually congenital and have an epithelial lining. These must be differentiated from echinococcal cysts, which should be removed, and liquification of a post-traumatic splenic hematoma, which will usually resolve over time. Symptomatic epithelial cysts should be removed by partial splenectomy if possible, or total splenectomy if partial splenectomy is not technically feasible. Asymptomatic epithelial cysts can be managed expectantly with serial imaging, but should be removed if they become symptomatic, or if they enlarge beyond 5 cm in diameter. Techniques such as unroofing or marsupialization, although less invasive, are associated with a very high incidence of recurrence.

15. **How should solid splenic masses be managed?**

Solid splenic masses are rare, and usually represent benign lesions such as hemangioma or hamartoma. These can be managed expectantly if they are asymptomatic, but excision with partial or total splenectomy should be considered if they become symptomatic or enlarge under observation.

16 **Are there any other indications for splenectomy?**

Occasionally splenectomy will be indicated for hypersplenism due to portal hypertension, splenic vein thrombosis, HIV infection, glycogen storage disease, or idiopathic splenomegaly. In some cases of lymphoproliferative disease the diagnosis of lymphoma or leukemia will be suspected, and the spleen will be removed for a tissue diagnosis. Splenic abscess can usually be managed with antibiotics, but occasionally will require splenectomy.

17. **What is post-splenectomy sepsis and how can it be prevented?** [4]

The spleen is involved in preventing infection with encapsulated organisms like Streptococcus pneumoniae, Haemophilus influenzae, and Neisseria meningitidis. Splenectomy increases the risk of overwhelming post-splenectomy infection (OPSI), which is fatal in more than 50% of cases. Because of this, all patients undergoing splenectomy should be immunized prior to the operation against all three organisms, and should take prophylactic antibiotics after splenectomy. Patients who have a splenectomy for trauma should be immunized after they have recovered from their injuries.

18. **What are the risks of thrombosis after splenectomy?** [5]

Early after total splenectomy the platelet count in most patients becomes markedly elevated, although this improves over time. There may be a role for anti-platelet therapy if it exceeds 1,000,000. There is also a recognized risk of portal vein thrombosis early after splenectomy, a risk which appears to be higher in adults than in children. Recent long-term follow-up studies have also suggested that there may be an increased risk of thrombotic complications, including thromboembolic pulmonary hypertension, in adults who have had a previous splenectomy.

References

1. Gates RL, Price M, Cameron DB, Somme S, Ricca R, Oyetunji TA, Guner YS, Gosain A, Baird R, Lal DR, Jancelewicz T, Shelton J, Diefenbach KA, Grabowski J, Kawaguchi A, Dasgupta R, Downard C, Goldin A, Petty JK, Stylianos S, Williams R. Non-operative management of solid organ injuries in children: an American Pediatric Surgical Association Outcomes and Evidence Based Practice Committee systematic review. J Pediatr Surg. 2019; 54:1519–26.
2. Khurmi N, Gorlin A, Misra L. Perioperative considerations for patients with sickle cell disease: a narrative review. Can J Anaesth. 2017;64:860–9.
3. Englum BR, Rothman J, Leonard S, Reiter A, Thornburg C, Brindle M, Wright N, Heeney MM, Jason Smithers C, Brown RL, Kalfa T, Langer JC, Cada M, Oldham KT, Scott JP, St Peter SD, Sharma M, Davidoff AM, Nottage K, Bernabe K, Wilson DB, Dutta S, Glader B, Crary SE, Dassinger MS, Dunbar L, Islam S, Kumar M, Rescorla F, Bruch S, Campbell A, Austin M, Sidonio R, Blakely ML, Rice HE; Splenectomy in Congenital Hemolytic Anemia Consortium. Hematologic outcomes after total splenectomy and partial splenectomy for congenital hemolytic anemia. J Pediatr Surg 2016;51:122–27.
4. Salvadori MI, Price VE, Canadian Pediatric Society Infectious Diseases and Immunization Committee. Preventing and treating infections in children with asplenia or hyposplenia. Paediatr Child Health 2014;19:271–74.
5. Kimmig LM, Palevsky HI. Review of the association between splenectomy and chronic thromboembolic pulmonary hypertension. Ann Am Thorac Soc. 2016;13:945–54.

Chapter 41
Pancreas

Elke Zani-Ruttenstock and Agostino Pierro

Abstract Disorders of the pancreas can origin from congenital structural abnormalities such as annular pancreas, pancreas divisum and pancreaticobiliary malunion and may require surgical interventions. Congenital hyperinsulinism (CHI) is a rare and complex genetic disorder, that can present with a focal, diffuse or atypical lesion. Near-total pancreatectomy is the procedure of choice for diffuse CHI, whereas a localized resection is curative for focal CHI. An increasing incidence of pancreatitis in children has been reported recently—likely due to the increased incidence of obesity, drug associated pancreatitis and improvements in detection. Benign and malignant pancreatic tumors are relatively uncommon in children, thus making diagnosis, classification and management challenging.

Keywords Annular pancreas · Pancreas divisum · Pancreaticobiliary malunion · Congenital hyperinsulinism (CHI) · Acute pancreatitis · Chronic pancreatitis · Pancreatic tumors

1. **What are the surgical conditions affecting the pancreas in infants and children?**

   – congenital anomalies
   – inflammatory conditions
   – neoplasms
   – trauma (see Chap. 56 on abdominal trauma)

E. Zani-Ruttenstock · A. Pierro (✉)
Division of General and Thoracic Surgery,
Department of Surgery, University of Toronto, Toronto, ON M5S, Canada
e-mail: agostino.pierro@sickkids.ca

M. Lacher et al. (eds.), *Pearls and Tricks in Pediatric Surgery*,
https://doi.org/10.1007/978-3-030-51067-1_41

2. **What are the most common congenital anomalies of the pancreas?**

Annular pancreas: caused by incomplete migration of the ventral pancreatic anlage (annular part encircles the second portion of the duodenum and drains independently into the duodenum or into Wirsung's duct); associated with Down's syndrome, malrotation, intrinsic duodenal obstruction, esophageal atresia and heart defects; duodenal obstruction should be bypassed by performing duodenoduodenostomy or duodeno-jejunostomy without resecting the pancreatic tissue.

Pancreas divisum: pancreatic buds are not fused and the two ducts are separate with majority of the pancreatic secretions draining from the minor papilla; most patients are asymptomatic; stenosis of the minor papilla may lead to recurrent acute pancreatitis and may be treated with sphincteroplasty.

Pancreaticobiliary malunion: common channel between the pancreatic and biliary ducts above the duodenal wall; this anatomy is common in choledochal cysts; channel may become clogged with stones or plugs causing obstruction and dilation, resulting in pancreatitis and sometimes jaundice.

Congenital hyperinsulinism (CHI): inappropriate insulin secretion by the pancreatic β-cells secondary to various genetic disorders; recurrent episodes of hyperinsulinemic hypoglycemia imply high risk of brain damage.

3. **What is the incidence of CHI?**

CHI is most frequent cause of persistent hypoglycemia in neonates and infants; estimated incidence is 1 in 50.000 live births, but can be as frequent as 1 in 500 in countries with high rate of consanguinity.

4. **What are the different histological forms of CHI?**

Focal CHI: consists of focus of adenomatous islet cell hyperplasia surrounded by normal pancreatic tissue; focal lesions vary in size from a few millimeters to greater than a centimeter or more; can be located in the surface of the pancreas or deep within the organ.

***Diffuse* CHI**: primary histological hallmark feature is beta cell nucleomegaly; in the vast majority of cases abnormal beta cells are distributed homogeneously throughout the pancreas.

In addition to the two major forms, there are rare ***atypical*** histological cases of CHI that are neither focal nor diffuse.

5. **How is CHI diagnosed?**

Valuable diagnostic information is obtained from a blood sample drawn during hypoglycemia:

- Fasting and/or post-prandial hypoglycemia (<2.5–3 mmol/L)
- abnormal detectable amounts of insulin and inappropriately low levels of free fatty acids and ketones
- high requirement for intravenous glucose to maintain adequate glucose levels (>8–10 mg/kg/min)

- rise of the glucose level after injection of glucagon.
- genetic test for variants related to focal or diffuse CHI (see below)
- PET scan using 18F-DOPA (see below).

6. **What techniques are used to determine whether the patient has focal or diffuse CHI, and how can focal lesions be localized?**

Combination of genetic testing and/or imaging studies are needed to determine if patient has focal or diffuse CHI:

When genetic testing confirms diffuse CHI (one mutation on the maternal allele plus one mutation on the paternal allele)—no imaging studies are necessary;

When genetic testing is suggestive of focal CHI, a 18F-DOPA PET/CT scan must be done to confirm the diagnosis of focal CHI and localize the lesion.

7. **What are the most common presenting symptoms of CHI?**

Neonates present with poor feeding, perioral cyanosis, lethargy, hypotonia, irritability and seizures. Unfortunately, untreated neonates can develop neurological abnormalities due to hypoglycemia. Older patients can present with typical clinical features of hypoglycemia like pallor, sweat and tachycardia.

8. **What strategies are used for the medical treatment of CHI?**

Hypoglycemia must be rapidly treated to prevent irreversible brain damage (glucose load and/or a glucagon injection), followed by treatment to prevent recurrence of hypoglycemia (frequent and glucose-enriched feeding, diazoxide, nifedipine and octreotide).

9. **Describe the surgical treatment of focal and diffuse CHI?**

Focal CHI: localized resection of the focal lesion is curative;

Head or neck focal lesions: open resection of the lesion with small rim of surrounding normal pancreatic tissue and pancreatico-jejunostomy to allow drainage of the distal pancreas.

Distal focal lesions: distal pancreatectomy (open or laparoscopically).

Diffuse CHI: open or laparoscopic near-total pancreatectomy (95%) is considered as gold standard; (tail, body, uncinate process and part of pancreatic head are resected, leaving a rim of pancreatic tissue surrounding the common bile duct and along the duodenum); long-term outcome is characterized by a high risk of diabetes [1].

10. **What are the causes and findings of acute pancreatitis in children?**

Most common causes: trauma, choledocholithiasis, congenital structural abnormalities of pancreatic and/or biliary system (choledochal cyst), systemic illness, drugs, familial or idiopathic.

Clinical findings: abdominal pain, vomiting, jaundice, fever, diarrhea, back pain, irritability and lethargy; in severe cases: shock, multiorgan failure including dyspnea, oliguria, hemorrhage and mental status change

Laboratory findings: elevated amylase and lipase are commonly found, but normal values do not rule out pancreatitis.

Radiographic findings:

Plain abdominal X-ray: paralytic ileus, colon cut-off sign, sentinel loop sign, calcified gallstones or pancreatic stones;
Plain chest X-ray: pleural effusion, ARDS, pneumonia
Abdominal ultrasound (US): pancreatic abnormalities, inflammation, free fluid, pseudocysts, dilated biliary or pancreatic ducts, gallstones
Abdominal computer tomography (CT) (95% sensitivity): pancreatic enlargement/mass/trauma, fluid collections, necrosis, hemorrhage
Magnetic resonance cholangiopancreatography (MRCP): delineating ductal anatomy

11. **How is acute pancreatitis treated in children?**

Medical treatment: mainly supportive with fluid and electrolyte supplementation, enteral feeding and analgesia [2]; antibiotic prophylaxis is not recommended [3].

Surgical treatment:

Infected pancreatic necrosis: extensive drainage for source control; in case of insufficient response—open surgical debridement or necrosectomy is rarely performed.

Symptomatic pseudocysts: drainage procedure after a cyst wall has formed (4–6 weeks); done by endoscopic drainage or surgical cystgastrostomy, cystduodenostomy, or cystjejunostomy (open or laparoscopic)

If drainage is needed prior to maturation of the cyst wall: external drainage (open or percutaneously) may be required; complications: fistula formation and recurrences.

Ductal obstruction: endoscopic retrograde cholangiopancreatography (ERCP) for clearance of stones, or stenting of ductal disruption.
ERCP with sphincterotomy for stricture at the ampulla to allow improved pancreatic fluid drainage.

12. **How is chronic pancreatitis defined?**

Irreversible structural damage to the pancreas with or without exocrine and endocrine insufficiency; may be the result of acute recurrent pancreatitis.

13. **How does chronic pancreatitis present in children?**

Presenting symptoms: recurrent or persistent abdominal pain associated with nausea, vomiting, anorexia, weight loss and malnutrition; pancreatic endocrine insufficiency may lead to diabetes; pancreatic exocrine insufficiency may lead to maldigestion with diarrhea, steatorrhea, gas bloating, intermittent abdominal distention and vitamin deficiency (AEDK) [4].

14. **What are the appropriate imaging studies in a child with chronic pancreatitis?**

US: inflammation, fluid collections, pseudocysts, gallstones
CT: pancreatic atrophy, dilated pancreatic ducts, calcifications, masses, fluid collections, necrosis and hemorrhage, guidance of interventions (drain placement or vessel embolization)
MRCP: delineating ductal anatomy and evaluating for strictures, stones, tumors and ductal anomalies.
ERCP: stone removal, stricture dilation or stenting, stricture or mass biopsy, sphincterotomy
Endoscopic ultrasound: pancreas visualization, biopsies of the mucosa, masses, strictures, lymph nodes, pseudocyst aspiration or drainage.

15. **How is chronic pancreatitis treated?**

Medical treatment:

Endocrine insufficiency: monitoring and treatment for diabetes
Exocrine insufficiency: supplementation of pancreatic enzymes, antacids, fat soluble vitamins (AEDK)

Surgical treatment:

Indications:

- failure of medical and endoscopic management of chronic pain
- complications such as pseudocysts, strictures or obstructing stones.

Pseudocysts: see surgical treatment of acute pancreatitis

Obstructions and strictures: ERCP to clear stones, protein plugs or to stent a ductal disruption; endoscopic or open sphincterotomy for stricture of the ampulla

Stenotic sphincter: sphincteroplasty

Multiple ductal strictures: side-to-side longitudinal pancreatico-jejunostomy (Puestow procedure)

"Head-dominant" disease: combination of Puestow procedure with partial resection of pancreas head in case of duct dilation;

pancreaticoduodenectomy (Whipple procedure) in case of non-dilated pancreatic duct

"Tail-dominant" disease: distal pancreatectomy.

16. **How can pancreatic tumors be classified?**

Pancreatic tumors can be classified as malignant or benign, cystic or solid and of exocrine versus endocrine origin [5].

Classification of pancreatic tumors

Primary pancreatic tumors	Tumors of the ***exocrine*** pancreas	**Benign**: *serous cystadenoma (microcystic/oligocystic), mucinous cystadenoma, mature cystic teratoma*
		Borderline malignant: *solid pseudopapillary neoplasm (SPN; previously known as Frantz tumor)*
		Malignant: *pancreatoblastoma mucinous cystadenocarcinoma acinar cell carcinoma pancreatic ductal adenocarcinoma*
	Tumors of the ***endocrine*** pancreas	**Benign**: *insulinoma sporadic gastrinoma VIPomas*
		Borderline to frankly malignant: *multiple endocrine neoplasia (MEN) associated insulinoma and gastrinoma*
Non-epithelial pancreatic tumors		**Benign**
		Malignant

17. **What is the most common pancreatic tumor in children?**

Solid pseudopapillary tumor of the pancreas: most commonly affects older adolescent females; tumor has both, cyst-like and solid parts; tumor is unlikely to spread; Very good prognosis.

18. **Which tumor is associated with Beckwith-Wiedemann and familial adenomatous polyposis (FAP)?**

Pancreatoblastoma: usually occurs in children aged 10 years or younger; tumor may produce adrenocorticotropic hormone (ACTH) and antidiuretic hormone (ADH); may spread to the liver, lungs, and lymph nodes; good prognosis

19. **Which tumors are associated with MEN1 syndrome?**

Islet cell tumors: rare in children; can be benign or malignant; most common types: insulinomas and gastrinomas.

20. **What are the presenting symptoms of pancreatic tumors in children?**

Most pancreatic tumors are slowly growing with few specific symptoms in the early phases: epigastric abdominal pain, palpable abdominal mass, jaundice, pruritus

Rarely severe abdominal pain or acute abdomen due to acute hemorrhage into tumor or tumor rupture

Endocrinologically active tumors (insulinoma/gastrinoma): signs and symptoms related to the effects of the hypersecretion of the active hormone.

21. **What are the most useful diagnostic studies for pancreatic tumors in children?**

Transabdominal ultrasonography: first choice, accurate in the initial delineation of most pancreatic lesions.

Magnetic resonance imaging (MRI) (gold standard): advantage of providing very precise anatomic differentiation between the various tissues; multiplanar capabilities

Abdominal CT: provides precise multiplanar information; many tumors have characteristic appearance on CT.

Endoscopic ultrasound: visualization of very small lesions (too small to be seen adequately on CT/MRI); fine needle aspiration or biopsy

22. **How are tumors of the pancreas treated in children?**

Treatment of pancreatic tumors is individualized. In general, operative exploration is mandated to obtain tissue diagnosis and to determine resectability.

Benign tumors

Benign lesions of exocrine pancreas: resection

Endocrine tumors of the pancreas (malignant or benign)

Functional lesions should be treated by enucleation from the pancreatic head and body or distal pancreatic resection of the tail; additional peri-pancreatic lymph node resection (to avoid small deposits of tumor cells, that can continue to produce active hormones); additional duodenotomy for hormonally active lesions in the submucosa of the duodenu [6].

Malignant tumors: resection—even in the presence of local invasion;

Long-term survival is expected for solid and cystic tumors of the pancreas, which metastasize infrequently and represent the most common histologic variant in children.

Distal lesion (body and tail of pancreas) are treated by distal pancreatectomy.

Tumors in head and neck can be enucleated with duodenal preserving operation followed by pancreatico-jejunostomy. Alternatively, a Whipple procedure (pancreatico-duodenectomy with removal of the head of the pancreas, duodenum, portion of the common bile duct, gallbladder, ±part of the stomach) is required [6].

References

1. Pierro A, Nah SA. Surgical management of congenital hyperinsulinism of infancy. Semin. Pediatr Surg. 2011;20(1):50–3.
2. Márta K, Farkas N, Szabó I, Illés A, Vincze Á, Pár G, Sarlós P, Bajor J, Szűcs Á, Czimmer J, Mosztbacher D, Párniczky A, Szemes K, Pécsi D, Hegyi P. Meta-analysis of early nutrition: The benefits of enteral feeding compared to a nil per os diet not only in severe, but also in mild and moderate acute pancreatitis. Int J Mol Sci. 2016;17(10).
3. Villatoro E, Mulla M, Larvin M. Antibiotic therapy for prophylaxis against infection of pancreatic necrosis in acute pancreatitis. Cochrane Database Syst Rev. 2010.
4. Gariepy CE, Heyman MB, Lowe ME, Pohl JF, Werlin SL, Wilschanski M, Barth B, Fishman DS, Freedman SD, Giefer MJ, Gonska T, Himes R, Husain SZ, Morinville VD, Ooi CY, Schwarzenberg SJ, Troendle DM, Yen E, Uc A. Causal evaluation of acute recurrent and chronic pancreatitis in children: Consensus from the INSPPIRE group. J Pediatr Gastroenterol Nutr. 2017;64(1):95–103.
5. Johnson PR, Spitz L. Cysts and tumors of the pancreas. Semin Pediatr Surg. 2000;9(4):209–15.
6. Nasher O, Hall NJ, Sebire NJ, de Coppi P, Pierro A. Pancreatic tumours in children: diagnosis, treatment and outcome. Pediatr Surg Int. 2015;31(9):831–5.

Chapter 42
Pearls for Pediatric Head and Neck Masses

Julie L. Wei

Abstract Pediatric head and neck masses can be broadly categorized as congenital versus non-congenital, the latter being most often infectious in etiology. Surgical precision and pearls minimize recurrence or persistence for both categories. Differential diagnosis for most common congenital neck masses can be based on location, with midline or lateral neck position being the most relevant information. Complete surgical excision when possible is especially critical when dealing with nontuberculous mycobacterial lymphadenitis. While excision of thyroglossal duct cysts is a very safe operation, rare devastating complications may occur if the cricoid is mistaken for the hyoid cartilage.

Keywords Neck mass · Cervical lymphadenitis · Branchial cleft cysts · Thyroglossal duct cyst

1. **What congenital head and neck masses are most common in infants and children?**

Dermoid cyst, benign lymph node, thyroglossal duct cyst (TGDC), cysts associated with 1st, 2nd or 3rd branchial cleft cysts (BCC) are the most common. Often they do not present at birth but later in childhood, especially after a viral URI (TGDC or BCC). Once present the mass may be persistent. Unless actively infected, rarely acute increase in size, or have any signs such as overlying skin erythema and/or fluctuance. Rarely will these cause airway compromise, dysphagia, or pain.

J. L. Wei (✉)
Pediatric Otolaryngology/Audiology, Nemours Children's Hospital, 13535 Nemours Parkway, Orlando, FL 32827, USA
e-mail: julie.wei@nemours.org

M. Lacher et al. (eds.), *Pearls and Tricks in Pediatric Surgery*,
https://doi.org/10.1007/978-3-030-51067-1_42

2. **What non-congenital neck masses are most common in infants and children?**

Torticollis (hematoma in sternocleidomastoid muscle) can occur in newborns as a classic firm "mass" in lateral neck noticeable shortly after birth, especially difficult vaginal birth of large size infant, forcep or vacuum delivery. Non-congenital masses are commonly secondary to infectious etiology and reactive. As lymph nodes enlarge there is central necrosis of the hilum due to inadequate blood supply to the entire node. Reactive lymphadenitis also occurs with acute streptococcal pharyngitis/tonsillitis or mononucleosis. Primary infectious lymphadenitis presenting on face or neck is rare but differential diagnosis should include non-tuberculous mycobacterial (NTM) lymphadenitis, bartonella or "Cat-Scratch", especially if there is positive history of recent cat scratch. Malignant masses are rare by always possible, including lymphoma, soft tissue sarcomas, and others.

3. **How should location of mass influence one's differential diagnosis?**

Midline versus lateral neck should dictate differential diagnosis. Midline neck mass is typically either a dermoid or TGDC, while lateral neck masses, especially anterior or medial to anterior border of sternocleidomastoid (SCM) muscle are likely BCC. Reactive lymph nodes are rarely midline but if midline it's most commonly a submental node above the hyoid cartilage. Posterior or levels 2, 3, and 4 of neck are likely reactive lymph nodes, and supraclavicular is rare and can be lipoma if soft, vascular malformation, or rare malignant masses. Often what feels like a larger node is a group of smaller accessory chain benign nodes.

4. **What is the typical presentation of pediatric neck masses?**

Most are asymptomatic and noticed by parents incidentally. Acute lymphadenitis of lateral, posterior neck, or retropharyngeal space are not painful, but can decrease neck range of motion. Lymphadenitis is very firm and are rarely fluctuant until the absolute late stages of abscess. Do NOT decide on whether to consult otolaryngology or consider need for incision and drainage of based on "feel" or presence of fluctuance. Decision for surgical intervention and timing should be based on clinical severity (fever, elevated WBC, ultrasound confirmation of central necrosis and phlegmon evolving to necrosis, etc.) and not based on "rim enhancement" on CT imaging with contrast as the "gold standard". Phlegmon versus actual abscess are simply spectrum of the process. Unless lymphadenitis is small and ultrasound confirms no drainable "fluid" collection, earlier surgical I&D provides early resolution of fever, minimize duration of hospitalization and need for systemic antibiotics.

5. **What specific questions should be included when obtaining history for pediatric neck masses?**

Ask if masses presented during concomitant acute illness, duration of mass, single or multiple, overlying skin discoloration, pain, size change, then always ask about exposure history such as exotic travel, exposure to tuberculosis, and recent cat scratches. For those who live in rural areas or farm, ask if they use well water (risk for NTM). Actinomycosis is a rare cause of neck masses which can mimic rhabodomyosarcoma, more common in the Midwest.

Ask for history of purulent drainage through skin indicating now a fistula, any recurrence of mass if intermittent, prior I&D by ED or others, prior surgery, history of MRSA, constitutional symptoms like night sweats, weight loss, and family history (especially preauricular pits, fistulas, BCC and BC fistulas).

6. **Which are the predominant sites of NTM involvement?**

Mandibular border, submandibular area, and preauricular area.

7. **What are the characteristic pathologic skin changes of NTM?**

NTM has a characteristic "bluish" or "dusky" pink hue of the skin over the lymphadenitis, and often the lymph node is immediately subcutaneous, so skin is "stuck" to the infectious tissue.

8. **What does histologic sectioning of NTM lesions show?** [1]

Pseudoepitheliomatous epidermal hyperplasia, intraepithelial abscesses, transepidermal elimination and dermal granulomatous inflammation accompanied by necrosis and suppuration are likely seen on histopathology of immunocompetent patients. For immunocompromised patients, there may be suppurative inflammation.

9. **What to do during actual NTM cervical lymphadenitis "excision"?**

Mark out an elliptical area carefully including involved discolored skin. Injecting local may introduce acid fast bacilli (AFB) into deeper tissue. Plan incisions to allow primary closure with minimal tension. Send tissue from the very periphery of lesion for AFB culture, not the central necrotic material. After gentle dissection to create skin flaps, debride granulomatous unhealthy tissue manually using moist raytec and rub until health tissue remains. Use 4-0 Polyglactin in interrupted fashion to close the subcutaneous layer, then 5-0 Poliglecaprone in running subcuticular fashion to close the skin without tension. No drains needed.

10. **Is there a difference between incisional versus excisional biopsy and outcomes?** [2]

Complete excision is best whenever possible to reduce persistence or recurrence. If not possible still remove as much as possible without risking marginal mandibular branch of facial (if submandibular location).

11. **Medical treatment of NTM cervical lymphadenitis pre, intraop, and post op?**

May treat pre- and post-operatively based on infectious disease consultation, but typically macrolide (azithro- or clarithromycin), add rifampin and even ethambutol for disseminated or systemic infections specifically pulmonary NTM. For face and neck NTM, macrolide is sufficient if there is residual disease after excision.

12. **What are complications of Sistrunk procedure or TGDC excision?** [3, 4]

In a NSQIP review of adult cases from 2005 to 2014, 48/793 (6.1%) underwent reoperation. Wound infection rates were higher in revision cases compared with primary operations (8.3% and 0.9%)

In a review of 99 pediatric TGDC excision cases from 2005 to 2015 from two university hospitals, with mean age of 4.4 years, seven were referred for recurrent TGDC. Overall complication found in 24/99 (26.4%). Hemorrhage and resection of thyroid cartilage were the most severe complications. Recurrence and wound infection (both n = 7, 7.7%) were most common.

Most devastating complication ENT sees that are not reported in literature, are rare cases performed by pediatric or general surgeons when there has been removal of the central portion of the cricoid instead of the hyoid cartilage. This will result in potential life threatening subcutaneous emphysema and airway distress, and remedied by laryngotracheal reconstruction and repair of defect using costochondral rib cartilage.

Make a horizontal incision along natural neck skin crease line that is wide enough (usually medial to anterior SCM border from side to side) and across apex of TGDC or slightly above. Elevate skin flaps and platysma, identify midline raphe, and lateralize strap muscles. Expose and identify thyroid notch in order to dissect superiorly and find hyoid cartilage. If you do not see the thyroid cartilage you may be too low. Dissect TGDC first then follow superiorly all the way to the hyoid. The cricoid is the hardest tracheal ring on palpation. Hyoid cartilage should be palpable at the level where soft tissue of jaw ends and most superior aspect of neck begins. Dissect suprahyoid and infrahyoid muscles off of the midportion prior to removal, and never resect lateral to the greater horn of hyoid cartilage to ensure no injury to superior laryngeal nerve which enters lateral and inferior to the greater horn.

13. **What if there has been significant infection of TGDC pre op?**

Treat with systemic oral antibiotics (amoxicillin/clavulanate, or clindamycin) for 7–10 days and let infection “cool”. Then expect and prepare for a more difficult dissection with poor tissue planes. Be patient, elevate skin flaps and strap muscles, perform gentle dissection using a baby Jake, “peanuts”, which will help, remove all soft tissue outside of well-defined TGDC wall.

14. **TGDC—What to do if there is a “fistula” and prior “drainage”?**

Treat preoperatively as above. Mark and make an elliptical excision surrounding the “fistula”, so that superior and inferior incisions are part of the skin flaps elevated. Dissect superiorly following the fistula and all unhealthy tissue for an “en bloc” excision of entire fistula, all the way up to the mid portion of the hyoid cartilage.

15. **Which masses will imaging be indicated and helpful? Which imaging studies?** [5]

TGDC—Clinical diagnosis, no routine CT or ultrasound necessary

BCC—CT with contrast

Preauricular pit/fistula with recurrent swelling and infection—MRI face/neck with gadolinium

3rd BCC are rare, presents typically with neck swelling at level of thyroid gland and even abscess. CT with contrast is helpful, but diagnosis is definitive when ENT performs microlaryngoscopy and finds a sinus opening at base of pyriform aperture. CT with contrast may show air in the sinus and track from pyriform sinus to the neck.

Neck masses—CT with contrast, and/or MRI with gadolinium for solid tumors

Suspected infectious lymphadenitis—ultrasound ONLY for uncomplicated lateral neck, and CT if limited neck ROM as need to rule out retropharyngeal/parapharyngeal phlegmon/abscess.

16. **Pearls for lateral neck/branchial cleft anomalies**

Do not perform needle aspiration of suspected BCC (often perfectly "round" on CT with contrast). Doing so creates a fistula to the outside and persistent drainage of serous mucous-like material, and will make future excision incredibly difficult.

17. **Rare diagnosis for large lateral neck masses**

Castlemann's disease, lymphoma, ganglioneuroblastoma, ganglioneuroma, neurofibroma fibrosarcoma.

18. **To drain or not to drain?**

Avoid I&D of acutely infected congenital masses like preauricular pit/cysts, TGDC and BCC whenever possible, but for acute lymphadenitis appropriate aggressiveness leads to fast recovery. Stab incision of 3–4 mm at apex of "mass", followed by curved mosquito clamps, gentle but fearless entry through capsule of lymph node, will release purulence. If only "dishwater" is encountered, proceed to use clamp tips to manually debride all central necrosis, irrigate with saline or bacitracin solution, then can pack using ½ inch plain gauze or leave ¼ in Penrose in for 12–24 hours.

19. **Peri and postoperative considerations**

After I&D of cervical lymphadenitis, expect resolution of fever within 12 hours, often can discharge to home next day on oral broad spectrum antiotic for 3–5 days or less. Excision of dermoid or preauricular lesions, and NTM excisional biopsies may go home same day. Sistrunk procedures deserve overnight observation, removal of "rubber band" or Penrose drain the next morning and discharge to home.

20. **How to treat post op fistula?**

Depending on fistula, extent, moist to dry packing (1/4 in plain gauze in saline) changed twice a day by parents at home may or may not be an option. If so, pack daily for 7–10 days until fistula heals by secondary intention. If packing not indicated, clean area with gentle soap and water twice daily or more, cover loosely with gauze or telfa dressing. Apply Desitin (diaper rash cream) to fistula opening 2–3 times daily for one week, often it can dessicate fistula and allow complete healing. May add oral antibiotics if there is associated soft tissue erythema, inflammation, or purulent drainage from fistula.

21. **When to consider re-excision of recurrent fistula?**

If despite all efforts listed above, and period of reasonable observation a fistula persists consider MRI with gadolinium if no imaging was done preop.

22. **When to ask for help from ENT colleagues—ANYTIME!**

References

1. Li JJ, Beresford R, Fyfe J, Henderson C. Clinical and histopathological features of cutaneous nontuberculous mycobacterial infection: a review of 13 cases. J Cutan Pathol. 2017;44(5):433–43.
2. Wei JL, Bond J, Sykes KJ, Selvarangan R, Jackson MA. Treatment outcomes for nontuberculous mycobacterial cervicofacial lymphadenitis in children based on the type of surgical intervention. Otolaryngol Head Neck Surg. 2008;138(5):166–71.
3. Anderson JL, Vu K, Haidar YM, Kuan EC, Tjoa T. Tisks and complications of thyroglossal duct cyst removal. Laryngoscope. 2019 Mar 13. https://doi.org/10.1002/lary.29818 [Epub ahead of print].
4. Lekkerkerker I, van Heurn EL, van der Steg AF, Derikx JP. Pediatric thyroglossal duct cysts: post-operative complications. Int J Pediatr Otorhinolaryngol. 2019;24(124):14–7.
5. Sajedi P, Shet N. Imaging of pediatric neck masses. Int J Head Neck Surg. 2016;7(2):89–96.

Chapter 43
Thyroglossal Duct Cysts and Sinuses

Priscilla P. L. Chiu

Abstract Thyroglossal duct cysts and sinuses are the remnants of thyroid development occurring along the path of descent of the thyroid anlage from the foramen cecum to the neck in the midline. It is the most common midline neck lesion in children and generally presents as an asymptomatic mobile mass that elevates with protrusion of the tongue or swallowing. The most common indications for surgical excision is infection and risk of malignancy. Surgical excision by Sistrunk procedure is the standard of care and is associated with minimal morbidity. Long-term outcomes are excellent following complete excision with a low risk of recurrence.

Keywords Thyroglossal duct cyst · Thyroglossal duct sinus · Thyroglossal duct · Neck cyst · Sistrunk procedure

1. **What are thyroglossal duct cysts (TGDC) and sinuses (TGDS)?**

Thyroglossal duct cysts are remnants of thyroid development. The thyroglossal duct marks the course as the thyroid anlage descends from the foramen cecum, tracking anteroventral to the hyoid bone before resting at the thyroid cartilage. TGDC result from failure of the thyroglossal duct to obliterate [1]. A TGDC with a skin opening (usually following infection with drainage) is known as TGDS.

2. **What are the histological features of TGDC and TGDS?**

TGDC are lined with respiratory columnar epithelium, squamous epithelium or both and contain microscopic foci of thyroid tissue within the cyst wall in 70% of cases [2]. More substantial thyroid tissue may be present within TGDC-resulting in hypothyroidism post excision if no other thyroid gland is present in the patient.

P. P. L. Chiu (✉)
Division of General and Thoracic Surgery, the Hospital for Sick Children,
Department of Surgery, University of Toronto, Toronto, ON, Canada
e-mail: priscilla.chiu@sickkids.ca

M. Lacher et al. (eds.), *Pearls and Tricks in Pediatric Surgery*,
https://doi.org/10.1007/978-3-030-51067-1_43

3. **How common are TGDC?**

TGDC are the most common midline neck lesions in the pediatric population. TGDC are present in approximately 7% of adults worldwide with 2.2/100,000 population at risk per annum. TGDC have a bimodal age distribution, presenting commonly in early childhood (more commonly among males) but also in adulthood in the fifth decade (more commonly females).

4. **What are the clinical features of TGDC?**

TGDC are typically found in four locations-at the base of the tongue or intra-lingual, in the midline of the neck with 20–25% supra-hyoid or submental, 15–20% thyro-hyoid and 45–65% sub-hyoid/supra-sternal [1]. Once infected, the sinus opening of the TGDS may be in the midline or slightly off midline with intermittent drainage. On palpation, TGDC not previously infected are mobile cysts that elevate with tongue protrusion or swallowing, indicating their proximal fixation to the base of the tongue.

5. **What are the symptoms associated with TGDC and TGDS?**

TGDC most commonly present in children as asymptomatic midline lesions of the neck that enlarge over time but 10–28% of patients present with infected TGDC with painful, erythematous midline lesion. Once the cyst drains to the skin, the TGDS or fistula tract is formed with drainage. Recurrent infections may occur. Large, lingual TGDC may cause airway obstruction in infants and in adults; lingual TGDC may present with dysphagia and pharyngeal discomfort.

6. **How can one distinguish TGDC from other cysts or masses of the neck?**

Epithelial inclusion cysts (i.e. dermoid cysts) are also commonly found in the midline of infants and children. Clinically, dermoid cysts may have a slightly more bright yellow colour compared to TGDC and should not move with swallowing. Lymph nodes are also commonly found in the neck and also should not move with swallowing. Type 2 branchial cleft cysts are usually situated laterally along the anterior border of the sternocleidomastoid muscle. Ectopic thyroid tissue may also present as a mass in the midline above the thyroid cartilage due to incomplete descent and can be found anywhere along the thyroglossal duct.

7. **How can one distinguish TGDS from other lesions with sinuses of the neck?**

For TGDS, the sinus opening is generally in or near the midline and commonly near the hyoid, whereas type 2 branchial cleft sinus openings are localized in the lower lateral neck region in close relation to the clavicular head of the sternocleidomastoid.

8. **What imaging is best for distinguishing TGDC from other neck cysts?**

Ultrasound (US) is the best imaging modality. Three US features most strongly predictive of TGDC are internal septae, irregular wall and presence of solid components [3]. Other helpful features include distance from the base of the tongue, location of the cyst relative to the hyoid bone, presence or absence of the tract, margin definition and intra-lesional Doppler flow.

9. **Are there other investigations that can help with TGDC diagnosis?**

CT and MRI imaging may also help to determine the diagnosis but these involve exposing children to ionizing radiation (CT) and/or general anesthetic/sedation (CT/MRI). Nuclear medicine scans of the thyroid are not routinely performed in children but would reveal a "cold" nodule. Routine thyroid function tests are not generally useful in the diagnosis of TGDC.

10. **What complications commonly arise from thyroglossal duct remnants?**

Infection is the most common complication and also the most common indication for the surgical excision of TGDC.

11. **Can TGDC become cancerous?**

The incidence of cancer in TGDC is 1%. Thyroid papillary carcinomas and follicular carcinomas have been found in TGDC in children and adults. The cancer is usually completely excised with TGDC excision but thyroidectomy is recommended in adults age >45 years due to the risks of cancer recurrence [4].

12. **What are the symptoms associated with a lingual TGDC?**

Very large, lingual TDGC can be a cause of upper airway obstruction, presenting with stridor and/or dyspnea, even mimicking an upper respiratory tract infection. More dramatically, there are case reports of asphyxia resulting in sudden deaths of infant and adults with the autopsies revealing the presence of the TGDC obstruct ing the upper airway at the epiglottis [5, 6].

13. **What is the treatment for TGDC and TGDS?**

Antibiotics are required to treat infected TGDC and TGDS. Surgery remains the most definitive treatment option as complete excision of the entire thyroglossal duct remnant eliminates both the infection and cancer risks. The standard of care is surgical excision of TGDC and TGDS using the Sistrunk procedure. Simple excision of the cyst alone is associated with a 45–55% recurrence rate whereas the Sistrunk procedure is associated with <10% recurrence rate [1].

14. **What are the steps in the Sistrunk procedure?**

The Sistrunk procedure involves *en bloc* resection of:

- the cyst
- the central third of the hyoid bone and
- the thyroglossal duct from the cyst up to the base of the tongue.

More than one duct or tract may be associated with a single cyst, further emphasizing the need for clearly visualizing the cyst and tract(s) as the mobilization proceeds through the midline.

15. **What are the manoeuvres to optimize surgical management of TGDC?**

Surgical considerations should include: pre-operative confirmation of the presence of an orthotopic thyroid (usually by US), extinguish any active infections prior to surgery (generally 3 months following infection), positioning the patient with a substantial under shoulder roll to allow good extension of the neck to aid exposure, nasal intubation to allow manual access into the oral cavity at the base of the tongue to push down during the cephalad dissection of the thyroglossal duct and inclusion of an ellipse of skin around the sinus opening of the TGDS to ensure complete TGDS excision.

16. **What are the complications from surgery for TGDC/TGDS?**

The most common complications following TGDC excision are wound infection, seroma, incomplete resection with recurrence, fistula, abscess, hematoma, hypoglossal nerve palsy (resulting in immobility of half of the tongue), hypothyroidism. Less common but devastating complications include resection of the thyroid cartilage, airway compromise and severe hemorrhage requiring multiple transfusions.

17. **Can TGDC/TGDS recur following surgery? What are the management options for recurrent TGDC/TGDS?**

Recurrence affects approximately 10% of cases and generally occurs within 1 year of the initial surgery. Recurrences manifest as persistent ± enlarging neck mass. Re-excision should include the previous incision, incorporate any sinus openings, wider excision down to the thyroid isthmus between the strap muscles, and include the medial margins of the strap muscles and the remaining hyoid bone remnants.

References

1. Amos J, Shermetaro C. Thyroglossal duct cyst. [Updated 2019 Feb 23]. In: **StatPearls [Internet]**. Treasure Island (FL): StatPearls Publishing; 2019. Retrieved from https://www.ncbi.nlm.nih.gov/books/NBK519057/.
2. Thompson LDR, Herrera HB, Lau SK. A clinicopathologic series of 685 thyroglossal duct remnant cysts. Head Neck Pathol. 2016;20:465–74.
3. Inarejos Clemente EJ, Oyewumi M, Propst EJ, Ngan B, Greer ML. Thyroglossal duct cysts in children: sonographic features every radiologist should know and their histopathological correlation. Clin Imaging. 2017;46:57–64.
4. Rayess HM, Monk I, Svider PF. Thyroglossal duct cyst carcinoma: a systematic review of clinical features and outcomes. Otolaryngol Head Neck Surg. 2017;156(5):794–802.
5. Byard RW, Bourne AJ, Silver MM. The association of lingual thyroglossal duct remnants with sudden death in infancy. Int J Pediatr Otorhinolaryngol. 1990;20:107–12.
6. Sauvageau A, Belley-Cote EP, Racette S. Fatal asphyxia by a thyroglossal duct cyst in an adult. J Clin Forensic Med. 2006;13:349–52.

Chapter 44
Branchial Clefts and Arch Anomalies

Reto M. Baertschiger and Lourenço Sbragia

Abstract Branchial arch and cleft anomalies are congenital malformation of the first, second, third and fourth branchial arch and most frequently present as cysts, sinuses or fistulae in the auricular, mandibular or cervical areas. Good knowledge of embryological development helps to understand the anatomy and relationships of branchial anomalies with surrounding structures, especially the laryngeal nerves (superior and recurrent) and vascular structures. Diagnostic work up includes a good physical exam, ultrasonographical evaluation as well as MRI for cross-sectional imaging in more complicated cases. Fistulogram and endoscopy can also be helpful, especially in third and fourth branchial cleft anomalies. Surgical excision is usually the treatment of choice, on an elective basis. If the cervical cyst, sinus or fistula are infected, incision and drainage and antibiotic treatment are recommended, followed by elective excision when the inflammation has resolved.

Keywords Branchial cleft anomalies · Branchial arch anomalies · Branchial sinus · Branchial fistula · Cervical cysts · Neck cysts · First branchial anomaly · Second branchial anomaly · Third branchial anomaly · Branchial clef remnants · Branchio-oto-renal syndrome (BOR) · Treacher collins syndrome · DiGeorge anomaly · Pierre robin sequence · Goldenhar's syndrome

R. M. Baertschiger (✉)
Division of General and Thoracic Surgery, The Hospital for Sick Children, Department of Surgery, University of Toronto, 555 University Ave, Toronto, ON M5G 1X8, Canada
e-mail: reto.baertschiger@sickkids.ca

L. Sbragia
Division of Pediatric Surgery, Department of Surgery and Anatomy, Ribeirao Preto Medical School, University of Sao Paulo, Ribeirao Preto, Sao Paulo, Brazil

M. Lacher et al. (eds.), *Pearls and Tricks in Pediatric Surgery*,
https://doi.org/10.1007/978-3-030-51067-1_44

1. **How many branchial clefts and arches are clinically relevant?**

The face, neck, pharynx and multiple glandular component develop from branchial arches and clefts (pouches) in the human embryo. There are six branchial arches that appear between the fourth and seventh week of gestation and form the precursors to the ear, muscles, blood vessels, bones, cartilage and glandular structures of the face, neck and superior thorax (see Table 44.1, reproduced with permission [1]). The branchial arches give rise to an arch, a cleft and a pouch, forming ectodermal, mesodermal and endodermal structures, respectively.

The first 4 branchial arches and clefts are the most clinically relevant for congenital malformations of the head and neck for which pediatric surgeons are involved. The fifth branchial arch is almost inexistent in humans. A branchial anomaly and its associated sinus usually lies caudally to the derivatives of the arch. The malformations are therefore divided into the first to the fourth branchial anomalies, including arches and clefts.

2. **What is the incidence of congenital branchial cleft anomalies?**

Branchial anomalies are the second most common congenital malformations of the head and neck, after thyroglossal duct cysts, and encompass approximately 20% of all congenital head and neck masses. Second branchial cleft anomalies are the most frequent subtype of anomalies amongst the branchial malformations. There is a slight female preponderance and up to 20% of sinuses are bilateral.

3. **How are the different branchial clefts defined and anatomically located?**

The first branchial arch gives rise to the maxilla, and mandible as well as the external auditory structures, and two ossicles (incus and malleus). The second branchial arch forms part of the hyoid bone, middle structures including the stapes and the supratonsillar fossa as well as the palatine tonsils. The third branchial structures give raise to the greater horn of the hyoid bone, the thymus and the inferior parathyroid glands. And the fourth branchial arch and cleft form the laryngeal cartilaginous structures, the superior parathyroid glands as well as the C-cells of the thyroid. See Table 44.1 for full details.

First branchial anomalies

4. **How does a first branchial cleft anomaly present?**

First branchial cleft anomalies are rare. The first branchial arch and cleft are involved in the development of the external ear, middle ear auditory tubes, as well as the incus and malleus. Remnant of the first branchial cleft can present with lesions located between the external auditory canal and the submandibular area. They can be mistaken for pre-auricular pits or sinuses. The first cleft anomalies may be closely associated with the parotid gland. The first branchial clefts are divided into type 1 and type 2, type 1 being a duplication of the membranous external auditory canal and type 2 being of ectodermal and mesodermal origins and may include cartilage. Type 2 lesions pass medial to the facial nerve and can present at pre-auricular, infra-auricular, or post-auricular locations. They can present as masses, infected lesions, cysts, draining sinuses or otorrhea.

Table 44.1 Derivatives of the branchial clefts and pouches. Arch 5 does not form structures in humans and is, therefore, not listed in table (Adams et al., Branchial cleft anomalies: a pictorial review of embryological development and spectrum of imaging findings. Insights Imaging. 2016;7:71—reproduced with permission—open access—creative commons license)

	Pharyngeal arch	Aortic arch artery	Cranial nerve	Muscular structures	Skeletal structures	Adult structures
External auditory meatus	I (Mandibular arc)	Maxillary artery	Trigeminal (V)	Mandibular prominence: muscles of mastication, anterior belly of digastric, tensor tympani, tensor veli palatini, mylohyoid. Maxillary prominence: none	Mandibular prominence: mandible, incus, malleus, Meckel's cartilages, Maxillary prominence: maxilla, zygomatic bone, squamos temporal bone, palatine bone, vomer	Middle ear auditory tube, tympanic activity
	II (Hyoid arch)	Stapedial artery, hyoid artery	Facial nerve (VII)	Muscles of facial expression, (buccinator, platysma, auricularis, frontalis, orbicularis oris, orbicularis oculi) stylohyoid, posterior belly of digastric, stapedius	Lesser horn of the hyoid bone, superior half of hyoid body, stapes, styloid process	Supratonsillar fossa, crypts of palatine tonsils
Cervical sinus of His	III	Common carotid, internal carotid artery	Glossopharyngeal (IX)	Stylopharyngeus	Grater horn of hyoid bone, inferior half of hyoid body	Thymus, inferior parathyroid glands
	IV	Right—Proximal subclavian artery Left—Aortic ach	Vagus nerve (X), superior laryngeal nerve	Intrinsic muscles of soft palate, levator veli palatini, cricothyroid	Laryngeal cartilages: thyroid cartilage, cricoid cartilage, arytenoid cartilage, corniculate cartilage, cuneiform cartilage, epiglottic cartilage	Superior parathyroid glands, C-cells of thyroid
	VI	Right—proximal pulmonary artery Left—proximal pulmonary artery an ductus arteriosus	Vagus nerve, recurrent laryngeal nerve	Intrinsic muscles of the larynx, (not cricothyroid)	Laryngeal cartilages: thyroid cartilage, cricoid cartilage, arytenoid cartilage, comiculate cartilage, cuneiform cartilage	

5. **What work up is performed?**

A careful physical exam of the lesion and its location is necessary. Any sinus, mass, or cyst within the pre-, infra- or post-auricular area, as well as submandibular space should be suspicious for a first branchial anomaly. An ultrasound and careful otoscopic evaluation should be performed. Cross-sectional imaging for large lesion can be helpful to better delineate the relationship of the cyst or sinus with the facial nerve [2].

6. **How is a first branchial cleft managed?**

Surgical excision is the treatment of choice. Careful dissection of the lesion is performed with special attention to the facial nerve. Superficial parotidectomy has been recommended to decrease the risks of injury to the facial nerve. It is necessary to excise the skin or associated cartilaginous anomalies if the external auditory canal is involved.

7. **Are there any complications or associated features to be concerned about?**

Injuries to the facial nerve are the most feared complication during excision of the first branchial cleft anomalies. Temporary facial nerve paralysis has been reported in up to 21% of cases, with 1% of permanent palsy. Rare injuries to the parotid gland with salivary fistula can also happen. If there was previous infection of the lesion, the scar tissue increases the difficulty of the dissection, as the planes might have been distorted.

Second branchial anomalies

8. **How does a second branchial cleft present?**

The second branchial cleft anomalies are the most frequent congenital branchial anomalies, with an incidence of 40% to 95%, varying between studies. They usually present as an asymptomatic neck mass or sinus along the anterior border of the sterno-cleido-mastoid muscle. The second branchial cleft anomalies can also present acutely after an upper respiratory infection with acute enlargement of the lesion. Cystic lesions are more frequent than sinuses. Sinuses can present with a small opening draining clear fluid, near the base of the neck, anterior to the sterno-cleido-mastoid muscle. Sinuses are more frequent on the right side and bilateral sinuses can be found in up to 10 percent. Less common symptoms include odyno- or dysphagia, stridor or cranial nerve palsies in case of infected lesions [2, 3].

9. **What work up is performed?**

A careful clinical exam of the neck is critical. Sinuses and cyst are found anterior to the sterno-cleido-mastoid muscle. Sometimes the tract can be palpated going cephalad. Cysts are usually mobile and non-tender. Some clear fluid can sometimes be expressed from sinuses, as they communicate with the tonsillar fossa.

Ultrasonography of the neck is recommended as initial imaging, even though a draining sinus in the correct location narrows the diagnosis. For large or symptomatic lesions, an MRI may better delineate the cyst or sinus and allow for better surgical planning. Rarely a sinogram can be performed but is currently more of historical interest [2].

10. **How is a second branchial cleft managed?**

As branchial clefts can become infected, and there is a reported potential long-term risk of malignant transformation, elective excision of second branchial cysts and sinuses is recommended. The procedure is performed under general anesthesia and the head slightly turned to the contralateral side. The sinus is excised with the skin opening and some surgeons use a small catheter, probe or dye to be able to follow the track cephalad. Good knowledge of the embryology and neck anatomy is required. Second branchial cleft sinuses or cysts track cephalad and end up in the tonsillar fossa, after having crossed the internal carotid artery antero-superiorly to the carotid bifurcation. Wide skin preparation is mandatory and sometimes a second counter-incision is needed for safe excision of the sinus [3].

11. **Are there any complications or associated features to be concerned about?**

Incomplete resection increases the risk of recurrence or infection. The risk of injuring neck structure is low if the dissection is accomplished close to the sinus tract. There is a reported low risk of malignant transformation in adults.

Third branchial anomalies

12. **How does a third branchial cleft anomaly present?**

Third branchial cleft anomalies have an incidence of less than 10% of all branchial clefts and extend medially between the bifurcation of the internal and external carotid arteries, lateral to the pharyngeal wall. They are more commonly found on the left side in the lower portion of the anterior neck. Third and fourth branchial cleft anomalies are very similar to second branchial cleft anomalies externally with a cutaneous opening in the supraclavicular area; however, internally, the third and fourth enter the pharynx through the pyriform sinus below the hyoid bone. Both are distinguished anatomically by their relationship to the superior laryngeal nerve with third pharyngeal cleft anomalies being above and fourth pharyngeal cleft anomalies being caudal to the superior laryngeal nerve. Anatomically, the third branchial cleft remnants pass through the thyrohyoid membrane cephalad to the superior laryngeal nerve and open into the upper piriform sinus. Third branchial cleft cysts present in the posterior cervical space more frequently, posterior to the sternocleidomastoid muscle as a painless, fluctuant mass that may enlarge and become tender if infected. Abscesses in the posterior triangle of the neck should be considered as an infected third branchial cleft cyst. Recurrent episodes of abscess can also promote thyroiditis [4].

13. **What work up is performed?**

There are many different forms of presentation of third branchial anomalies including fistulas, cysts or sinuses. A classic third branchial fistula opens in the pyriform sinus and exits at the skin, which makes it an epithelized tract. A cyst has no opening and sinus has an opening in direction of skin or pyriform sinus but not both. Repeated procedures of drainage and incision may convert a sinus to a fistula [2, 3].

The diagnostic investigation should include a careful physical exam, and an Ultrasound. Possible further investigation with magnetic resonance imaging (MRI) can be helpful to better delineate the anatomy. Further fiberoptic endoscopy could be necessary to identify the entry point of a third and fourth branchial sinus at the level of the pyriform sinus. In that case, the orifice of the sinus or fistula can be identified, and cannulation or injection of the tract can be helpful for surgical dissection.

14. **How is a third branchial cleft anomaly managed?**

Elective surgical resection is necessary to treat third branchial cleft anomalies. As mentioned above, upper endoscopy can be helpful to identify the internal pyriform sinus opening. The operation is performed under general anesthesia and the neck is widely prepped. The dissection must respect the anatomic structures in order to avoid any damage and perform a complete resection of the cyst, sinus or fistula to its origin. Very careful attention to the superior and recurrent laryngeal nerves are necessary to prevent injury, as these nerves are closely associated with a third branchial cleft anomaly. Rarely, these cysts can extend into the chest. Previous infections can make the dissection more difficult, secondary to scar tissue. If the cyst or sinus is infected, drainage and antibiotic therapy are recommended followed by an elective excision once the infection and inflammation have resolved.

15. **Are there any complications or associated features to be concerned about?**

During the dissection, injury to the superior and recurrent laryngeal nerves has been documented. Patients are also at risk of recurrence of cervical abscesses and mediastinitis, more commonly observed in incomplete excision of the sinus tract or cyst.

Fourth branchial anomalies

16. **How does a fourth branchial cleft anomaly present?**

A fourth branchial cleft fistula/sinus tract arises from the apex of the pyriform sinus and descends inferiorly to the mediastinum in the path of the tracheo-esophageal groove. Fourth branchial anomalies can therefore present as lower cervical masses as third branchial cysts, but also with thyroiditis, dyspnea or dysphagia and rarely with chest pain. Similarly to the third branchial anomalies, fourth branchial malformations are more frequent on the left side and their overall incidence is 1–4% of all congenital neck anomalies. The fourth branchial sinus runs caudal to the superior laryngeal nerve and over the recurrent laryngeal nerve [4].

17. **What work up is performed?**

The diagnostic work up should include a careful physical exam, and an Ultrasound. Possible further investigation with magnetic resonance imaging (MRI) can be helpful to better delineate the anatomy, especially if one suspects an extension into the chest. Further fiberoptic endoscopy could be necessary, similarly to the third branchial anomalies to identify the entry point of a sinus at the level of the pyriform sinus. In that case, the orifice of the sinus or fistula can be identified, and cannulation or injection of the tract can be helpful for surgical dissection.

18. **How is a fourth branchial cleft anomaly managed?**

Most of fourth branchial anomalies present as a cervical inflammatory process located at the left side, and half of them have associated acute suppurative thyroiditis or recurrent neck abscesses. Elective surgical excision is recommended after drainage and treatment of the infection with resolution of the inflammation. Fiberoptic endoscopy with possible catheterization of the fistula can facilitate the dissection.

19. **Are there any complications or associated features to be concerned about?**

Fourth arch anomalies with thyroiditis and abscess formation may require ipsilateral hemithyroidectomy for complete excision of the tract as well as partial resection of the thyroid cartilage to provide adequate exposure of the pyriform sinus. As for third arch anomalies, careful attention to the recurrent laryngeal nerve is recommended, to prevent its injury. As fourth branchial anomalies may extend into the chest, the surgeon and anesthesiologist need to be prepared for that possibility.

20. **Are there any special considerations—syndromes in branchial cleft anomalies and their treatment?**

Common syndromes associated with branchial cleft anomalies include Branchio-oto-renal syndrome (BOR), Treacher Collins Syndrome, DiGeorge Anomaly, Pierre Robin Sequence, Goldenhar's Syndrome and Hemifacial Microsomia [5].

BOR syndrome is an autosomal dominant disorder and is characterized by branchial arch anomalies (branchial clefts, fistula, cysts), hearing impairment (malformations of the auricle with preauricular pits, conductive, or sensorineural hearing impairment), and renal malformations (urinary tract malformation, renal hypoplasia, or agenesis, renal dysplasia, renal cysts). Treacher Collins Syndrome (mandibulofacial dysostosis, Franceschetti-Zwahlen syndrome) is an autosomal dominant genetic disorder, characterized by bilateral, symmetric abnormalities of first and second branchial arch structures. DiGeorge Anomaly is a congenital disorder of the third and fourth branchial pouches in which there is abnormal development of the thymus and the parathyroid glands. Pierre Robin sequence is characterized by micrognathia, glossoptosis, and a U-shaped cleft soft palate. Goldenhar's Syndrome and Hemifacial Microsomia are also called oculo-auriculo-vertebral syndrome and the anomaly is characterized by impaired development of eyes, ears (with or without hearing loss), lip, tongue, palate, mandible, maxilla and deformations of the teeth structures.

Recurrent cervical abscesses, on the lateral and posterior side, as well as thyroiditis in children associated with a cervical inflammatory process should raise suspicion about congenital branchial anomalies. The most important recommendation is a correct location of the lesion, including sinus, cyst or fistula that therefore define the anatomy and allows the classification of a brachial cleft defect.

References

1. Adams A, Mankad K, et al. Branchial cleft anomalies: a pictorial review of embryological development and spectrum of imaging findings. Insight Imaging. 2016;7:69–76.
2. Goff C, Allred C, et al. Current management of congenital branchial cleft, cysts, sinuses and fistulae. Curr Opin Otolarygol Head Neck Surg. 2012;20:533–9.
3. Lillehei C. Branchial anomalies. In: Pediatric surgery, 7th edn, vol. 1. Elsevier Saunders Publishers, Chapter 59. pp. 757–61.
4. Nicoucar K, Giger R, Pope HG Jr, Jaecklin T, Dulguerov P. Management of congenital fourth branchial arch anomalies: a review and analysis of published cases. J Pediatr Surg. 2009;44:1432–9.
5. Mandell DL. Head and neck anomalies related to the branchial apparatus. Otolaryngol Clin North Am. 2000;33:1309–32.

Chapter 45
Torticollis

Jill M. Arganbright and Jason R. Brown

Abstract Torticollis is a clinical sign of ipsilateral head tilt with contralateral rotation. There are several causes of torticollis, the most common of which is congenital muscular torticollis. While no imaging is required, ultrasound is useful to aid in the diagnosis. Treatment is primarily conservative with physical therapy encompassing the bulk of treatment modalities. Adjunctive therapies, including botulinum toxin and surgical release, can be performed in refractory cases.

Keywords Torticollis · Congenital · Sternocleidomastoid · Pediatric · Fibromatosis coli · Physical therapy · Botulinum toxin

1. **What is torticollis?**

The term 'Torticollis' is derived from two Latin root words 'tortus' and 'collum' that together mean 'twisted neck'. Torticollis is not a specific diagnosis but rather a clinical sign of ipsilateral head tilt with contralateral rotation [1].

Although it has been known since ancient times, it was first defined by A. H. Tubby in 1912. Interestingly, some portraits and statues of Alexander the Great depict him with his head tilted or twisted, which has led some medical researchers to believe he suffered from ocular torticollis.

2. **What is congenital muscular torticollis?**

There are many presentations of torticollis, however, the most prevalent is congenital muscular torticollis (CMT). CMT is defined as a musculoskeletal deformity observed at birth or infancy, characterized by a persistent head tilt toward the

J. M. Arganbright (✉) · J. R. Brown
Department of Pediatric Surgery, Division of Pediatric Otolaryngology, University of Missouri - Kansas City, Children's Mercy Hospital, 2401 Gillham Road, Kansas City, MO 64108, USA
e-mail: jarganbright@cmh.edu

M. Lacher et al. (eds.), *Pearls and Tricks in Pediatric Surgery*,
https://doi.org/10.1007/978-3-030-51067-1_45

involved side with the chin rotated toward the contralateral shoulder. Classically, the sternocleidomastoid muscle (SCM) in involved.

3. **How common is congenital muscular torticollis?**

Historically, the incidence of CMT was reported to be 0.3–2% with overall incidence that can be as high as 1 in 250 live births. It is the third most common congenital pediatric musculoskeletal deformity, behind hip dysplasia and talipes equinovarus.

4. **What are 3 different types of congenital muscular torticollis?**

Congenital muscular torticollis can be divided into 3 groups based on presentation:

Group 1: Infants with sternocleidomastoid tumor. This group consists of torticollis with range of motion limitations and a palpable pseudotumor or swelling in the body of the SCM. The pseudotumor, also called fibromatosis colli, is a hard, immobile mass within the substance of the SCM and is noted at birth. It is usually located in the middle to lower third of the sternal portion of the SCM. This type occurs in 33–47% of cases.
Group 2: Muscular torticollis. This group consists of torticollis with limitations in active and passive range of motion secondary to tightness or contracture of the SCM, but no palpable intramuscular mass is present
Group 3: Postural torticollis. This group includes patients with clinical torticollis, in which there is no presence of SCM mass and no passive range of motion restrictions [2]

5. **Describe hypotheses for possible causes of congenital muscular torticollis**.

The exact cause of CMT is still unknown, however, there are a variety of hypotheses. Many revolve around in utero positioning or trauma during delivery. One theory suggests that CMT is caused by a congenitally shortened SCM torn at birth, resulting in the formation of a hematoma that underwent fibrous contracture. Ischemia within the SCM produced by possible venous occlusion has also been posited. Another hypothesis is intrauterine or perinatal compartment syndrome involving the SCM. Less likely causes have also been described, such as infection and heredity. Despite these hypotheses insufficient evidence has been found to definitively identify a cause for CMT.

6. **What are the three strongest negative prognostic factors for congenital muscular torticollis treatment outcomes?**

   1. Sternocleidomastoid mass present
   2. >15 degrees passive range of motion deficit in cervical rotation
   3. Physical therapy treatment started >3 month of age.

These three factors contribute to patients requiring a longer duration of physical therapy, having an increased need for surgical intervention, and having an overall poorer outcome

7. **If left untreated, what sequelae can develop from congenital muscular torticollis?**

Secondary sequelae from the presence of CMT include plagiocephaly and facial asymmetry. This is primarily caused by the forces of gravity pulling unevenly on a baby's tilted head, causing a flattened appearance on one side of the skull or face. This emphasizes the importance of early identification and treatment to prevent the development of these secondary issues.

8. **What are non-muscular causes of torticollis?**

It is imperative that congenital muscular torticollis is differentiated from other congenital or acquired types of torticollis [3]. There are a variety of known non-muscular causes of torticollis in children and can include:

- Osseous: includes Klippel-Feil anomalies, scoliosis, clavicle fracture, and atlantoaxial rotatory subluxation
- Ocular: includes 4th cranial nerve palsy and resulting strabismus, Brown's syndrome, and gaze dysfunction
- Neurologic: includes brachial plexus palsies and central nervous system lesions
- Otologic: includes saccular dysfunction
- Inflammatory: includes Grisel's syndrome after adenoidectomy
- Gastrointestinal: includes Sandifer syndrome.

9. **How common is non-muscular torticollis in children?**

Non-muscular causes were thought to be rare compared to CMT, however, recent studies have shown this may be occurring more frequently than initially thought; showing that approximately 20% of torticollis is non-muscular in nature. This highlights the need for providers to be well educated in the differential diagnosis for torticollis, as misdiagnosis can cause a delay in appropriate treatment.

10. **In the 2018 clinical practice guidelines for the management of congenital muscular torticollis, why is there such an emphasis on early referral to physical therapy and a physician for evaluation?**

Early intervention has shown to require a shorter duration of physical therapy and a higher chance of reaching complete resolution of the torticollis [4]. More than 98% of infants with torticollis treated before 1 month of age recover by 2.5 months of age. Infants treated between 1 and 6 months usually require about 6 months of treatment. After that point, therapy will take closer to 9 months, and it is less likely that the torticollis will be fully resolved, resulting in the need for surgical intervention. Early identification, referral, and intervention are key to obtaining the best possible outcome for the child.

11. **What is recommended if the patient does not progress with 4–6 weeks of intensive physical therapy?**

Recommendations are for therapist to refer to a physician for re-evaluation and assessment for non-muscular causes of the torticollis.

12. **What is the preferred radiological modality in the diagnosis of torticollis?**

Due to its low cost and non-invasive nature, ultrasonography can be used to aid in the diagnosis of CMT. For CMT, ultrasound has been shown to correlate with the severity of disease but is not sensitive enough to determine changes in the muscular architecture [5]. Other imaging modalities such as computerized tomography (CT) and magnetic resonance imaging (MRI) are not necessary for the initial work-up and management of CMT, however they may be useful when investigating non-muscular causes of torticollis.

13. **Describe the ultrasound features of normal sternocleidomastoid muscle.**

The normal SCM on ultrasound presents as a hypoechoic mass with echogenic lines, indicating muscle fascicles running throughout its length.

14. **What are characteristic features on ultrasound for patients with congenital muscular torticollis and sternocleidomastoid pseudotumor?**

The presence of a SCM pseudotumor affects not only the size of the muscle, but also its signal intensity. For patients with CMT, the involved SCM tends to be larger and will appear more hyperechoic on ultrasound.

15. **Describe the primary therapy modality for congenital muscular torticollis.**

Physical therapy is the primary treatment modality for CMT. The 2018 Clinical Practice Guidelines outline five main areas of therapy intervention: passive neck range of motion exercises, cervical and trunk muscle strengthening, development of an infant's symmetrical movement, environmental adaptations, and parent education. The frequency of treatment can be based on the age at presentation, the presence of a fibrotic mass in the sternocleidomastoid, and the infant's neck rotational deficit.

16. **What medical therapies can be used as an adjunct therapy for congenital muscular torticollis?**

Botulinum toxin type A has been shown to be beneficial as an adjunct therapy in patients with CMT and is to be used in conjunction with physical therapy. Systemic medical therapies such as muscles relaxants have shown no benefit and are to be avoided [6].

17. **In the event of medical and therapy failure, what surgical interventions can be employed to treat congenital muscular torticollis?**

Surgical release of the sternocleidomastoid muscle is used mainly in cases of severe CMT that are unresponsive to more conservative therapies. Surgical intervention involves a unipolar or bipolar approach. For the unipolar approach, the sternocleidomastoid muscle is released from either its mastoid or sternum/clavicular insertions, whereas a bipolar approach releases the SCM from both insertion points.

18. **Which patients tend to require surgical intervention?**

- Persistent sternocleidomastoid muscle contracture limiting head movement
- Persistent sternocleidomastoid muscle contracture accompanied by progressive facial hemihypoplasia
- Torticollis in untreated children older than 12 months of age.

19. **List some potential complications of surgical management of congenital muscular torticollis.**

- Hematoma
- Wound dehiscence or infection
- Non-resolution of torticollis
- Vascular injury to the carotid artery, internal jugular vein, or brachiocephalic artery
- Neural injury to the spinal accessory nerve or the brachial plexus.

20. **What are the histologic findings of congenital muscular torticollis?**

Histologic studies of the resected surgical specimens have demonstrated edema, degeneration of the SCM muscle fibers, and fibrosis.

References

1. Nilesh K, Mukherji S. Congenital muscular torticollis. Ann Maxillofac Surg. 2013;3(2):198–200.
2. Cheng JC, Tang SP, Chen TM, Wong MW, Wong EM. The clinical presentation and outcome of treatment of congenital muscular torticollis in infants - a study of 1,086 cases. J Pediatr Surg. 2000;35(7):1091–6.
3. Ballock RT and Song KM. The prevalence of nonmuscular causes of torticollis in children. J Pediatr Orthop. 1996;16(4):500–4.
4. Kaplan SL, Coulter C, Sargent B. Physical therapy management of congenital muscular torticollis: a 2018 evidence-based clinical practice guideline from the apta academy of pediatric physical therapy. Pediatr Phys Ther. 2018;30(4):240–90.
5. Suhr MC, Oledzka M. Considerations and intervention in congenital muscular torticollis. Curr Opin Pediatr. 2015;27(1):75–81.
6. Oleszek JL, Chang N, Apkon SD, Wilson PE. Botulinum toxin type a in the treatment of children with congenital muscular torticollis. Am J Phys Med Rehabil. 2005;84(10):813–6.

Chapter 46
Renal Cystic Diseases

Alexandra Rehfuss, Christina Ching, Daniel DaJusta, and Molly Fuchs

Abstract Renal cystic diseases may be inherited or acquired. The most common renal cystic disease is multicystic dysplastic kidney, which is essentially a nonfunctioning kidney. Most renal cysts and cystic diseases do not require intervention, with the exception of multilocular cystic nephroma. Cases of multilocular cystic nephroma cannot be differentiated from malignant tumors (ex: cystic Wilm's tumor) and therefore must undergo nephrectomy. Autosomal dominant polycystic kidney disease and autosomal recessive polycystic kidney disease are both inherited renal cystic diseases, with the latter more commonly presenting in the neonatal period. These inherited renal cystic diseases should be managed in conjunction with nephrology given their sequelae of renal dysfunction.

Keywords Multicystic dysplastic kidney · Polycystic kidney disease · Multilocular cystic nephroma

1. **What is the most common renal cystic disease diagnosed in childhood?**

   - Multicystic dysplastic kidney (MCDK) is the most common renal cystic disease diagnosed in childhood, with an incidence of approximately 1 in 2,500 [1]. MCDKs occur sporadically and are more common in males than females. They are usually unilateral (left more common than right) and asymptomatic. Most cases are diagnosed on prenatal ultrasound.

2. **Does a MCDK have any function?**

   - Multicystic dysplastic kidneys are non-functional and associated with ureteral atresia. There are two main theories as to why MCKDs form. One theory is that renal pelvic ureteral atresia results in severe hydronephrosis and MCKD

A. Rehfuss · C. Ching · D. DaJusta · M. Fuchs (✉)
Department of Pediatric Urology at Nationwide Children's Hospital, Columbus, OH 43206, USA
e-mail: Molly.fuchs@nationwidechildrens.org

M. Lacher et al. (eds.), *Pearls and Tricks in Pediatric Surgery*,
https://doi.org/10.1007/978-3-030-51067-1_46

[2]. The other theory is that there is a disruption in the interaction between the metanephric blastema and the ureteric bud during development, which results in failure of the kidney and ureter to develop normally [2].

3. **How can you differentiate between multicystic dysplastic kidney and a severely hydronephrotic kidney** [3]?

- **Appearance on renal ultrasound**: The MCDKs have multiple small cysts among larger cysts, the cysts do not communicate, and there is no large central cyst. In kidneys with severe hydronephrosis the dilated calyces appear as cysts, and are organized around the periphery. In hydronephrosis there appears to be a central cyst, which is the dilated renal pelvis. Normal reniform shape is preserved in hydronephrosis but not in MCDKs.
- **Radionuclide scan**: Nuclear imaging studies to look at the function of the cystic kidney are helpful in differentiating between MCDK and hydronephrosis. Using either dimercaptosuccinic acid (DMSA) or technetium-99 m mercaptoacetyltriglycine (MAG3), there will be no radiotracer uptake in a MCDK, while a kidney with hydronephrosis will usually show some uptake.

4. **Do patients with MCDKs need a voiding cystourethrogram (VCUG)?**

- No. It is known that vesicoureteral reflux to the contralateral kidney occurs in 17–43% of patients with MCDKs. However, studies have shown that VCUG results do not impact management and that the use of VCUG does not prevent febrile urinary tract infections [4].

5. **Do MCDKs need to be removed?**

- The natural history of MCDKs is that they will involute over time, and therefore the current standard is non-operative management of these kidneys. Follow up renal ultrasound can confirm involution and compensatory hypertrophy of the contralateral kidney. Nephrectomy is performed in the setting of enlarging MCDKs, especially if symptomatic. For children with MCDKs who develop hypertension, some studies have shown that hypertension can be cured by nephrectomy.

6. **What cystic renal lesions require nephrectomy?**

- Patients with a benign multilocular cyst, or multilocular cystic nephroma, must undergo nephrectomy. Although it is a benign lesion, multilocular cystic nephroma cannot be differentiated on imaging from malignant cystic renal tumors (for example: cystic Wilms tumor, mesoblastic nephroma, clear cell sarcoma) [3].

7. **How can you tell the difference between MCDK and multilocular cystic nephroma?**

   - While MCDK is a dysplastic kidney, a multilocular cystic nephroma is a complex multicystic mass with uniformly thin septa between the cysts that arises from the kidney.

8. **How do you manage a simple renal cyst?**

   - A simple renal cyst is a solitary thin walled cyst with no septations or nodules. They occur in less than 0.3% of children, and are more common in adults. The most common location is the right upper pole, which can make it hard to distinguish from upper pole hydronephrosis related to an obstructed ureterocele or ectopic ureter. If needed, the cyst can be aspirated to aid with diagnosis (cyst fluid has the same BUN and creatinine as the patient). Simple renal cysts are usually discovered incidentally and are asymptomatic. It is important to obtain a family history, as patients with autosomal dominant polycystic kidney disease may only have a single cyst in childhood.
   - If the cyst is large and symptomatic, treatment options include percutaneous drainage with a sclerosing agent (or they will recur) or surgical marsupialization.

9. **Is autosomal dominant polycystic kidney disease (ADPKD) diagnosed in childhood?**

   - Not typically. In contrast to autosomal recessive polycystic kidney disease (ARPKD), patients with ADPKD most commonly present in adulthood, between 30 and 50 years old. However, there have been a few reported cases of early-onset ADPKD.

10. **How do you differentiate between ARPKD and early-onset ADPKD** [1]**?**

    - While early-onset ADPKD is rare, it can be challenging to differentiate it from ARPKD. Obtaining a family history aids in differentiating the two. A history of oligohydramnios supports ARPKD. A liver biopsy can be obtained, which will always show congenital hepatic fibrosis in ARPKD, and almost never in ADPKD [1]. A biopsy of the kidney in ARPKD would show cysts arising from the collecting ducts only that remain connected to the nephron of origin. Meanwhile, a biopsy of the kidney in ADPKD would show cysts arising from all segments of the tubule that are not connected to the nephron of origin. There are commercially available tests for the ARPKD mutation, but these are unreliable. Commercially available tests also exist for the ADPKD mutation, but there are false negatives.

11. **What are the key differences between ADPKD and ARPKD** [1]?

	ADPKD	ARPKD
Incidence	1:400–1:1,000	1:6,000–1:55,000
Inheritance	Autosomal dominant	Autosomal recessive
Gene mutation	Chromosome 16 (PKD1 gene), Chromosome 4 (PKD2 gene)	Chromosome 6 (PKHD1 gene)
Usual age at presentation	Adult	Perinatal
Appearance of kidneys on ultrasound	Enlarged kidneys with random cysts	Enlarged hyperechoic kidneys with no discrete cysts

12. **What are the clinical features of ARPKD?**

- ARPKD is diagnosed by bilaterally enlarged kidneys in infants, due to numerous microscopic collecting duct cysts. It can be detected as early as 24 weeks gestation on ultrasound, which will demonstrate bilateral enlarged echogenic kidneys with poor corticomedullary differentiation. There may be oligohydramnios due to poor renal function. ARPKD has a spectrum of severity, with the most severe forms appearing at birth. The most common presentation is respiratory failure due to pulmonary hypoplasia, volume overload, or poor diaphragm function due to the enlarged kidneys. It is always associated with congenital hepatic fibrosis, which causes portal hypertension. Clinical features of portal hypertension include esophageal varices, splenomegaly and dilated biliary ducts which can predispose to cholangitis.

13. **When do patients with ARPKD require nephrectomy?**

- Patients with significant respiratory distress can benefit from unilateral or bilateral nephrectomies. If unilateral nephrectomy is performed, renal function should first be assessed to determine which kidney provides greater function and should therefore be left in situ. If bilateral nephrectomy is performed, peritoneal dialysis (PD) catheter should be placed simultaneously. If a PD catheter is to be placed, it is recommended that nephrectomy be approached extraperitoneally [1]. The size of these kidneys not only compromises the respiratory system, but can also have a significant impact on feeding tolerance and therefore nephrectomy is sometimes indicated in these cases.

14. **How do you treat an infected renal cyst?**

- In the setting of an infected cyst, the urine culture may be negative. Thus patients with signs and symptoms of infection should be treated accordingly. Patients should be treated with lipid soluble antibiotics that can penetrate the cysts, such as trimethoprim-sulfamethoxazole or ciprofloxacin [3]. Rarely, infected cysts will need to be percutaneously aspirated.

References

1. George R, Greenbaum L. Cystic Kidney Disease. In: Docimo S, editor. The Kelalis-King-Belman textbook of clinical pediatric urology. 6th ed. Boca Raton: CRC Press; 2019. p. 381–97.
2. Cardona-Grau D, Kogan BA. Update on multicystic dysplastic kidney. Curr Urol Rep. 2015;16(10):67.
3. Pope J. Renal dysgenesis and cystic disease of the kidney. In: Wein A, editor. Campbell-walsh urology. 11th ed. Philadelphia: Elsevier; 2016. p. 3006–42.
4. Brown C, McLeod D, Ching C. Knowledge of vesicoureteral reflux obtained by screening voiding cystourethrogram in children with multicystic dysplastic kidney does not change patient management or prevent febrile urinary tract infection. J Pediat Urol. 2019;15(3):267.

Chapter 47
Obstructive Uropathy

Alexandra Rehfuss, Molly Fuchs, Daniel DaJusta, and Christina Ching

Abstract Obstructive uropathy is the leading cause of chronic kidney disease in children. It may be caused by upper or lower urinary tract obstruction and most often hydronephrosis on renal ultrasound is the first indicator of obstruction. The key in management of these patients is determining if hydronephrosis is due to obstruction, and this can be done with further imaging such as a nuclear scan or magnetic resonance urography. Once obstruction is confirmed, the crucial step is to bypass the level of obstruction and drain the urinary tract so as not to compromise renal function.

Keywords Hydronephrosis · Posterior urethral valves · Ureteropelvic junction obstruction · Ureterocele · Ectopic ureter

1. **What is the leading cause of chronic kidney disease in children?**

Congenital urinary tract obstruction is the #1 cause of chronic kidney disease in males under 1 year old, and is one of the most common diagnosis in children undergoing renal transplant for end stage renal disease [1].

2. **What are common causes of pediatric obstructive uropathy?**

   a. Ureteropelvic junction obstruction
   b. Ureterovesical junction obstruction
   c. Ureterocele
   d. Ectopic ureter
   e. Posterior urethral valves.

A. Rehfuss · M. Fuchs (✉) · D. DaJusta · C. Ching
Department of Pediatric Urology at Nationwide Children's Hospital, Columbus, OH 43206, USA
e-mail: Molly.fuchs@nationwidechildrens.org

M. Lacher et al. (eds.), *Pearls and Tricks in Pediatric Surgery*,
https://doi.org/10.1007/978-3-030-51067-1_47

3. How is obstruction diagnosed?

Hydronephrosis on renal ultrasound (RUS) is usually the first indication of underlying urinary tract obstruction.

The Society for Fetal Urology (SFU) developed a grading system for reporting hydronephrosis on RUS [2]. The higher the grade, the worse the hydronephrosis.

Grade	Renal pelvis	Renal parenchyma
0	No splitting	Normal
1	Splitting	Normal
2	Dilated renal pelvis and major calyces	Normal
3	Dilated renal pelvis, major and minor calyces	Normal
4	Dilated renal pelvis, major and minor calyces	Thinned

The Urinary Tract Dilation (UTD) classification system risk stratifies based on prenatal and postnatal RUS characteristics and anterior-posterior renal pelvis diameter (AP RPD) [3].

Prenatal UTD classification	AP RPD (mm)	RUS characteristics
UTD A1 (low risk)	16–27 wk: 4 to $\leq$7 $\geq$28 wk: 7 to $\leq$10	Central or no calyceal dilation
UTD A2–3 (increased risk)	16–27 wk: $\geq$7 $\geq$28 wk: $\geq$10	Peripheral calyceal dilation Parenchymal thickness abnl Parenchyma appearance abnl Ureters abnormal Bladder abnormal Unexplained oligohydramnios

Postnatal UTD classification	AP RPD (mm)	RUS characteristics
UTD P1 (low risk)	10 to $<$15	Central calyceal dilation
UTD P2 (intermediate risk)	$\geq$15	Peripheral calyceal dilation Ureters abnormal
UTD P3 (high risk)	$\geq$15	Peripheral calyceal dilation Parenchymal thickness abnl Parenchyma appearance abnl Ureters abnormal Bladder abnormal

4. How do you determine if hydronephrosis is due to obstruction?

Renal function and drainage must be assessed. This can be done with a MAG3 diuretic renal scan or with magnetic resonance urography (MRU).

The MAG3 scan requires an IV and a urinary catheter if not toilet trained. The radiotracer is injected intravenously and within the first 2–3 minutes radiotracer uptake by the renal parenchyma is detected (radiotracer binds to the proximal tubules). The differential renal function is determined at this point. Normal differential renal function should be 50/50, with an accepted error of ±5%. At approximately 20 minutes, furosemide is administered intravenously and the drainage curves are analyzed. The time is takes for half of the radiotracer to clear the renal pelvis is called the "t 1/2". An obstructed kidney will have a flat, or plateaued, drainage curve, and a t 1/2 > 20 minutes. An unobstructed kidney will have a down-slopping drainage curve and a t1/2 < 15 minutes.

Magnetic resonance urography (MRU) is a newer imaging modality that utilizes gadolinium-dTPA. The advantage of MRU is that in addition to determining function and drainage, it also provides excellent anatomical evaluation. The disadvantages of MRU are the need for sedation, cost, and limited availability.

5. **What is the Whitaker test [4]?**

The Whitaker test measures the pressure needed to propel fluid through the upper urinary tract at a fixed rate. Under anesthesia, a nephrostomy tube is inserted into the renal pelvis and the collecting system is perfused at a continuous rate while simultaneously measuring the pressure in the renal pelvis. In an obstructed system, renal pelvis pressures measure > 20 cmH_2O. The invasiveness of this procedure has resulted in its limited use, however it can be helpful in equivocal cases. Additionally, if performed in the fluoroscopy suite, simultaneous antegrade imaging studies can be obtained to help further assess the anatomy.

6. **When should a voiding cystourethrogram (VCUG) be obtained in a patient with hydronephrosis?**

According to the American Urological Association guidelines, a VCUG is recommended in children with SFU grade 3 or 4 hydronephrosis [5]. This recommendation is based not only on the risk of vesicoureteral reflux (VUR), but also the potential for bladder outlet obstruction. One should have a high index of suspicion for posterior urethral valves (PUV) if a male infant has a thickened trabeculated bladder with bilateral hydroureteronephrosis. VCUG is the gold standard for diagnosing PUV, and imaging will show a dilated posterior urethra that funnels abruptly at the valves and a trabeculated bladder with a hypertrophied bladder neck. Approximately 50% of patients with PUV will also have high grade VUR.

Patients with prenatally diagnosed hydronephrosis without PUV have an incidence of vesicoureteral reflux (VUR) of 16%. VUR coexists with UPJ obstruction in approximately 10% of children.

7. **What is the incidence of prenatal hydronephrosis?**

Due to the increased use of ultrasound screening in the second trimester, the incidence of prenatal hydronephrosis is 1:100 to 1:500 [2].

8. **What are antenatal signs of obstructive uropathy?**

Prenatal ultrasound may show hydronephrosis, a distended bladder, and dilated posterior urethra ("keyhole" sign). After 16 weeks gestation, amniotic fluid is mostly comprised of fetal urine, therefore fetuses with obstructive uropathy may have oligohydramnios. Since amniotic fluid is vital to pulmonary development, oligohydramnios can result in pulmonary hypoplasia and there may be significant respiratory distress at birth. Oligohydramnios can also result in Potter facies, club-feet and deformed hands, and poor abdominal muscle tone.

9. **What is the timeline for postnatal imaging in a patient with prenatal hydronephrosis?**

RUS should be obtained after 48 h of life. If the RUS is performed too early, it may underestimate hydronephrosis due to the relative oliguria shortly after birth. If prenatal imaging in boys shows bilateral hydroureteronephrosis and/or thickened bladder with "keyhole" sign, a VCUG should be performed as soon as possible to evaluate for PUV.

For patients with hydronephrosis that do not have PUV, a follow up RUS can be performed in 3–6 months to reassess the degree of hydronephrosis. If hydronephrosis is persistent or worsening, a MAG-3 and/or VCUG can be ordered at this time. Imaging can be ordered sooner if there is a clinical change, such as a febrile urinary tract infection.

10. **What is the initial management for a patient with PUV?**

First, a catheter (small feeding tube or coude catheter) should be placed to drain the bladder. The balloon should not be inflated as this can obstruct the ureteral orifices in these small hypertrophied bladders. Once the child is stable, they can be taken to the operating room for cystoscopy and valve ablation. Ablation can be performed with a cold knife, bugbee, or laser. A catheter is left in place for 24 hours after the procedure and a VCUG is performed one month after ablation to confirm success. An alternative to valve ablation is creation of a vesicostomy. This allows for decompression of the upper tracts and bladder, and valve ablation can be performed when the child is bigger.

Children with PUV have a 50–60% risk of UTI, therefore circumcision is recommended to reduce this risk.

11. **What are the clinical outcomes of PUV?**

Patients with PUV have renal dysplasia and require long term monitoring of renal function. Studies have shown that the serum nadir creatinine level in the first year of life correlates with the need for renal replacement therapy (RRT), with 100% of patients with Cr > 1 requiring RRT by 10 years old [6]. Patients with PUV also have significant polyuria that worsens bladder dysfunction, and 26% of patients will require intermittent catheterization [6].

12. **What causes UPJ obstruction?**

In infants, the most common cause of UPJ obstruction is an intrinsic narrowing of the UPJ. In older children and adolescents, the most common cause is extrinsic compression from a crossing lower pole vessel.

13. **What is the management of UPJ obstruction?**

Dismembered pyeloplasty is the gold standard for the treatment of UPJ obstruction. This can be performed open, laparoscopically, or robotically. If a patient initially presents with uncontrollable pain or acute infection, a nephrostomy tube can be placed to decompress the collecting system until definitive surgery.

14. **What are the principles of management for an ectopic ureter or ureterocele?**

Ectopic ureters and ureteroceles are commonly associated with the upper pole of a duplex collecting system, which is evident on RUS as upper pole hydronephrosis. The goals of management are to preserve renal function, prevent infection or reflux, and maintain urinary continence. If there is adequate upper pole function, ureteroureterostomy or common sheath ureteral reimplant can be performed. If there is no upper pole function, upper pole heminephrectomy is an option.

15. **How does management of ureterocele differ from ectopic ureter?**

Ureteroceles can be large and result in obstruction of the lower pole or contralateral ureter. They can also prolapse and cause bladder outlet obstruction. If the ureterocele is causing obstruction or if the patient is acutely ill from infection, they should be punctured endoscopically.

References

1. Peters C. Congenital urinary obstruction: pathophysiology. In: Wein A, editor. Campbell-Walsh urology. 11th ed. Philadelphia: Elsevier; 2016. p. 3040–56.
2. Nguyen HT, Herndon CD, Cooper C, et al. The society for fetal urology consensus statement on the evaluation and management of antenatal hydronephrosis. J Pediatr Urol. 2010;6(3):212–31.
3. Nguyen HT, Benson CB, Bromley B, et al. Multidisciplinary consensus on the classification of prenatal and postnatal urinary tract dilation (UTD classification system). J Pediatr Urol. 2014;10(6):982–98.
4. Farrugia MK, Whitaker RH. The search for the definition, etiology, and effective diagnosis of upper urinary tract obstruction: the Whitaker test then and now. J Pediatr Urol. 2019;15(1):18–26.
5. Peters CA, Skoog SJ, Arant Jr. BS, Copp HL, Elder JS, Hudson RG, et al. Management and screening of primary vesicoureteral reflux in children. 2010. Available from http://www.auanet.org/guidelines/vesicoureteralreflux-(2010-reviewed-and-validity-confirmed-2017.
6. McLeod DJ, Szymanski KM, Gong E, et al. Renal replacement therapy and intermittent catheterization risk in posterior urethral valves. Pediatrics. 2019;143(3).

Chapter 48
Vesicoureteral Reflux (VUR)

Xiaoyan Feng, Prem Puri and Martin Lacher

Abstract Vesicoureteral reflux (VUR) is the most common disease of the urinary tract in children, occurring in 1 to 2% of the pediatric population and in 30 to 40% of children presenting with a urinary tract infection (UTI). The familial nature of VUR is well recognized. Siblings of children with VUR are at a much higher risk for reflux than the general pediatric population with a reported prevalence between 25 and 50%. The association of VUR, febrile UTI, and renal parenchymal damage is well recognized. Reflux nephropathy is a cause of childhood hypertension and chronic renal failure. The diagnosis is made by voiding cystourethrogram (VCUG) which allows grading of the VUR. The main goals of treatment of children with VUR are to prevent renal parenchymal damage and morbidity associated with recurrent febrile UTIs. Treatment options for children with VUR include non-surgical and surgical management. The various treatment options currently available for VUR are: (1) long term antibody prophylaxis; (2) minimally invasive endoscopic treatment; (3) ureteral reimplantation by open, laparascopic or robotic-assisted procedures; and (4) observation or intermittent therapy with management of bladder/bowel dysfunction (BBD) and treatment of UTI as they occur.

Keywords Vesicoureteral reflux (VUR) · Urinary tract infection (UTI) · Antibiotics · Voiding cystourethrogram (VCUG) · Bulking agents · Ureteral reimplantation

X. Feng · M. Lacher (✉)
Department of Pediatric Surgery, University of Leipzig, Leipzig, Germany
e-mail: martin.lacher@medizin.uni-leipzig.de

P. Puri
National Children's Research Centre, Our Lady's Children's Hospital, Dublin, Ireland

M. Lacher et al. (eds.), *Pearls and Tricks in Pediatric Surgery*,
https://doi.org/10.1007/978-3-030-51067-1_48

1. **What is the pathophysiology of VUR?**

Normally, urine flows down the urinary tract, from the kidneys, through the ureters, to the bladder. In VUR, there is retrograde flow of urine up through one or both ureters and kidneys.

2. **What is the etiology of VUR?**

VUR in children can be divided into primary and secondary. In primary VUR, the valve between the ureter and the bladder does not close well, so urine flows back into the ureters; in secondary VUR, there is an anatomical or functional blockage in the posterior urethra, which stops some of the urine from leaving the bladder, so the urine flows back into the upper urinary tracts. Not infrequently the patient may have neuropathic bladder in which nerves to the bladder may not work well, preventing the bladder from relaxing and contracting normally to release urine.

3. **What is the prevalence of VUR in normal children?**

As VUR can resolve spontaneously with age it is difficult to accurately determine the exact prevalence of VUR. The reported prevalence of VUR is 0.4–1.8%.

4. **What is the incidence of VUR in children with urinary tract infection (UTI)?**

The incidence declines with age. Among infants less than 1 year of age presenting with UTI, the incidence of reflux is as high as 70%, those less than 5 years of age have an estimated incidence of 25–40% [1].

5. **Which individual risk factors for UTI (with or without VUR) in children do you know?**

Individual risk factors include white race, age<12 months, bladder/bowel dysfunction (BBD), and structural anatomical abnormality of the urinary tract [2].

6. **What is the probability of VUR among febrile infant girls and infant boys?**

Girls are more likely than boys to have VUR. However, when a UTI is diagnosed, boys are more likely than girls to have VUR (29% versus 14%). Furthermore, a child is more likely to have VUR if a brother, sister, or parent was diagnosed with VUR. Finally, in children with BBD, VUR is commonly seen.

7. **Do children who present with their first febrile UTI have to be evaluated for VUR?**

This is still an ongoing controversy. According to the American Academy of Pediatrics (APP) 2011 clinical practice guidelines, a voiding cystourethrography (VCUG) is not recommended routinely after the first UTI. In contrast, the EAU (European Association of Urology) Guidelines 2012 advocate a VCUG at age 0–2 after the first proven UTI. There is a consensus that VCUG is indicated if renal and bladder ultrasonography reveals hydronephrosis, scarring, or other findings that would suggest either high-grade VUR or obstructive uropathy and in other atypical or complex clinical circumstances. VCUG should also be performed in cases of recurrent febrile UTIs [2].

8. **Does every child with VUR have symptoms?**

No, many children with VUR do not have symptoms.

9. **If a child is symptomatic, what are the most common symptoms?**

UTI is the most common symptom at presentation with or without fever, dysuria, urgency and frequency of micturition, daytime dribbling and abdominal pain.

10. **What are the most common complications of VUR?**

Refux nephropathy which may lead to childhood hypertension and chronic renal failure.

11. **How do you make the diagnosis of VUR?**

Voiding cystourethrogram (VCUG) is the gold standard test to detect the backflow of urine from the bladder to the kidneys (Fig. 48.1). Abdominal ultrasound is used to rule out structural abnormalities (upper urinary tract obstruction, dilated ureters) as well as renal scarring. Recently a new technique called contrast-enhanced voiding urosonography (ceVUS) has been proposed as an alternative to the VCUG without radiation.

12. **Describe the procedure of a VCUG**

The child lies down on the fluoroscopy table with the legs in butterfly position. A transurethral catheter is then placed in the bladder. After emptying, the bladder is filled with contrast media to evaluate for abnormalities of the bladder wall and possible VUR. When the bladder is filled with contrast the older child may be able to tell the technologist when he/she is not able to hold it any longer. Infants and young children will not be able to communicate this to the technologist. Then the child micturates under fluoroscopy. The purpose is to detect a possible VUR and to assess the bladder and urethra during urination. Finally, complete bladder emptying is confirmed. The catheter is removed as soon as the x-ray is taken.

13. **How is VUR graded?**

Refux is graded according to the International Reflux Classification (Fig. 48.2). In grade I, the urine flows back into one or both nondilated ureters but does not reach the kidney. Grade II demonstrates a urinary flow back into the kidney, but does not cause dilation of the renal pelvis. In grade III there is mild to moderate dilation of the ureter and the renal pelvis. Finally, in grade IV, the ureter is dilated and tortuous, the renal pelvis and calyces are dilated with blunting of fornices. In grade V there is severe dilation of the ureters, renal pelvis and calyces with loss of papillary impressions.

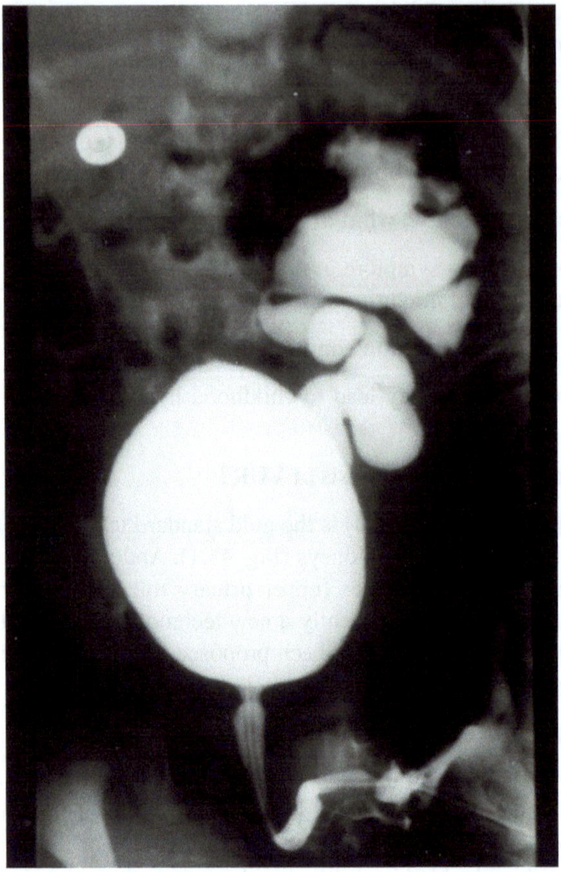

Fig. 48.1 VCUG shows grade V left vesicoureteral reflux in a male infant. Source: Author

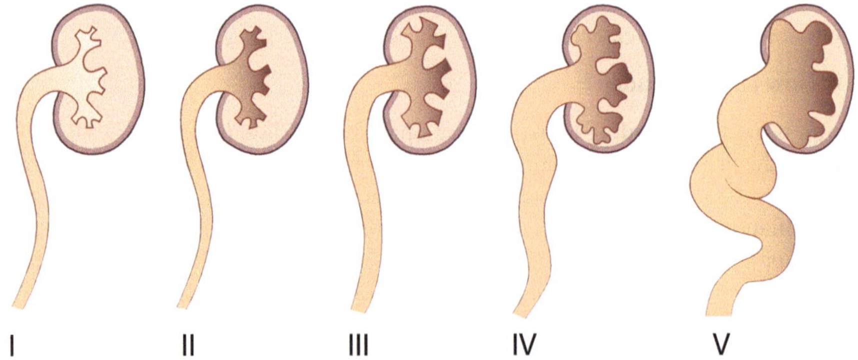

Fig. 48.2 Grading of VUR into five grades according to International Reflux Scale (IRS) in children system. Images are origin of Pediatric Radiology from Springer

14. **Can VUR resolve spontaneously?**

Yes. When UTIs are prevented by continuous antibiotic prophylaxis (CAP), as many as 87% of grade I, 63% of grade II, 53% of grade III, 33% of grade IV and only approximately 9% of grade V may spontaneously resolve over time [3].

15. **How long does it take for VUR to resolve spontaneously?**

The mean time for spontaneous resolution from the initial presentation is about 3 years [3].

16. **Can sterile reflux lead to renal damage?**

Sterile reflux usually does not cause kidney damage, but high-grade sterile reflux may contribute.

17. **Which conditions are required to produce renal scarring?**

VUR, bacterial infection and intrarenal reflux.

18. **How long does the renal parenchyma take to develop renal scarring?**

Scarring can take as long as 5 months to 2 years from the time of the acute urinary tract infection to evolve [4], but the proportion varies in different studies.

19. **What is the most common method to detect renal scarring?**

Dimercaptosuccinic acid (DMSA) scintigraphy. Recently contrast-enhanced ultrasound (CEUS) has also been verified as a highly sensitive, rapid and radiation free technique to evaluate renal scars.

20. **What are the treatment options for children with VUR?**

Non-surgical and surgical management.

21. **Which non-surgical treatments do you know?**

As in some cases VUR resolves spontaneously surveillance and prophylactic antibiotics are the first line treatment.

22. **What is the current concept of continuous antibiotic prophylaxis (CAP)?**

Several well-conducted trials have been carried out with the intent to define the role of CAP in the management of VUR, but no definite conclusion could be drawn from the data. Currently CAP is recommended mainly in patients diagnosed with VUR within the first year of life as well as in girls with high-grade (III-V) VUR and recurrent febrile urinary tract infections.

23. **Can antibiotic prophylaxis prevent renal scarring?**

Antibiotic prophylaxis does not prevent renal scarring according to a recent meta-analysis.

24. **What are the indications for surgical treatment?**

Surgery is indicated in children with a low probability of spontaneous resolution, recurrent pyelonephritis, and breakthrough febrile UTI while on CAP, renal scarring, grade IV–V reflux, VUR into complete duplex systems and parental preference.

25. **What are the surgical options to treat VUR?**

Endoscopic injection of bulking agents and ureteral reimplantation by open, laparoscopic or robotic–assisted procedures.

26. **What is the incidence of ureteral obstruction (UO) after endoscopic bulking agent injection for VUR?**

Less than 1% of treated cases.

27. **Does the type of injected bulking agent influence the incidence of ureteric obstruction (UO) after endoscopic injection?**

No. The incidence of UO is independent of the injected substance, volume, and technique [5].

28. **Which factors influence the success of the bulking agent injection?**

Pre-operative reflux grade, presence of functional or anatomic bladder abnormalities such as voiding dysfunction and duplicated collecting systems, surgeon experience, and injection technique.

29. **Which techniques for injecting a bulking agent are used nowadays?**

The most commonly used bulking agent for endoscopic injection is Dextranomer/Hyaluronic Acid. In STING technique, the bulking agent is injected 2 to 3 mm distal to the ureterovesical junction after advancement of the needle in the submucosal plane for 4 to 5 mm. A correctly placed injection creates the appearance of a nipple, on the top of which is a slit-like orifice. The Hydrodistention-implantation technique (HIT) describes a method in which the needle is inserted into the floor of the distal ureter. "Double HIT" means proximal and distal intraluminal injection sites that coapt both the ureteral tunnel and orifice. HIT/STING are also performed in combination.

30. **What are the most common surgical techniques to correct VUR?**

The principle of surgical ureteral reimplantation is creating a ureteral tunnel between the bladder mucosa and bladder muscle, which allows ureteral compression with bladder filling and contraction.

The most widely used surgical approaches include intra-vesical (Politano-Leadbetter, Cohen) and extra-vesical (Lich-Gregoir) ureteral reimplantation (Fig. 48.3).

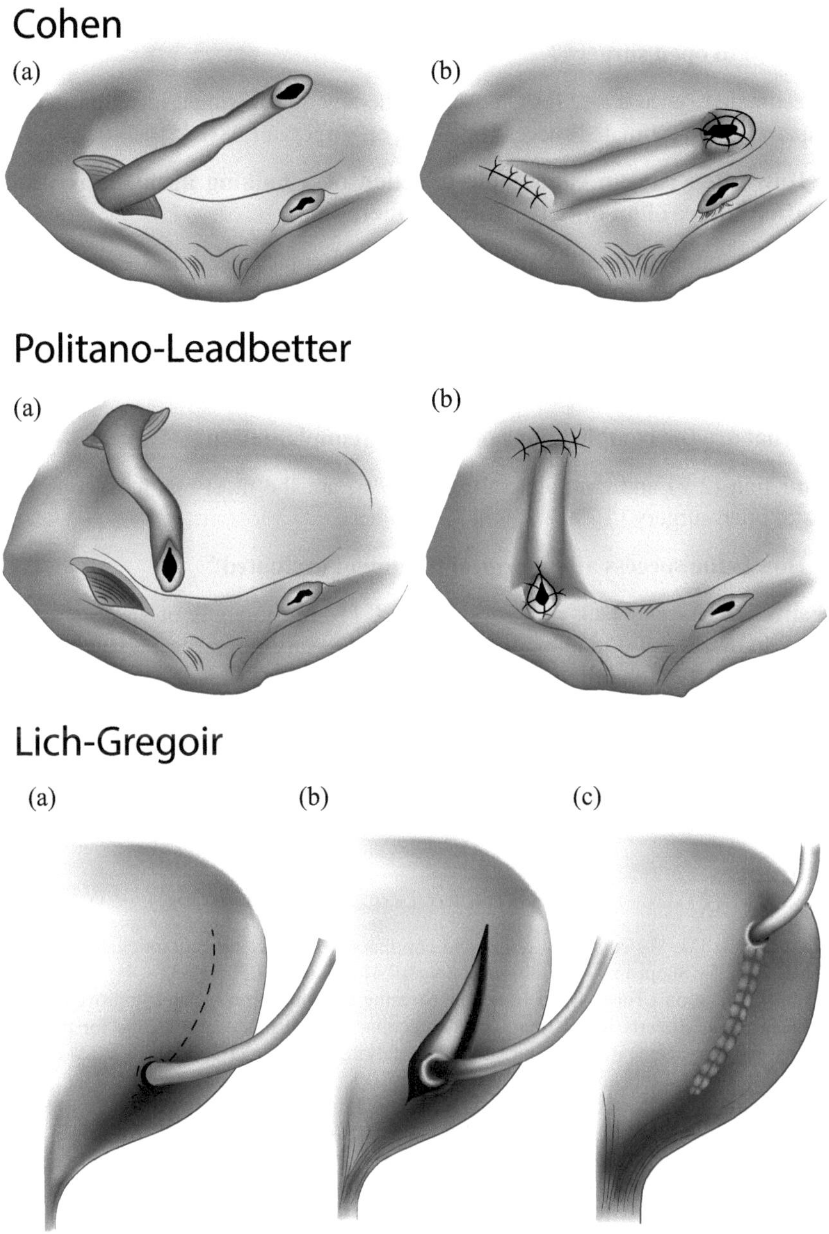

Fig. 48.3 Different surgical procedures of ureteral reimplantation

31. **What is the success rate of endoscopic injection of bulking agents compared to open surgery?**

The estimated success rate for endoscopic therapy after a single injection is 83%, compared to the estimated success rate of open surgery of 98% [5].

32. **How often can an endoscopic injection of a bulking agent be repeated after failure of an initial endoscopic therapy?**

The most commonly used bulking agent for endoscopic injection is Dextranomer/Hyaluronic Acid. One or two repeated injections may be needed if the initial injection fails to correct reflux. A recent study reported that the overall resolution rate after the first endoscopic injection in grade IV–V reflux was 70% and after the second injection 90%.

33. **What are the complications of ureteral reimplantation?**

Obstruction (2%) and contralateral reflux (9%) are the most common complications of open surgery [5].

34. **How is the success after surgical treatment evaluated?**

Negative VCUG and lack of postoperative UTI are the signs of success after a follow-up of at least 3 months. Whether it is necessary to perform a routine postoperative VCUG is controversial. Unless indicated by high-grade, young age, clinical failure, or family/surgeon preference, consideration should be given to make postoperative VCUG an option rather than a recommendation in children undergoing endoscopic treatment of primary VUR [6].

References

1. Lee T, Park JM. Vesicoureteral reflux and continuous prophylactic antibiotics. Investig Clin Urol. 2017;58(Suppl 1):S32–7. https://doi.org/10.4111/icu.2017.58.S1.S32.
2. Subcommittee on Urinary Tract Infection, Steering Committee on Quality Improvement and Management, Roberts KB. Urinary tract infection: clinical practice guideline for the diagnosis and management of the initial UTI in febrile infants and children 2 to 24 months. Pediatrics. 2011;128(3):595–610. https://doi.org/10.1542/peds.2011-1330.
3. Robinson J. Antibiotic prophylaxis in vesicoureteral reflux: a practice revisited. Can Pharm J (Ott). 2013;146(2):84–7. https://doi.org/10.1177/1715163513481570.
4. Swerkersson S, Jodal U, Sixt R, Stokland E, Hansson S. Urinary tract infection in small children: the evolution of renal damage over time. Pediatr Nephrol. 2017;32(10):1907–13. https://doi.org/10.1007/s00467-017-3705-5.
5. Sung J, Skoog S. Surgical management of vesicoureteral reflux in children. Pediatr Nephrol. 2012;27(4):551–61. https://doi.org/10.1007/s00467-011-1933-7.
6. Wang PZT, Abdelhalim A, Walia A, Wehbi E, Dave S, Khoury A. Avoiding routine postoperative voiding cystourethrogram: Predicting radiologic success for endoscopically treated vesicoureteral reflux. Can Urol Assoc J. 2019;13(5):E119–24. https://doi.org/10.5489/cuaj.5589.

Chapter 49
Circumcision and Disorders of the Penis

Bristol B. Whiles and Alonso Carrasco Jr.

Abstract Circumcision is one of the most common procedures performed on newborns and children. Substantial controversy exists surrounding indications to perform a circumcision. Providers should be aware of the normal penile anatomy as well as the potential disorders or abnormalities of the penis commonly seen in pediatric patients.

Keywords Circumcision · Hypospadias · Phimosis · Epispadias · Meatal stenosis

1. **Describe the anatomical components of the penis.**

The penis is composed of paired corpora cavernosa and a corpus spongiosum (Fig. 49.1). Corpora cavernosa are comprised of spongy erectile tissue surrounded by the tunica albuginea. The corpus spongiosum is located ventrally and surrounds the urethra. These structures are surrounded by Buck's fascia, dartos fascia, and skin.

2. **Define the blood and nerve supply to the penis.**

Penile blood supply originates from the internal pudendal artery which gives rise to the bulbar artery, urethral artery, and common penile artery. The common penile artery branches into the dorsal penile artery as well as the cavernosal artery (Figs. 49.1 and 49.2). The penile skin and prepuce are supplied by the external pudendal artery. The dorsal neurovascular bundle contains the deep dorsal vein, the dorsal penile artery, and the dorsal nerves of the penis (Fig. 49.1).

B. B. Whiles
Department of Urology, The University of Kansas, Medical Center, Kansas City, KS, USA

A. Carrasco Jr. (✉)
Department of Pediatric Urology, Children's Mercy, Kansas City, MO 64108, USA
e-mail: acarrasco@cmh.edu

M. Lacher et al. (eds.), *Pearls and Tricks in Pediatric Surgery*,
https://doi.org/10.1007/978-3-030-51067-1_49

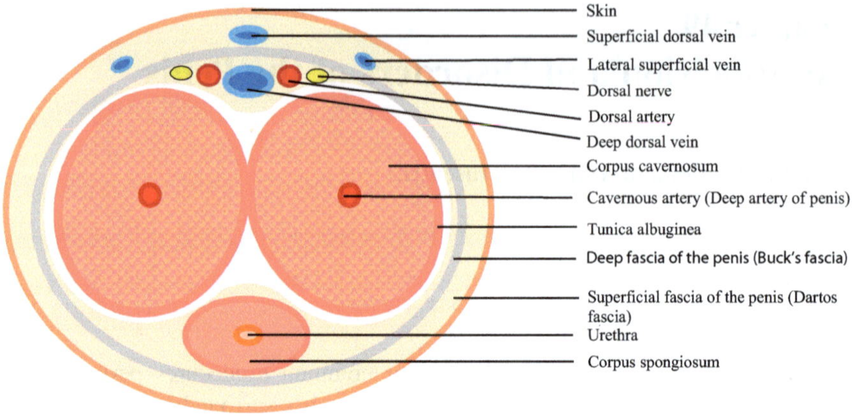

Fig. 49.1 Penile anatomy

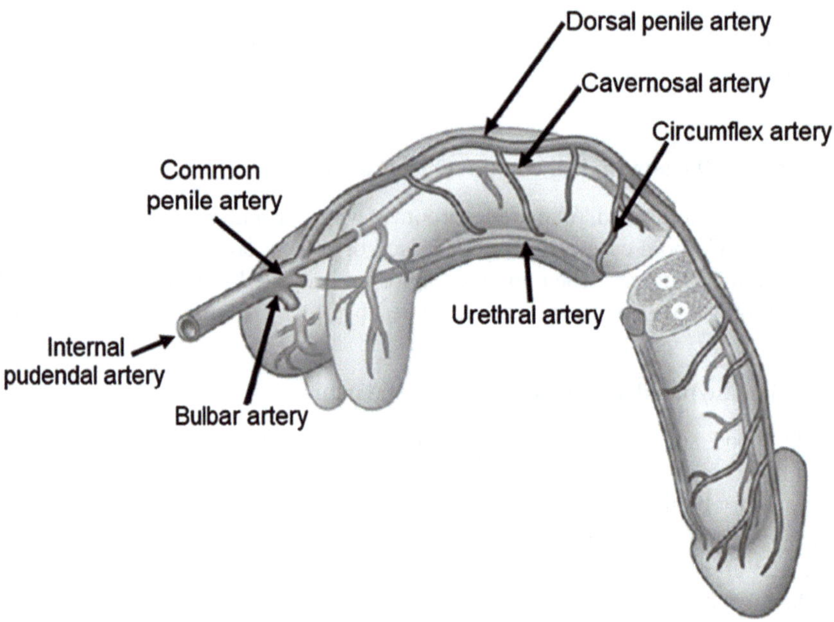

Fig. 49.2 Blood supply to the penis

3. **What are the medical indications for circumcision?**

Circumcision is commonly performed for the management of phimosis, recurrent episodes of inflammation/infection of the prepuce (e.g. balanoposthitis, posthitis, or balanitis), penile cancer, and balanitis xerotica obliterans (BXO). Non-medical reasons include religious or parental preference.

4. **Should neonatal circumcision be performed routinely?**

This is a controversial topic with practices varying widely. The benefits and potential risks to circumcision are important to discuss. One benefit of neonatal circumcision is decreased risk of UTI within the first year of life and a decreased risk of penile cancer in circumcised men. In addition, population-based studies have demonstrated protective effect towards sexually transmitted infections in circumcised men and their female partners [1, 2]. The American Academy of Pediatrics recognizes these health benefits but states that circumcision requires a shared decision-making process with the parents.

5. **What are the major contraindications to newborn circumcision?**

- Abnormal prepuce (e.g. incomplete foreskin)
- Hypospadias
- Significant chordee or angulation of penis
- Penoscrotal webbing
- Congenital concealed penis
- Small anatomy so commonly used clamps do not fit well (e.g. prematurity, micropenis)
- Coagulopathy (hemophilia, Von Willebrand's disease, omission of newborn vitamin K administration).

6. **What are the risks of circumcision?**

- Bleeding
- Infection
- Removing too much or too little skin
- Secondary phimosis or scar formation
- Meatal stenosis
- Poor cosmetic outcome
- Injury to the glans or urethra
- Penile adhesions.

7. **How is circumcision performed?**

Neonatal Circumcision is performed using a Gomco clamp, Mogen clamp, or Plastibell typically prior to 6 weeks of life (Fig. 49.3). Local anesthesia for this procedure includes a dorsal penile block. Free hand circumcision is the most common method utilized outside of the neonatal period, typically completed after 6 months of age under general anesthesia in conjunction with caudal block or penile block.

8. **What is chordee?**

Chordee is defined as ventral (downward) or dorsal (upward) curvature of the penis, typically due to disproportionate growth of the corporal bodies. It is often

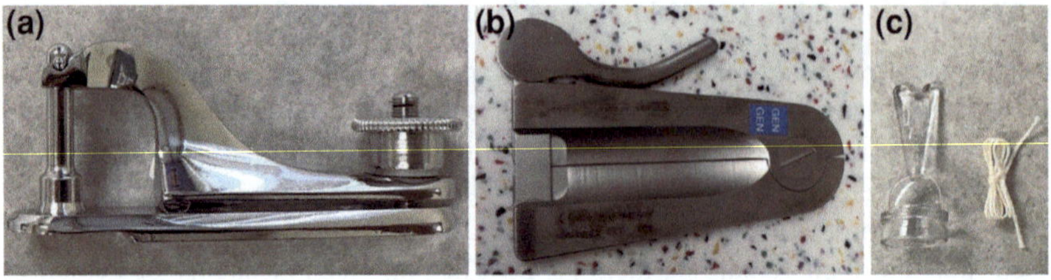

Fig. 49.3 Instruments commonly used in newborn circumcision. **a**—Gomco clamp, **b**—Mogen clamp, and **c**—Plastibell

associated with hypospadias but can be an isolated finding. Lateral penile curvature (i.e. left or right) is typically due to corpora cavernosa length disproportion. The need to treat chordee is based on the degree of penile curvature, particularly if functional limitations are likely (e.g. inability to direct the urinary stream, unable to participate in penetrative intercourse later in life).

9. **Describe penoscrotal webbing.**

Penoscrotal webbing occurs when the ventral junction of the scrotum and penis meets distally along the penile shaft, rather than the normal anatomic location at the base of the penis (Fig. 49.4). This is often a congenital finding, but can be seen with hypospadias, or as a result of excessive removal of ventral penile shaft skin during circumcision.

10. **What is a micropenis? Contrast this to a buried or concealed penis?**

Micropenis is defined as a penile length measuring more than 2.5 standard deviations below the mean in a newborn male. In a term newborn male, this equates to a stretched penile length of less than 2 cm [3]. Newborn babies with micropenis require endocrine evaluation as this is typically due to an endocrinopathy (hypogonadotropic or hypergonadotropic hypogonadism). In contrast, a buried penis is one that appears small but has a normal stretched penile length. The most common etiology of buried/concealed penis is a large prepubic fat pad. To accurately measure the penile length, the prepubic fat must be pushed back prior to measuring.

11. **What is Phimosis?**

Phimosis is defined as the inability to retract the foreskin (Fig. 49.5). Phimosis is a normal finding in newborns and requires no intervention. When the phimotic ring is significantly tight, it can lead to ballooning of the foreskin during voiding, chronic irritation, and/or recurrent infections. Foreskin should probably be retractable by the time a child is fully potty trained, so as to encourage good voiding and hygiene habits.

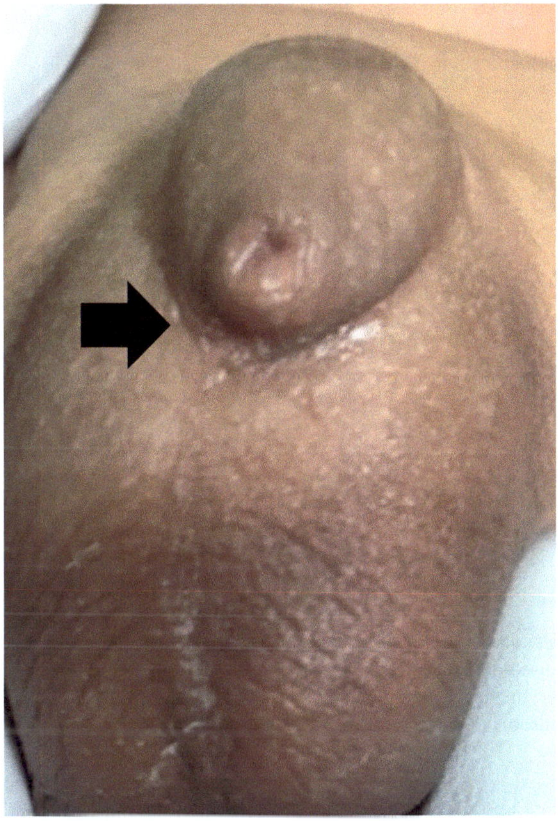

Fig. 49.4 Penoscrotal webbing. Arrow points to the penoscrotal junction, note lack of ventral penile shaft skin

12. **What are the treatment options for phimosis?**

Treatment options for phimosis include observation for spontaneous resolution, application of topical steroid cream, a dorsal slit procedure, or circumcision. If parents/patients wish to avoid a procedure, a trial of topical steroids cream may facilitate the foreskin to become more elastic and allow for resolution of phimosis in over 75% of patients [4].

13. **What is paraphimosis?**

Paraphimosis is when the foreskin is stuck in the retracted position and cannot be pulled forward/reduced due to distal penile edema. This is an emergency. Paraphimosis causes a tourniquet effect on the distal penis which can result in tissue ischemia. The goal of treatment is to reduce the foreskin into its normal position via manual compression and reduction, a dorsal slit, or emergent circumcision.

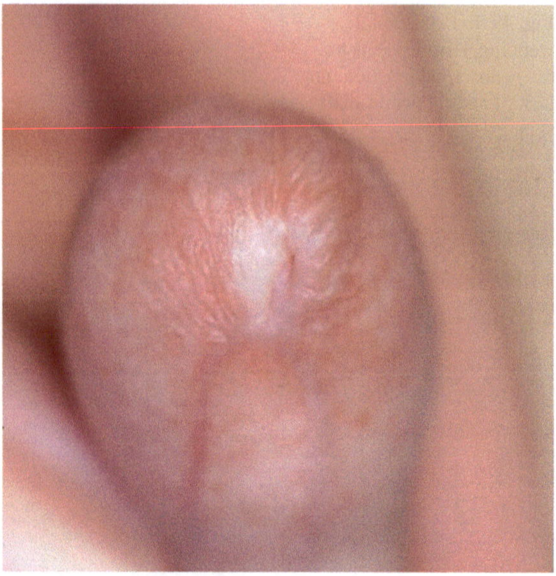

Fig. 49.5 Phimosis with scar formation due to chronic inflammation

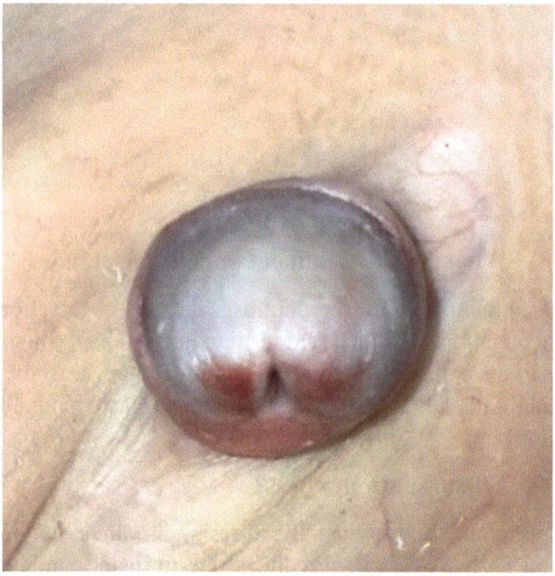

Fig. 49.6 BXO with white discoloration of the glans and erythema adjacent to urethral meatus

14. **What is balanitis xerotica obliterans (BXO)?**

Balanitis xerotica obliterans, or lichen sclerosis, is a chronic, inflammatory vasculitis. It is most often associated with chronic inflammation secondary to phimosis. It results in white discoloration of the involved tissues, which can include the prepuce, glans, meatus, and urethra (Fig. 49.6). Treatment involves surgical excision of the affected skin (circumcision) or application of steroid cream to decrease the inflammatory response. When BXO involves the meatus or urethra, this can lead to urethral stricture disease.

15. **What is meatal stenosis?**

Meatal stenosis, narrowing of the urethral meatus, is thought to be due to chronic irritation of the urethral meatus. It is most often observed in circumcised patients. The most common symptom of meatal stenosis is change in urinary stream such as spraying or deviation of the stream. Treatment is recommended when changes in the urinary stream are noted and bothersome. This involves either a meatotomy or a meatoplasty.

16. **What is hypospadias?**

Hypospadias is the second most common congenital abnormality of the urinary tract. It is seen in approximately 1 in 300 live birth males. It is characterized by a urethral meatus which opens on the ventral surface of the penis (Figs. 49.7 and 49.8). The etiology of hypospadias is multifactorial with genetic factors, inadequate hormonal stimulation, maternal/placental factors, and environmental factors implicated.

17. **What are the typical physical findings in patients with hypospadias?**

- Urethral meatus located in an abnormal location on the ventral surface of penis
- Dorsally hooded foreskin (with deficiency of ventral foreskin) (Fig. 49.9)
- Chordee.

18. **What is epispadias?**

Epispadias is defined as a urethral meatus that opens on the dorsal aspect of the penis. The opening can be as distal as the dorsal aspect of the glans and as proximal as the bladder neck (Fig. 49.10).

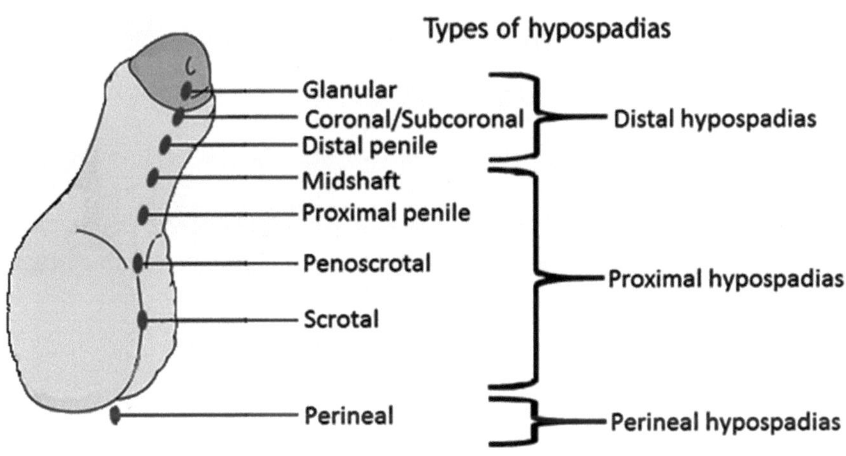

Fig. 49.7 Meatal location in hypospadias

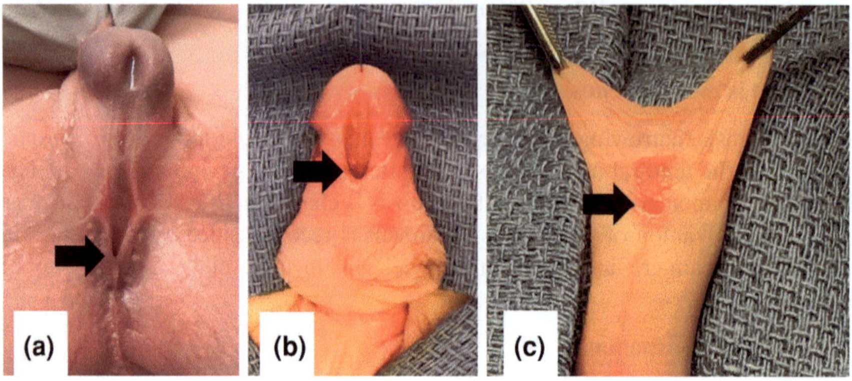

Fig. 49.8 Examples of different locations of urethral meatus (black arrow) seen in hypospadias. **a**—Scrotal hypospadias, **b**—Distal penile hypospadias, **c**—Subcoronal hypospadias

Fig. 49.9 Dorsally hooded foreskin

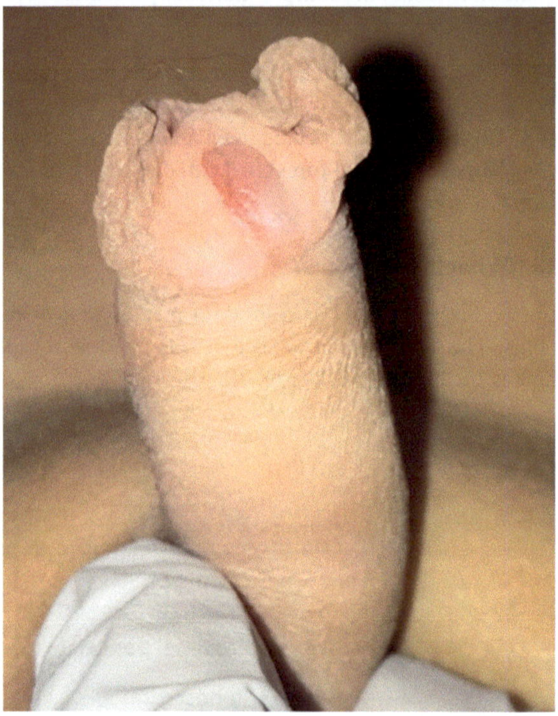

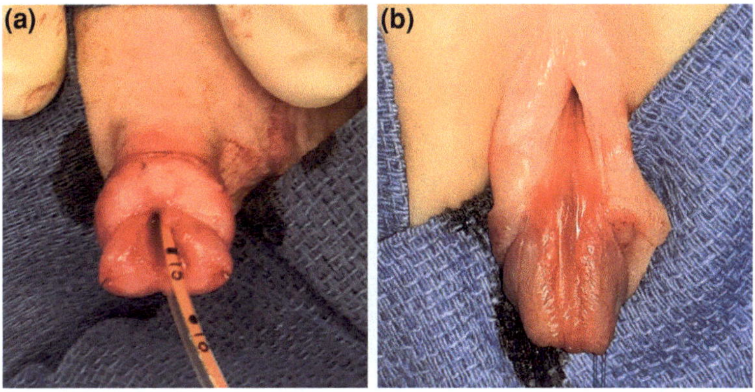

Fig. 49.10 Examples of epispadias, **a**—Distal epispadias and **b**—Penopubic epispadias

Mnemonic to differentiate hypospadias versus epispadias: The urinary stream is directed toward the heels in hypospadias and toward the eye in epispadias.

19. **What congenital anomalies are associated with epispadias?**

- Diastasis of the symphysis pubis
- Bladder exstrophy
- Renal agenesis
- Ectopic/pelvic kidneys
- Vesicoureteral reflux.

20. **What is urethral duplication?**

Urethral duplication is a congenital anomaly in which two urethras developed. There are multiple types of configurations (Fig. 49.11). The ventral urethra is usually normal caliber and location, and the dorsal urethra is typically an accessory urethra that is stenotic/hypoplastic.

21. **What is aphallia?**

Aphallia, or penile agenesis, is a rare congenital absence of the penis with an estimated incidence of 1 in 10 to 30 million live births. This is due to maldevelopment of the genital tubercle. The urethral meatus is often times located in the scrotum, perineum, or within the anal ridge. It is commonly associated with other genitourinary and anorectal abnormalities.

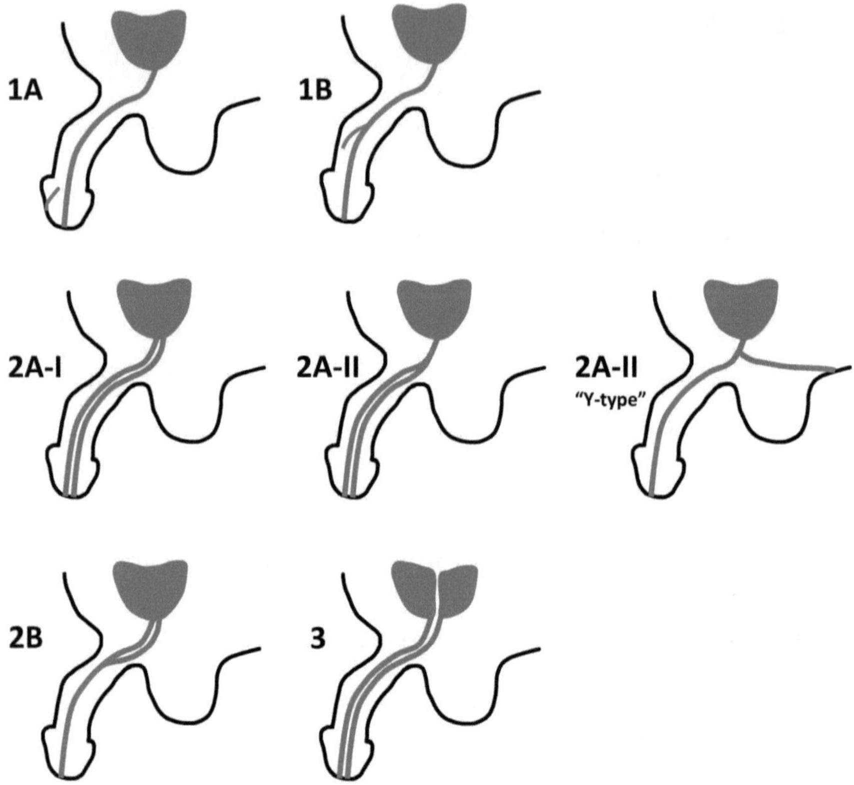

Fig. 49.11 Types of urethral duplication

22. **What is diphallia?**

Diphallia, penile duplication, is a rare congenital malformation with estimated incidence of 1 in 5 million live-births. Diphallia is classified into true diphallia or a bifid phallus. Each classification is further divided into complete or partial duplication (Fig. 49.12).

23. **What is priapism? What is the most common cause?**

Priapism is a prolonged erection lasting more than 4 hours. The most common cause of priapism in children is sickle cell disease. Additional etiologies include other hemoglobinopathies, leukemia, and trauma.

24. **What size Foley catheter should be used in a child?**

Either weight or age are typically used to determine the appropriately sized Foley catheter to use in children. Table 49.1 demonstrates one method for determining catheter size. One formula to estimate catheter size in children is [5]:

$$\text{Uninary catheter (FR)} = (\text{Weight(kg)}/3) + 4$$

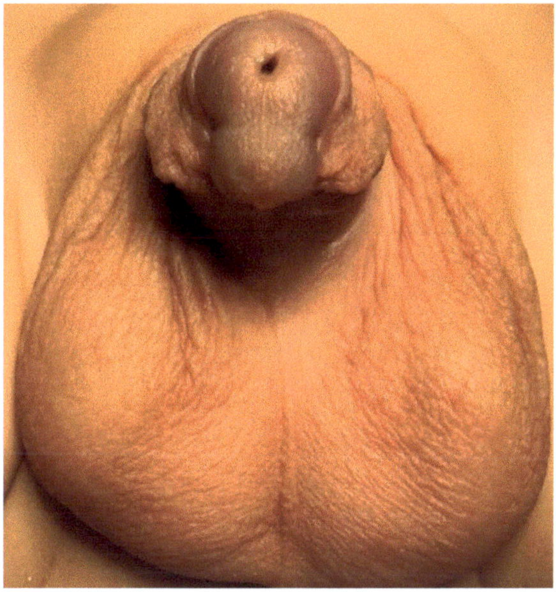

Fig. 49.12 True partial penile duplication with dominant glans located dorsally

Table 49.1 Recommended catheter size for children

Age	Weight (Kg)	Catheter size (F)
Term newborn—6 months	0–6	6
6–9 months	5–9	6–8
1–6 years	10–20	8–10
8–12 years	20–40	10–12
14+ years	45+	12–14

References

1. Friedman B, Khoury J, Petersiel N, Yahalomi T, Paul M, Neuberger A. Pros and cons of circumcision: an evidence-based overview. Clin Microbiol Infect Off Publ Eur Soc Clin Microbiol Infect Dis. 2016;22(9):768–74. https://doi.org/10.1016/j.cmi.2016.07.030.
2. Grund JM, Bryant TS, Jackson I, et al. Association between male circumcision and women's biomedical health outcomes: a systematic review. Lancet Glob Health. 2017;5(11):e1113–22. https://doi.org/10.1016/S2214-109X(17)30369-8.
3. Hatipoğlu N, Kurtoğlu S. Micropenis: etiology, diagnosis and treatment approaches. J Clin Res Pediatr Endocrinol. 2013;5(4):217–23. https://doi.org/10.4274/Jcrpe.1135.
4. Elmore JM, Baker LA, Snodgrass WT. Topical steroid therapy as an alternative to circumcision for phimosis in boys younger than 3 years. J Urol. 2002;168(4 Pt 2):1746–1747; discussion 1747. https://doi.org/10.1097/01.ju.0000027260.18990.9b.
5. Kopac M. Formula estimation of appropriate urinary catheter size in children. J Pediatr Intensive Care. 2013;2:177–80.

Chapter 50
Testicular Problems and Varicocele

Karen Milford and Armando Lorenzo

Abstract This chapter addresses the presentation, investigation, diagnosis and management of the most common scrotal pathologies in children. Topics covered in this chapter include the differential diagnosis of groin swellings and the acute scrotum, as well as the investigation and management of hydrocele, undescended testes and varicocele.

Keywords Hydrocele · Acute scrotum · Testicular torsion · Epididymitis · Undescended testicle · Orchidopexy · Varicocele · Pediatrics

1. **What is the differential diagnosis for groin and scrotal swellings in children?**

It is broad. Includes inguinal hernia, hydrocele, infections (such as epididymitis), testicular tumors, inguinal lymphadenopathy or abscess, and medical causes of scrotal swelling such as Henoch-Schönlein Purpura.

2. **What should be established on history in children with groin or scrotal swelling?**

In babies, gestational age at birth should be determined as inguinal hernias are more common in premature infants. Acuity of the swelling should be established, as well as a history of change in swelling size. It should be determined if there is any associated pain.

K. Milford · A. Lorenzo (✉)
Division of Urology, the Hospital for Sick Children, University of Toronto, Toronto, ON, Canada
e-mail: armando.lorenzo@sickkids.ca

M. Lacher et al. (eds.), *Pearls and Tricks in Pediatric Surgery*,
https://doi.org/10.1007/978-3-030-51067-1_50

3. **What should be established during examination?**

Clinicians should confirm that the child is clinically well, with no systemic evidence of infection, abdominal distension or bowel obstruction. The swelling should be assessed for its relationship to the inguinal crease, the external inguinal ring and the testicle. Lymphadenopathy tends to occur lateral to the inguinal crease, and inguinal hernias will be apparent at the inguinal ring, occasionally descending into the scrotum. It should be established whether or not the swelling is reducible into the abdomen, which is diagnostic of hernia. Hydroceles transilluminate. A painless mass within the scrotum should raise suspicion of a possible neoplasm.

4. **What is the cause of a hydrocele?**

In children, a partially patent processus vaginalis, with fluid trapped between the layers of the tunica vaginalis is the most common cause.

5. **How is the diagnosis of hydrocele made?**

Hydrocele is a clinical diagnosis. On history there may be swelling of the scrotum that may be static in size, or increase with ambulation. Findings on examination consist of a simple cystic structure in the scrotum or related to the spermatic cord, which typically cannot be reduced, and transilluminates.

6. **Is imaging necessary in cases of suspected hydrocele?**

Imaging is not generally indicated, although ultrasound should be utilized if there is a suspicion of an intra-scrotal mass

7. **When is surgery indicated in hydrocele?** [1]

Most hydroceles will close spontaneously by two years of age. If a hydrocele persists beyond this age, surgery may be offered. There is no evidence that hydroceles cause testicular damage or other morbidity and the natural history of hydroceles beyond 2 years of age is poorly documented. As such, it is safe to observe hydroceles if surgical correction is not desired. An absolute indication for repair is ipsilateral inguinal hernia.

8. **How are hydroceles repaired?**

By ligation of the processus vaginalis (usually through an inguinal incision) and wide opening of the distal sac. Cord hydroceles should be deroofed or excised. Secondary or non-communicating hydroceles may be addressed through a scrotal approach with opening and eversion of the sac.

9. **What is the definition of an acute scrotum?**

Acute scrotal pain with or without swelling or erythema.

10. **What is the differential diagnosis for the acute scrotum?**

Testicular torsion, torted appendix testis, epididymitis or viral orchitis, pain following scrotal or testicular trauma, incarcerated inguinal hernia and some medical conditions such as idiopathic scrotal oedema and rheumatoid purpura.

11. **What should be established during history taking in these patients?**

Acuity of pain, history of previous symptoms, history of recent groin trauma, the presence of a current or recent systemic illness and a history of urinary tract infections or conditions that may predispose to these.

12. **How does clinical examination help in determining the cause of acute scrotum?**

It can be difficult to differentiate between causes of acute scrotum on clinical examination. Clinicians should assess patients for evidence of systemic illness or fever. A horizontal-lying testicle and absence of cremasteric reflex favours testicular torsion. Relief of pain with elevation of the scrotum favours epididymitis. In the early stages, patients with epididymitis may have pain localized to the epididymis.

13. **What additional testing can be employed in the investigation of acute scrotum?**

Urinalysis may be useful in identifying patients with epididymitis, although abnormal analysis does not exclude torsion, and bland urine does not exclude orchitis.

Doppler ultrasound may exclude some patients with epididymitis, but is operator dependent and the presence of arterial flow may be falsely reassuring in cases of early or intermittent torsion. High-resolution ultrasound may be useful in visualizing a twist in the spermatic cord.

Importantly, rapid detorsion improves testicular salvage, and so transfer to the operating room should not be delayed to seek imaging in cases where the index of suspicion for torsion is high.

14. **What is the treatment of testicular torsion?**

Early scrotal exploration, detorsion and pexy of the affected testicle, and contralateral fixation. Fasciotomy and tunica vaginalis flap may be considered in borderline cases. In cases of frank testicular necrosis, orchiectomy should be considered.

15. **What is the fate of the torted testicle?**

Torsion results in impaired blood flow to and ischaemia of the testicle. Overall, the rate of testicular loss following torsion may be as high as 60%, once accounting for early orchiectomy and late atrophy. It is reasonable to counsel families that there is concern for testicular loss if exploration occurs more than 6 hours after onset of pain, and significant concern for loss at 10 hours after onset of pain [2].

16. **What is the management of epididymitis?**

In cases of positive urine bacterial culture, children should be treated and investigated as for a UTI. Most cases, however, are self-limiting and no organisms are identified on urine culture.

17. **What is the definition of an undescended testicle?**

A testicle that is not present in the scrotum and cannot be brought into the scrotum with manipulation, or does not remain in the scrotum for any length of time after exhaustion of the cremaster.

18. **How can undescended testicles be classified?**

They may be palpable or impalpable. Palpable testes may be in the groin in the expected path of descent between the inguinal canal and the scrotum, they may be ectopic, or they may be retractile. Impalpable testes may be intra-abdominal, or absent entirely.

19. **What is a retractile testis?**

A testicle that can be manipulated into the scrotum and remains there for a period of time, but that returns to the groin due to an overactive cremasteric reflex. Orchidopexy is not indicated in retractile testes but their position should be monitored as they may become undescended.

20. **What investigations should be performed in children with undescended testes?**

Imaging is not indicated to confirm testicular position.

Children with features to suggest a difference in sexual differentiation (such as bilateral impalpable testes, proximal hypospadias, bifid scrotum) should be investigated accordingly.

21. **What is the treatment for undescended testicles?**

Orchidopexy is surgical placement of the testicle within the scrotum. This may be performed through a scrotal or inguinal approach in the case of palpable testes, or as a single- or two-stage laparoscopic procedure in the case of abdominal testes.

22. **When should orchidopexy be performed?**

Ideally, orchidopexy should be performed between the ages of 6 and 18 months [3].

23. **What are the reasons for performing orchidopexy?** [3]

Undescended testicles may result in sub-fertility. Early orchidopexy, prior to 12 months of age, is recommended in order to improve preservation of fertility.

Boys with undescended testes also have increased risk for testicular malignancy. There is evidence that pre-pubertal orchidopexy may decrease the risk of malignancy, while also facilitates self-examination.

24. **What is a varicocele?**

The abnormal dilatation or tortuosity of the veins of the pampiniform plexus.

25. **What is the cause of a varicocele?**

The etiology of a varicocele is usually multifactorial. It is probably related to increased hydrostatic and venous pressure within the left gonadal vein, due to the fact that this vein is longer than the right and drains into the renal vein at a right angle. Additionally, gonadal veins associated with varicoceles have been shown to often have absent or incompetent valves [4].

Isolated right-sided varicoceles are unusual, and this finding should always prompt imaging of the retroperitoneum to exclude a mass causing compression of the right gonadal vein.

26. **What problems do varicoceles cause?** [4]

Besides discomfort and concerns regarding cosmetic appearance, varicoceles are associated with testicular atrophy and dysfunction. Varicocele may cause loss of testicular volume as well as areas of testicular dysfunction on biopsy, and semen analysis may reveal decreasing sperm density and motility over time.

27. **By what mechanism do varicoceles cause testicular dysfunction and subfertility?** [4]

Through testicular hyperthermia, a varicocele interferes with the mechanisms that usually allow the scrotum to be 1–2° Celsius cooler than body temperature, thereby interfering with spermatogenesis. It is also possible that varicoceles cause hypoxia and oxidative stress in testes, and that renal and adrenal metabolites may reflux into the spermatic vein.

28. **How should a clinician examine a patient with suspected varicocele?**

The patient should be made comfortable, and examined in a warm room, in both the recumbent and upright positions, and should be asked to perform a valsalva manoeuvre if the varicocele is not apparent. The testicular cord should be palpated directly above the testis, with the clinician specifically looking for dilated veins above the testicle. The testes should be examined for size discrepancies.

29. **What imaging modalities can be used in the investigation of varicocele?**

Colour Doppler ultrasound is not indicated routinely, however can be used when the examination is equivocal. Ultrasound is also useful in obtaining an objective assessment of testicular volume. In pre-pubertal boys and in cases of right-sided varicocele, the abdomen should be imaged to exclude a retroperitoneal mass or Wilm's tumour. Venography is highly sensitive but also invasive, and is generally only used when there is an intention to treat the varicocele with thromboembolism in the same setting.

30. **How are varicoceles classified?** [5]

There are 3 grades:
Grade I—palpable with Valsalva manoeuvre only
Grade II—palpable without Valsalva manoeuvre
Grade III—visible at a distance.

31. **What are the indications for treatment of varicocele in adolescents?** [6]

In adolescents, indications for treatment include a discrepancy in testicular volume of more than 20%, pain that cannot be explained by other pathology and that does not respond to conservative therapy, the presence of an additional testicular condition which may predispose to sub-fertility, and bilateral varicoceles. Additionally, males with decreasing sperm counts over serial samples should be offered treatment.

32. **What are the goals of treatment of varicocele?**

To cause disruption of the internal spermatic drainage of the testicle, whilst preserving the spermatic artery, vasal and differential vessels, and lymphatics.

33. **What are the options for treatment of varicocele?**

Varicocelectomy can be performed through surgical ligation of the internal spermatic vein, or by radiographic venous embolization. This may be performed through and inguinal or sub-inguinal approach, or laparoscopically. Magnification should be used, and intra-operative Doppler is useful to differentiate between venous structures and the artery.

References

1. Hall NJ, Ron O, Eaton S, Pierro A. Surgery for hydrocele in children—an avoidable excess? J Pediatr Surg. 2011;46(12):2401–5. https://doi.org/10.1016/j.jpedsurg.2011.07.029.
2. Macdonald C, Kronfli R, Carachi R, O'Toole S. Review article a systematic review and meta-analysis revealing realistic outcomes following paediatric torsion of testes. J Pediatr Urol. 2018;14(6):503–9. https://doi.org/10.1016/j.jpurol.2018.09.017.
3. Chan E, Wayne C, Nasr A. Ideal timing of orchiopexy : a systematic review. 2014:87–97. https://doi.org/10.1007/s00383-013-3429-y.

4. Masson P, Brannigan RE. The varicocele. Urol Clin North Am. 2014;41:129–44. https://doi.org/10.1016/j.ucl.2013.08.001.
5. Amelar R, Dubin L. The varicocele and infertility. In: Amelar RD, Dubin L, Walsh PC, editors. Philadelphia: Saunders; 1977.
6. Radmayr C, Bogaert G, Dogan HS, Koc R, Associates G, Hoen LA. EAU guidelines on paediatric urology. 2018.

Chapter 51
Gynaecological Problems

Tazim Dowlut-McElroy

Abstract Pediatric surgeons may be consulted regarding the management of gynecological problems. This chapter provides an overview of diagnosis and management of the following gynaecolgical problems: Ovarian/Adnexal Torsion, Ovarian Cysts, Ectopic pregnancy, Hydrometrocolpos, Uterine and Vaginal Agenesis, and Pelvic Inflammatory Disease.

Keywords Ovarian torsion · Ovarian cysts · Ectopic pregnancy · Hydrometrocolpos · Uterine and vaginal atresia · Pelvic inflammatory disease

Ovarian/Adnexal Torsion

1. **What is the incidence of adnexal torsion in the pediatric population?**

Adnexal torsion accounts for 2.7% of cases of children with acute abdominal pain [1]. Within children ages 1 to 20 years, the incidence of adnexal torsion has been estimated at 4.9:100,000 [2].

2. **What are the typical clinical findings in a child with ovarian torsion?**

Sudden onset of severe unilateral pain in the lower abdomen or pelvic area. Pain is commonly associated with nausea and/or vomiting. If the torsion remains untreated, the child may develop leukocytosis and a low-grade fever [1].

T. Dowlut-McElroy (✉)
Pediatric and Adolescent Gynecology, Department of Surgery, Children's Mercy Hospitals, Gillham Rd 2401, Kansas City, MO 64113, USA
e-mail: tazimdowlut@gmail.com

M. Lacher et al. (eds.), *Pearls and Tricks in Pediatric Surgery*,
https://doi.org/10.1007/978-3-030-51067-1_51

3. **What ultrasound findings suggest ovarian torsion?**

The hallmarks of ovarian torsion on Doppler ultrasound are ovarian enlargement and absent Doppler arterial flow [3, 4]. However, as venous flow is affected first, the presence of arterial flow does not exclude torsion [5].

4. **What is the recommended treatment of ovarian torsion?**

Ovarian torsion is a surgical emergency. Laparoscopic detorsion with ovarian tissue conservation is favored over oophorectomy to preserve ovarian function even if the ovary appears necrotic (blue-black) [1]. The risk of malignancy is low (0.4 to 5%) and oophorectomy should only be performed if there is clear evidence of malignancy [2, 6]. More than half of torsions in post-pubertal patients occur in the setting of an adnexal mass. Concurrent cystectomy can be performed in these patients to decrease the need for repeated surgery [1].

5. **Should oophoropexy be routinely performed?**

Routine oophoropexy is controversial. The risk of recurrence of ovarian torsion is 2 to 12%, with higher risk in cases of spontaneously torsed normal ovaries [7]. Oophoropexy does not eliminate the risk of recurrence of ovarian torsion with a reported rate of approximately 9% after ovarian fixation [8]. Oophoropexy can be offered in the setting of repeated ipsilateral torsion, absent contralateral ovary, elongated ovarian ligament and torsion of a normal ovary [1]. Laparoscopic oophoropexy can be performed by shortening the ovarian ligament with permanent suture or fixing the ovary to the round ligament, uterosacral ligament or the posterior uterus [9].

Ovarian Cysts

1. **What is the incidence of fetal ovarian cysts?**

Ovarian cysts occur in approximately 1 in 2500 fetuses and are the most common abdominal anomalies diagnosed in female fetuses [10]. They are categorized by their sonographic appearance as simple cysts (thin-walled, round, anechoic, unilocular cysts measuring>2 cm) or complex cysts (thick-walled, heterogeneous, containing hyperechoic components) [11].

2. **What are the risks associated with fetal ovarian cysts?**

Fetal ovarian cysts may develop intracystic hemorrhage, rupture and ovarian torsion [11].

3. **What is the management of a fetal ovarian cyst greater than 5 cm?**

Consideration should be given to antenatal percutaneous aspiration to decrease the risk of ovarian torsion. In utero aspiration of anechoic ovarian cysts has been shown to increase the incidence of in utero cyst involution and to decrease the rate of oophorectomy [12].

4. **What ultrasound findings of ovarian cysts in children and adolescents are concerning for malignancy?**

Ovarian mass size≥8 cm with complexity [13].

5. **What is the most common ovarian tumor in children?**

The most common ovarian tumor in children, a mature cystic teratoma (dermoid cyst), is also the most common germ cell tumor in children. Germ cell tumors are the most common ovarian tumors in children and adolescents [13]. The majority of ovarian tumors in children and adolescents are benign. Only from 4% to 11% of adnexal masses are malignant [14].

Ectopic Pregnancy

1. **What is the prevalence of ectopic pregnancy?**

Ectopic pregnancy has been reported in upwards of 18% of women presenting to an emergency department for first trimester vaginal bleeding, abdominal pain or both [15]. Ectopic pregnancy occurs in 1.5 to 2% of all pregnancies and ruptured ectopic pregnancy accounts for 6% of maternal deaths [16].

2. **What risk factors increases an adolescent's risk of ectopic pregnancy?**

Previous ectopic pregnancy, prior history of pelvic inflammatory disease, early initiation of oral contraceptives (at age ≤ 16 years), use of intrauterine device for contraception, smoking (current or previous use), consumption of ≥ 10 Grams per day of alcohol, previous tubal surgery, in utero exposure to DES (diethylstilbestrol), history of infertility, use of assisted reproductive technology.

3. **How is ectopic pregnancy diagnosed?**

By confirming pregnancy (with serum hCG level) and transvaginal ultrasound. Sonographic visualization of a gestational sac with a yolk sac, an embryo, or both in the adnexa definitively diagnoses an ectopic pregnancy.

4. **Where are ectopic pregnancies most frequently located?**

More than 95% of ectopic pregnancies are located in the fallopian tube. The remaining are interstitial (2 to 4%), ovarian (<1%), cervical (<1%), abdominal (<1%), and along a previous cesarean section uterine scar (<1%). Of ectopic pregnancies that occur in the fallopian tube, 70 to 80% occur in the ampulla, 12% are isthmic and 5% are located on the fimbria.

5. **What are the contraindications to treating ectopic pregnancy with methotrexate and when is surgery indicated?**

Surgery is indicated if the patient is hemodynamically unstable, has signs of intraperitoneal bleeding or symptoms of ongoing ruptured ectopic pregnancy such as pelvic pain. In addition the following absolute contraindications to the use of methotrexate require the surgical treatment of ectopic pregnancy: evidence of immunodeficiency; moderate to severe anemia, leukopenia or thrombocytopenia; sensitivity to methotrexate; active pulmonary or peptic ulcer disease; clinically important hepatic dysfunction or renal dysfunction; breastfeeding; inability to participate in follow up. Surgical management can also be considered in the setting of the following relative contraindications to methotrexate therapy: embryonic cardiac activity detected by transvaginal ultrasonography; high initial hCG concentration (>5000 mIU/mL); ectopic pregnancy>4 cm in size as imaged by transvaginal ultrasonography; refusal to accept blood transfusion.

Hydrometrocolpos

1. **What are possible etiologies of hydrometrocolpos?**

Hydrometrocolpos may result from imperforate hymen, transverse vaginal septum, vaginal atresia in the setting of a functional uterus, OHVIRA(obstructed hemivagina with ipsilateral renal anomaly) or cloacal anomaly.

2. **What are the typical presenting symptoms of hydrometrocolpos?**

Progressively worsening, episodic lower abdominal cramping and pelvic pain after onset of puberty. Less common symptoms include back pain, urinary retention, urinary incontinence and constipation. A partial or microperforate transverse vaginal septum allows for some egress of menstrual blood. The patient usually reports dysmenorrhea. In the case of OHVIRA, regular periods from the unobstructed hemivagina are associated with progressively worsening dysmenorrhea.

3. **What complications can occur as a result of hydrometrocolpos?**

The distended vagina can cause mass effect on other pelvic structures leading to hydronephrosis and urinary retention.

4. **How is an imperforate hymen diagnosed?**

On physical examination, an abdominal/pelvic mass may be palpable and the hymen bulges and may appear bluish. Ultrasound imaging shows a cystic structure in the lower abdomen and pelvis (representing the distended vagina) with the uterus at the cranial end of the structure. An MRI is typically not necessary for diagnosis.

5. **How is imperforate hymen treated?**

Surgically with cruciate of annular hymenal incisions. The evacuation of blood from the vagina leads to the resolution of symptoms. Less commonly, imperforate hymen may be diagnosed in infancy. In infants, surgical intervention is reserved for symptomatic patients (as with hydronephrosis) due to the risk of reclosure and infection.

6. **How is a transverse vaginal septum diagnosed?**

In contrast to an imperforate hymen, examination reveals no bulging noted at the introitus and the external genitalia is normal in appearance. The vagina appears to end in a blind pouch with no visualization of the cervix. As with imperforate hymen, pelvic ultrasound shows a cystic pelvic mass with a uterus at the cranial end. Ultrasound or MRI may help delineate the thickness and location of the vaginal septum. Approximately 46% of transverse vaginal septa occur in the upper vagina, 40% in the mid vagina and 14% in the lower vagina.

7. **How is a transverse vaginal septum treated?**

The septum is surgically resected and the upper and lower vagina are anastomosed in an end-to end fashion. An indwelling stent or vaginal mold is typically left in place in the immediate postoperative period. Thereafter, the use of vaginal dilators are recommended to prevent stricture.

8. **How is vaginal atresia diagnosed?**

Physical examination of the external genitalia reveals lack of a vaginal orifice or a vaginal dimple. On rectal examination, the distended upper vagina may be palpable. Transperineal ultrasound or MRI are useful to assess the distance between the hymenal tissue and the proximal aspect of the obstructed vagina.

9. **How is vaginal atresia treated?**

Pull-through vaginosplasty with a perineal flap is performed to anastomose the distal aspect of the obstructed upper vagina to the perineum. For high atresias, additional graft using bowel, skin, or buccal mucosa may be needed.

10. **How is OHVIRA (obstructed hemivagina with ipsilateral renal anomaly) diagnosed?**

Digital vaginal examination reveals a mass felt to bulge from the lateral wall of the vagina to the midline. In addition to hematometrocolpos, ultrasound may reveal a uterine didelphys with ipsilateral renal agenesis (Herlyn-Werner-Wunderlich syndrome).

11. **How is OHVIRA treated?**

The longitudinal vaginal septum is resected to relieve the obstruction and create a single vaginal vault. Postoperative vaginal dilation is not typically indicated.

Uterine and Vaginal Agenesis

1. **What are conditions associated with uterine and vaginal agenesis?**

Uterine and vaginal agenesis is typically one symptom of broader conditions involving abnormalities of the reproductive system such as MRKH

(Meyer-Rokintanski-Kuster-Hauser) syndrome and AIS (Androgen Insensitivity Syndrome).

2. **What other anomalies are associated with uterine and vaginal agenesis?**

Up to 50% of mullerian anomalies are associated with renal anomalies including renal agenesis, malrotation or ectopic kidney. Fewer have cervical somite anomalies (MURCS, mullerian duct aplasia, renal dysplasia and cervical somite anomalies.

3. **What are the typical presenting symptoms of MRKH and AIS?**

Primary amenorrhea after normal development of secondary sexual characteristics. The external genitalia in both MRKH and AIS appears phenotypically normal female. The vagina may appear as a dimple or short and blind-ending without a palpable cervix.

4. **What are the differences between MRKH and AIS?**

Women with AIS have decreased or absent axillary and pubic hair and testosterone levels in the normal male range. Karyotype analysis is 46 XX with MRKH and 46XY with AIS. There is an approximately 2% risk of gonadoblastoma of the intraabdominal testes in women with AIS. Prophylactic gonadectomy is typically delayed until after puberty when the patient can participate in decision making and understands risks and benefits including use of hormone replacement therapy.

5. **What are methods of creating a vagina in the absence of a functional uterus?**

Vaginal elongation with vaginal dilators is successful in 90% of patients. Surgical techniques vary and require the postoperative use of dilators or intercourse to maintain the neovagina. Various tissue including split-thickness skin grafts, peritoneum, bowel, buccal mucosa and human amion have been used to create a vagina.

Pelvic Inflammatory Disease

1. **What clinical symptoms are associated with PID?**

90% of patients have lower abdominal pain. 55% have vaginal discharge. 45% have nausea. 20% have vomiting. 40% have back pain. Only 25% report fever.

2. **What are the 3 major sequelae of PID?**

Chronic pelvic pain, ectopic pregnancy, infertility.

3. **Does negative testing for gonorrhea and chlamydia exclude the diagnosis of PID?**

No. PID is generally polymicrobial in nature. Anaerobic and facultative bacteria with and without *N. gonorrhea* and *C. trachomatis* have been isolated from the upper genital tract in up to 70% of women with PID. In 30% of cases only anaerobic and/or facultative bacteria such as bacterial vaginosis and Mycoplasma genitalium have been isolated.

4. **Can PID be diagnosed in a child/adolescent who is not sexually active?**

Yes. PID can occur in non-sexually active children and adolescents. Patients have been noted to have concurrent illnesses such as inflammatory bowel disease. Microbial etiology differs from that of sexually active adolescents. Documented micro-organisms include Escherichia Coli, Alpha-Hemolytic Streptococci, Coagulase Negative Staphylococcus, Streptococcus, Abiotrophia and Granulicatella.

5. **What is the role of surgical intervention in the diagnosis and treatment of PID?**

When compared to laparoscopy, the diagnosis of PID based on clinical criteria has an accuracy of only 65 to 90%. Only 20% of patients with laparoscopically confirmed PID present with the classic symptoms of acute salpingitis including lower abdominal pain, vaginal/cervical discharge, fever, leukocytosis and increased ESR. Due to the risk of major sequelae, the CDC recommends initiating empiric treatment for PID in patients at risk who have no identifiable cause for illness and cervical motion tenderness or uterine tenderness or adnexal tenderness. Diagnostic laparoscopy is considered in patients who do not respond to antimicrobial therapy and in whom other diagnoses such as endometriosis or ovarian torsion are being considered. Laparoscopy is 100% specific for the diagnosis of PID.

Up to 40% of patients with TOA do not respond to broad-spectrum antibiotic therapy within 48 to 72 hours as evidenced by persistent fever and leukocytosis and increasing size of the abscess. Surgical intervention includes percutaneous drainage with CT or ultrasound guidance or laparoscopy or laparotomy with incision and drainage of the abscess. An effort is made to preserve fertility in children and adolescents with conservative surgical approaches that preserve the uterus, fallopian tubes and ovaries if possible.

6. **What is Fitz-Hugh-Curtis syndrome?**

Perihepatic inflammation in the setting of PID leads to the formation of adhesions between the liver capsule and the anterior abdominal wall. The patient may report pleuritic right upper quadrant abdominal pain. Fitz-Hugh-Curtis syndrome has been reported in approximately 14% of patients with PID but may be less common in adolescents.

7. **Does an IUD need to be removed when a patient is diagnosed with PID?**

The IUD does not need to be removed prior to initiation is antimicrobial therapy except for patients with actinomyces and PID. IUD removal should be considered for patients who fail to respond to antimicrobial therapy.

References

1. Adeyemi-Fowode O, Lin EG, Syed F, Sangi-Haghpeykar H, Zhu H, Dietrich JE. Adnexal torsion in children and adolescents: a retrospective review of 245 cases at a single institution. J Pediatr Adolesc Gynecol. 2019;32(1):64–9.
2. Guthrie BD, Adler MD, Powell EC. Incidence and trends of pediatric ovarian torsion hospitalizations in the United States, 2000-2006. Pediatrics. 2010;125(3):532–8.
3. Servaes S, Zurakowski D, Laufer MR, Feins N, Chow JS. Sonographic findings of ovarian torsion in children. Pediatr Radiol. 2007;37(5):446–51.
4. Linam LE, Darolia R, Naffaa LN, Breech LL, O'Hara SM, Hillard PJ, et al. US findings of adnexal torsion in children and adolescents: size really does matter. Pediatr Radiol. 2007;37(10):1013–9.
5. Lourenco AP, Swenson D, Tubbs RJ, Lazarus E. Ovarian and tubal torsion: imaging findings on US, CT, and MRI. Emerg Radiol. 2014;21(2):179–87.
6. Ashwal E, Krissi H, Hiersch L, Less S, Eitan R, Peled Y. Presentation, diagnosis, and treatment of ovarian torsion in premenarchal girls. J Pediatr Adolesc Gynecol. 2015;28(6):526–9.
7. Bertozzi M, Esposito C, Vella C, Briganti V, Zampieri N, Codrich D, et al. Pediatric ovarian torsion and its recurrence: a multicenter study. J Pediatr Adolesc Gynecol. 2017;30(3):413–7.
8. Comeau IM, Hubner N, Kives SL, Allen LM. Rates and technique for oophoropexy in pediatric ovarian torsion: a single-institution case series. J Pediatr Adolesc Gynecol. 2017;30(3):418–21.
9. Fuchs N, Smorgick N, Tovbin Y, Ben Ami I, Maymon R, Halperin R, et al. Oophoropexy to prevent adnexal torsion: how, when, and for whom? J Minim Invasive Gynecol. 2010;17(2):205–8.
10. Trinh TW, Kennedy AM. Fetal ovarian cysts: review of imaging spectrum, differential diagnosis, management, and outcome. Radiographics. 2015;35(2):621–35.
11. Bascietto F, Liberati M, Marrone L, Khalil A, Pagani G, Gustapane S, et al. Outcome of fetal ovarian cysts diagnosed on prenatal ultrasound examination: systematic review and meta-analysis. Ultrasound Obstet Gynecol. 2017;50(1):20–31.
12. Bagolan P, Giorlandino C, Nahom A, Bilancioni E, Trucchi A, Gatti C, et al. The management of fetal ovarian cysts. J Pediatr Surg. 2002;37(1):25–30.
13. Rogers EM, Casadiego Cubides G, Lacy J, Gerstle JT, Kives S, Allen L. Preoperative risk stratification of adnexal masses: can we predict the optimal surgical management? J Pediatr Adolesc Gynecol. 2014;27(3):125–8.
14. Bergeron LM, Bishop KC, Hoefgen HR, Abraham MS, Tutlam NT, Merritt DF, et al. Surgical management of benign adnexal masses in the pediatric/adolescent population: an 11-year review. J Pediatr Adolesc Gynecol. 2017;30(1):123–7.
15. Barnhart KT, Sammel MD, Gracia CR, Chittams J, Hummel AC, Shaunik A. Risk factors for ectopic pregnancy in women with symptomatic first-trimester pregnancies. Fertil Steril. 2006;86(1):36–43.
16. Barnhart KT. Clinical practice ectopic pregnancy. N Engl J Med. 2009;361(4):379–87.

Chapter 52
Disorders/Differences of Sex Development (DSD)

Kathleen van Leeuwen

Abstract Disorders of sex development (DSD), sometimes called *differences* of sex development are conditions that affect reproductive organs and can include alterations of chromosomal, metabolic, gonadal or anatomical function. Some of the conditions result in genital ambiguities that are noted in newborns and some are not discovered until adolescence. There have been rapid shifts in the understanding of these conditions with strong support from advocacy organizations allowing more self-direction from patients affected by DSD. A multidisciplinary team is essential to the comprehensive care these patients will need over their lifetime and the team should include psychosocial providers, endocrinologists, geneticists, gynecologists, social workers and surgeons. Peer support is also a key part of the care, especially during adolescence, and attention to age-appropriate education and cultural sensitivity can customize the care for each individual patient and their needs. Fertility issues should be a part of the discussion from an early age, especially when decisions are being made about irreversible surgery and/or gonadectomy. Shared decision making tools have been developed to help address all of these issues for individuals affected by DSD.

Keywords Disorders of sex development · Congenital adrenal hyperplasia · Androgen insensitivity syndrome · Vaginal agenesis · Mayer-Rokitansky-Kuster-Hauser syndrome · Mixed gonadal dysgenesis

1. **What are the categories of DSD?**

The 2006 consensus statement from the Lawson Wilkins Pediatric Endocrine Society and the European Society for Paediatric Endocrinology helped defined nomenclature and established the term disorder of sex development [1]. Table 52.1

K. van Leeuwen (✉)
Colorectal/DSD Clinic at Phoenix Children's Hospital, 1919 E Thomas Rd, Phoenix, AZ 85029, USA
e-mail: kvan@phoenixchildrens.com

M. Lacher et al. (eds.), *Pearls and Tricks in Pediatric Surgery*,
https://doi.org/10.1007/978-3-030-51067-1_52

Table 52.1 Categories of disorders/differences of sex development [2]

46, XX DSD	46, XY DSD	Gonadal ambiguities or absence	Anatomical/developmental anomalies
Congenital adrenal hyperplasia	Androgen insensitivity syndrome (AIS)	Mixed gonadal dysgenesis (MGD) or chromosomal mosaicism (45, X/46, XY)	Cloacal anomalies
			Bladder exstrophy
	Partial AIS		
	Complete AIS		
21-hydroxylase deficiency	Insufficient testosterone production	Pure gonadal dysgenesis (46, XX or 46, XY)	Caudal regression syndrome
11-hydroxylase deficiency	Inability to convert testosterone to dihydrotestosterone	Ovotesticular DSD (46, XX or 46, XY)	VACTERL synd
3β-hydroxysteroid deficiency			Persistent mullerian duct syndrome
Aromatase deficiency			Mayer-Rokitansky-Kuster-Hauser syndrome/vaginal agenesis
			Urogenital sinus

shows the categories which are based on chromosomal makeup and anatomical findings.

2. **What is the current nomenclature used to describe patients with DSD?**

Patients with DSD are described by the chromosomal makeup, e.g. XY, DSD, as well as their descriptive diagnosis, e.g. complete androgen insensitivity. The word 'differences' has been suggested instead of 'disorders.' Older terms that are not used include hermaphrodite, pseudohermaphrodite and the use of the word 'virilized' is discouraged. Describing an individual as intersex or as having intersex traits has become more acceptable.

3. **How is gender of rearing determined?**

Most infants with DSD will have a gender assigned that is in line with what is expected as they grow but in some cases a gender of rearing may be deferred.

4. **When are patients with DSD diagnosed?**

Diagnosis can be made prenatally when there is discordance between a cell-free fetal DNA test and the appearance of the genital structures on ultrasound. More frequently, newborns with genital differences will be identified postnatally. Adolescents can also be diagnosed with DSD during a work up for amenorrhea.

5. **What is the most common DSD?**

Congenital adrenal hyperplasia is the most common DSD with a worldwide incidence estimated to be 1 in 14,000–15,000 live births.

6. **What is involved in the evaluation of a newborn with a DSD?**

Newborns with genital differences should be evaluated by a pediatrician or neonatologist with the goal of ruling out any life-threatening conditions such as salt-wasting congenital adrenal hyperplasia or any associated cardiac or renal anomaly. Consultation with a multidisciplinary team including genetics and endocrinology is essential. Labs and imaging in the nursery can help narrow the differential.

7. **Are these diagnoses picked up prenatally?**

Evaluation of the gender of a fetus involves ultrasound imaging of the genitalia and, in some cases, cell-free fetal DNA detected in the mother's blood stream. There can be limited views of the fetus due to positioning. If there is a concern for genital ambiguity on prenatal imaging, referral to a center with a DSD clinic is indicated.

8. **Are there any prenatal therapies available for DSD?**

For families with a previous history of congenital adrenal hyperplasia, a possible therapy for future pregnancies involves early steroid therapy for the mother to mitigate the effects of excess androgens and potentially limit the virilizing effects on the genitalia of the fetus. This therapy has come under question due to the need to treat all fetuses, even when it is not known if the fetus is affected by CAH. The steroids may be related to cognitive deficits long term. [3]

9. **What types of chromosomal differences are seen in patients with DSD?**

Patients with DSD can have normal chromosomes that do not match their phenotypic sex or gender identity. They can also have a chromosomal mosaicism. Providers should first order a standard karyotype and depending on the results, more sophisticated studies should be pursued and that may include a chromosomal microarray.

10. **What medical and anatomical findings are expected on a newborn with congenital adrenal hyperplasia** (CAH)**?**

Infants with CAH can be expected to have elevated levels of hormones depending on which enzyme deficiency is present. In the most common form of the disease, 21-hydroxyprogesterone deficiency, the excess androgen is 17-beta-hydroxyprogesterone. This level should be checked in an infant with XX chromosomes and genital difference, especially in the setting of an enlarged clitorophallic structure and nonpalpable gonads.

11. **What is the medical and surgical management of a newborn with CAH?**

Initial medical management of a newborn diagnosed with CAH is support in terms of treatment with steroids. Infants are given a form of cortisol called hydrocortisone. Patients with classic CAH also require fludrocortisone to replace aldosterone. No surgical intervention is indicated in a newborn with CAH unless there is urinary obstruction from the urogenital sinus, which is rare.

12. **How does a shared decision making process affect the care of a newborn or adolescent with DSD?**

Patient centered care has been an initiative of recent efforts to decrease complications and costs in medicine. Families of patients with DSD are suited to this type of decision making since many crossroads in care are encountered that require careful education and weighing of options. Involving the patients themselves in any irreversible decision is especially important.

13. **What other diagnoses are seen in newborns?**

Other that CAH, infants can have genital difference due to chromosomal mosaicism or mixed gonadal dysgenesis. This can result in a variable upper reproductive tract anatomy that can included dysgenetic gonads or discordant gonads (testis or ovotestis on one side and ovary or streak gonad on the other) and variable lower reproductive tract anatomy including an enlarged clitorophallic structure and urogenital opening. Many infants with cloacal anomalies also have genital differences.

14. **Which DSDs present in older patients?**

Part of the workup of primary amenorrhea in an adolescent teen may reveal chromosomal or anatomical reasons that end up being a DSD. Patients with androgen insensitivity syndrome (AIS) will be found to have XY chromosomes and retained testicles. Patients with vaginal agenesis or Mayer-Rokitansky-Kuster-Hauser (MRKH) syndrome are often diagnosed in this time period and will be found to have XX chromosomes.

15. **What is the medical and anatomical evaluation of an older child with DSD?**

Older patients should be seen by a DSD team and undergo a medical evaluation that includes basic labs and hormone levels, chromosomal studies, and imaging to evaluate upper and lower reproductive tract anatomy. A complete psychosocial evaluation can guide the patient's understanding of the diagnosis and desired goals.

16. **How are the gonads managed in an adolescent with androgen insensitivity syndrome (AIS)?**

Historically, the gonads or retained testicles were removed after AIS patients reached puberty due to a perceived risk of malignancy. That risk may have been overstated and now options including gonad retention and/or preservation of genetic material for fertility should be discussed. Some patients may wish to avoid gonadectomy so they can continue to have their endogenous hormone production as long as possible. [4]

17. **If gonadectomy is perfomed in a patient with AIS, what are recommendations for hormone replacement?**

Patients with AIS who opt for gonadectomy would benefit from hormone replacement with estrogen and some patients have sought testosterone supplementation as well. Hormone levels can be followed and the goal of therapy should be to avoid symptoms that mimic those of post-menopausal women.

18. **How is partial androgen insensitivity syndrome (PAIS) different from complete androgen insensitivity syndrome (CAIS)?**

PAIS is a diagnosis of exclusion in that patients may not have a detectable defect in the androgen receptor gene. Anatomy is variable but usually involves genital differences, a urogenital sinus and/or utricle, and retained gonads consistent with testicles. Malignancy risk is unknown for retained gonads.

19. **What is Mayer-Rokitansky-Kuster-Hauser (MRKH) syndrome and how is it managed?**

Patients with MRKH or vaginal agenesis have an XX chromosomal makeup and normal ovaries. The uterine anatomy is variable and they may have rudimentary uterine tissue but no vagina. A dimple of hymenal tissue on the perineum is usually present. Diagnosis is made by physical exam, chromosome and/or lab evaluation, and ultrasound imaging of the upper reproductive tract anatomy.

20. **What is the treatment for adolescents and young adults with MRKH?**

Decision making tools can be helpful in guiding patients with MRKH. Understanding the diagnosis and options for fertility is the first step and vaginal anatomy is assessed when the patient is ready. In most cases, nonoperative therapy with progressive perineal dilation can establish a vaginal canal. Coital dilation and reconstructive vaginoplasty are other options [5].

21. **What are options for patients with mixed gonadal dysgenesis (MGD) or chromosomal mosaicism?**

Due to the variable nature of the chromosomal makeup and upper/lower reproductive tract anatomy in patients with DSD, careful consideration should be made to delaying irreversible procedures. CAH should be ruled out since anatomy can be similar but patients with CAH may need steroid therapy.

22. **How are the gonads managed for patients with MGD or chromosomal mosaicism?**

The malignancy risk may relate to the amount of virilization and families of patients with chromosomal mosaicism should be educated on ways to perform surveillance on retained gonads. Allowing the patient to make any decisions about reconstructions, if desired, is ideal.

23. **What psychosocial support is suggested for patients and families affected by DSD?**

An essential part of the DSD team is the psychosocial provider. Psychology support as well as clinical counselor and social workers can help monitor anxiety, depression, adjustment disorder, body self-image issues and help recommend therapies that build confidence and resilience.

24. **How does public opinion and changes in the way society sees gender affect the care of patients with DSD**

Attention from the media toward patients with gender differences can be a positive force that helps society accept a wide range of gender identities. Providers can be part of a process that allows patient autonomy and self-direction while emphasizing medical and anatomical priorties.

References

1. Lee PA, Houk CP, Ahmed SF, Hughes IA. In collaboration with the participants in the International Consensus Conference on Intersex organized by the Lawson Wilkins Pediatric Endocrine Society and the European Society for Paediatric Endocrinology. Consensus statement on management of intersex disorders. Pediatrics. 2006;118:e488–e500.
2. Graziano K, Fallat ME. Using shared decision-making tools to improve care for patients with disorders of sex development. Adv Pediatr. 2016;63(1):473–80.
3. Dreger A, Feder EK, Tamar-Mattis A. Prenatal dexamethasone for congenital adrenal hyperplasia: an ethics canary in the modern medical mine. J Bioeth Inq. 2012;9(3):277–94.
4. Weidler EM, et al. A management protocol for gonad preservation in patients with androgen insensitivity syndrome. J Pediatr Adolesc Gynecol. 2019;S1083–S3188(19):30217–27.
5. Gargollo PC, et al. Should progressive perineal dilation be considered first line therapy for vaginal agenesis? J Urol. 2009;182(4 Suppl):1882–9.

Chapter 53
Trauma–General Considerations

Christian J. Streck Jr

Abstract Injury is a leading cause of morbidity and mortality in children. While the priorities for trauma evaluation and management are similar in children relative to adults, unique anatomic, physiologic and mechanistic differences in pediatric trauma should be considered.

Keyword Pediatric trauma

1. **What is the most common cause of death in childhood?**

Trauma is the most common cause of death and disability in childhood.

2. **What is the most common mechanism of injury in children?**

Falls are the most common mechanism of injury in children but rarely result in mortality.

3. **What is the most common mechanism of injury associated with death in children?**

Injuries related to motor vehicles, including automobile passengers as well as bicyclists and pedestrians struck by automobiles are the most common cause of death in children.

4. **What is the most common cause of homicide in children**?

Firearm related death is the most common cause of homicide in children and adolescents while child abuse accounts for the most common cause of homicide in infants [1].

C. J. Streck Jr (✉)
Division of Pediatric Surgery, Medical University of South Carolina, Charleston, SC, USA
e-mail: streck@musc.edu

M. Lacher et al. (eds.), *Pearls and Tricks in Pediatric Surgery*,
https://doi.org/10.1007/978-3-030-51067-1_53

5. **What are the leading causes of failed resuscitation in pediatric patients following severe trauma?**

The leading causes of failed resuscitation is failure to control an airway and support breathing.

6. **What is the leading cause of death in injured children who arrive to the Hospital alive?**

The leading cause of death in children who arrive to the Hospital with a pulse is traumatic brain injury [2].

7. **What are the major anatomic and physiologic considerations for pediatric trauma?**

Children have smaller body mass, less fat, less connective tissue, a more pliable skeleton and relatively larger heads than adults. These factors contribute to higher frequencies of multi-system injury, rapid thermal injury loss with resultant hypothermia, significant internal organ damage, and traumatic brain injuries and ligamentous cervical spine injuries without associated bony injury. The major anatomic considerations include a larger occiput resulting in passive flexion of the cervical spine leading to an "anterior airway", relatively larger pharyngeal soft tissues (tongue and tonsils), and a more anterior and a funnel-shaped larynx and vocal cords.

8. **What sized endotracheal tube should be used in a child?**

Endotracheal tube (ETT) size selection is based on the child's weight, which can be estimated with a Broselow tape. A general rule to estimate ETT size is the diameter of the child's pinky finger. Cuffed ETT's are recommended, even in infants and small children, to improve ventilation management [3].

9. **What are the major anatomic differences in the pediatric cervical spine?**

Children have relatively larger heads, more flexible interspinous ligaments, flatter facet joints and anteriorly wedged vertebral bodies. These factors contribute to a higher angular momentum and a propensity for higher cervical spine injuries in young children. Unique radiologic considerations include pseudosubluxation in up to 40% of younger children, increased distance between the dens and anterior arch of C1 and skeletal growth centers.

10. **What is SCIWORA?**

SCIWORA is the acronym for spinal cord injury without radiographic abnormality in children. A normal cervical spine series may be seen in up to 2/3 of children with spinal cord injury. With improvement in CT imaging quality and increased availability of MRI, demonstrable injury to the spinal cord, soft tissue (ligaments and muscles) and vertebral body endplate in patients with normal plain radiographs is much more common.

11. **How do you clear the cervical spine following trauma in children?**

When in doubt, cervical spine precautions, including a properly fitting pediatric c-collar, should be maintained. Multiple clinical guidelines for evaluation of the pediatric c-spine following trauma exist including the National Emergency X-radiography Utilization Study (NEXUS) criteria, the Canadian C-spine Rule (CCR) and the Pediatric Emergency Care Applied Research Network (PECARN) c-spine decision rule. Blunt cerebrovascular injury (BCVI) is rare (0.1–1%), but potentially underdiagnosed, in children.

12. **Which pediatric patients should be screened for blunt cerebrovascular injury?**

Major risk factors for BCVI include Basilar skull fracture, Le Fort II/III facial fractures, unexplained neurological abnormality, arterial epistaxis, high cervical spine fracture and neck soft tissue injuries. Cervical CT-Angiography should be considered in high-risk patients.

13. **What are the important considerations in children with thoracic trauma?**

The chest wall is more pliable in children, which allows kinetic energy from blunt mechanisms to be transmitted to the underlying lung and mediastinal structures. Rib fractures are rarer than in adults and are associated with significant force. The mobility of mediastinal structures makes children more susceptible to tension pneumothorax, the most immediate life-threatening thoracic injury. Most thoracic injuries in children can be identified with plain radiographs and children rarely require chest CT.

14. **Do pediatric trauma patients benefit from emergency department thoracotomy (EDT)?**

Survival following EDT for blunt trauma in the pediatric population is extremely rare and should be discouraged without compelling evidence of a reversible cause of extremis.

15. **When should CPR be stopped in children who present in "pulseless arrest" following a traumatic mechanism of injury?**

Patients who undergo CPR for more than 15 minutes and who remain pulseless following trauma rarely survive [4].

16. **How is shock secondary to circulatory compromise recognized in children?**

Children have increased physiologic reserve and maintain cardiac output with increased heart rate and vasoconstriction. A normal blood pressure (BP) is maintained with up to 30% circulating blood volume loss at which point blood pressure may precipitously drop.

17. **What are normal blood pressure values in children?**

The lower limit of normal BP is 70 mm Hg + two times age (years).

18. **How is volume resuscitation performed in children?**

Early subtle signs of shock include tachycardia and poor skin perfusion, which can be missed secondary to pain/anxiety and exposure in the trauma bay. A narrowed pulse pressure (<20 mm), lethargy and mottled skin are other early signs of shock. Intravenous access in young children can be challenging. Intraosseous access, commonly in the proximal tibia or distal femur is an excellent alternative. Some children require central venous access either percutaneously or via saphenous vein cutdown. Volume resuscitation begins with a warm isotonic crystalloid bolus of 20 mL/kg. If there is continued hypotension or evidence of ongoing bleeding 10 mL/kg of packed red blood cells (PRBC) are transfused. The principles of "damage control resuscitation" include addressing hemorrhage early with restrictive use of crystalloid and early administration of balanced ratios of blood products (PRBC, fresh frozen plasma and platelets), typically as a part of a mass transfusion protocol (MTP). Further investigation of goal-directed therapy, which includes point of care testing to analyze clot formation and strength kinetics, like rotational thromboelastometry (ROTEM) or thromboelastography (TEG), is needed in children. Medical adjuncts to bleeding control, which are components of a MTP, may include Tranexamic acid (TXA), [5] Aminocaproic acid and activated Factor VII.

19. **What are the modifications to the Glasgow Coma Scale (GCS) in children under age 4 years?**

The verbal component of the GCS scale must be modified in children less than age 4 years. Common modifications to the verbal score are 5 (coos/babbles, words, social smile), 4 (cries but consolable), 3 (Persistently crying or irritable), 2 (Grunts, restless/agitated), 1 (None).

20. **What are the most important priorities in management of pediatric Traumatic Brain Injury (TBI) in the Trauma Bay**

Attention to the primary survey (ABCDE's) are important to decrease morbidity from head trauma in children. Children are particularly susceptible to secondary brain injury that results from hypoxia and hypovolemia. Rapid intubation and oxygen delivery in patients with GCS <8 secondary to TBI and restoration of intravascular volume to improve cerebral perfusion are critical components of pediatric TBI management.

21. **What are the unique mechanisms of injury and injury patterns that should be considered in pediatric blunt abdominal trauma?**

Most intra-abdominal injuries (IAI) in children result from blunt mechanisms. Motor vehicle collisions remain the most common cause of IAI in children; however children are more commonly involved as pedestrians or bicyclists struck by automobiles as well. The most significant risk factor for an IAI requiring an intervention (transfusion, angiography or surgery) is an abnormal abdominal physical exam. The presence of a lap seatbelt or handlebar contusion on the abdominal wall are significant risk factors for IAI.

22. **What are the major risk factors for intra-abdominal injury and when can an abdominal CT scan be safely avoided?**

Patients with no complaint of abdominal pain, a normal abdominal physical exam, a normal chest x-ray, AST and amylase are at very low risk for IAI and an abdominal CT scan can typically be safely avoided [6].

23. **What is the value of Focused Assessment Sonography in Trauma (FAST) in children?**

Although FAST has shown significant promise in adult trauma patients, FAST alone is not sensitive for identification of IAI. FAST can be particularly useful in determining whether there is a significant amount of intra-peritoneal blood in hemodynamically unstable patients.

24. **When should child maltreatment be considered based on the patients provided history?**

A thorough history and exam should be performed on all children with suspected non-accidental trauma (NAT). Suspicious history includes discrepancies between the stated mechanism of injury and physical exam findings, prolonged interval of time between injury and presentation for medical care, repeated visits for trauma or burn evaluations, changing or evolving stories from different caregivers, and injuries that are implausible based on the child's developmental age.

25. **What physical exam findings suggest child maltreatment?**

Physical exam findings include evidence of previous injuries (healed fractures, old scars, bruises in different stages of healing), perioral/genital/perianal injuries, subdural hematomas or abdominal solid organ injuries without antecedent trauma, long bone fractures in young children, retinal hemorrhages and rib fractures.

26. **How common is child abuse in the United States? What is the impact of child maltreatment on morbidity and mortality?**

Child abuse is very common in the U.S. (>1.2 million reported cases/year), particularly in children younger than age 2 years. In many pediatric trauma centers, screening for NAT is performed on all young children who present with blunt injuries that do not involve a motor vehicle. Children who present following NAT have a significantly higher morbidity and mortality than children who sustain accidental injuries.

References

1. Centers for Disease Control and Prevention, National Centers for Injury Prevention and Control. Web-based injury statistics query and reporting system (WISQUARS). Available at www.cdc.gov/injury/wisqars.
2. Rotondo MF, Cribari C, Smith RS (Eds.). Resources for optimal care of the injured patient. Am Coll Surg. 2014.
3. Vogel A, Escobar MA, Edwards MJ. Trauma resuscitation and initial evaluation. Pediat Surg Natl Am Pediat Surg Assoc. 2019.
4. Flynn-O'Brien KT, Stewart BT, Fallat ME, et al. Mortality after emergency department thoracotomy for pediatric blunt trauma: analysis of the national trauma data bank 2007–12. J Pediatric Surg. 2015.
5. Eckert MJ, Wertin TM, Tyner SD, et al. Tranexamic acid administration to pediatric trauma patients in a combat setting: the pediatric trauma and tranexamic acid study (PED-TRAX). J Trauma Acute Care Surg. 2014.
6. Arbra CA, Vogel AM, Zhang J, et al. External validation of a 5-variable clinical prediction rule for identifying children at very low risk for intra-abdominal injury following blunt abdominal trauma. J Trauma Acute Care Surg. 2018.

Chapter 54
Pediatric Traumatic Brain Injury and Cervical Spine Injuries

Matthias Krause

Abstract Pediatric brain trauma and cervical spine trauma are often associated. Brain trauma is the leading cause of death in children below the age of 4. The Glasgow Coma Scale is the most important clinical score to evaluate patients after brain trauma. There are guidelines of the Brain Trauma Foundation and PECARN for assessing, diagnosing and treating children with brain and spine traumas. Esp. indications for CT scans and X-radiographs in children differ from adult patients.

Keywords Pediatric brain trauma · Cervical spine injury · NEXUS · Glasgow coma scale · SCIWORA

1. **What is a pediatric head trauma?**

A head trauma is a trauma caused by an undue external force onto the head resulting in an injury of the scalp and the cranial bone. A traumatic brain injury (TBI) more specifically involves the central nervous system (meninges, brain itself and adjacent structures).

2. **How does the head trauma and cervical spine injuries connect?**

Combined traumata of the brain and cervical spine are much more common in children than in adults due to the imbalance between head and body as well as lower muscular strength to sustain an impact. Pediatric patients are reported to suffer from combined trauma in up to 20% of the accidents. Thus, the clinical examination should always expect spinal cord injuries as cause for neurological deficits.

M. Krause (✉)
Consultant Pediatric Neurosurgeon, Department of Neurosurgery, University of Leipzig, Leipzig, Germany
e-mail: m.krause@medizin.uni-leipzig.de

M. Lacher et al. (eds.), *Pearls and Tricks in Pediatric Surgery*,
https://doi.org/10.1007/978-3-030-51067-1_54

3. **How is the severity of a pediatric TBI evaluated?**

Glasgow Coma Scale (GCS). It is applied in children older than 2 years of age. For younger children, the GCS is modified to a pediatric GCS in terms of language evaluation. This classification of head trauma is widely used and sub grouped into: mild TBI (GCS 15-14), moderate (GCS 13-9) and severe (GCS 8-3).

4. **What is the outcome and mortality of pediatric head trauma?** [1]

Pediatric TBI is associated with a significant mortality that increases with its severity. Below the age of 4 years, it is the leading cause of death (6%) of all hospitalizations for TBI). Mild TBI usually has a good outcome with no or minor *sequelae* in neurocognitive outcome. Moderate and severe TBI is suggested to have a long-term impact on neurodevelopment reflecting in functional, cognitive and behavioral impairment. It is correlated to the severity of trauma (initial GCS) and white matter injury.

5. **What are specific signs of a pediatric head trauma?**

Pediatric TBI is only proven by the following signs and symptoms: Open wound with direct loss of CSF or brain herniation (direct open TBI) or liquorrhea via ear, nose, mouth (indirect open TBI). Common indicators for a possible TBI are: headache, repetitive vomiting, nausea, dizziness, reduced level of consciousness, neurological deficits, seizures, Battle's sign, raccoon sign.

6. **Is the age of the patient important?**

For evaluation and decision-making in TBI, children below 2 years of age are distinguished from older children in the following aspects:

- Clinical assessment is more difficult
- Infants with intracranial injuries are frequently asymptomatic
- Skull fractures or clinically important traumatic brain injury may occur despite minor trauma
- Inflicted injuries occur more frequently.

7. **When do I need to call the radiologist?** [1–4]

In pediatric TBI, there is a paucity of guidelines and recommendations for CT and X-Ray examinations and no recommendation for MRI. X-Ray examinations of the skull are considered obsolete because they can neither rule out fractures nor detect intracranial pathologies.

Because of the low incidence of surgically managed intracranial injuries in mild TBI, there is no indication for CT scans in children with GCS 15-14. Exceptions are children with a history of neurosurgical interventions, hemophilia etc. and children that present with seizures or neurologic deficits. According to a PECARN study, the following criteria have been suggested for a low risk group of children that do not require imaging:

Age	Clinical criteria
<2	Normal mental status
	Normal behavior per routine caregiver
	No LOC
	No severe mechanism of injury
	No nonfrontal scalp hematoma
	No evidence of skull fracture
≥2–18	Normal mental status
	No LOC
	No severe mechanism of injury
	No vomiting
	No severe headache
	No signs of basilar skull fracture

In children with moderate and severe TBI an initial CT is obtained acutely to evaluate intracranial injury, need for neurosurgical procedures, and for signs of intracranial hypertension. The incidence of intracranial hematoma increases with lower GCS. If available, CT scans can be substituted with MRI scans at the discretion of the physicians' team.

8. **When do I need imaging of the spine?**

Cervical spine injuries can be ruled out solely by clinical examination in older and alert children above the age of 2 years. In cases with neurological deficits, pain during distraction or compression maneuvers or restricted range of motion the following radiographs should be obtained: plain lateral, anterior-posterior view and—if possible—open-mouth view. CT scans should be done in severe cases or with neurological deficits. MRI scans have a high rate of false positive findings and should be used in selected case of physicians' discretion, especially when a spinal cord injury is suspected.

9. **What intracranial lesions have to be expected?**

Intracranial lesions in pediatric TBI are usually epidural and subdural hematomas, brain edema, intracerebral hemorrhages (brain contusions) and posttraumatic hydrocephalus. Severe traumas can also present as diffuse axonal brain damage with multiple small, not space-occupying intracerebral hemorrhages. They are distributed throughout the brain with predominance in the corpus callosum, brain stem and subcortical structures.

10. **How do I treat patients with a mild TBI?**

Children have a higher risk for intracranial injury after mild TBI than adults. Therefore, children with mild TBI that need to admitted should be monitored closely either on an ICU or IMC unit with hourly assessment of the neurological status. Deterioration of the GCS is suspicious for an increasing intracranial pressure and necessitates further workup. In most institutions children undergo in-patient observation for 48–72 hours due potential delayed onset of brain edema.

11. **Is there a need for repeated CT scans?**

An initial CT is obtained to assess intracranial injury, need for neurosurgical procedures, and intracranial hypertension. However, routine repeated CT imaging is very controversial and indicated mostly in children with severe TBI only. Repeating CT scan is usually considered when there is (1) no neurologic improvement (2) persistent or increasing ICP or (3) inability to assess the neurologic status because of sedation or paralytic agents.

12. **What is an epidural hematoma?**

Epidural hematomas usually arise from a linear skull fracture with or without laceration of a meningeal artery. Typically, patients present with a short period of unconsciousness and secondary deterioration due to growing size of the hematoma. This "symptom-free interval" is the reason for clinical observation of patients with TBI. Rapid increase of intracranial pressure can lead to rapid neurological deterioration especially in small children. The incidence of epilepsy after conservative treatment is unknown.

13. **What is a subdural hematoma?**

Subdural hematomas are located between the dura mater and the brain itself. They can be acute after trauma or chronic. Typically, acute subdural hematomas arise from ruptured cortical arteries or veins on the surface due to direct impact. Chronic subdural hematomas are encountered mostly in children that sustained mild traumas or repetitive injuries (shaken-baby syndrome, non-accidental head trauma). Chronic hematomas may arise from a tear of bridging veins and a chronic inflammation within the subdural space. Usually, there is a long delay in the onset of symptoms making it difficult to elucidate the incident of the impact.

14. **How do I monitor unconscious patients with TBI?**

In unconscious or sedated and/or ventilated patients that cannot be monitored sufficiently by neurological examination, additional neuromonitoring with intracranial pressure (ICP) monitors is advocated. CT scans do not help in estimating intracranial pressure even in children with normal initial CT scan.

The Gold standard is external ventricular drainage (EVD), but intraparenchymatous probes are also available. Successful control of intracranial hypertension with ICP monitoring demonstrated some evidence to improve survival and neurological outcome.

15. **Does delay of neurosurgical intervention in TBI affect outcome?**

Time between onset of neurological symptoms of raised ICP and surgical evacuation of the hematoma is crucial for the patient's outcome. The "Golden Hour of Neurosurgery" indicates that neurosurgical intervention beyond that time has a significant worse prognosis.

16. **Are there treatment thresholds for intracranial hypertension in children?**

There are no generally accepted normal values for ICP in children. Subsequently, there are no treatment thresholds for intracranial hypertension. A generally accepted treatment threshold is 20 mmHg. However, it is believed that brief episodes less than 5 minutes are insignificant. This belief has been recently challenged for adults.

17. **Is there a recommendation for adequate of cerebral perfusion?**

The CPP is defined as difference between mean arterial pressure (MAP) and ICP. There is a recommendation to maintain a cerebral perfusion pressure (CPP) at range between 40–50 mmHg in infants. Very young children and adolescents should have higher CPP around 60 mmHg.

18. **Is seizure prophylaxis initiated?**

Children have a lower threshold for seizures. In severe TBI in children, studies found a frequency of up to 70% of electrographic seizures is described. The prophylactic use of phenytoin or levetiracetam may reduce the risk for posttraumatic seizures within the first seven days.

19. **When do I discharge patients with a mild TBI?** [2]

Children after mild TBI with a **low risk** for intracranial injury can be discharged after an observational interval of 4–6 hours. Children within the **non-low risk** group for intracranial injury that showed a normal CT or MRI scan can also be discharged home instead of admission. Both groups have to fulfill the following clinical criteria:

- No suspicion of inflicted injury
- Easily aroused with light touch with a normal neurologic examination (GCS = 15)
- Return to baseline level of function
- Toleration of oral fluids/feeds after initial vomiting,
- No extracranial injuries warranting admission
- Capable caretakers who can reliably observe the child and who can return for care if indicated.

20. **What are the NEXUS criteria in C-spine injury?** [3]

NEXUS (National Emergency on X-Radiographic Utilization Study) criteria are well-validated criteria for avoiding unnecessary X-Radiography by clinically ruling out relevant cervical spine injury. If all criteria are met, imaging is not required in order to exclude clinically relevant injury of the cervical spine. The NEXUS study group also found, that the criteria can be applied in children, but did not recommended usage in small children, toddlers and babies.

Criteria	Explanation
1. No posterior midline cervical tenderness	Midline posterior bony cervical spine tenderness is present if the patient complains of pain on palpation of the posterior midline neck from the nuchal ridge to the prominence of the first thoracic vertebra, or if the patient reports pain with direct palpation of any cervical spinous process
2. No evidence of intoxication	Patients should be considered intoxicated if they have either of the following: (a) a recent history, by the patient or an observed intoxication or intoxicating ingestion; or (b) evidence of intoxication on physical examination, such as odour of alcohol, slurred speech, ataxia, dysmetria, or other cerebellar findings, or any behavior consistent with intoxication. Patients may also be considered to be intoxicated if tests of bodily secretions are positive for drugs that affect level of alertness, including a blood alcohol level greater than 0.08 mg/dL
3. Normal level of alertness	An altered level of alertness can include any of the following: (a) Glasgow Coma Scale score of 14 or less; (b) disorientation to person, place, time, or events; (c) inability to remember 3 objects at 5 minutes; (d) delayed or inappropriate response to external stimuli; or (e) other
4. No focal neurological deficit	Any focal neurological complaint (by history) or finding (on motor or sensory examination)
5. No painful distracting injuries	No precise definition for distracting painful injury is possible. This includes any condition thought by the clinician to be producing pain sufficient to distract the patient from a second (neck) injury. Examples may include, but are not limited to, the following: (a) a long bone fracture; (b) a visceral injury requiring surgical consultation; (c) a large laceration, degloving injury, or crush injury; (d) large burns; or (e) any other injury producing acute functional impairment. Physicians may also classify any injury as distracting if it is thought to have the potential to impair the patient's ability to appreciate other injuries

21. **What are criteria for X-radiographs in C-spine injury in children?** [4]

According to the PECARN study (pediatric emergency care research network), the following criteria in clinical examination should trigger plain X-radiographic examination in children:

- Neck pain
- Midline posterior neck tenderness
- Decreased neck range of motion
- Torticollis
- Altered mental status either due to trauma or intoxication
- Focal neurologic finding
- Substantial co-existing injury, especially torso injuries
- Predisposing conditions e.g. Down syndrome, cervical arthritis, Ehlers-Danlos syndrome

- High-risk mechanisms:
  - MVC where patient partially or completely ejected from vehicle, passenger death, or passenger compartment intrusion > 12 inches at roof and/or > 18 inches at any site
  - Diving
  - Hanging
  - Axial load force
  - Clotheslining force

22. **What is SCIWORA?**

SCIWORA is an acronym for spinal cord injury without radiographic abnormalities. Cervical spine fracture, dislocation, or subluxation are differential diagnoses that are ruled out by imaging studies performed during the acute phase of management and evaluation. When children present with transient neurologic symptoms and normal neurologic exams, it may be difficult to distinguish between cervical brachial plexus injuries (burners or stingers) and SCIWORA. Patients with SCIWORA usually have neck pain with reduced range of motion, and bilateral paresthesias or weakness that can involve the lower extremity. Findings can progress to flaccid paralysis and quadriparesis.

23. **Should steroids be given after spinal cord injury?** [5]

The National Acute Spinal Cord Injury Study (NASCIS) II investigated the use of methylprednisolone (30 mg/kg IV, followed by 5.4 mg/kg per hour over 23 more hours). At one year, there was a modest better motor outcome. Therefore, early administration of glucocorticoids after spinal cord injury is advocated by most clinicians.

24. **What about immobilization of the cervical spine after injury?** [6]

The pediatric techniques for spinal motion restriction should be used until about 16 years of age as they are influenced by their developmental anatomy. Compared to adults, children younger than eight years have proportionally larger heads and weak cervical muscles that make them more prone to axial cervical spine injury. The neck is placed in a cervical collar, and the body is positioned supine, preferably on a soft surface with attention to the head-body relation: Infants and young children warrant a cut out in the board or padding under the shoulders to maintain neutral position.

References

1. Kochanek PM, Tasker RC, Carney N, Totten AM, Adelson PD, Selden NR, Davis-O'Reilly C, Hart EL, Bell MJ, Bratton SL, Grant GA, Kissoon N, Reuter-Rice KE, Vavilala MS, Wainwright MS. Guidelines for the management of pediatric severe traumatic brain injury,

third edition: update of the brain trauma foundation guidelines, executive summary. Pediatr Crit Care Med. 2019;20(3):280–9.
2. Kuppermann N, Holmes JF, Dayan PS et al. Identification of children at very low risk of clinically-important brain injuries after head trauma: a prospective cohort study. Lancet. 2009;374:1160.
3. Hoffman JR, Mower WR, Wolfson AB, Todd KH, Zucker MI. Validity of a set of clinical criteria to rule out injury to the cervical spine in patients with blunt trauma. National emergency X-radiography utilization study group. N Eng J Med. 2000;343:94–9.
4. Leonard JC, Kuppermann N, Olsen C, Babcock-Cimpello L, Brown K, Mahajan P, Adelgais KM, Anders J, Borgialli D, Donoghue A, Hoyle JD Jr, Kim E, Leonard JR, Lillis KA, Nigrovic LE, Powell EC, Rebella G, Reeves SD, Rogers AJ, Stankovic C, Teshome G, Jaffe DM. Pediatric emergency care applied research network. Factors associated with cervical spine injury in children after blunt trauma. Ann Emerg Med. 2011;58(2):145.
5. Bracken MB, Shepard MJ, Collins WF Jr, Holford TR, Baskin DS, Eisenberg HM, Flamm E, Leo-Summers L, Maroon JC, Marshall LF. Methylprednisolone or naloxone treatment after acute spinal cord injury: 1-year follow-up data. Results of the second national acute spinal cord injury study. J Neurosurg. 1992;76(1):23.
6. Herzenberg JE, Hensinger RN, Dedrick DK, Phillips WA. Emergency transport and positioning of young children who have an injury of the cervical spine. The standard backboard may be hazardous. J Bone Joint Surg Am 1989;71:15.

Chapter 55
Thoracic Trauma

Maeve O'Neill Trudeau, Joshua Ramjist, and Paul W. Wales

Abstract Pediatric thoracic trauma accounts for about 5–10% of injuries in children, but relative to other body symptoms, the mortality is relatively higher at 15–20%. Most thoracic injuries can be managed with supportive care including oxygen support, good analgesia, and possible tube thoracostomy. Surgical intervention is uncommon.

Keywords Trauma · Injury · Pediatrics · Thoracic · Pediatric surgery

1. **In a child with documented chest injury, what should the trauma surgeon suspect?**

Chest injury is often a marker for other injuries. More than two-thirds of children with chest injury have other organ system injuries, including closed-head injury, extremity fractures, and intra-abdominal solid-organ damage [1].

2. **What is the significance of rib fractures in children?**

Less bone mineralization in children, is associated with increased pliability of a child's chest wall relative to an adult [2]. Therefore, pulmonary contusions can occur without overlying rib fractures. When rib fractures do occur, they are an indication of severe impact. *Posterior rib fractures are very specific for non-accidental trauma.* In one large study, all children with four or more rib fractures had at least one other injured chest organ.

M. O. Trudeau · J. Ramjist · P. W. Wales (✉)
Division of General and Thoracic Surgery, The Hospital for Sick Children, Rm 1526, 555 University Avenue, Toronto, ON M5G 1X8, Canada
e-mail: paul.wales@sickkids.ca

M. O. Trudeau · J. Ramjist · P. W. Wales
Department of Surgery, University of Toronto, Toronto, ON, Canada

M. Lacher et al. (eds.), *Pearls and Tricks in Pediatric Surgery*,
https://doi.org/10.1007/978-3-030-51067-1_55

3. **What type of thoracic injury is common in children?**

Contusions are most common, followed by pneumo/hemothorax. Rib fractures are more common in adolescents.

4. **What clinical signs raise the suspicion of a pulmonary contusion?**

Evidence of a shunt with resultant hypoxia, indicative of a ventilation-perfusion mismatch.

5. **What are the complications of pulmonary contusion?**

- **Pneumonia** may develop in the injured lung *segment and is the most common complication of a contusion*. Frequent suctioning and physiotherapy may prevent the development of pneumonia.
- **Posttraumatic pneumatoceles**. In children, posttraumatic pneumatoceles typically resolve over time; however, they may become infected and form lung abscesses.
- Chest tube insertion may be necessary if the contusion leads to secondary pneumothorax, hemothorax, pleural effusion or, rarely, a bronchopleural fistula.

6. **What are the signs and symptoms of a tension pneumothorax?**

Chest pain, respiratory distress, hemodynamic compromise (tachycardia, hypotension), tracheal deviation, ipsilateral reduced or absent breath sounds, and neck vein distension.

7. **What hemodynamic changes occur with a tension pneumothorax?**

The mediastinum shifts away from the collapsed lung, compresses the contralateral lung, and displaces the diaphragm downward. This shift of the mediastinum results in an angulation of the inferior vena cava with decreased systemic venous return to the heart and cardiac output, and increased central venous pressure. It may result in cardiovascular collapse.

8. **Describe the treatment of a tension pneumothorax.**

Immediate decompression by a large-bore (14 Ga) needle inserted into the second intercostal space in the mid-clavicular on the side of the chest with absent breath sounds. *Tension pneumothorax is a clinical diagnosis*. Valuable time may be lost in obtaining a chest film. Once the patient is stabilized it is always necessary to insert a chest tube in the affected hemithorax.

9. **What is a "sucking" chest wound?**

Penetrating trauma may cause an open pneumothorax. The opening of the chest wall allows air to enter and escape the thorax, resulting in paradoxical respirations.

10. **How does an open pneumothorax compromise ventilation?**

The chest wall can no longer generate a negative intrathoracic pressure, and ventilation is severely compromised. Treatment requires occlusion of the wound and chest tube insertion.

11. **What is Beck's triad? Is it present in small children?**

Beck's triad represents the three physical findings associated with adult cardiac tamponade: (1) markedly diminished heart sounds, (2) venous distention in the neck, and (3) decreased arterial pressure. In a child or infant cardiac tamponade may be difficult to assess, and must be suspected when mediastinal trauma and hypotension or shock are present. Jugular venous engorgement and pulsus paradoxus can also indicate cardiac tamponade.

12. **What chest x-ray findings suggest pericardial effusion or hemorrhage?**

Increase in size of cardiac silhouette and overall profile of the heart appearing more rounded than normal.

13. **Describe the *immediate* treatment for suspected cardiac tamponade.**

If tamponade is suspected, pericardiocentesis should be performed. An angiocatheter is passed upward and to the left of the xyphoid process. After a flash of blood the needle is removed, and a syringe is attached for aspiration. Aspiration of as little as 15–20 ml of blood results in immediate improvement.

14. **What is indicated by the aspiration of blood that "clots" during pericardiocentesis?**

The blood is from an intracardiac chamber rather than the pericardial space. Intracardiac blood forms a clot, whereas pericardial aspirate should not form a clot due to the fibrinolytic and anticlotting activities of the pericardial mesothelium [3].

15. **When should cardiac contusion be suspected?**

Patients with blunt injuries to the anterior chest associated with diminished cardiac output despite adequate blood volume and fluid resuscitation should be suspected of having cardiac contusion. Important clinical signs and symptoms of cardiac contusion include hypotension, significant conduction abnormalities on EKG, or wall motion abnormalities on echocardiography. Troponin levels in children can aid in diagnosing cardiac injuries [4].

16. **How long should a patient with mild cardiac contusion be monitored?**

Patients with mild cardiac contusion (diagnosed by conduction abnormalities) are at risk for sudden dysrhythmias and should be monitored for the first 24 hours after injury. After 24 hours the risk of sudden dysrhythmia decreases substantially.

17. **What is the speculated mechanism of sudden death in a young athlete who sustained a blow to the chest from a projectile object (e.g., a baseball)?**

Sudden death is most likely due to ventricular dysrhythmia induced by an abrupt blow to the chest, presumably delivered at an electrically vulnerable phase of ventricular excitation (thought to be during cardiac repolarization, specifically immediately prior to the peak of the T wave). This is also referred to as "commotio cordis".

18. **Aortic injury in children is rare. Name two situations in which it may be suspected?**

Deceleration injuries such as (1) motor vehicle crash with unrestrained adolescent driver and (2) fall from a great height [5].

19. **Where does the aorta usually lacerate?**

At the level of the ligamentum arteriosum where the aorta is fixed.

20. **What is the gold standard for diagnosis of aortic injury?**

Computed Tomography Angiography (CTA). Historically aortograms were employed, however the improved imaging and rapidity of obtaining a CTA mean that aortograms are now usually only necessary for an interventional procedure, if at all.

21. **What chest film findings indicate a possible thoracic aortic disruption?**

- Widened mediastinum
- Obliteration of the space between the pulmonary artery and the aorta
- Depression of the mainstem bronchus
- Deviation of the esophagus (nasogastric tube) to the right
- Fractures of the first or second rib or scapula.

22. **When should a tracheobronchial injury be suspected in a child?**

Tracheobronchial injuries are rare in children. Tracheal and bronchial tears occur after high energy mechanism injuries, such as motor vehicle collisions or heavy objects falling onto the chest/crush injuries. Clinical presentation may include subcutaneous emphysema, tension pneumothorax, hypoxia and/or hemoptysis. Chest tube placement indicates a massive air leak that does not resolve.

23. **Which tracheobronchial injuries require direct repair?**

Tears of the intrathoracic trachea and major bronchi require direct repair.

24. **What is the treatment of basilar bronchi tears?**

Rents of basilar bronchi frequently respond to high-frequency, low-pressure ventilation. Distal bronchial leaks may be occluded with fibrin glue selectively placed via bronchoscopy. When these measures fail, segmental resection or lobectomy is required.

25. **What is the most common cause of esophageal injury in infancy and childhood?**

Iatrogenic injuries secondary to endoscopic or dilatation procedures are most common, followed by injuries from caustic ingestion and penetrating injuries [6].

26. **What findings on a chest film may indicate esophageal injury?**

Pneumomediastinum, subcutaneous emphysema, pneumothorax, hemothorax, pleural effusion and mediastinal widening.

27. **Name the best study for esophageal injury.**

Esophagram with a water-soluble contrast material, and consideration of intraoperative or rigid esophagoscopy.

28. **What is the treatment of an acute esophageal injury?**

If diagnosed within 12 hours of injury, primary repair, administration of broad-spectrum antibiotics and wide mediastinal drainage are indicated for significant injuries. If there is a delay in diagnosis, proximal salivary diversion, placement of a gastrostomy tube and drain placement may be necessary. An intercostal muscle pedicle flap may be used to buttress a primary esophageal repair. Stents may present alternatives for specific circumstances.

29. **How is diaphragmatic rupture diagnosed in children? How is blunt diaphragmatic injury repaired?**

Plain chest films showing evidence of the nasogastric tube above the diaphragm or viscera in the chest. The repair is done via laparotomy, which provides access to possible concomitant injury to abdominal viscera.

30. **What is the indication for emergency thoracotomy in a pediatric trauma setting?**

Penetrating thoracic injury with signs of life witnessed by health care workers (pre- or in-hospital). The use of ED thoracotomy for blunt trauma, only when arrest occurs in the emergency department, remains highly controversial.

References

1. Bliss D, Silen M. Pediatric thoracic trauma. Crit Care Med. 2002;30(11 Suppl):S409–15 [PMID:12528782].
2. Garcia VF, Gotschall CS, Eichelberger MR, et al. Rib fractures in children: a marker of severe trauma. J Trauma. 1990;30:695–700.
3. Spodick DHW. Bloody pericardial effusion: clinically significant without intrinsic diagnostic specificity. Chest. 1999;116(6):1506–7.

4. Hirsch R, Landt Y, Porter S, et al. Cardiac troponin I in pediatrics: normal values and potential use in the assessment of cardiac injury. J Pediatr. 1997;130(6):872–7 [PMID:9202607].
5. Heckman SR, Trooskin SZ, Burd RS. Risk factors for blunt thoracic aortic injury in children. J Pediatr Surg. 2005;40(1):98–102.
6. Eroglu A, Can Kürkçüogu I, Karaoganogu N, et al. Esophageal perforation: the importance of early diagnosis and primary repair. Dis Esophagus. 2004;17(1):91–4 [PMID:15209749].

Chapter 56
Abdominal Trauma

Raphael H. Parrado and David M. Notrica

Abstract Abdominal trauma is a common source of morbidity and mortality in the pediatric population. Early evaluation and early detection of any injuries and vital in the treatment of this patients. Evaluation includes the use of ultrasound and computed tomography. In the last decade there has been a recent development of an algorithmic non-operative management strategy for solid organ injury that is based on the physiological status of the child and not the grade of the injury. This management if effective in over 90% of the patients. Recently, there has been increased use of laparoscopy, endoscopic measures and angioembolization for the treatment of this patients depending the injury. This evidence-based management provides shorter hospital stay and reduces the need of more invasive measures. Surgical exploration remains the choice in presenting unstable patients or who fail non-operative management.

Keywords Abdominal trauma · Penetrating trauma · Laparoscopy · Blunt trauma · Blunt splenic injury · Blunt liver injury · Pancreatic injury · Renal injury

1. **How common is pediatric abdominal trauma? [1, 2]**

In the US, 1 in 10,000 children sustain abdominal trauma each year with 85% of injuries due to blunt trauma.

R. H. Parrado
Phoenix Children's Hospital, Phoenix, AZ, USA

D. M. Notrica (✉)
Phoenix Children's Hospital, Mayo College of Medicine,
University of Arizona College of Medicine Phoenix,
1919 E Thomas Rd, Phoenix, AZ 85016, USA
e-mail: dnotrica@phoenixchildrens.com

M. Lacher et al. (eds.), *Pearls and Tricks in Pediatric Surgery*,
https://doi.org/10.1007/978-3-030-51067-1_56

2. **How do pediatric and adult blunt abdominal trauma patients differ?**

Children and have less soft tissue protecting their internal organs. As a result, the organs are often in close proximity to the abdominal wall increasing the force transmission and risk of injury. The reported success rates of nonoperative management are higher in children. Children who fail nonoperative management (NOM) fail early (within 4 hours), and rebleeding is very uncommon (<0.2%).

3. **What is the most commonly injured organ?**

The liver is the most common injured organ (50%) followed by the spleen (41%). Ten percent of patients have injuries of both the liver and spleen.

4. What is the most common mechanism of pediatric abdominal trauma?

Fall from a height is the most common mechanism, but motor vehicle collisions account for a larger number of serious injuries. Child abuse is a major source of trauma mortality in children under 3 years of age.

5. **What finding on physical exam is most correlated with abdominal injury in a pediatric patient? [2]**

Abdominal contusions such as "seat-belt" signs or "handle bar" marks carry a 19% risk of internal injury. Seat belt signs are associated with hollow viscus injuries and Chance fractures of the spine (11%). Pain to palpation in the alert child is moderately sensitive (79%) for intraabdominal injury in children who are fully alert and cooperative, but specificity is low.

6. **What are the radiographic adjuncts for evaluation of pediatric abdominal trauma?**

Focused abdominal ultrasonography for trauma (FAST) is a non-invasive, inexpensive and portable technique that assesses for the presence of free fluid (presumably blood) in the abdominal cavity and pericardium. Approximately 40% of patients with intra-abdominal injury do not have free fluid, so sensitivity for minor injury is low. The true usefulness appears to be in unstable pediatric patients. Computed Tomography with IV contrast remains the preferred modality for solid organ injury.

7. **When can the Computed Tomography be omitted in the evaluation of pediatric abdominal trauma? [3]**

The Pediatric Emergency Care Applied Research Network (PECARN) suggests that computed tomography may be omitted if 7 conditions are met (See Table 56.1).

8. **What are the indications for non-operative management (NOM) of pediatric abdominal trauma? [5]**

Most children with blunt liver or spleen injury stop bleeding, or never bleed at all. The management of pediatric abdominal trauma is based on hemodynamic

Table 56.1 Pecarn criteria for omitting abdomen computed tomography [4]

• Glasgow comma scale > 14
• No complaints of abdominal pain
• No vomiting
• No abdominal tenderness
• No thoracic wall trauma
• No abdominal wall bruising ("Seat belt Sign"/ "Handle Bar Injury")
• No absent or decreased breath sounds.

Reprinted with permission from Notrica [2]

status, not the injury grade. Non-operative management has become the standard for treatment of injured children with isolated liver or spleen injuries, with over 96% of children managed without a surgical intervention. The ATOMAC guideline for the treatment of blunt liver and spleen injury provides an evidence-based algorithm for management (see Fig. 56.1).

9. **What are the indications for surgery in a child with blunt abdominal trauma?**

   – Failure to stabilize after a transfusion or early recurrent shock.
   – Bleeding requiring more than 40 ml/kg of packed red blood cells (PRBCs) or >4 units of PRBCs.
   – Free intraperitoneal air.

10. **What is the role of laparoscopy in pediatric abdominal trauma?**

Laparoscopy has a role in stable patients with persistent abdominal tenderness or peritonitis suspicious for bowel injury. Laparoscopy is also an effective way to perform distal pancreatectomy in cases of complete transection of the main pancreatic duct or to evaluate and/or repair a diaphragm injury. Delayed laparoscopy with drain placement has been employed in cases of significant intraperitoneal blood to decrease abdominal pressure and reduce pain. In penetrating trauma, laparoscopy may be useful to confirm peritoneal penetration and evaluate and/or repair the bowel repair.

11. **What is the grading for liver and splenic injuries (Table** 56.2)**?**

12. **What is the hemoglobin threshold for initiating blood transfusion for children with liver or spleen injuries who are not in shock?**

Children with an acute liver or spleen injury should have a transfusion threshold of 7.0 g/dL. This has been shown to be safe in multiple prospective studies, and higher thresholds show no increased benefit.

13. **How often does the hemoglobin (Hb) level need to re-checked?**

In the past, hemoglobin was rechecked at a scheduled frequency of every 4 to 6 hours. New data suggests the hemoglobin only needs to be re-evaluated if the

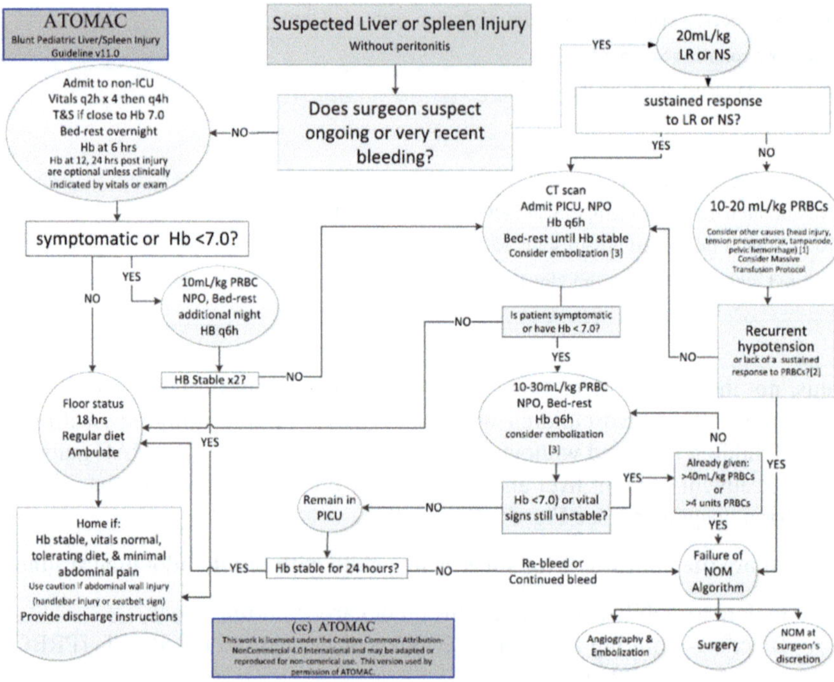

Fig. 56.1 ATOMAC guideline for management of pediatric BLSI. (1) More than 50% of injured children with hypotension have no significant intra-abdominal bleeding but do have severe traumatic brain injury. (2) Recurrent hypotension within the first hour because of intra-abdominal bleeding or an SBP of less than 50 mm Hg after transfusion is an ominous sign, and strong consideration should be given to operative or angiographic intervention. (3) Embolizing CT blush may be considered, but more than 80% of children with blush do not require angiography for successful NOM. (4) Interventional modalities such as ERCP, laparoscopy, angiography, or percutaneous drainage may be required to manage complications of bile leak or hemobilia. Hb, hemoglobin; NPO, "non per os" or nothing per mouth; PICU, pediatric ICU; PRBC, packed red blood cell; q6h, every 6 hours; SBP, systolic blood pressure. Reprint with permission from the ATOMAC Research Network [5]

vital signs or clinical condition suggest bleeding. Vitals and clinical exam assessment will detect ongoing bleeding. In fact, hemoglobin drops in the absence of clinical signs should be verified prior to transfusion.

14. **What are the options for patients not responding to resuscitation in the setting of a liver/spleen injury?**

Initial failure to respond to transfusion warrants surgical exploration, with rare exceptions (non-survivable brain injury). In the setting of a patient failing NOM (persistent hemodynamic instability and signs of ongoing hemorrhage) options are urgent angioembolization and/or surgical exploration.

Table 56.2 Classification of spleen and liver injuries in trauma

Grade	Type	Description
I	Hematoma	Subcapsular, <10% surface area
	Laceration	Capsular tear, <1 cm depth
II	Hematoma	Subcapsular, 10–50% surface area, intraparenchymal <5 cm (Spleen), <10 cm (liver) diameter
	Laceration	Capsular tear, 1–3 cm depth, does not involve trabecular vessel (spleen), <10 cm length (liver)
III	Hematoma	Subcapsular, >50% surface area, intraparenchymal >5 cm (spleen), >10 cm (liver) diameter
	Laceration	>3 cm depth, involves trabecular vessel (spleen)
IV	Laceration	Spleen: Segmental or hilar vessels producing >25% devascularization/ Liver: 25–75% hepatic lobe or >3 Couinaud's segments
V	Hematoma	Spleen: Completely shattered or hilar injury resulting in Devascularization
	Vascular	Liver: >75% of hepatic lobe or >3 Couinaud's segments Juxtahepatic venous injuries, retrohepatic vena cava/central major hepatic veins
VI	Vascular	Complete hepatic avulsion

Adapted from Becker C, Mentha G, Terrier F. Blunt abdominal trauma in adults: role of CT in the diagnosis and management of visceral injuries. Part 1: liver and spleen. Eur Radiol. (1998);8:553

15. **What is the role of angioembolization in the setting of a liver/spleen/renal injury?**

Approximately 5–15% of patients with splenic injuries have contrast extravasation on CT, but very few of these require angioembolization. Unlike adults, angioembolization is generally reserved for patients otherwise failing NOM. Spleen rebleeding in children is very uncommon, making the need for AE rare. AE for liver injury may be slightly more common, and AE for renal injury may also have a role.

16. **What are the operative steps in surgical management of blunt liver injury?**

The abdomen is explored, blood clots are extracted, and all 4 quadrants of the abdomen are packed. The packs are then removed sequentially. Bleeding is surgically controlled if mild. If bleeding is not controlled, the abdomen is re-packed. If packing controls the bleeding, the patient should be transferred for angioembolization with packs in place. If not controlled, a Pringle maneuver should be performed. If bleeding is controlled the source is likely the hepatic artery or a portal vein branch which can be treated with selective ligation. If not controlled, the bleeding is most likely from an inferior vena cava (IVC) injury or hepatic veins for which vascular repair is needed. The mortality from retrohepatic caval injury remains high.

17. **What is the role of endoscopic retrograde cholangiopancreatography (ERCP) in liver trauma?**

Biloma is initially treated with US or CT-guided external drainage. In severe biliary injury, endoscopic retrograde cholangiopancreatography (ERCP) has been used to identify the source of leak and improve drainage through a sphincterotomy with stenting. Additionally, a biliary stent past the biliary injury by be beneficial. The rate of bile leak after high grade liver injuries is about 4%.

18. **After injury recovery when can patients with liver/spleen injuries be discharged?**

Historically, the length of stay was equal to the injury grade +1 day, however recent studies have shown that patients without clinical signs of bleeding can be safely discharged after 18 hours of observation. Post-discharge activity should be restricted for grade of injury +2 weeks.

19. **What is the grading for renal injury (Table** 56.3)**?**

20. **What is the management of a renal injury? [6]**

NOM is advocated for most injuries. Even high grade injuries (IV–V) in children have 80 to 100% success rates of NOM. Failure of nonoperative management has been related to collecting system hematomas, urinomas greater than 4 cm, dissociated renal fragments and interpolar extravasation. Adjunctive procedures such as stenting, percutaneous drainage and angioembolization can be performed to improve renal preservation.

21. **How are pancreatic injuries graded?**

Injury grade is determined by the extent, location, and status of the main pancreatic duct (see Table 56.4).

Table 56.3 Organ injury scale for renal injuries

Grade	Type	Description
I	Contusion	Microscopic or gross hematuria, urologic studies normal
	Hematoma	Subcapsular, nonexpanding without parenchymal laceration
II	Hematoma	Nonexpanding perirenal hematoma confined to renal retroperitoneum
	Laceration	<1.0 cm parenchymal depth of renal cortex without urinary extravasation
III	Laceration	>1.0 cm parenchymal depth of renal cortex without collecting system rupture or urinary extravasation
IV	Laceration	Parenchymal laceration extending through renal cortex, medulla, and collecting system
	Vascular	Main renal artery or vein injury with contained hemorrhage
V	Laceration	Completely shattered kidney
	Vascular	Avulsion of renal hilum with kidney devascularization

From Chiron P, Hornez E, Boddaert G et al. Eur J Trauma Emerg Surg. (2016);42:237

Table 56.4 Pancreas injury scale

Grade	Type	Description
I	Hematoma	Minor contusion without duct injury
	Laceration	Superficial laceration without duct injury
II	Hematoma	Major contusion without duct injury or tissue loss
	Laceration	Major laceration without duct injury or tissue loss
III	Laceration	Distal transection or parenchymal injury with duct injury
IV	Laceration	Proximal? transection or parenchymal injury involving ampulla
V	Laceration	Massive disruption of pancreatic head

From Debi U, Kaur R, Prasad KK, Sinha SK, Sinha A, Singh K. Pancreatic trauma: a concise review. World J Gastroenterol. 2013;19(47):9003–11. https://doi.org/10.3748/wjg.v19.i47.9003. Reprinted with permission from Campbell R, Kennedy T. The management of pancreatic and pancreaticoduodenal injuries. Br J Surg. 1980;67:845–50. https://doi.org/10.1002/bjs.1800671203

22. **How are pancreatic injuries managed?**

There is general agreement that low-grade injuries (grade I and II) do not benefit from surgery. The treatment for patients with ductal transection treatment varies, with many major centers recommending laparoscopic distal pancreatectomy without splenectomy. For proximal complete ductal transection Roux-en-Y pancreatojejunostomy or pancreaticogastrostomy is recommended. In contrast, high grade injuries without ductal transection may be managed non-operatively.

23. **Are there any special considerations regarding diaphragmatic injury?**

Diaphragmatic rupture is an uncommon and frequently missed injury. Laparoscopy has been successfully used in in acute, but stable patients, Thoracoscopy is recommended when the diaphragm injury is identified late. Thoracoscopy allows lysis of thoracic adhesions and easier repair of the defect than laparoscopy.

References

1. Notrica, DM. Abdominal and renal trauma. In: Ashcraft KW, Holcomb GW, Murphy JP, St. Peter SM (eds.). Ashcraft's pediatric surgery (7th ed.). Philadelphia: Saunders/Elsevier; 2020.
2. Notrica DM. Pediatric blunt abdominal trauma: current management. Curr Opin Crit Care. 2015;21(6):531–7.
3. Acker SN, Stewart CL, Roosevelt GE, et al. When is it safe to forgo abdominal CT in blunt-injured children? Surgery. 2015;158:408–12.
4. Holmes JF, Lillis K, Monroe D, et al. Identifying children at very low risk of clinically important blunt abdominal injuries. Ann Emerg Med. 2013;62:107–16.
5. Notrica DM, Eubanks JW, Tuggle DW, Maxson, RT, Letton RW, Garcia NM et al. Nonoperative management of blunt liver and spleen injury in children: evaluation of the ATOMAC guideline using GRADE. J Trauma Acute Care Surg. 2015;79(4):683–93.
6. Notrica DM, Linnaus ME. Nonoperative management of blunt solid organ injury in pediatric surgery. Surg Clin North Am. 2017;97(1):1–20.

Chapter 57
Soft Tissue Injuries

Aaron T. Scott and Bindi Naik-Mathuria

Abstract Soft tissue injuries are among the most common traumatic injuries sustained by children and vary in severity from minor cuts and scrapes that require no intervention to severe, life-threatening injuries requiring emergent surgical intervention. A brief summary of the epidemiology, evaluation, management, and outcomes of soft tissue injuries is given.

Keywords Soft tissue injuries · Wounds · Compartment syndrome · Bites

Questions:

General:

1. **What types of soft tissue injuries are typical in children?**

Common injuries include lacerations, contusions, and superficial injuries. Compared to adults, wounds in children are more likely to be on the head, more likely to be linear, more likely to be smaller, less likely to be contaminated, and more commonly caused by blunt trauma. In the outpatient setting, sports injuries, falls, or animal/insect bites are the mechanism in 50% of cases. In the emergency setting, falls are the most common cause of injuries in children younger than 10 years old and motor-vehicle collisions are the most common mechanism in children aged 10 and above. Penetrating trauma increases in frequency with age.

A.T. Scott
Michael E. DeBakey Department of Surgery, Baylor College of Medicine, Houston, TX, USA

B. Naik-Mathuria (✉)
Trauma Medical Director, Texas Children's Hospital, Houston, TX, USA
e-mail: bnaik@texaschildrens.org

M. Lacher et al. (eds.), *Pearls and Tricks in Pediatric Surgery*,
https://doi.org/10.1007/978-3-030-51067-1_57

2. **What are the priorities in the management of soft tissue injuries?**

After addressing immediately life-threatening injuries by ATLS protocol, soft tissue injuries should be addressed. Efforts should focus on achieving hemostasis, restoring perfusion if compromised, and preventing infection.

3. **How should life-threatening bleeding from soft tissue injuries be managed in the pre-hospital and hospital settings?**

   a. In the pre-hospital setting, the Stop the Bleed campaign (bleedingcontrol.org) offers a concise strategy for achieving hemostasis with three methods of hemorrhage control. When no other material is available, direct pressure is indicated. When packing material is available, wounds should be packed with gauze followed by direct pressure. If a tourniquet is available, the wound is on an extremity, and bleeding cannot be controlled with pressure alone, the tourniquet should be applied.
   b. In the hospital setting, direct pressure, packing, and tourniquets can all be used, but an emphasis should be placed on rapidly identifying the source of bleeding and then obtaining hemostasis. For life-threatening bleeding, intervention in the OR is often required.

4. **Why is depth an important factor in pediatric injuries?**

An apparent soft tissue injury may involve deeper structures. Given the smaller size/thickness of anatomic structures in children, deep organs are more likely to be injured than in adults.

5. **Which wounds are prone to infection?**

Risk factors for infection of traumatic wounds include location (higher in lower extremity), wound contamination, wound size, wound mechanism, shock, blood loss, older age, diabetes mellitus, and number of associated organs injured [1].

6. **Which injuries require tetanus vaccination?**

Tetanus vaccination depends on both the wound and the patient's prior vaccinations. For clean, minor wounds where the patient is known to have completed a primary tetanus-diphtheria series (minimum of three doses) with the last dose within the last 10 years, no further vaccine is needed. If the patient has not completed a primary series, does not know if they have completed a primary series, or last received a vaccine more than 10 years ago, they should be given an age appropriate vaccine. For more complex wounds (contaminated, puncture, avulsions, crush, devitalized tissue, etc.), if the patient is known to have completed a primary series with the last dose within the last five years, no further vaccine is needed. If the patient has completed the primary series, but the last dose was more than five years prior, an age appropriate vaccine should be given. If the patient has not completed the primary series or does not know their status, both the vaccine and human tetanus immune globulin should be given.

7. **What adjunctive studies should be considered when evaluating soft tissue injuries?**

For simple, minor injuries, physical exam alone is adequate. When there is concern of contamination, radiographs and ultrasound can help identify foreign bodies, but plain films do not rule out the presence of radiolucent foreign bodies. In the setting of crush injuries and envenomation, CK can be useful for identifying rhabdomyolysis. Venomous bites indicate the need for a CBC and coagulation studies.

Open Wounds

8. **Which wounds should be left open?**

Wounds should be left open at the time of initial management when there is inadequate tissue for primary closure, when delayed assessment of the tissue for viability and or debridement is required, and when there is active infection or concern for a high risk of infection. Delayed presentation/management has classically been considered a contraindication to wound closure, but evidence for this practice is lacking.

9. **What steps should be taken to clean wounds?**

Open wounds should be irrigated and any foreign bodies removed. High pressure irrigation should be avoided in puncture wounds as it may force foreign bodies deeper into the tissue. Antiseptic solutions should not be used as it may impede wound healing. For grossly contaminated wounds and deep abrasions with a high volume of impacted debris, mechanical agitation with a brush may be needed. Debridement of large areas of necrotic tissue should be performed.

10. **Should prophylactic antibiotics be administered when closing lacerations?**

For minor, non-bite wounds in otherwise healthy children, prophylactic antibiotics are not needed when undergoing laceration repair. The data are less clear for large, complex, or contaminated wounds [2].

11. **What is the role of negative pressure wound therapy (NPWT) in the management of traumatic wounds?**

In adults, NPWT has shown benefits in increasing abdominal fascia closure rates, decreasing time to healing of open wounds, decreasing pain associated with dressing changes, decreasing hospital length of stay, and decreasing costs associated with wound management compared to traditional dressings. Although there is a paucity of randomized trials in children, multiple series have reported good outcomes with NPWT in children. NPWT devices provide effective coverage of large, complex wounds which are not amenable to primary closure.

12. **What is a mangled extremity and how does its management differ from lower severity injuries?**

A mangled extremity is an extremity that has sustained injury to multiple organ systems (soft tissue, bone, vessel, nerve). Management requires a multidisciplinary approach and prediction of functional outcomes to avoid salvage of a non-functional limb with eventual delayed requirement for amputation. Multiple clinical scoring systems, such as the Mangled Extremity Severity Score and Predictive Salvage Index have been developed for adults, but have shown variable performance in children. More recent studies, possibly effected by advances in microsurgical techniques, have shown that predictive scores may overestimate the need for primary amputation.

Compartment Syndrome

13. **What injuries predispose children to developing compartment syndrome?**

Compartment syndrome is a clinical entity which occurs when the pressure within an enclosed fascial space rises high enough to prevent adequate perfusion. Amongst children, the most common mechanisms of injury are auto-pedestrian collisions, falls, sports injuries, and motor-vehicle collisions. The peak incidence is in children aged 10–14, with boys effected in a 4:1 ratio compared to girls. The majority of cases of acute compartment syndrome occur following a fracture (85%), with the majority of those fractures being in the forearm or leg. The overall incidence of compartment syndrome with fractures is low, occurring in 1% of forearm fractures and 3.3% of leg fractures. Other high risk injuries known from the adult literature include crush injury and vascular injury, particularly combined arterial and venous injuries where the incidence of compartment syndrome is over 40% [3].

14. **What are the symptoms and physical exam findings of compartment syndrome?**

Compartment syndrome is classically described as causing the 6 P's—pain, paresthesias, paresis, pallor, poikilothermia, and pulselessness. These findings have relatively poor sensitivity for the diagnosis and may not be present until late in the disease process. Pain is often exacerbated by passive stretch of the effected compartment. Palpation of the compartment often elicits tenderness and the compartment may feel tense or firm, but these examination findings also have poor sensitivity.

15. **How are compartment pressures measured and used to guide management of suspected compartment syndrome?**

Intra-compartmental pressures can be measured by introducing a needle into the compartment and transducing the pressure using a hand-held solid-state manometer designed for this purpose. If compartment syndrome is suspected, pressures should be measured in all suspected compartments. Classically, an absolute intra-compartmental pressure of 30 mmHg has been used as an indication for surgical release. Given variations in baseline compartment and blood pressures between individuals, however, a differential pressure rather than an absolute pressure can be used. A differential pressure (diastolic blood pressure—intra-compartmental pressure) less than 30 mmHg is an indication for surgical release [3].

16. **What is the surgical management of acute compartment syndrome?**

The presence of compartment syndrome is an indication for emergent fascial release. Any constricting dressings/casts should be immediately removed and hypotension corrected. For compartment syndrome in the leg, two longitudinal incisions are performed to achieve release of the four compartments: an lateral incision to release the anterior and lateral compartments and a medial incision to release the deep and superficial posterior compartments. In the forearm, the volar compartment is released with a lazy-S incision that extends across the carpal tunnel and the dorsal compartment can be released by a longitudinal incision.

17. **What are the long-term sequelae of compartment syndrome?**

Morbidity is related to muscular necrosis and fibrosis, nerve injury, renal injury from elevated myoglobin levels, and poor cosmesis. Morbidity is minimized by prompt recognition and surgical release. Notable injuries include foot drop from anterior compartment ischemia related to tibial fractures and Volkmann's contracture (claw deformity of fingers, hand, and wrist) from flexor compartment ischemia secondary to compartment syndrome or compromise of brachial arterial flow due to a supracondylar humerus fracture.

Bites

18. **What patterns of injury are characteristic of animal bites in children?**

Children are more likely to sustain dog bites than adults. The highest incidence of bites is in children aged five to nine years old. Two-thirds of all bites to the face occur in children under the age of 10, with pre-school age children the group most likely to sustain bites to the head/face. Three-quarters of bites occur on the extremities; the majority to the hand. Females are more often injured by cats than males; dog bites are twice as common in males as females.

19. **Should prophylactic antibiotics be used after bites?**

a. For human bites that break the skin, prophylaxis should be given. Amoxicillin-clavulanate is the agent of choice, with a three to five-day course.
b. For animal bites, antibiotic prophylaxis should be given for high risk wounds. High risk wounds include those on the face, hands, and genitals; wounds in immune compromised patients; deep puncture wounds and wounds that approach joint capsules; and wounds associated with crush injury. Amoxicillin-clavulanate is the agent of choice, with a three to five-day course. Alternative therapies should have good coverage of *Pasteurella multocida* (e.g. avoid macrolides) [4].

20. **How should bite wounds be closed?**

All wounds should be washed out as quickly as possible. Deep or wide wounds may require sedation or anesthesia to be adequately irrigated. Wounds can then generally be closed primarily or managed with NPWT. Consider closing larger wounds over a penrose drain or vessel loop to limit infection risk.

21. **When should rabies prophylaxis be administered?**

Healthy domestic animals that are available for 10 days of observation: propylaxis only if animal develops signs of rabies. Rabid, suspected or unknown: immediate immunization and Rabies Immunoglobulin (RIG). All bites by bats, skunks, racoons, foxes, woodchucks and most wild carnivores should be regarded as rabid until proven otherwise and immunization with RIG administered. Livestock, rodents or other bites should be considered immediately and consultation with public health officials should be sought regarding immunization.

Morell-Lavalle Lesions

22. **What causes these lesions?**

Blunt trauma with tangential impact causing shearing forces that result in a closed soft tissue degloving injury. This causes skin and subcutaneous tissue to separate from the underlying fascia and fluid accumulation that forms a pseudocyst.

23. **How do these lesions present?**

They most commonly present over the trochanteric region and proximal thigh as a soft, fluctuant area with a contour deformity, bruising, skin hypermobility or a palpable bulge. When diagnosed late, they present as contour deformities from chronic fluid collections or infected cysts.

24. **What is the best imaging modality?**

MRI is the modality of choice, but CT or ultrasound can also demonstrate the lesions.

25. **What are the treatment options?**

Lesions diagnosed early can often be treated with compression ± sclerotherapy, or cryotherapy may also be considered. If no resolution, then percutaneous drainage or open debridement may be necessary. Chronic lesions generally require surgical debridement or excision with primary or secondary closure [5].

References

1. Quinn JV, Polevoi SK, Kohn MA. Traumatic lacerations: what are the risks for infection and has the 'golden period' of laceration care disappeared? Emerg Med J. 2014;31(2):96–100. https://doi.org/10.1136/emermed-2012-202143.

2. Stevens DL, Bisno AL, Chambers HF, Dellinger EP, Goldstein EJ, Gorbach SL, Hirschmann JV, Kaplan SL, Montoya JG, Wade JC. Practice guidelines for the diagnosis and management of skin and soft tissue infections: 2014 update by the infectious diseases society of America. Clin Infect Dis. 2014;59(2):147–59. https://doi.org/10.1093/cid/ciu296.
3. Gottlieb M, Adams S, Landas T. Current approach to the evaluation and management of acute compartment syndrome in pediatric patients. Pediatr Emerg Care. 2019;35(6):438–9.
4. Bula-Rudas FJ, Olcott JL. Human and animal bites. Pediatr Rev. 2018;39(10):490–500. https://doi.org/10.1542/pir.2017-0212.
5. Dawre S, Lamba S, Harinatha S, Gupta S, Gupta A. The Morel-Lavellee lesion: a review and a proposed algorithmic approach. Europen J Plast Surg. 2010;35(7):489–94. https://doi.org/10.1007/s00238-012-0725-z.

Chapter 58
Orthopedic Trauma and Sports Injuries

Kevin H. Latz

Abstract Pediatric and adolescent multi-skeletal injuries are common in trauma patients and student athletes that participate in sports. Awareness of these unique injuries can lead to prompt recognition and better outcomes.

Keywords Chance fracture · Tibial tubercle fracture · Tibial spine fracture and shoulder dislocation pulseless · Supracondylar fracture · Pelvic apophyseal fractures

1. **What is a physeal fracture, and how are they classified?**

Physis (growth plates) are located at the top and bottom of the long bones of the upper and lower extremity. The Salter-Harris classification (1–5) has both descriptive and prognostic value with regards to the probability of growth plate closure as a result of the injury.

2. **What is the role of Vitamin D in trauma?**

Vitamin D levels have been found to be deficient or insufficient in 77% of orthopedic trauma patients [1].

3. **What is an open fracture, and how are they managed?**

An open fracture is a fracture that generally occurs in association with a laceration of the overlying skin. These fractures can be associated with delayed healing and an increased risk of infection. Successful treatment of these fractures includes provision of antibiotics, irrigation and debridement of the wound and bone. There

K. H. Latz (✉)
Children's Mercy Hospital, Department of Orthopaetic Surgery, 2401 Gillham Road, Kansas City, MO 64108, USA
e-mail: klatz@cmh.edu

M. Lacher et al. (eds.), *Pearls and Tricks in Pediatric Surgery*,
https://doi.org/10.1007/978-3-030-51067-1_58

may be a role for provision of antibiotics and irrigation of the fracture in the outpatient (ED) setting for certain open fractures [2].

4. **What is the concept of fracture remodeling?**

Children and adolescents can straighten a mal-aligned fracture over time. Younger patients with fractures close to the physis and a deformity in the plane of motion of the adjacent joint remodel more quickly.

5. **What types of fractures occur in the spine with various ages?**

Upper cervical spine fractures occur in younger children due to the head (large) to body (small) ratio as well as perhaps due to laxity and cervical facet orientation. Children older than 10 sustain injuries to the lower aspect of cervical, and thoracic and lumbar spine in a pattern similar to adults [3].

6. **Why are odontoid fractures relatively common in children under 6 years of age?**

The synchondrosis of the odontoid fuses at approximately 6 years of age thus this area is vulnerable with flexion injuries of the C spine in children under 6 years of age. The anteriorly displaced dens can usually be identified via radiographs or CT.

7. **Why are children with cervical spine injuries or suspected cervical spine injuries difficult to transport?**

A child's relatively large head places a young child at risk for a flexion injury of the cervical spine during transport unless the backboard has an occipital recess, or the body is elevated relative to the head.

8. **Describe the etiology and management of atlantoaxial rotatory subluxation?**

Atlantoaxial rotatory subluxation can occur with trauma or infection. This condition is identified on clinical exam and confirmed via CT. Instances of subluxation associated with infection or low velocity trauma often can be effectively treated with a soft collar and anti-spasm medication. Rotatory subluxation that results from a high velocity mechanism often requires an MRI to evaluate for a posterior ligamentous injury and a C1–C2 fusion when identified.

9. **What is SCIWORA, and why is it more common in children?**

Spinal cord injury without radiographic abnormality most commonly occurs in the cervical spine secondary to the elasticity of a child's spine and the inelasticity of the spinal cord. An MRI can be useful to detect spinal cord injury.

10. **Describe Chance fractures, and why do they happen in children?**

Chance fractures occur via a flexion injury of the spine often from sudden deceleration mechanism on a child with an incorrectly applied seat belt. The injury entails a flexion—compression injury to the anterior column and a distraction injury to the posterior column. These injuries can occur in combination with intra-abdominal visceral and vascular injuries thus a high suspicion for these injuries is paramount. Chance fractures typically occur in the upper lumbar spine, and can be ligamentous, bone or mixed [4].

11. **What is the presentation and management of pars interarticularis fractures?**

Pars fractures or spondylolysis occur in the lumbar spine. Patients present with low back pain which is exacerbated with extension. These injuries can typically be diagnosed with AP, lateral, and oblique lumbar sacral radiographs. There may be a role for CT to distinguish acute vs. chronic injuries and MRI to identify stress injuries. Adolescents who perform repetitive extension of the lumbar spine are at risk for developing these injuries e.g. offensive lineman in football and gymnasts. Most of these patients can be treated with activity modification, physical therapy ± spinal orthotics with few going on to require surgery.

12. **Which clavicle fractures may benefit from surgery?**

Most clavicle fractures are treated without surgery. Clavicle fractures which are open or are associated with a floating shoulder require surgery. Additionally, some young adults who sustain a displaced clavicle fractures may benefit from surgery to maintain shoulder biomechanics, provide a quicker time to fracture union and potentially a quicker return to sports. The benefit of surgery for clavicle fractures in adolescents is not clear [5].

13. **What is a SC dislocation, and how are they managed?**

Sternoclavicular dislocations can occur with the clavicle dislocating anteriorly or posteriorly relative to the sternum. Anterior dislocations are at risk for recurrence. Posterior dislocations can involve injury to adjacent neurovascular structures, trachea or esophagus, and mandate urgent or emergent reduction either via open or closed techniques.

14. **What is unique about adolescent shoulder dislocations?**

Adolescents who sustain a shoulder dislocation are at significant risk for recurrence. Surgical stabilization of first-time shoulder dislocation has been advocated to prevent recurrence and avoid injury to the articular cartilage of the glenoid and humeral head.

15. **What is the mechanism of injury and classification for supracondylar humerus fractures?**

Supracondylar fractures are described as extension (majority) or flexion type based on the position of the fracture fragment relative to the shaft of the humerus. Extension supracondylar fractures result from a hyperextension injury of the elbow via a fall on an outstretched arm. Extension supracondylar fractures can result in a neurological injury (anterior interosseous nerve) approximately 10% of the time. Flexion injuries occur as a result of a fall onto a flexed elbow [6].

16. **How should a pulseless supracondylar humerus fracture be managed?**

Significantly displaced extension supracondylar humerus fractures can present to the ED with a pulseless limb. These fractures should be reduced promptly in the operating room. There is no consensus on how to manage a pulseless supracondylar fracture that has been reduced with a return of doppler signal but not palpable pulses or a hand which is well perfused but pulseless following reduction.

17. **How do medial epicondyle fractures occur, and what are the treatment options?**

Medial epicondyle fractures can occur in isolation or in combination with elbow dislocations. An elbow dislocation should be considered with those fractures accompanied by global elbow swelling rather than isolated medial elbow swelling and ecchymosis. Fractures which are open or that remain incarcerated following reduction of elbow dislocations require surgery. Medial epicondyle fractures that occur in dominant limbs and those fractures that occur in combination of elbow dislocations may benefit from surgery. Loss of elbow motion following both operative and non-operative management is not unusual.

18. **Describe the characteristics and management of lateral condyle fractures of the elbow.**

Lateral condyle fractures are intra-articular fractures. Fractures with more than 2 mm of intraarticular displacement require surgery. Non or minimally displaced fractures should be followed with internal oblique radiographs in addition to AP/lateral radiographs out of plaster.

19. **Which forearm fractures are more likely to displace following reduction?**

Most forearm fractures can be treated with closed reduction and casting. Displacement after reduction and casting is more common in patients greater than 10-years-old, fractures which involve the proximal third of the bone, and those casted with poor casting technique. Open reduction and internal fixation can be accomplished with plates and screws or intramedullary fixation (single or both bone).

20. **How common are pelvic fractures in children?**

Pelvis fractures can be classified as stable or unstable. Unstable pelvis fractures are relatively rare and can be associated with visceral, neurovascular, and spinal injuries and should be evaluated by the trauma team. Stable pelvic fractures include apophyseal fractures which often occur in adolescent athletes. Apophyseal fractures occur as a result of muscle traction on the apophysis and include anterior superior iliac spine (ASIS) fractures–tensor, sartorius, anterior inferior iliac spine fractures (AIIS)–rectus, ischial tuberosity fractures–hamstring, and lesser trochanter fractures–psoas, and can often be treated non operatively. These fractures are typically treated without surgery

21. **What risks are associated with femoral neck fractures?**

Femoral neck fractures require prompt anatomic reduction and often require internal fixation. These challenging fractures can be complicated by non-union, malunion, and AVN.

22. **What radiographs should be obtained in an obese patient with acute or chronic thigh and knee pain who present to the ED with the inability to stand or walk?**

Slipped Capital Femoral Epiphysis (SCFE), a fracture of the proximal femoral physis, should be considered in any adolescent patient that presents with groin, thigh or knee pain. AP and frog pelvis radiographs should be obtained in any patient with a suspected SCFE.

23. **How are fractures of the femur managed?**

Femur fractures in children can be managed with closed reduction and spica casting, intramedullary fixation (flexible or rigid), or submuscular plates. External fixation has been utilized historically and may still have a role in the management of open fractures. Rigid intramedullary nails should be placed via the greater trochanter rather than the piriformis fossa to avoid the development of AVN.

24. **What is injured in a patella dislocation, and who is likely to experience a recurrence?**

Patella dislocations in which the patella dislocates laterally with respect to the trochlea are common injuries and can result in injury to the articular cartilage of the medial patella facet and both the anterior aspect and the weight bearing aspect of the lateral femoral condyle. Recurrence is more common in those patients with open growth plates and valgus lower extremity alignment.

25. **What condition is associated with a knee "clunk"?**

A patient with a misshapen (discoid) lateral meniscus can demonstrate a visible and audible shift of the knee (clunk) with active range of motion of the knee.

26. **What is a tibial spine fracture, and how are they managed?**

A tibial spine fracture occurs in children and adolescents as the result of a traction injury on the medial tibial spine by the ACL. These fractures can be minimally displaced (type 1), posteriorly hinged (type 2), or displaced (type 3) and comminuted (type 4). Tibial spine fractures can be associated with articular cartilage and meniscus injuries, and thus if treated in a closed manner an MRI should be considered. Type 1 fractures are treated with immobilization, type 2 fractures can be treated with closed or arthroscopic/open reduction, type 3 and 4 fractures are treated with arthroscopic/open reduction and fixation. These injuries can be complicated by arthrofibrosis and laxity.

27. **A 14-year-old male attempts to dunk a basketball during basketball try-outs for his 8th grade team, and develops pain, swelling, and the inability to weight bear. What is his likely injury?**

Tibial tubercle fractures result from a forceful contraction of the quadriceps often during sports. Type 1 fractures are non-displaced and are treated with immobilization. Type 2 fractures are displaced tubercle apophysis fractures and are treated with open reduction and internal fixation. Type 3 fractures extend into the knee joint and are treated with open reduction and internal fixation and consideration of an arthrotomy or arthroscopy to ensure anatomic intra articular reduction. Displaced tubercle fractures can be associated with compartment syndrome of the leg.

28. **What are transitional ankle fractures?**

Triplane and juvenile tillaux fractures are transitional ankle fractures that occur in adolescents with closing growth plates. Triplane fractures appear as Salter Harris (SH) 2 fractures on the lateral ankle radiograph and SH 3 fractures on the AP ankle x-ray. Juvenile tillaux fractures are SH 3 fractures that occur via traction of the anterior tibiofibular ligament on an incompletely closed distal tibia physis. These fractures are treated with anatomic intra articular reduction, and rarely result in a significant leg length inequality given the maturity of the patients that sustain these injuries.

29. **What complications are associated with medial malleolus fractures?**

Medial malleolus fractures are SH 3 or 4 fractures which often result in an arrest of the distal tibia physis. Fractures with significant initial displacement and those reduced without anatomic reduction are more likely to result in a growth plate arrest.

References

1. Hood, MA, Murtha YM. Prevalence of low vit D LEVELS in patients with orthopedic trauma. Am. J. Orthopedics 2016;45(7):522–6.
2. Lobst CA, Spurdle C, Baitner AC, et al. A protocol for the management of pediatric type 1 open fractures. J Child Orthop. 2014;8(1):71–6.
3. Knox JB, Schneider JE, Cage JM, et al. Spine trauma in very young children: a retrospective study of 206 patients presenting to a level 1 pediatric trauma center. J Pediatr Orthop. 2014;34(7):698–702.
4. Arkader A, Warner WC Jr, Tolo VT, et al. Pediatric chance fractures: a multicenter perspective. J Pediatr Orthop. 2011;31(7):741–4.
5. Canadian Orthopaedic Trauma Society. Nonoperative treatment compared with plate fixation of displaced midshaft clavicular fractures: a multicenter, randomized clinical trial. J Bone Joint Surg Am. 2007;89(1):1–10.
6. Babal JC, Mehlman CT, Klein G. Nerve injuries associated with pediatric supracondylar humeral fractures: A meta-analysis. J Pediatr Orthop. 2010;30(3):253–63.

Chapter 59
Pediatric Burns

Eduardo I. Gus, Joel Fish, and Charis Kelly

Abstract Pediatric Burn Injury in developed countries are common with the majority of these injuries being under the age of 5 due to scalding with hot liquids. The diagnosis, treatment and outcomes are covered in this chapter highlighting the pediatric specific burn care issues. Extensive burns involving fifty percent body surface area or greater are rare. This chapter therefore focusses on the more common injury where less than 15% of the skin surface is injured emphasizing the importance of pain control, proper wound assessment and wound care.

Keywords Burn · Thermal injury · Lund and browder diagrams · Advanced burn life support

E. I. Gus
Victorian Adult Burns Service, The Alfred Hospital, Melbourne, VIC, Australia

J. Fish (✉)
FRCS(C) Medical Director Burn Program, The Hospital for Sick Children, 555 University Ave, M5G1X8 Toronto, ON, Canada
e-mail: joel.fish@sickkids.ca

C. Kelly
Nurse Practitioner Burn Program, The Hospital for Sick Children, Toronto, ON, Canada

M. Lacher et al. (eds.), *Pearls and Tricks in Pediatric Surgery*,
https://doi.org/10.1007/978-3-030-51067-1_59

1. **Who manages Pediatric Burn Injuries?**

Pediatric Burn Care in developed countries is practiced in dedicated programs with the full spectrum of caregivers providing interprofessional care including emergency management and resuscitation, nursing, wound care, pain control, acute and reconstructive surgical management, psychosocial support and reintegration into school/activities for children. It is for this reason that many pediatric centers in North America are part of a verification system run by the American Burn Association to ensure that children with a thermal injury are treated with resources and personnel specific to pediatrics.

2. **What is unique about the acute pediatric burn injury?**

There are many differences between adult and pediatric care including the fact that most injuries in children are scalding injuries (70% of occurrences) with high levels of smaller burns (less than 15% body surface area) with an emphasis on short-term admissions to control pain, provide expert wound care, ensure the child is able to eat and then transition quickly to an outpatient model of care. Rates of acute surgery vary but are between 10–20% of pediatric cases in larger centers. Even though many pediatric burn wounds will heal without surgery, the need for scar management is common requiring burn team care. Infants in the acute phase of burn injury require special care in terms of airway management, infectious practices, nutritional metabolic requirements.

3. **What are the specific key points in the initial emergency room management of a child with a burn injury?**

Primary survey for burned children follows the same *Advanced Burn Life Support* (ABLS) protocol than adults and after other forms of injury are cleared the burn is considered for care. Nonetheless, pediatric patients have special considerations:

A. **Airway maintenance**

Burn size greater than 20% body surface area needs to consider prophylactic intubation to protect the airway from the extensive swelling that ensues as fluid resuscitation commences. Burn size of 15–20% BSA can be monitored for fluid requirements in a unit where intubation is immediately available sometimes avoiding intubation.

B. **Breathing and ventilation**

If inhalation injury is suspected, start high flow 100% oxygen.

Circumferential full-thickness burns of the trunk and chest should be closely monitored, and may require escharotomies if mean airway pressures are high in the face of compromised tidal volumes.

Children have more compliant chests, and tend to use the abdominal muscles for breathing.

C. **Circulation and cardiac status, with hemorrhage control**

Insert a large bore intravenous catheter (2 catheters if TBSA > 20%) and indwelling urinary catheters to measure urine output. If IV lines are difficult to obtain, intraosseous infusion (distal femur or proximal tibia) may be lifesaving.

"Initial fluid rates", for patients with visibly large burns, before proper assessment of TBSA during short term transport (less than one hour):

5 years old and younger: Ringer's lactate (RL), 125 ml/h
6–13 years old: RL 250 ml/h
14 years old and older (considered adults): RL 500 ml/h.

Definitive calculation of hourly fluid rates ("adjusted fluid rates") will occur after TBSA calculation Acute burns do not bleed. If bleeding, rule out associated trauma.

D. **Disability, neurological deficit and gross deformity assessment**

Burn patients should be initially alert and oriented. If not, consider carbon monoxide intoxication, substance abuse (adolescents), hypoxia, or pre-existing comorbidities.

E. **Exposure and environmental control**

Completely undress the patient (remove diapers), examine for associated injuries, and maintain a warm environment.

Infants are particularly prone to hypothermia in the emergency room and during transport therefore digital pictures of the injury should be acquired ensuring the entire surface of the patient skin is visualized and then quickly covered to prevent ongoing losses.

All burned areas can be covered with warm, dry surgical towels and then transport safely rather than wasting time applying dressings which are going to be removed when the child arrives at a burn unit.

F. **Pain Control**

Intravenous narcotics are the ***first line treatment*** for acute burn pain and should be dosed according to pediatric guidelines based on weight which guide the dose. Anti-inflammatories should also be administered.

G. There is no role for prophylactic antibiotics in initial acute burn care.

4. **What influences the depth of a burn wound and how can depth be determined?**

Burn depth is classified into superficial, superficial partial, deep partial and full-thickness burns. It is common for emergency room personnel to comment that pediatric scald burns "are not that deep" but clinical predications have low accuracy (60–70% correct) in the first three days.

Burn wound progression, or "declaration", **refers to the natural evolution of a burn wound, meaning that it tends to progress to deeper tissues in the first 48–72 h. What a health care practitioner may see at time of presentation is not what will appear 48–72 hours later.** The depth of the tissue damage depends on temperature of offending agent, duration of contact, thickness of the skin affected, and blood supply to the area. Children under the age 2 years have thinner skin and are more prone to full-thickness burns at lower temperatures, or shorter duration of contact [1]. Laser Doppler imaging is used in many pediatric burn centers on day three to improve the clinical accuracy of burn depth prediction to 93%.

5. **What are the clinical characteristics of scald burns?**

Hot water can burn like fire! It is a common misconception that hot water burns could never be very deep. The majority of scald burns in the first 24–72 are categorized as "indeterminate depth". This means that they are typically a mixture of superficial burns (which might splatter to small areas), partial thickness and possibly full thickness components. It is difficult to predict which burned areas will heal without surgery.

Burn-injured areas where the hot water first contacts the skin is where one would expect to find the deepest burn (*hottest* water in contact with the skin for the *longest* duration of time). Deeper burn s might demonstrate physical characteristics such as no blanching with pressure, firmer skin (similar to a rubbery egg white that has been cooked), and possibly dry, non-exudative wound bed. The presence of hemorrhage in the dermis (likely non-blanching) also would indicate a deeper burn injury. Affected areas that are less deep may be uniformly pink, blanching, soft to touch, and have an obvious amount of exudate leaking from the burn wound.

6. **How can the extent of a burn body surface area be determined in children?**

Small children have a larger surface area on the head and a smaller surface area on the lower extremities; the Lund and Browder diagrams offers a more accurate determination of % TBSA based on the ages of the child to account for this difference. These charts are readily available on the internet.

The most practical method for burn determination in pediatrics is the palmar method of estimation of burn size; the area of the hand, *including the fingers and thumb*, being 1% TBSA, regardless of age. This is used to estimate the body surface area of injured skin.

7. **Once the burn depth and extent have been determined, how should fluid resuscitation be calculated for pediatric patients ("adjusted fluid rates")?**

Burn injury will result in a controlled and predictable inflammatory response which results in leaky capillaries and loss of fluid from the intravascular space to the interstitium. The degree to which this process occurs will be modulated by the depth of injury with deeper injuries having more fluid loss for a longer duration. In order to combat the expected drop in intravascular volume, burn fluid resuscitation formulae are used worldwide which represent a starting point for fluid needs based on body weight and burn size.

The various formulae used represent a *starting point only* for fluid requirements.

The 2018 edition of the Advanced Burn Life Support manual recommends, 3 ml x Body Weight (Kg) × Body Surface Area Burned (%) to calculate the total fluid for the first 24 hours, in the form of ***Ringers Lactate*** [2]. Only partial-thickness and full-thickness burns should be taken into consideration when calculating fluids.

Fluid resuscitation needs to be started for any pediatric injury totaling 15% Body Surface area or larger.

The parkland formula suggests administering 50% of the calculated volume in the first 8 h, and the remaining 50% in the next 16 h. Hourly titration according to urinary output (aim for 0.5–1 ml/Kg/h in children < 30 kg and 0.5 ml/Kg/h in patients > 30 kg).

Children with < 30 kg should also receive maintenance fluids, D5-RL being the fluid of choice. The maintenance fluid rate should be decided based on the weight of the patient, and should be continuous, not being titrated according to urine output. Infants have glycogen deposits depleted faster than adults and older children, and may become hypoglycemic very quickly.

8. **When should a pediatric patient be referred to a burn center?**

- >10% TBSA partial-thickness burns
- Full-thickness burns of any size and location
- Burns of face, hands, feet, genitalia or perineum
- Inhalation injury
- Chemical injuries
- Electrical injuries, including lightning injuries
- Associated traumatic injuries
- Associated comorbidities
- Special social situations (abuse/neglect)
- Children in hospitals without qualified personnel or equipment for the care of pediatric patients.

9. **What are the concerns about temperature regulation in pediatric burned patients?**

Hypothalamic dysregulation induced by various inflammatory cytokines and pain causes elevation of core body temperature after a significant thermal injury. Commonly referred to the hypermetabolic state following major thermal injury. Thus, fevers in acutely burned patients tend to be inflammatory in nature. Nevertheless, persistent fevers, or elevated temperature later in the course of a burn should be considered infection-related, as wounds that are infected or highly-contaminated tend to take longer to heal, increasing the risk of developing hypertrophic scars. The commonly accepted definition for SIRS in the general critical care population is not accepted for burn cases as the criteria are always met based on the hypermetabolic response.

Nonetheless, the augmented heat loss secondary to epidermal loss, makes conventional methods of heat conservation dysfunctional. Particularly in young children, low muscle mass limits their shivering capacity, making them more prone to hypothermia than adults. Maintaining normal body temperature is also affected by the greater BSA-to-weight ratio. Thus, temperature for this age group depends highly on environmental control. Heated rooms are essential for safe care for major burn injury.

10. **What are the metabolic consequences in children who sustained a significant thermal injury?**

Inflammatory mediators released secondary to major thermal injuries (TBSA > 40%) induce profound metabolic derangements, resulting in an abnormal "stress-induced" hormonal environment, typically characterized by higher serum levels of catecholamines and cortisol and lower serum levels of human growth hormone and testosterone. These derangements result in supraphysiologic metabolic rates, including accelerated proteolysis, lipolysis, glycolysis, liver dysfunction, insulin resistance, and loss of total and lean body mass. As a result, children with burns greater than 40% TBSA show a growth delay of height and weight, and a decrease in exercise capacity, which may persist up to three years post-injury.

11. **How should the metabolic derangements of a thermal injury be managed?**

Nutritional support is essential in the management of pediatric burn patients. Pediatric patients admitted to the ICU should have a nasogatric tube inserted shortly after admission, and a high-protein, high-calorie diet should be started to ameliorate the hypermetabolic state. In addition, early enteral nutrition preserves gut mucosal integrity, and improves blood flow and motility, decreasing the risk for bacterial translocation and sepsis. Patients with smaller burns should also receive nutritional support to enhance calorie and protein intake. For children with growth delay, several pharmacological interventions have been tested, and the literature supports administration of propranolol and oxandrolone in the long-term.

12. **How is pain managed in acute burn injury?**

Pain and anxiety in children is underreported and mismanaged in pediatric burn patients. Repeated procedures and hospitalizations coupled with the initial trauma from the burn injury cause acute stress disorder and can evolve into post-traumatic stress disorder if there is inadequate attention and care. The WHO guidelines also refer to a standard of care where no child should have a pain score greater than 4/10. There are a variety of pain scales (FLACC, VAS, FACES) that can be used to assess pain and narcotics are the mainstay for acute burn care management. Doses are based on the child's weight and can be modified based on the child's response.

Pain can be separated into background, procedural and post-operative pain. There are also policies in many health care institutions/burn programs that may address these different kinds of pain and starting points for narcotic doses/infusions based on location/extent of injury.

Providing sedation in addition to analgesia is crucial in burn care. Burns are extremely painful and require these in combination to ensure the child is comfortable and unaware of the painful procedure thus minimizing the chance of contributing to a post-traumatic response. This will also allow the health care practitioner to adequately assess and clean the wounds and ensure appropriate dressings have been applied and they are effectively secured.

13. **What are the essential steps in acute burn wound care?**

- Burn wounds need to be initially cleaned with warm, soapy water which removes the non-viable dermal/epidermal components to help prevent infection. This is a clean procedure, not sterile! Removing any blisters will allow the health care practitioner an opportunity to assess the wound bed and apply an appropriate dressing to facilitate wound healing.
- Any burn wound that heals within 2 weeks can expect minimal scarring. Burn wounds that heal within 14–21 days (a deep partial thickness burns) is at a higher risk of leaving permanent scars. Any wound that takes longer than 3 weeks to will result in permanent scars. If burns are determined to be full thickness within the first 1–2 weeks, the outcomes are almost always better with excision and skin grafting to provide a better quality scar, especially over a functional area.
- Burns that are full thickness should always be referred to a specialized burn center for appropriate surgical management and scar rehabilitation.
- **Closed dressing technique:** The advent of silver-based dressings with prolonged release of silver has changed the model of pediatric burn wound care. These products are applied after sedating the child and carefully and completely cleaning the wound and then applying a dressing, which is designed to stay in place for 5–7 days thus eliminating the need for daily wound care. By adopting the model of closed-dressings, most smaller burns that do not require hospitalization can be treated as an outpatient with weekly dressing changes under sedation.
- **Conservative management for many scald injuries allowing** the full 2–3 weeks for indeterminate depth burns to heal before making a decision for grafting is a common practice. Most scald burns can heal well within 2 weeks and do not require surgical intervention which exposes them to other co-morbidities at the donor site.
- **No Surgery does not mean no ongoing care is not required.** Children that heal without surgery still may have pigmentation or subtle textural issues with their skin. There also may be pruritus that can last for months affecting their quality of life. These are constant reminders to the parents and the child of the traumatic injury. Although the medical condition has been treated,

the psychological aspects of the burn injury may require support long-term. Ensuring appropriate psychosocial supports such as social work, child life and peer support are integral to ensuring these potential concerns are addressed.

14. **How are the burn scars managed?**

Following burn injury, if the deep dermis is injured there will be a high likelihood of burn scars forming. Burn scar physical characteristics are easily measured and clinically followed by burn rehabilitation therapists (occupational and physiotherapists) measuring the scar stiffness, pain, itch and erythema. Standard therapies for scars following burn injury include moisturizers for the skin which is dry and prone to become pruritic. Range of motion exercises and splinting to maintain and regain full active range of all major joints. Massage therapy for scars symptoms (hypersensitivity, pruritis and pain) and to help soften and flatten the scars. Silicone products in the form of sheets or liquid applications have shown effectiveness as well as pressure garment therapy. The newest form of burn hypertrophic scar therapy is the combined use of fractionated laser and pulsed dye laser therapy which has demonstrated efficacy in treating the physical characteristics and symptoms of burn hypertrophic scars in children. The overall outcome of scars in children are not correlated to anatomic location, gender or extent of injury but are more predicted based or caregiver acceptance, positive coping strategies, supports by family and skilled burn team members all of whom model positive strategies for coping with the visible injury.

15. **Special Pediatric Burn Care requirements**

Child life specialists are unique to the pediatric hospital environment. They are trained in child development and behavior and aim to help support children and their siblings throughout their hospital journey. They support the children through procedural pain, medical play to prepare them for procedures/surgeries and can even help children learn how to take troublesome medications. They help normalize the hospital experience and provide suggestions to staff on how to best support a child through their admission and return visits. They are invaluable for burn patients and their families to ensure they are coping well.

School Reintegration: A burn injury affects a child for life. Depending on the child's age, returning to school can be quite challenging. The child may have differences in the color of their skin or have life-long scars that they may never accept. They may have limitations in function as a result of thick, firm scars and wear pressure garments that make them feel different. Loss of identity and/or a multitude of questions upon returning to a classroom full of new and old friends can be overwhelming for everyone. Supporting a child transition back to the classroom with a visit from the health care team can diffuse the tension and excitement in the room and also help support the teacher answer questions they are not knowledgeable about.

Burn Camps: There may be a Burn Camp accessible to families/kids within your facility. It is worth looking into. This is an invaluable experience that allows children who have sustained a burn injury to meet other children with a similar past. This is the true meaning of peer support and allows children to learn from each other, share with each other and provide each other with support.

16. **Outcomes**

Survival rates of pediatric burn injuries are almost 100% for all burn injuries below 50% body surface area with 50% mortality with extensive burns or greater than 70–80%. With this in mind, mortality rates do not reflect outcomes. Reported rates of reintegration following major burn injury are very favorable in the pediatric population. Outcomes can be measured using commonly accessible reporting such as the POSAS and SCAR Q and for older children Burn Specific Outcomes. There is an emphasis in modern burn care programs to ensure that outcomes are measured in order to ensure high quality of care. (Ref verification).

References

1. Lopes ON, Norbury WB, Herndon DN, Lee JO. Special considerations of age. In: DN Herndon editor. Total Burn Care, fifth edition. Elsevier. p. 372–80.
2. American Burn Association. 2018 advanced burn life support—2018 provider manual update.
3. Sheridan RL, Hinson MI, Liang MH, Nackel AF, Schoenfeld DA, Ryan CM, Mulligan JL, Tompkins RG. Long-term outcome of children surviving massive burns. Jama. 2000 Jan 5;283(1):69–73.

Chapter 60
Neuroblastoma

Jochen Hubertus and Dieterich von Schweinitz

Abstract Neuroblastoma is the most frequent extracranial solid malignancy in children less then 5 years of age and accounts for 6–10% of all pediatric malignancies and accounts for about 15% of cancer death in children. It arises from the sympathetic nervous system, most likely from the adrenal gland but also from sympathetic side chain. 40% of neuroblastomas are incidental findings. Most patients with clinical signs present with abdominal distention. The most common localization of neuroblastoma is the adrenal glands. Metastatic spread to the lymph nodes and bone marrow is common. MYCN is an oncogene and the most important molecular marker for poor prognosis. Image defined Risk Factors (IDRF) describe the extent and invasive/extrusive growth of neuroblastoma in different anatomical areas, such as neck, thorax or abdomen. Primary complete resection should be attempted if no IDRF are present. Although complete resection (R0) is the goal in surgical oncology, recent studies indicate that < 10% of residual tumor after resection (gross total resection) can be tolerated does not affect outcome.

Keywords Neuroblastoma · MYCN · Image defined risk factors (IDRF) · Resection · Surgery

1. **At what age is neuroblastoma most likely to occur?**

90% of neuroblastomas affect children less than 5 years of age with the highest incidence in infancy. Less than 2% of patients are older than 18 years at diagnosis.

2. **How do patients present clinically?**

40% of neuroblastomas are incidental findings. Most patients with clinical signs present with abdominal distention. Fatigue, fever and/or loss of appetite are

---

J. Hubertus (✉) · D. von Schweinitz
Department of Pediatric Surgery, Dr. von Hauner Children's Hospital, Ludwig-Maximilians-University, Lindwurmstrasse 4, 80337 Munich, Germany
e-mail: jochen.hubertus@med.lmu.de

M. Lacher et al. (eds.), *Pearls and Tricks in Pediatric Surgery*,
https://doi.org/10.1007/978-3-030-51067-1_60

unspecific symptoms. Other frequently observed symptoms include constipation, dyspnea, ostealgia, local or generalized pain, pallor from aplastic anemia, limping, Horner syndrome, hypertension, treatment resistant diarrhea, and/or ataxia. About 2–4% present with dancing eye-dancing feet syndrome (opsoclonus myoclonus syndrome). 5% of cases have a transverse myelopathy due compression of the myelon. This can cause palsy, fecal and/or urinary disorders. Myelopathy is an emergency and requires rapid diagnosis and induction therapy.

3. **Where are neuroblastomas located anatomically?**

The most common localization of neuroblastoma is the adrenal glands. These are involved in 40% of localized and in 60% of widespread tumors. Moreover, neuroblastoma can arise from sympathetic side chain of the neck to the pelvis in decreasing frequency: abdomen (non-adrenal) 30%, chest 19%, neck and pelvis 1% each. In rare cases the site of the primary tumor remains unknown.

4. **To which sites does neuroblastoma metastasize?**

Metastatic spread in neuroblastoma is common. In up to 60% of cases, metastases are present at diagnosis and most commonly found in lymph nodes and bone marrow. Liver, bones, other solid organs, and/or the skin can be affected as well. Lung metastases are very rare.

5. **What classification system is used for neuroblastoma?**

There are different levels of classification for neuroblastoma.

- **International Pathology Classification (INPC) system** defines the different subtypes of so-called neuroblastic tumors. These range from classical neuroblastoma with small-round-blue cells to ganglioneuroma, differentiated tumors with mature ganglion cells [1].
- **International Neuroblastoma Staging System (INSS)** represents the main staging system. Stage 1 are localized tumors with complete gross excision with or without microscopic residual disease. Stage 4 is any primary tumor with dissemination to distant lymph nodes, bone, bone marrow, liver, skin and/or other organs except as defined for stage 4 s. Stage 4 s is any primary tumor but with dissemination to the liver, skin and minimal bone marrow (<10%). Age at diagnosis is restricted to infants<1 year of age. The main difference between stage 2 and 3 tumors is the tumor extension across the midline [2].
- **International Neuroblastoma Risk Group (INRG)** described in 2009 defines the INRG staging system (INRGSS). It estimates the surgical risk of tumor resection prior to surgery using “Image Defined Risk Factors (IDRF)”. The INRGSS distinguishes between localized L1 tumors without image-defined risk factors, localized L2 tumors with image-defined risk factors making initial complete resection unlikely, stage M metastatic disease and stage MS disease with metastases restricted to skin, liver and/or bone marrow. Based on these parameters, neuroblastoma is categorized in low, intermediate and high risk tumors.

6. **What is MYCN?**

MYCN is an oncogene and the most important molecular marker for poor prognosis. MYCN amplification always means a classification as high risk tumor. Besides the INRGSS and the IDRF, molecular markers are important factors for risk stratification, first of all MYCN. Other markers such as 1p and/or 11q copy number are even considered to be standard diagnostic markers. ALK amplification is recommended as well in refractory or relapsed neuroblastoma.

7. **What prognostic factors are clinically used for risk stratification?**

The combination of age, INSS, INRG and molecular markers, such as MYCN and 1p copy number stratify neuroblastoma in different risk groups (Fig. 60.1).

8. **What is the diagnostic work-up for neuroblastoma?**

Besides the general and neurologic clinical assessment blood/urine samples (Neuron-Specific Enolase (NSE), Lactate Dehydrogenase (LDH) and urine catecholamine excretion for vanillylmandelic (VMA) and homovanilic (HVA) acids), ultrasound of the neck, mediastinum, and abdomen as well as chest X-ray are first line diagnostics. Contrast-enhanced magnetic resonance imaging (MRI) and 123I-meta-iodobenzylguanidine (123I-mIBG) scintigraphy performed with or without single-photon emission computed tomography (SPECT) or 18F-fluorodeoxyglucose positron emission tomography-computed tomography (18F-FDG PET-CT) are conducted if either clinical, radiological or ultrasound examinations return with positive finding.

9. **What are Image Defined Risk Factors (IDRF) and what do they indicate?**

Image defined Risk Factors (IDRF) describe the extent and invasive/extrusive growth of neuroblastoma in different anatomical areas, such as neck, thorax or

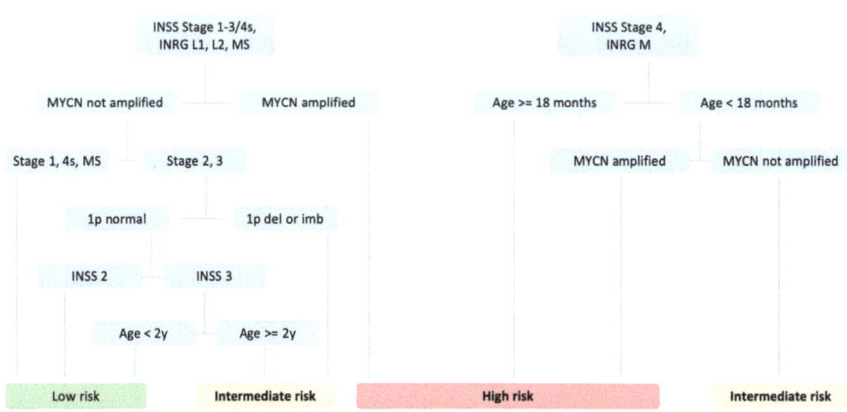

Fig. 60.1 Treatment stratification according to the *2017 GPOH Guidelines for Diagnosis and Treatment of Patients with Neuroblastic Tumors* (Simon T et al. Klin Padiatr. 2017)

abdomen. This may be tracheal compression or encasement of the aorta. IDRF are part of the risk stratification system and indicate a surgical risk during frontline resections.

10. **Is there a central organization coordinating the treatment of neuroblastomas?**

The International Society of Paediatric Oncology European Neuroblastoma (SIOPEN) is a subgroup of the International Society of Paediatric Oncology (SIOPE). SIOPEN is coordinating treatment and scientific work in Europe. In North America, this function is at the Children Oncology Group (COG).

11. **Is a biopsy needed prior to induction therapy?**

Since the bone marrow is not homogenously infiltrated by neuroblastoma, aspirates from four different puncture sites are mandatory. Additionally, tumor histology and molecular markers are crucial for risk stratification. These biopsies can be done openly or if possible, with a true cut needle. However, the amount of harvested tissue should allow not only histological but also molecular studies. It is recommended to send all biopsies to a reference pathologist to validate the diagnosis.

In children below 3 months of age with a perinatal detected small lesion can be observed by ultrasound only. If needed, a biopsy can be obtained at the age of 3–6 months.

12. **When should you consider surgical resection?**

Primary complete resection should be attempted if no IDRF are present. If the tumor is positive for IDRF or the patient is in poor condition, resection should be delayed until two, four, or six cycles of neoadjuvant chemotherapy have been given. The goal of surgery is to achieve complete tumor resection if no IDRF are present. But surgery should avoid mutilation since radiation is highly efficient in treating the remaining tumor in intermediate or high risk tumors.

13. **What is the role of minimal invasive surgery (MIS) in treating neuroblastomas?**

MIS is only justified to take biopsies and to resect smaller tumors in the absence of IDRF [3].

14. **What are major challenges during surgical resection?**

Complexity of surgical resection depends on different factors such as tumor stage, localization, response to neoadjuvant chemotherapy, infiltration of surrounding tissues, encasement of major vessels and/or other critical structures, and/or main patient's constitution. Since resection of stage 1 or 2 neuroblastomas is feasible without major difficulties, resection of stage 3 and 4 neuroblastomas can be extremely challenging and should be done by experienced oncosurgeons only. Most common complications include lymphatic leakage due to widely involvement of lymphatic vessels. If the tumor arises from the sympathetic trunk, patients and parents need to be counselled preoperatively that the ipsilateral leg may be warmer and hyperperfused due to sympathectomy. Some neuroblastomas tend to infiltrate major vessels such as the aorta, the vena cava and their major branches. Therefore, it can be extremely challenging to dissect the tumor off these vessels. Another vulnerable organ is the pancreas with the risk of pancreatic fistula after tumor resection. Since a minimal remaining tumor tissue can be tolerated (R1-resection), mutilation must be avoided.

15. **Is it possible to achieve complete resection of neuroblastoma?**

Although complete resection (R0) is the goal in surgical oncology, recent studies indicate that<10% of residual tumor after resection (gross total resection) can be tolerated does not affect outcome. Of note, stage 4 tumors are defined as a systemic disease without any chance for complete resection. In these cases, surgical strategy is tumor debulking and resection of the primary tumor.

References

1. Shimada H, et al. The international neuroblastoma pathology classification (the Shimada system). Cancer. 1999;86:364–72.
2. Brodeur GM, et al. Revisions of the international criteria for neuroblastoma diagnosis, staging, and response to treatment. J Clin Oncol. 1993;11:1466–77.
3. Fuchs J. The role of minimally invasive surgery in pediatric solid tumors. Pediatr Surg Int. 2015;31(3):213–28.

Chapter 61
Wilms Tumor

Denis A. Cozzi and Silvia Ceccanti

Abstract Wilms tumor, or nephroblastoma, is the most frequent primary renal tumor in the pediatric age group, accounting for 5% of all childhood cancers and affecting one in about 10,000 children. Clinical onset tends to occur between ages 1 and 5 years, with 90% of new cases diagnosed before age 7 years. Despite its malignant nature, long term survival rate after treatment is excellent, being greater than 90% for localized disease and 75% for metastatic disease. Most of the dramatic improvements in survival of these children have been achieved by results from randomized clinical studies conducted by the two largest collaborative groups from both sides of the Atlantic, namely the Children's Oncology Group (COG—formerly the National Wilms Tumor Study [NWTS]) and the Société Internationale d'Oncologie Pédiatrique (SIOP). Surgery still plays a pivotal role in the multimodal treatment strategy of Wilms tumor, which also includes chemotherapy, and, in certain circumstances, radiation therapy according to patient stratification into well-defined risk groups. Future goals will focus on further reduction in frequency and intensity of acute and late toxicity while maintaining current high rate of cure. Additionally, the use of biomarkers for patient risk stratification and the introduction of newer molecular targeted therapies will hopefully improve prognosis and treatment of the high risk patients.

Keywords Wilms tumor · Kidney cancer · Nephroblastoma · Nephron-sparing surgery

D. A. Cozzi (✉) · S. Ceccanti
Pediatric Surgery Unit, Sapienza University of Rome, AOU Policlinico Umberto I, Viale Regina Elena, 324, 00161 Rome, RM, Italy
e-mail: da.cozzi@uniroma1.it

M. Lacher et al. (eds.), *Pearls and Tricks in Pediatric Surgery*,
https://doi.org/10.1007/978-3-030-51067-1_61

1. **How frequent is Wilms tumor (WT)?**

WT is a specific childhood cancer, with 90% of new cases diagnosed before seven years of age and with a median age at diagnosis of 3.5 years. On exceedingly rare occasions, it is also seen in adults, accounting for less than 1% of renal tumors in this age group. Girls are slightly more affected than boys. Only about 5% of WT patients have a relative with the disease, but typically not a parent. The incidence varies among ethnic groups, being more common in Africans, while it is least common in Asians. European and North American rates are about the same. This variation is mostly related to racial/ethnic categories rather than geographic areas, suggesting that genetic factors play the most important role in the etiology of the tumor.

2. **What is known about WT etiology?**

The cause of WT is not precisely known, but it is believed to be due to genetic alterations that deal with the normal embryological development of the genitourinary tract.

3. **What are the genomic alterations that contribute to WT formation?** [1]

Some of the genetic markers that have been associated with WT include WT1, WT2, FBXW7, GPC3, and WTX gene alterations that have been found in about 1/3 of all cases. Other genes associated with WT include TP53 and MYNC. In addition to specific genes implicated in its tumorigenesis, whole and partial chromosomal gains and losses, as well as loss of heterozygosity (LOH) are commonly seen in WTs, particularly gains of chromosomes 1q, 2, 7q, 8, 12 and 13 and losses of chromosomes 1p, 7p, 16q and 22q.

4. **What are the WT1-related WT syndromes?**

The WT1-related WT syndromes are a group of genetically determined disorders caused by alterations in a tumor-suppressor gene known as WT1. This group of disorders includes WAGR (Wilms tumor-Aniridia-Genitourinary malformation-Retardation) syndrome, Denys-Drash syndrome, Frasier syndrome and genitourinary anomalies. Children with these syndromes have a chance of developing WT ranging between 30 and 90%. Other WT predisposing conditions include Beckwith-Wiedemann syndrome (linked with LOH of the WT2 locus on chromosome 11p15) and rarely Sotos syndrome, Perlman syndrome, Trisomy 18 (Edwards syndrome), Bloom syndrome, Li-Fraumeni syndrome and Simpson-Golabi-Behmel syndrome. All these patients should be screened for WT by renal ultrasonography performed every 3 months until the patient is 5–7 years of age.

5. **What is hyperplastic perilobar nephroblastomatosis?** [2]

This condition is another known disorder predisposing to WT, which is characterized by residual embryonal cells known as nephrogenic rests. These cells form multiple unilateral or bilateral renal masses, lying along the peripheral renal cortex and appearing homogeneous on imaging. Chemotherapy is the recommended treatment, given with curative intent until complete regression of the lesions. Stabilization or progression of the lesions, as well as heterogeneous changes on imaging, should prompt surgical treatment using a nephron-sparing approach.

6. **What are the clinical features of WT?**

The most common presentation is an asymptomatic abdominal mass. Associated signs and symptoms such as malaise, pain, and either microscopic or gross hematuria are found in approximately 20–30% of the children. Hypertension, which may occur as a direct effect of the presence of a renal mass, is present in approximately 25% of children with Wilms tumor, and usually resolves after nephrectomy. Occasionally, a child may present with an acute abdomen (rapidly enlarging abdominal mass, anemia, hypertension, pain and fever) due to tumor rupture or under assessment of varicocele or other genitourinary abnormalities.

7. **What investigations are needed to make WT diagnosis?**

An abdominal ultrasonography is the most useful initial investigation to confirm the presence of a primary intrarenal mass. Second-line imaging studies include computed tomography (CT) or magnetic resonance imaging (MRI) scan of the abdomen and pelvis. Recently, MRI diffusion studies have shown to allow better differentiation between WT and neuroblastoma, which is the other common abdominal malignancy in children. This differentiation is critical as the treatments for these two tumors are different. Additionally, CT and MRI accurately demonstrate intravascular tumor extension, which occurs in approximately 11% of WT patients. Renal veins and inferior vena cava are involved the most, although the thrombus may reach the right atrium in about 1% of cases. Chest CT scan is increasingly being used as first-line modality to detect metastatic spread of WT in the lungs, occurring in 10–20% of children at the time of diagnosis. However, whether or not lesions visible only on chest CT should be treated is still a matter of debate. Metastases to bones are uncommon but ominous, and typically develop as late distant recurrence.

8. **What are the histopathological characteristics of WT?**

The classic WT exhibits the so-called triphasic appearance, consisting of cells in variable proportions of blastemal, stromal, and epithelial lineage. However, they are not all present in every case. Blastemal cells are foci of abnormally persistent nephrogenic cells, which are thought to be the precursor lesions of WT. In the SIOP classification, where histology is assessed after chemotherapy, WT are sub-classified and risk stratified based on the percentage of each of these types of cells. Survival of a high proportion of blastemal cells is classified as high-risk. In contrast, the COG classification is based on histological assessment of the chemotherapy-naive tumor, and does not take the predominant cell type into account for risk-stratification purposes, but recognizes only two distinct WT histopathologic types - favorable and unfavorable. The unfavorable group comprises WTs with anaplasia. Notably, the presence of diffuse anaplasia is considered high-risk in both the SIOP and COG protocols. However, the two groups differ in how they classify focal anaplasia, which is considered intermediate risk by the SIOP and has recently been placed in the high-risk category by the COG.

9. **What are the non-Wilms pediatric renal tumors?**

These less common pediatric renal tumors include clear cell sarcoma of the kidney (CCSK), renal cell carcinoma (RCC), malignant rhabdoid tumor of the kidney (MRTK), and congenital mesoblastic nephroma (CMN). CMN occurs mainly in early infancy. It has been associated with a very good prognosis, and surgery alone may be curative in most cases. By contrast, patients with MRTK have overall survival rates of only 20–25%, even with intensive multimodality treatment regimens. The outcomes of CCSK and RCC are intermediate between CMN and MRTK.

10. **What substantial differences exist between the SIOP and COG treatment protocols?**

The principal difference is that the SIOP protocol relies on imaging-based diagnosis and nephrectomy is postponed after neoadjuvant chemotherapy, that is given to all cases except for very young infants (<6 months of age). In contrast, the COG protocol advocates for primary surgery and adjuvant chemotherapy. Neoadjuvant chemotherapy is administered only in specific circumstances such as bilateral, multicentric, or bilaterally-predisposed unilateral WT. Despite the different policy of the initial approach, clinical outcomes are excellent in both cooperative group studies.

11. **What are the WT stage groupings?**

Table 61.1 summarizes stage systems for WT utilized by the SIOP and COG protocols. Tumor extension and histology are key components of patient stratification criteria for the ongoing WT clinical trials.

12. **How does lymph node (LN) sampling at the time of WT surgery affect disease control?**

LN involvement in children with WT has significant prognostic and therapeutic implications. The presence of nodal involvement is associated with an increased incidence of tumor relapse and a poorer prognosis. However, the magnitude of the effect of LN positivity on event free survival is more profound for patients with tumors of anaplastic histology rather than favorable histology. A good rule of thumb is to sample at least 5–7 LNs at the time of nephrectomy.

13. **What is the risk of vascular involvement in WT patients?** [3]

In 4–10% of cases, WT shows a propensity to invade blood vessels in the form of tumor thrombus. In addition to CT and MRI, Doppler ultrasonography is a reliable modality to demonstrate the presence and extent of tumor thrombus. The management of a WT patient presenting with intravascular tumor thrombus generally includes primary chemotherapy to decrease the extent of the vascular thrombus, thus facilitating surgical excision and minimizing the risk for surgical complications.

Table 61.1 Staging system for Wilms' tumor according to the SIOP and COG protocols

	SIOP	COG
Stage I	Tumor limited to kidney or surrounded with fibrous pseudocapsule and completely resected; intrarenal vessel involvement may be present; no involvement of renal sinus (its vessels and soft tissues); percutaneous cutting needle biopsy is allowed; presence of necrotic tumor in the renal sinus or peri-renal fat does not upstage to stage II providing it does not reach the resection margins	Tumor limited to kidney with intact renal capsule and completely resected, with no evidence of the tumor at or beyond the margins of resection; intrarenal vessel involvement may be present; no involvement of renal sinus vessels; no biopsy has been performed
Stage II	Tumor extension beyond kidney or renal pseudocapsule, but tumor is completely resected; infiltration of renal sinus and/or blood and lymphatic vessels outside renal parenchyma, but tumor is completely resected; local invasion of adjacent structures or extension into the vena cava is allowed providing resection is performed en bloc and there is no evidence of tumor at or beyond the resection margins	Tumor extension beyond kidney or penetration of renal capsule, but tumor is completely resected; local invasion of adjacent structures or extension into the vena cava is allowed providing resection is performed en bloc and there is no evidence of tumor at or beyond the resection margins; absence of tumor rupture of spillage, even confined to the flank; no biopsy has been performed
Stage III	Any of the following reasons, either individually or collectively, assign a tumor to stage III: (I) tumor extends to or beyond resection; margins microscopically or there is macroscopic incomplete excision; (II) positive abdominal lymph nodes; (III) tumor rupture before or intra-operatively including diffuse peritoneal contamination by the tumor or where peritoneal implants are present; (IV) piecemeal removal of intravascular tumor thrombus; (V) open biopsy prior to preoperative chemotherapy or surgery	Any of the following reasons, either individually or collectively, assign a tumor to stage III: (I) tumor extends to or beyond resection margins microscopically or there is macroscopic incomplete excision; (II) positive abdominal lymph nodes; (III) tumor rupture before or intra-operatively including spillage confined to the flank or diffuse peritoneal contamination by the tumor or where peritoneal implants are present; (IV) piecemeal removal of intravascular tumor thrombus; (V) any biopsy is performed prior to surgery
Stage IV	Hematogenous metastases or distant lymph node metastases	Hematogenous metastases or distant lymph node metastases
Stage V	Bilateral renal involvement at the time of initial diagnosis	Bilateral renal involvement at the time of initial diagnosis

SIOP Société Internationale d'Oncologie Pédiatrique (International Society of Paediatric Oncology); *COG* Children's Oncology Group

14. **What is the role of nephron-sparing surgery (NSS) in WT patients?** [4–6]

Synchronous bilateral tumor involvement (i.e., stage V), which is reported to occur in 3.6–8% of cases, represents the commonest absolute indication for NSS in WT patients. NSS is preceded by neoadjuvant chemotherapy in both SIOP and COG protocols. A similar approach (neoadjuvant chemo & NSS) is also recommended for multifocal, bilaterally-predisposed unilateral WT (see questions 4 and 5). In contrast, both protocols consider elective NSS for unilateral WT still investigational at present. However, the increasing awareness of the potential risk of renal dysfunction in nephrectomized children with normally functioning contralateral kidney, should likely extend the applications of NSS also to this subset of patients.

15. **What is the WT Prognosis?**

Despite its malignant nature, long-term survival rate after WT treatment is excellent, being greater than 90% for localized disease and 75% for metastatic disease, making this rare tumor one of the real successes of pediatric oncology. However, unfavorable histology (anaplasia) and recurrent disease still carry a dismal prognosis.

16. **What are the late effects after WT therapy?**

Long-term WT survivors are at increased risk of treatment related morbidity and mortality. The most common complications are cardiotoxicity (4.4%), musculoskeletal problems (3%), and the development of secondary malignant neoplasms (1%), such as soft-tissue sarcomas, breast cancer, lymphoma, leukemia, and melanoma. The antineoplastic agent doxorubicin and radiotherapy are the two most common treatment culprits. The cumulative incidence of end-stage renal disease caused by chronic renal failure at 20 years from WT diagnosis is considered low (3.1% for patients with bilateral WT, and less than 1% for unilateral WT). However, there is an increasing evidence that unilateral nephrectomy alone is an independent risk factor for increased all-cause mortality and cardiovascular accidents.

References

1. Dome JS, Graf N, Geller JI, Fernandez CV, Mullen EA, Spreafico F, Van den Heuvel-Eibrink M, Pritchard-Jones K. Advances in Wilms tumor treatment and biology: progress through international collaboration. J Clin Oncol. 2015;33:2999–3007.
2. Cozzi F, Schiavetti A, Cozzi DA, Morini F, Uccini S, Pierani P, Martino A. Conservative management of hyperplastic and multicentric nephroblastomatosis. J Urol. 2004; 172:1066–9; discussion 1069–70.
3. Morris L, Squire R, Sznajder B, van Tinteren H, Godzinski J, Powis M. Optimal neoadjuvant chemotherapy duration in Wilms tumour with intravascular thrombus: a literature review and evidence from SIOP WT 2001 trial. Pediatr Blood Cancer. 2019;24:e27930. https://doi.org/10.1002/pbc.27930.
4. Davidoff AM, Interiano RB, Wynn L, Delos Santos N, Dome JS, Green DM, Brennan RC, McCarville MB, Krasin MJ, Kieran K, Williams MA. Overall survival and renal function of patients with synchronous bilateral Wilms tumor undergoing surgery at a single institution. Ann Surg. 2015;262:570–6.
5. Cozzi DA, Zani A. Nephron-sparing surgery in children with primary renal tumor: indications and results. Semin Pediatr Surg. 2006;15:3–9.
6. Ceccanti S, Cozzi F, Cervellone A, Zani A, Cozzi DA. Volume and function of the operated kidney after nephron-sparing surgery for unilateral renal tumor. J Pediatr Surg. 2019;54:326–30.

Chapter 62
Hepatic Tumors

Michael Berger and Dietrich von Schweinitz

Abstract Hepatic tumors in children are rare. Malignant tumors are more common than benign lesions, and the aggressive hepatoblastoma is not only the most common malignant but also the most common liver tumor overall amongst children. Differential diagnoses of hepatoblastoma include hepatocellular carcinoma, undifferentiated embryonic sarcoma of the liver or rhabdomyosarcoma of the bile ducts. These tumors have a worse prognosis than hepatoblastoma because of their more aggressive biology. Fortunately, they are less common than hepatoblastoma. Despite their infrequency, malignant hepatic tumors attract substantial scientific attention because their therapy exemplifies innovative treatment approaches.

Keywords Hepatoblastoma · Liver tumors · Pediatric cancer · Pediatric oncology · Pediatric surgery · Tumor surgery · Liver surgery · Liver resection · Transplant surgery · Liver transplantation · Pediatric liver transplant · SIOPEL · Hedgehog-signaling

1. **What are typical hepatic tumors in children?**

Benign: Hepatic hemangioma, hepatocellular adenoma, mesenchymal hamartoma, and focal nodular hyperplasia (FNH).

Malignant: Hepatoblastoma, hepatocellular carcinoma (HCC), undifferentiated embryonic sarcoma of the liver, and rhabdomyosarcoma of the bile ducts.

M. Berger (✉) · D. von Schweinitz
Department of Pediatric Surgery, Dr. von Hauner Children's Hospital, Ludwig-Maximilians-University, Lindwurmstrasse 4, 80337 Munich, Germany
e-mail: michael.berger@med.uni-muenchen.de

D. von Schweinitz
e-mail: dietrich.schweinitz@med.uni-muenchen.de

M. Lacher et al. (eds.), *Pearls and Tricks in Pediatric Surgery*,
https://doi.org/10.1007/978-3-030-51067-1_62

2. **What age groups are typically affected by hepatic tumors?**

Hepatic tumors exhibit a variety of benign and malignant entities that correspond to typical age groups [1]. For example, most hepatoblastomas manifest before or around age 3 years. HCC, in contrast, usually affects older children and adolescence and is extremely rare in a young child. Most benign lesions such as hepatic hemangiomas are diagnosed before 6 months of age.

3. **How rare are hepatic tumors in children?**

Primary liver tumors embody the third most common abdominal childhood tumor (after neuroblastomas and kidney tumors). With an incidence of 0.5–2 to 1 million in Central Europe, they constitute approximately 0.3–2% of all pediatric tumors. Hepatoblastoma is the most common.

4. **How important is surgery in hepatoblastoma therapy?**

Surgical resection is crucial in hepatoblastoma therapy. As a matter of fact, unless hepatoblastoma is resected completely, it cannot be cured. Therefore, traditionally the prognosis for non-resectable hepatoblastoma was poor. For this reason, the use of primary liver transplant as a tool for achieving complete surgical resection has revolutionized hepatoblastoma therapy over the last decade.

5. **Does hepatoblastoma respond to chemotherapy?**

Like other embryonic tumors in children, hepatoblastomas respond well to chemotherapy. Typical agents that show a good response are cisplatin, carboplatin, doxorubicin, ifosfamide, etoposide, vincristine, and 5-fluorouracil. Importantly, following repeated administration of chemotherapy, hepatoblastoma-cells typically show a marked cytostatic resistance.

6. **What are risk factors for hepatoblastoma?**

The most important risk factors are extreme premature birth, the Wiedemann-Beckwith syndrome and other hemihypertrophy, and familial polyposis coli (FAP).

7. **A 2-year-old child treated for hepatoblastoma had a liver resection to remove the tumor. The pathology report of the specimen says "vital HCC". What is going on?**

This is a case of *pleomorphic epithelial hepatoblastoma*, formerly called *transitional liver cell tumor (TLCT)*. This tumor shows features of both hepatoblastoma and HCC. Due to the preoperative chemotherapy, the more responsive hepatoblastoma cells of the tumor have been killed off. This leaves vital HCC cells behind, which then give the false impression in the tumor specimen that this is HCC. Importantly, these children need to be treated as hepatoblastoma.

8. **Should you get a biopsy in all cases to know the exact diagnosis before instituting treatment?**

Yes, with one exception. In the old days (and unfortunately still ongoing), hepatic tumors that showed the typical signs of hepatoblastoma (large tumor, typical characteristics on imaging, young age, high AFP) were treated without biopsy. Today this approach is obsolete and all tumors should get a biopsy before starting chemotherapy. The only exception to this protocol is a PRETEXT I or II tumor with more than 1 cm margin to large vessels on imaging than can be removed with simple hemihepatectomy. These tumors may undergo an upfront resection without prior biopsy. All others need prior biopsy.

9. **How do you perform a biopsy for a suspected hepatoblastoma?**

The workup of a liver tumor typically does not entail extensive molecular genetic studies. Therefore, the US-guided percutaneous core biopsy of the tumor is the method of choice. If the tumor is poorly accessible percutaneously or very well perfused, an open biopsy may be indicated. Fine needle biopsy with cytology is insufficient in most cases and not standard of care. Primary resection of childhood liver tumors is only rarely indicated (see above).

10. **What can be typical symptoms of liver tumors?**

The majority of children with malignant hepatic tumors come to attention via a large palpable mass in the upper abdomen. Normally, the children are in a good clinical condition in early stages of the disease. Later, abdominal pain, weight loss, loss of appetite, anemia, and vomiting ensue. Ascites can rarely be present and is not a typical symptom of hepatic tumors in children. Liver function is characteristically preserved. Sometimes, there may be respiratory insufficiency due to prominent and diffuse lung metastases.

11. **How are hepatoblastomas worked up?**

In addition to routine blood count, CRP, and liver enzymes, the tumor markers AFP, β-HCG, ferritin, LDH, and CEA should be investigated. Malignant liver tumors in children usually have very high AFP levels, especially hepatoblastoma. Low AFP levels do not exclude the diagnosis of hepatoblastoma but rather indicate a poor prognosis. For imaging, in addition to ultrasound either a CT scan or an MRI is mandatory for PRETEXT grouping of the tumor.

12. **How is hepatoblastoma classified?**

The PRETEXT ("pre-treatment extension") system for staging malignant primary liver tumors of childhood was first conveyed by the *Société Internationale d'Oncologie Pédiatrique*—Epithelial Liver Tumor Study Group (SIOPEL) [2]. This grouping system respects pretherapeutic imaging and describes the extent of the tumor across the 4 surgical sectors of the liver. Additionally, it contains letter-defined PRETEXT risk factors (invasion of the tumor into one or more hepatic veins (V) or portal vein (P), extrahepatic tumor (E), tumor rupture (R) or multifocal tumor (F). This classification was found to have a high prognostic relevance and dominates international scientific literature regarding hepatoblastoma.

13. **What is the risk stratification in hepatoblastoma?**

Recently, a worldwide coalition for the study of hepatoblastomas was formed (Children's Hepatic Tumors International Collaboration (CHIC)). It newly engendered a risk stratification for hepatoblastoma based on data from more than 1,600 children treated for 25 years. It is based on PRETEXT, the initial AFP value at diagnosis, the presence of metastases, the presence of vascular invasion and the age of the child and characterizes four risk levels: very low, low, intermediate and high. This risk stratification is currently being used in the PHITT study [3].

14. **What is the PHITT study?**

The PHITT study is a global, multicenter, multinational treatment study for children with either hepatoblastoma or HCC. Both chemotherapeutic regimens as well as surgical guidelines for resection versus primary liver transplantation are being investigated (trial number: NCT03017326).

15. **What are typical scenarios in hepatoblastoma that warrant a liver transplant?**

From Meyers et al. [4].

1. Multifocal tumors, especially multifocal PRETEXT IV tumors that have multifocal tumor in all four liver sections at diagnosis
2. Unifocal PRETEXT IV, even if with neoadjuvant chemotherapy these tumors "downstage" to a Post-treatment Extent of Disease (POST-TEXT) III and become amenable to conventional resection by trisegmentectomy.
3. PRETEXT III+V, with proximity of the tumor to the vena cava or all three major hepatic veins that makes adequate tumor clearance doubtful.
4. PRETEXT III+P, with proximity of the tumor to the portal venous bifurcation or both major branches of the portal vein that makes adequate tumor clearance doubtful.
5. Intrahepatic relapse or residual tumor after previous attempt at resection or re-resection (called "rescue transplant").

16. **In adults, extrahepatic tumor extension is an absolute contraindication for liver transplantation. Is it the same for children with hepatoblastoma**?

No. In children with hepatoblastoma, extrahepatic tumor extension is <u>not</u> a contraindication for liver transplantation as long as all metastases can be eliminated either with surgery or chemotherapy.

17. **As liver transplant is very invasive and liver resection is easier to do—should you try a resection first and then do a liver transplant once the tumor comes back?**

While primary liver transplant for hepatoblastoma has excellent results with survival rates > 85%, salvage liver transplant has poor results with survival near 30%. Therefore, if complete surgical resection is doubtful, all efforts should be made to perform primary liver transplant as a means for surgical resection [5].

18. **If relapse in hepatoblastoma is so bad, how else can you avoid it?**

    1. *Don't improvise*—When considering resection versus transplant, stick to current guidelines brought forth by the SIOPEL.
    2. *Don't cowboy*—If complete resection seems doubtful or needs extraordinary measures like ex-vivo reconstruction or use of the heart–lung-machine, don't do it. The data is against you.
    3. *Don't worry*—Despite the many pitfalls that most certainly do exist in pediatric liver transplant, in experienced centers, pediatric liver transplant is standard therapy with excellent long-term results.
    4. *Don't delay*—A tumor that has not become resectable after the risk-stratified preoperative chemotherapy has been given will remain unresectable. Don't delay the liver transplantation by giving more chemotherapy in an ill-advised attempt to try to make it resectable. The tumor cells will have developed insensitivity against the chemotherapy and it will not work.

19. **What about hepatocellular carcinoma in children?**

HCC often grows multifocal in the liver. HCC infiltrates local lymph nodes and causes distant metastases. Both are absolute contraindications for liver transplantation because at this point the prognosis is dismal. Contrary to adulthood, HCC in children typically does not develop on the basis of liver cirrhosis. About 50% of HCC produce AFP.

20. **What do you need to know about benign liver tumors?**

The most common benign hepatic tumor in children is hepatic hemangioma. It is usually diagnosed early in life (<6 months) and hardly ever causes symptoms. If it does, it can often be treated successfully with propranolol. Very rarely, these tumors show an aggressive course and need to be resected. Nobody knows why a miniscule portion of these tumors shows aggressive behavior, but recently the hedgehog-signaling pathway was identified to be over-activated in specimen of such aggressive hemangiomas [6].

21. **Do hepatic hemangiomas cause the Kasabach-Merrit syndrome?**

Actually, despite many articles in the older literature saying otherwise, they do not. Rather, they cause a transient anemia and thrombocytopenia. The only known association with the Kasabach-Merrit syndrome is for the kaposiform hemangioendothelioma and the so-called tufted angioma.

22. **What other benign hepatic tumors are important in children?**

Focal nodular hyperplasia (FNH) and adenomas are more likely to occur in older children and adolescents. FNH can be seen as a reactive lesion, for example in glycogen storage disorders, after intensive chemotherapy or in children with poor or no portal flow (for example in Abernethy malformation). The hepatocellular adenoma is mainly found in young women who have been taking oral contraceptives for an extended time.

References

1. von Schweinitz D. Hepatoblastoma: recent developments in research and treatment. Semin Pediatr Surg. 2012;21(1):21–30.
2. Towbin AJ, Meyers RL, Woodley H, Miyazaki O, Weldon CB, Morland B, et al. 2017 PRETEXT: radiologic staging system for primary hepatic malignancies of childhood revised for the Paediatric Hepatic International Tumour Trial (PHITT). In: Pediatric radiology, vol. 48. Berlin, Heidelberg: Springer; 2018. p. 536–54.
3. Meyers RL, Maibach R, Hiyama E, Häberle B, Krailo M, Rangaswami A, et al. Risk-stratified staging in paediatric hepatoblastoma: a unified analysis from the Children's Hepatic tumors International Collaboration. Lancet Oncol. 2017;18(1):122–31.
4. Meyers RL, Tiao GM, Dunn SP, Langham MR. Liver transplantation in the management of unresectable hepatoblastoma in children. Front Biosci (Elite Ed). 2012;1(4):1293–302.
5. Trobaugh-Lotrario AD, Meyers RL, Tiao GM, Feusner JH. Pediatric liver transplantation for hepatoblastoma. Transl Gastroenterol Hepatol. 2016;1(3):44–54.
6. Wendling-Keim D, Vokuhl C, Walz C, Rieder L, Grantzow R, Schweinitz von D, et al. Activation of hedgehog signaling in aggressive hepatic hemangioma in newborns and infants. Anticancer Res. International Institute of Anticancer Research; 2019;39(5):2351–60.

Chapter 63
Endocrine Tumors

Mary Brandt

Abstract Endocrine tumors are an interesting spectrum of lesion that are hormone producing. They are frequently associated with syndromes and other conditions and have variable patterns of inheritance. These result in a wide spectrum of presentation and because of the associated conditions with each endocrine tumor, it is important that pediatric specialists possess full knowledge of these lesions to facilitate complete workups, provide adequate treatment and oversee anticipatory surveillance. This chapter outlines the more common and important endocrine tumors that pediatric surgeons should fully understand.

Keywords Endocrine tumors · Pediatric

1. **What are the six types of MEN (Multiple Endocrine Neoplasia) syndrome?**

MEN1 (also known as Wermer syndrome) is due to a mutation in the MEN1 tumor suppressor gene that encodes menin. The constellation of tumors in patients with MEN1 include pancreas islet cell tumors, tumors of the anterior pituitary, hyperparathyroidism and tumors of the adrenal cortex. The pancreatic neuroendocrine tumors associated with MEN1 are often microadenomas, rather than a single tumor [1].

MEN2a (often referred to as MEN2) is characterized by the trio of pheochromocytoma, medullary cancer of the thyroid and parathyroid adenomas.

MEN2b (also known as MEN 3 or Wagenmann–Froboese syndrome) includes pheochromocytomas and medullary thyroid cancer as well as a marfanoid habitus and neural dysfuntion leading to megacolon [2, 3].

Three additional MEN syndromes have been identified, in addition to MEN1, MEN2a and MEN2b:

M. Brandt (✉)
Houston, TX, USA
e-mail: mary.brandt@cmh.edu

M. Lacher et al. (eds.), *Pearls and Tricks in Pediatric Surgery*,
https://doi.org/10.1007/978-3-030-51067-1_63

- The Familial Medullary Thyroid Cancer (FMTC) consists of patients with medullary cancer of the thyroid without associated pheochromocytomas or other endocrine tumors.
- MEN 4 is due to mutations in the CDKN1B gene. These patients present with hyperparathyroidism and anterior pituitary tumors.
- The hyperparathyroidism-Jaw Tumor syndrome is also thought to be a possible MEN syndrome. This syndrome is due to inactivating mutations of the CDC73 gene. These patients have hyperparathyroidism, ossifying fibromas of the jaw and a variety of other associated tumors [2].

"Classic" presentations of the MEN syndrome

	MEN 1	MEN2a (can also be called MEN 2)	MEN2b (can also be called MEN 3)	MEN2-FMTC	MEN 4	HJT
Gene	MEN1	RET	RET	RET	CDKN1B	CDC73
Pheochromocytoma	No	Yes	Yes	No	No	Yes
MTC	No	Yes	Yes	Yes	No	No
Parathyroid	Yes	Yes	No	No	Yes	Yes
Pancreas (islet cells)	Yes half are gastrinomas, one-third are insulinomas and 05% are glucagonomas, vasoactive intestinal peptide (VIP)-omas or pancreatic polypeptide (PP)-omas	No	No	No	Yes	
Anterior pituitary	Yes	No	No	No	Yes	No
Other	Angiofibromas (88%), collagenomas (72%), multiple lipomas (33%), foregut carcinoids (15%), meningiomas (10%)	Marfanoid habitus, mucosal neuromas, thickened corneal nerve fibres and intestinal autonomic ganglion tumours that can lead to megacolon." [2]	Cutaneous neuroma Intestinal gangli-oneuroma			Ossifying jaw fibromas Tumors of the uterus, kidney, thyroid, testes, pancreas

2. **In addition to the MEN syndromes, what other genetic syndromes are associated with neuroendocrine tumors of the pancreas?**

There are four primary genetic syndromes other than the MEN syndromes which are associated with neuroendocrine tumors of the pancreas: von Hippel-Lindau (VHL) disease, neurofibromatosis type 1 (NF-1), Mahvash disease, and tuberous sclerosis (TS) [1].

Approximately 12% of patients with Von Hippel-Lindau disease will develop a pancreatic neuroendocrine tumor [1]. Approximately 10% of patients with NF-1 will develop a neuroendocrine tumor and these are almost exclusively duodenal (periampullary) somatostatinomas [4]. Tumors in Mahvash disease and Tuberous Sclerosis are exceedingly rare.

3. **When should prophylactic thyroidectomy be performed in a child with MEN2b to prevent medullary thyroid cancer?**

Patients with MEN2b can develop aggressive MTC as early as infancy, so early testing is essential to identify patients at high risk. Specific mutations in the RET proto-oncogene are associated with higher risk, which allows risk-stratification based on the genetic results [5]. There are four tiers of risk A, B, C and D. Mutations in codons 804, 883, and 918 represent the highest risk (group D). Children with the mutations in group D should undergo prophylactic thyroidectomy before age 1. Children in group C, the next highest risk group should undergo prophylactic thyroidectomy before age 5 [6].

4. **In addition to pheochromocytoma and medullary cancer of the thyroid, what other diseases are associated with specific mutations in the RET oncogene in patients with MEN2a?**

Hirschsprung disease, like MEN2a, is associated with exon 10 mutations in the RET proto-oncogene. It is rare (but not impossible) for MEN2a and Hirschsprung disease to occur in the same patient. In the presence of a family history suggestive of MEN2a, patients with Hirschsprung disease should undergo genetic testing for MEN2a.

Cutaneous lichen amyloidosis (CLA) is a pruritic skin lesion which manifests in the intrascapular region in up to a third of patients with MEN2a. In addition to the pruritis, this lesion typical has areas of depigmentation in the intrascapular region. It is associated with mutations in codon 634 of exon 11. The presence of CLA can be considered a marker for MEN2a, but does not appear to change prognosis.

5. **What are the symptoms associated with the most common functional pancreatic neuroendocrine tumor?**

It is not surprising that insulinomas are the most common pancreatic neuroendocrine tumor since beta cells are the most common cells of the pancreatic islets. Insulinomas represent almost half of all pancreatic neuroendocrine tumors. The symptoms of an insulinoma are related to the episodic secretion of insulin and are classically described by Whipple' triad: symptoms of hypoglycemia with fasting, documented hypoglycemia, and reversal of the symptoms with the administration of glucose [1, 4].

6. **What is the primary treatment for Zollinger-Ellison syndrome?**

Zollinger-Ellison syndrome is the clinical syndrome which is the result of high levels of gastrin secreted by a gastrinoma of the pancreas. The elevated gastrin levels result in over secretion of gastric acid, which results in peptic ulcers, symptoms of gastroesophageal reflux and/or abdominal pain. Therefore, the first step in treatment of ZE syndrome is to block acid secretion with a proton-pump inhibitor (PPI). The dose of the PPI should be titrated to achieve a pH of>5 rather than absence of symptoms [1]. These tumors tend to be more aggressive than other pancreatic neuroendocrine tumors with a third of patients presenting with metastatic disease [1]. For this reason, surgical resection should be offered to all patients with a solitary lesion and for any lesion>2 cm for patients with multiple tumors [1]. 70% of these tumors are located in the duodenum, 25% in the pancreas and 5% elsewhere [4].

7. **What is the pathognomonic symptom associated with glucagonomas?**

Patients with hypersecretion of glucagon from a glucagonoma may have glucose intolerance or diabetes mellitus, anemia, weight loss, proximal muscle weakness, ataxia and depression [4]. The presence of necrolytic migratory erythema (NME) is pathognomonic for glucagonoma. This dermatologic finding begins with erythematous macules that become pruritic. They may go on to become necrotic and secondarily infected [1].

8. **What neuroendocrine tumor is most commonly associated with neurofibromatosis Type 1 (von Recklinghausen disease)?**

Patients with NF Type 1 have a 4–25% lifetime risk for a gastrointestinal stromal tumor and a 1% risk of duodenal somatostatinomas, also referred to as carcinoid tumors in some reports. Although duodenal somatostatinomas are the most common neuroendocrine tumor in patients with NF1, pancreatic islet cell tumors have also been reported in patients with NF Type 1.

9. **What differentiates a paraganglioma from a pheochromocytoma?**

Histologically there is no difference between a pheochromocytoma and a paraganglioma which are distinguished by they anatomical location. Pheochromocytomas arise from the chromaffin cells of the adrenal medulla. Paragangliomas can be either sympathetic or parasympathetic in origin. Sympathetic paragangliomas arise from the sympathetic chain in the thorax, abdomen and pelvis. One of the classic locations for paragangliomas is in the organ of Zuckerkandl at the bifurcation of the aorta. Parasympathetic paragangliomas usually arise in the cervical region and, unlike pheochromocytomas and sympathetic paragangliomas, rarely secrete catecholamines.

10. **Which of the genetic disorders associated with pheochromocytomas has the highest risk for a malignant pheochromocytoma?**

All patients with suspected pheochromocytoma or paraganglioma should undergo genetic testing using established algorithms, since prognosis and, in some cases, tailored treatments can be established based on these results. There are at least 14 genetic disorders associated with pheochromocytomas/paragangliomas and up to 80% of patients less than 21 years of age will have a genetic mutation associated with pheochromocytomas. The most common of these disorders are MEN2A, MEB 2B, von Hippel Lindau syndrome, Neurofibromatosis Type 1, and Hereditary Paraganglioma-Pheochromocytoma syndrome (HPP). HPP is the result of mutations in the succinate dehydrogenase gene (SDH), with four mutations recognized: A, B, C and D. Of these, SDHB is the genetic disorder with the highest risk for malignancy.

11. **Which imaging modality is optimal for a patient with a suspected pheochromocytoma/paraganglioma?**

Ultrasound is not recommended as there is a significant risk for missing a lesion. Contrast enhanced CT scans are recommended as the first imaging study. MIBG and Functional imaging (^{18}F-FDG PET/CT, ^{18}F-FDOPA PET/CT, ^{18}F-FDA PET/CT and ^{68}Ga-DOTATATE PET/CT) can be tailored based on specific mutations and anatomic locations and is particularly helpful in identifying metastatic disease.

12. **When should cortical sparing resection of a pheochromocytoma be considered?**

80% of children with a pheochromocytoma have a germline mutation, and therefore are at risk for a future pheochromocytoma. In order to prevent the complications of a bilateral adrenalectomy, patients with low risk for malignancy such as MEN2 or Von Hippel Lindau syndromes, should undergo a cortical sparing adrenalectomy if technically possible. A complete adrenalectomy should be performed for patients with an SDHB mutation (29–74% risk of malignancy) or a MAX mutation (10% risk of malignancy).

13. **What is Mahvash disease?**

Mahvash disease results from a genetic mutation in the glucagon receptor gene (GCGR) which subsequently leads to alpha cell hyperplasia and hyperglucagonemia without the clinical manifestations of a high glucagon level. This is a very rare disorder which has not yet been seen in children, as the youngest patient reported is 25 years of age.

14. **How should a child be prepared for resection of a pheochromocytoma?**

The key to the perioperative management of a child with a pheochromocytoma is managing the very high levels of catecholamines and, once the tumor is removed, managing the sudden fall of catecholamines. The core of the pre-operative management is the use of phenoxybenzamine to provide α-blockade. The phenoxybenzamine should be started at 10 mg BID 3–4 weeks before surgery and slowly increased to 30–40 mg BID. Patients who are adequately blocked will experience orthostatic hypotension and significant nasal congestion. Metryrosine, which results in complete blockade of catecholamine release, can be added one week before surgery to reduce intra-operative hypertension as the tumor is resected. This drug is expensive and can have side effects so may not be indicated in all patients. A high salt, high-fluid diet is also started one week before surgery and this volume repletion is supplemented by a 2–3 day hospital stay before surgery for a saline infusion. Beta blockade is rarely needed, but can be used in patients who remain significantly tachycardic. Post-operatively, patients need careful ICU monitoring for hypotension and may require pressors until equilibrium of catecholamine levels is achieved.

References

1. Parbhu SK, Adler DG. Pancreatic neuroendocrine tumors: contemporary diagnosis and management. Hosp Pract. 2016;44:109–19.
2. Walls GV. Multiple endocrine neoplasia (MEN) syndromes. Semin Pediatr Surg. 2014;23:96–101.
3. McDonnell JE, Gild ML, Clifton-Bligh RJ, et al. Multiple endocrine neoplasia: an update. Intern Med J. 2019;49:954–61.
4. Anderson CW, Bennett JJ. Clinical presentation and diagnosis of pancreatic neuroendocrine tumors. Surg Oncol Clin N Am. 2016;25:363–74.
5. Prete FP, Abdel-Aziz T, Morkane C, et al. Prophylactic thyroidectomy in children with multiple endocrine neoplasia type 2: prophylactic thyroidectomy in children with multiple endocrine neoplasia type 2. Br J Surg. 2018;105:1319–27.
6. Wang TS, Opoku-Boateng A, Roman SA, et al. Prophylactic thyroidectomy: who needs it, when, and why: prophylactic thyroidectomy. J Surg Oncol. 2015;111:61–5.

Chapter 64
Germ Cell Tumors

Andrea Doud and Mary E. Fallat

Abstract Germ cell tumors (GCTS) arise from progenitor germ cells and comprise a very heterogenous group of neoplasms that differ substantially in histology. They occur in both in both sexes and in both gonadal and extra-gonadal sites due to arrested or abnormal migration of progenitor germ cells. GCTs predominate in those <20 years and are the most common solid tumor in those 15–19 years. Prognosis and treatment varies based on risk groups. Low risk groups typically require only surgery. Intermediate and high risk groups require surgical resection and chemotherapy. Age of presentation and symptoms vary substantially. Testicular tumors typically present as painless masses in those <4 years or after puberty. Ovarian GCTs present with vague abdominal pain and distension. Occurance increases with age until 20 years. Sacrococcygeal tumors present in utero as large external masses or early in life with bowel or bladder dysfunction and a presacral mass. Chemotherapy regimens are similar for the various GCTs and are platinum-based. Outcomes are favorable for low and intermediate risk groups but ongoing trials are working to improve outcomes for poor risk groups.

Keywords Germ cell tumors · Testicular tumors · Ovarian tumors · Sacrococcygeal teratomas

A. Doud (✉)
Division of Pediatric Surgery, Kentucky Children's Hospital,
University of Kentucky, Lexington, USA
e-mail: mefall01@louisville.edu

M. E. Fallat
Professor of Surgery, Hiram C Polk Jr Department of Surgery, University of Louisville,
315 E. Broadway Suite 565, Louisville, KY 40202, USA

M. Lacher et al. (eds.), *Pearls and Tricks in Pediatric Surgery*,
https://doi.org/10.1007/978-3-030-51067-1_64

1. **What are germ cell tumors (GCT)?**

GCTs are a diverse group of tumors that arise from progenitor germ cells. GCTs occur in both gonadal and extragonadal sites. They vary substantially in histology owing to the totipotent nature of the parent progenitor germ cells.

2. **What is the incidence of GCTs?**

GCTs represent 3.5% of all childhood cancers that occur before 15 years. Among those 15–19 years, GCTs are the most common solid tumor, accounting for 13.9%.

3. **How are GCTs classified?**

GCTs are classified according to site and histology. The primary site distinction is gonadal or extra-gonadal. Arrested or abnormal migration of germ cells from the yolk sac to the genital ridge results in extra-gonadal GCTs, namely sacrococcygeal, retroperitoneal and mediastinal GCTs. Normal migration with subsequent neoplastic transformation leads to ovarian and testicular GCTs.

GCTs are divided into seminomatous and nonseminomatous histologic types. Seminomatous GCTs arise directly from undifferentiated progenitor cells. These tumors are seminomas when arising in the testis, dysgerminomas when arising in the ovary and germinomas when found in extra-gonadal sites. Nonseminomatous GCTs arise from progenitor cells that have begun early embyronic or extra-embryonic differentiation. Nonseminomatous GCTs demonstrating early extra-embryonic differentiation include yolk sac tumors (YST) and choriocarcinomas. Nonseminomatous GCTs demonstrating early embryonic differentiation result in teratomas.

4. **What are the most common histologic types with respect to sex, site and age?**

Testicular GCTs have a small peak in infancy, at which time YSTs predominate, and a larger peak in adolescence, at which time mixed GCTs are most common. The incidence of ovarian GCTs increases with age until late adolescence. Over 90% are mature teratomas.

Sacrococcygeal and retroperitoneal GCTs are most often teratomas. When sacrococcygeal GCTs are malignant or recur, the histology is nearly always YST. Mediastinal GCTs are most commonly YSTs in girls and younger boys and mixed histology in older boys.

5. **What are GCT risk groups?**

Low, intermediate and high risk groups have been defined for GCTs based on tumor site and Children's Oncology Group (COG) Stage to guide therapy and address research questions. Low risk groups can be treated with resection and active surveillance alone. This group includes stage I ovarian, testicular and extra-gonadal GCTs. Intermediate risk groups require surgery and chemotherapy but have excellent outcomes with present therapy. This group includes stage II–III ovarian GCTs, certain stage II–IV testicular GCTs and stage II extragonadal

GCTs. High risk groups encompass those with poor outcomes with present regimens. This group includes stage IV ovarian GCTs, certain stage II–IV testicular GCTs and stage III–IV extra-gonadal GCTs [1].

6. **How do testicular GCTs present?**

Testicular GCTs usually present as a painless swelling of one testis, usually before 4 years or after puberty (bimodal distribution). 10% are associated with a hydrocele [1].

7. **What diagnostic tests should be performed?**

Tumor markers, including AFP (elevated in 70% of non-seminomatous GCTs) and HCG (elevated in 20% of seminomas and choriocarcinomas) should be obtained. Testicular ultrasound is mandatory. If tumor markers are elevated, CT chest, abdomen and pelvis should be obtained.

8. **What is the proper technique to biopsy testicular tumors?**

An inguinal approach should always be employed. Trans-scrotal approaches disrupt lymphatic channels and lead to an increased rate of recurrence.

9. **What is the role of retroperitoneal lymph node sampling or dissection in testicular GCTs?**

Current COG protocol recommends retroperitoneal lymph node sampling only if nodes are > 2 cm on CT scan. Lymph nodes > 4 cm are considered stage III disease and do not require sampling. There is no role for complete retroperitoneal lymph node dissection prior to chemotherapy [2].

10. **How are testicular tumors treated?**

Prepubertal boys with a normal AFP can have testis-sparing surgery with enucleation of the intact tumor. Prepubertal boys with an elevated AFP and postpubertal boys require radical orchiectomy. Cisplatin, etoposide and bleomycin (PEB) are administered with stage II–IV disease. After 3 cycles, tumor markers should achieve > 90% decrease. If not, patients may need further surgical debulking or additional chemotherapy.

11. **How do ovarian GCTs present?**

Ovarian GCTs typically present with gradual onset of abdominal distension or discomfort and a pelvic mass. Occasionally, a tumor can torse or rupture, leading to acute abdominal symptoms.

12. **What diagnostic tests should be performed?**

Tumor markers, including AFP, HCG, CA-125, Inhibin A and LDH, should be obtained. Initial evaluation is often with ultrasound. Malignancy is suspected with size > 8 cm and presence of solid components. These findings should prompt a CT scan of the chest, abdomen and pelvis. This is followed by surgical staging.

13. **What are the goals of surgical treatment/assessment for ovarian tumors?**

If an ovarian tumor is large, complex, solid, or associated with elevated tumor markers, operative conduct should proceed as if the lesion is malignant. This involves removal of the ovary and tumor, avoiding intraoperative spill. The COG germ cell committee recommends laparotomy when malignancy is expected. Laparoscopic options include using a retrieval bag and decompressing the cystic component within the retrieval bag prior to tumor removal. One might also consider gluing a bag to the cyst and decompressing the cystic component through the extraperitoneal bag.

After removal of the ovary and tumor, complete surgical staging is completed with collection of peritoneal fluid or washings for cytology and inspection of all peritoneal surfaces, the omentum, retroperitoneal lymph nodes and the contralateral ovary. Suspicious areas should be biopsied. Omentectomy is no longer routinely performed unless it is macroscopically involved with tumor.

Stage I tumors are treated with resection followed by observation. Stage II+ require postoperative chemotherapy (PEB) [2, 3].

14. **How should one proceed if bilateral ovarian tumors are present?**

Neoadjuvant chemotherapy with delayed resection may allow for fertility-sparing surgery.

15. **What are the two main clinical presentations of sacrococcygeal tumors (SCT)?**

There are 4 types of SCTs relating to their relative external and internal components. SCTs commonly present in one of two ways. The first is a large predominantly external lesion detected prenatally or at birth and is rarely malignant. The second is an older infant presenting with bladder or bowel involvement due to a less apparent presacral tumor. Such tumors have a very high rate of malignancy [4].

16. **What issues can arise in utero due to large SCTs?**

Large, vascular SCTs can consume a large percentage of cardiac output, ultimately leading to high output cardiac failure and, in late stages, hydrops fetalis. Large and vascular tumors can rupture in utero, leading to hemorrhage and death. Large and solid SCTs can compress the placenta, compromising fetal blood flow.

17. **When should prenatal resection be considered?**

In fetuses less <28 weeks with predominantly external SCTs (Type I and II) and progressive high output cardiac failure, prenatal resection of the tumor should be considered. In fetuses <28 weeks with predominantly internal SCTS (Type III and IV) and progressive high output cardiac failure, there is currently no successful prenatal fetal intervention and care should be directed toward supporting the mother. In a fetus>28 weeks with progressive cardiac failure secondary to any type of SCT, one should proceed with delivery [5].

18. **What are the surgical considerations for SCTs?**

Complete resection is required, including removal of the coccyx as this decreases recurrence. Bleeding risk is substantial. Laparoscopic ligation of the middle sacral artery prior to resection, and distal aortic occlusion techniques have been described. A purely sacral approach may be undertaken for predominately external tumors via an inverted V-shaped incision over the gluteal region. Laparotomy may be required if there is a significant internal portion.

19. **How does postoperative treatment vary based on histology?**

Mature teratomas are treated with surgery alone. Immature teratomas are graded 0–3 based on the amount of immature elements. These may or may not have a malignant component. If malignancy is present, postoperative chemotherapy is based on the type of malignancy. It is unclear if chemotherapy is helpful for immature teratomas without malignancy [1].

20. **How are children with SCTs followed?**

Recurrent tumors occur in 10–20% of initially benign tumors and 50% of malignant tumors. Postoperatively, AFP level should be obtained every 3 months to ensure normalization by 9 months. Rectal exam should be performed every 3 months until 3 years. Note that bowel and bladder dysfunction can occur in 11–41% [3].

21. **How do mediastinal GCTs present?**

In younger children, mediastinal GCTs typically present with respiratory distress or fevers. Older children tend to present with chest pain, superior vena cava syndrome and sometimes precocious puberty.

22. **What are the anesthetic considerations when dealing with a mediastinal GCT?**

Mediastinal GCTs are typically located in the anterior mediastinum. With the onset of anesthesia, patients lose spontaneous muscle tone and are at risk of airway/great vessel compression causing cardiorespiratory collapse [3].

References

1. Shaikh F, Murray M, Amatruda J, Coleman N, Nicholson J, Hal J, Pashankar F, Stoneham S, Poynter J, Olson T, Billmire D, Stark D, Rodriguez-Galindo C, Frazier L. Paediatric extracranial germ-cell tumors. Lancet Oncol. 2016;17(4):e149–62.
2. Horton Z, Schlatter M, Schultz S. Pediatric germ cell tumors. Surg Oncol. 2007;16(3):205–13.
3. Rescorla F. Pediatric germ cell tumors. Semin Pediatr Surg. 2012;21(1):51–60.
4. Pierce J, Frazier L, Amatruda J. Pediatric germ cell tumors: a developmental perspective. Adv Urol. 2018;2018(Article ID 9059382):8.
5. Roybal J, Moldenhauer J, Khalek N, Bebbington M, Johnson M, Hedrick H, Adzick S, Flake A. Early delivery as an alternative management strategy for selected high-risk fetal sacrococcygeal teratomas. J Pediatr Surg. 2010;2011(46):1325–32.

What are the surgical considerations for [illegible]

Chapter 65
Miscellaneous Tumors

Andrew J. Murphy and Andrew M. Davidoff

Abstract This objective of this chapter is to review key insights in rare pediatric tumors pertinent to the pediatric surgery board examination and clinical management of rhabdomyosarcoma, appendiceal carcinoid, pleuropulmonary blastoma, DICER1 syndrome, sacrococcygeal teratoma, desmoid-type fibromatoses, inflammatory myofibroblastic tumor, pediatric melanoma, and malignant peripheral nerve sheath tumor.

Keywords Rhabdomyosarcoma · Appendiceal carcinoid · Pleuropulmonary blastoma · DICER1 syndrome · Sacrococcygeal teratoma · Desmoid-type fibromatoses · Inflammatory myofibroblastic tumor · Pediatric melanoma · Malignant peripheral nerve sheath tumor

1. **What are the two main subtypes of rhabdomyosarcoma?**

Rhabdomyosarcoma is a mesenchymal embryonal tumor of childhood that was historically divided into two histopathologic subtypes: embryonal rhabdomyosarcoma and alveolar rhabdomyosarcoma. However, this classification has been replaced by *PAX3/PAX7-FOXO1* translocation status in current Children's Oncology Group risk stratification protocols, because the presence of these genetic translocations is a better predictor of outcome than histology. *PAX3/PAX7-FOXO1* translocation-positive rhabdomyosarcoma is strongly associated with alveolar

A. J. Murphy · A. M. Davidoff (✉)
Department of Surgery, St. Jude Children's Research Hospital, Memphis, TN 38105, USA
e-mail: Andrew.Davidoff@STJUDE.ORG

A. J. Murphy
e-mail: Andrew.Murphy@STJUDE.ORG

A. J. Murphy · A. M. Davidoff
Division of Pediatric Surgery, Department of Surgery, University of Tennessee Health Science Center, Memphis, TN 38105, USA

M. Lacher et al. (eds.), *Pearls and Tricks in Pediatric Surgery*,
https://doi.org/10.1007/978-3-030-51067-1_65

histology and is associated with less favorable clinical features (age<1 or>10, extremity primary site, and metastases at diagnosis) than translocation-negative disease [1].

2. **What primary sites of rhabdomyosarcoma are associated with favorable prognosis?**

Favorable rhabdomyosarcoma primary sites include nonparameningeal head and neck, genitourinary tract (other than kidney, bladder, and prostate), and biliary tract. All other sites are unfavorable. Rhabdomyosarcoma that occurs at favorable sites is typically translocation-negative with embryonal histology [1].

3. **How is the treatment plan for rhabdomyosarcoma selected?**

Treatment for rhabdomyosarcoma is based on risk group classification (low, intermediate, and high risk). Risk group classification is based on the following three components: *translocation, stage, and surgical-pathologic group*. The *translocation status* is determined by molecular testing of either a tumor biopsy or surgical resection specimen. The *pretreatment stage* (1–4) is determined according to favorable versus unfavorable primary site, absence (T1) or presence (T2) of invasion into surrounding tissue, tumor size (> or <5 cm), involvement of regional lymph nodes, and the presence or absence of distant metastases. The *surgical-pathologic group* (I–IV) is based on localized versus metastatic tumor, gross total resection versus incomplete resection or tumor biopsy, and microscopic assessment of surgical resection margins [1].

4. **What patients with paratesticular rhabdomyosarcoma should undergo retroperitoneal lymph node dissection?**

Pathologic evaluation of regional nodes, even if they are radiographically negative, is required in current COG protocols for boys with paratesticular rhabdomyosarcoma who are greater than 10 years old. This is because microscopic tumor is often found in these nodes in this age group even when they are not enlarged. If found, radiotherapy to these nodal basins is required. Previously, a template retroperitoneal lymph node dissection was recommended which included the ipsilateral iliac, paraaortic, paracaval, and aortocaval nodes up to the level of the renal vein. In future COG protocols, lymph node sampling (>6 nodes), rather than formal dissection, is likely to be advocated, as this procedure is designed to obtain adequate staging rather than provide definitive local control [1].

5. **How is a pediatric appendiceal carcinoid tumor treated?**

Pediatric appendiceal carcinoid tumors are typically unexpected, incidental neuroendocrine tumors discovered in appendectomy surgical resection specimens. Historically, tumors that were larger than 2 cm in diameter, located at the base of the appendix, demonstrated microscopic or gross invasion of the mesoappendix, or microscopic lymphovascular invasion were managed by reoperation with right hemicolectomy. These features continue to warrant right hemicolectomy in the adult population. However, recent studies have documented excellent long-term outcomes with expectant management of resected pediatric appendiceal carcinoid tumors, even when the above features are present. Therefore, the current recommendation is that most pediatric appendiceal carcinoid tumors discovered incidentally in surgical appendectomy specimens be managed by observation alone [2].

6. **What is the most common malignant primary tumor of the lung in childhood?**

Pleuropulmonary blastoma (PPB) is a sarcomatous malignant embryonal tumor of the lung parenchyma and pleural surfaces. Although PPB is the most common pediatric primary pulmonary malignancy, it is still very rare with an annual incidence of 25–50 cases per year in the United States. This tumor undergoes a well-documented progression through several forms from type I (cystic) to type II (cystic and solid) and type III (purely solid) disease. Type I disease is typically managed by complete surgical resection alone. Type II and III disease may require neoadjuvant chemotherapy followed by radical surgical resection or upfront radical surgical resection depending on the extent of disease at presentation. Types II and III PPB require adjuvant chemotherapy. Germline loss of function mutations in the microRNA processing gene *DICER1* (with accompanied somatic loss of the second copy of *DICER1* in the tumor) are found in approximately 70–80% of children with PPB. Nearly all patients with PPB and no germline *DICER1* mutation exhibit biallelic somatic loss of *DICER1* in the tumor [3].

7. **How can a pleuropulmonary blastoma be differentiated from a congenital pulmonary airway malformation?**

Congenital pulmonary airway malformations (CPAMs) are a group of non-malignant developmental pulmonary anomalies that typically present in infancy. Controversy exists whether these lesions should be surgically resected in asymptomatic patients. Symptomatic patients should undergo surgical resection. If a non-operative approach is chosen for an asymptomatic patient, it becomes critical to differentiate CPAMs from type I (cystic) PPB. Features which favor CPAM over type I PPB include the presence of a systemic feeding vessel seen on CT scan, prenatal detection of the lesion, regions of pulmonary hyperinflation, simple (versus complex) cyst architecture, and small size (<0.5 cm). DICER1 germline testing may inform this decision because presence of a *DICER1* germline mutation strongly favors type I PPB and would, therefore, lead to a recommendation for resection [4].

8. **What is DICER1 syndrome? What tumor types are associated with DICER1 syndrome?**

DICER1 syndrome is an autosomal dominant, familial cancer predisposition syndrome caused by loss of function mutations in the *DICER1* microRNA processing gene located on chromosome 14q32.13. Patients who present with pleuropulmonary blastoma, cystic nephroma, ovarian sex cord-stromal tumors (juvenile granulosa cell tumor and Sertoli-Leydig cell tumors), botryoid embryonal rhabdomyosarcoma, nasal ciliary body medulloepithelioma, nasal chondromesenchymal hamartoma, pituitary blastoma, and pineoblastoma, especially if these tumors occur with a thyroid neoplasm (adenomas and thyroid cancer), should undergo germline testing for *DICER1* mutations. DICER1 syndrome has also been weakly associated with neuroblastoma, Wilms tumor, and medulloblastoma, although the presence of these tumors alone should not provoke *DICER1* germline testing due the rarity of these associations [5].

9. **Which childhood tumors commonly metastasize to the lungs?**

The lungs are the most common site of distant metastasis of pediatric solid tumors. Nearly all solid tumors in children metastasize to the lung including Wilms tumor, rhabdomyosarcoma, osteosarcoma, Ewing sarcoma, non-rhabdomyosarcoma soft tissue sarcomas, hepatoblastoma, hepatocellular carcinoma, and adrenocortical carcinoma. The one exception is neuroblastoma, where lung metastases, particularly at diagnosis, are quite rare [6].

10. **Should lung metastases be surgically resected?**

Since lung metastases signify disseminated disease, a therapeutic role for pulmonary metastasectomy is not intuitive. Nevertheless, there are circumstances, generally histology-dependent, where surgery can play a therapeutic role. There may be a role for surgery in solid tumor histologies which are generally resistant to adjuvant therapies. This is most well-established for osteosarcoma, but also for other non-rhabdomyosarcoma soft tissue sarcomas, adrenocortical carcinoma and hepatocellular carcinoma. In general, operative removal of metastatic disease should be undertaken in the context of a significant tumor response at the primary site. Pulmonary metastasectomy is an important part of a multimodal treatment approach to many pediatric malignancies and should be discussed by a multidisciplinary tumor board as part of a comprehensive treatment strategy [6]. A diagnostic role for pulmonary metastasectomy is common, however.

11. **What is a teratoma?**

Teratomas are embryonal neoplasms derived from totipotential cells that contain tissue from at least two and more often all three germ layers (ectoderm, endoderm, mesoderm). Teratomas can be benign but can also undergo malignant degeneration and, therefore, harbor malignant elements.

12. **How are sacrococcygeal teratomas (SCT) classified?**

The American Academy of Pediatrics Section on Surgery has classified SCT as follows:

Type I—Tumors are predominantly external, attached to the coccyx, and may have a small presacral component (46% of cases).

Type II—Tumors have both an external mass and significant presacral pelvic extension (34% of cases).

Type III—Tumors are visible externally, but the predominant mass is pelvic and intraabdominal (9% of cases).

Type IV—Tumors are not visible externally but are entirely presacral (10% of cases).

13. **What are the operative principles for removing a sacrococcygeal teratoma?**

Treatment of a SCT is complete excision. Malignant degeneration is typical in SCTs that are resected after eight weeks of life. Baseline alpha fetoprotein (AFP) level is determined for postoperative comparison and follow-up. Blood is cross-matched with a low threshold for early transfusion. Large-bore intravenous lines should be placed in the upper extremities as opposed to the groin or lower extremities. The use of an intraoperative harmonic scalpel or electrocoagulation device may help decrease intraoperative blood loss. For large tumors, or tumors with a significant intraabdominal component, laparotomy or laparoscopy with tumor mobilization and ligation of the middle sacral vessels may be required prior to the prone portion of the procedure [7]. In this case, a circumferential prep of the chest and entire lower body can facilitate positioning transition during the operation for the infant population. An inverted-V incision is made in the skin over the lower sacrum although other types of incisions have been functionally and cosmetically useful. The dissection is continued in the midline directly down to the fourth or fifth sacral vertebra. The sacrum is divided to perform a coccygectomy and the tumor is displaced inferiorly to expose, ligate, and divide the middle sacral vessels. Failure to remove the coccyx is associated with a 35% recurrence rate. The normal anatomy is often distorted and the presacral mass often pushes the perineal structures forward. The rectum must be delineated during dissection with a rectal pack or Hegar dilator. The tumor is dissected outside the capsule from the thinned levator and gluteus muscles and then out of the pelvis. The pelvic floor is reconstructed with muscle and fascia.

14. **What is the appropriate follow-up plan for a patient who has undergone resection of a sacrococcygeal teratoma?**

Serum AFP should be measured and rectal exams should be performed every 3 months for 1 year. An MRI should be obtained at 1 year. If this MRI is normal, the patient should be followed every six months with rectal exams and serum AFP for two additional years, with a second MRI performed at the end of this three-year period. Most recurrences occur within 3 years. The patient should be followed clinically at least through the period of toilet training, since bowel and bladder functional abnormalities are found in up to 30% of patients with this disease [8]. More recent reports describe late recurrence of disease and advocate for follow-up until adulthood and an additional MRI when the child can undergo this imaging procedure without sedation [9].

15. **What is desmoid-type fibromatosis and how is it treated?**

Desmoid-type fibromatosis (previously called desmoid tumor or aggressive fibromatoses) is an intermediate (locally aggressive) fibroblastic tumor with an extremely low potential to metastasize. Mutations in exon 3 of the *CTNNB1* gene cause WNT pathway activation and are found in 80% of desmoid-type fibromatoses. Alternatively, the disease may be associated with *APC* gene mutation and Familial Adenomatous Polyposis (FAP) syndrome. Common sites for FAP-associated desmoid-type fibromatosis include the abdomen or abdominal wall. Optimal treatment consists of complete surgical resection with negative margins. Observation, chemotherapy, targeted therapies (tyrosine kinase inhibitors sorafenib or pazopanib), and external beam radiotherapy are all options for recurrent or unresectable tumors [10].

16. **What is an inflammatory myofibroblastic tumor, what is the responsible genetic driver of this tumor type, and how is it treated?**

Inflammatory myofibroblastic tumor (IMT) is an intermediate (rarely metastasizing) soft tissue or visceral organ fibroblastic tumor that most frequently presents in children or adolescents. These tumors may be locally invasive. IMT are characterized by aberrations in the *ALK* gene and are typically strongly positive for ALK by immunohistochemistry. Complete surgical resection with negative margins is the optimal treatment. For recurrent or unresectable tumors, ALK inhibitor therapies such as crizotinib may achieve complete or partial tumor response [11].

17. **What is the appropriate management of a large chest wall Ewing sarcoma?**

CT, MRI and/or PET should be performed for anatomic characterization of the primary tumor and possible metastases. Biopsy of the lesion can usually be easily be performed by core needle. Bone marrow aspiration and biopsy should be performed given the propensity of Ewing sarcoma to metastasize to this site. Neoadjuvant chemotherapy to shrink the tumor, improve the chance of negative surgical margins, and reduce the morbidity and disfigurement of surgical resection is generally the standard approach for the treatment of Ewing sarcoma, as it is generally very sensitive to chemotherapy. Therefore, morbid, pre-chemotherapy resections should be avoided. The goal of surgical resection of the primary tumor is to achieve negative margins, although resection of a rib above and/or below the primary site is generally not supported by current evidence. Chest wall reconstruction may be required after chest wall resection, if a flail segment is likely to result. Radiotherapy is usually administered if surgical margins are positive. Definitive radiotherapy can be administered in place of surgical resection for unresectable disease [12, 13].

18. **When should a thoracotomy versus a thoracoscopic approach be utilized for the resection of osteosarcoma pulmonary metastases?**

The approach to pulmonary metastasectomy is controversial. The dogma for the management disseminated osteosarcoma is that all disease must be cleared surgically in order to have a chance at cure. This would suggest that open thoracotomy should be the approach, as it allows careful palpation of the lung and identification of lesions that were not detected on pre-operative chest CT. These lesions would likely be missed with a thoracoscopic approach in which tactile sensation is largely lost. However, the survival benefit of open thoracotomy has not been definitively demonstrated and the minimal approach of thoracoscopy (possibly repeated) might, therefore, be favored [14].

19. **What is the most common pediatric malignancy that exhibits aggressive peritoneal dissemination and what are the treatment options for this disease?**

Desmoplastic small round cell tumor (DSRCT), characterized by the presence of the t(11;22)(p13;q12) *EWS-WT1* translocation, is the most common malignancy with aggressive peritoneal spread that presents in children and young adults. The overall prognosis is extremely poor. DSRCT has a predilection for male patients (85%) and dozens to hundreds of intraperitoneal deposits are commonly found. Neoadjuvant chemotherapy should be administered. Complete surgical resection should be attempted in patients with no PET-avid extra-abdominal disease and no intraparenchymal liver disease after neoadjuvant chemotherapy. Complete surgical resection is associated with improved outcomes and typically entails cytoreductive surgery, which may require en-bloc resection of intraabdominal organs and peritonectomy. Hyperthermic intraperitoneal chemotherapy (HIPEC) with cisplatin may improve survival in carefully selected patients, but following a defined renal protection strategy is imperative. Whole abdominal radiotherapy has also been independently associated with improved overall survival in the context of a multimodal treatment approach [15, 16].

20. **What is the surgical approach to pediatric gastrointestinal stromal tumor? What are the responsible genetic drivers of this disease in children?**

Pediatric gastrointestinal stromal tumors (GIST) are characterized by loss of function alterations in the *SDH* gene, either by mutation or silencing via promoter methylation. In contrast to adult GIST, which is characterized by *c-KIT* mutations in 85% of cases and *PDGFR* mutations in 5–10% of cases, pediatric GIST is typically wild type for *c-KIT* and *PDGFR*. Because pediatric GIST has an extremely high rate of chronic, recurrent relapse regardless of the status of microscopic surgical resection margins, a non radical complete resection with negative margins should be targeted, but is not mandatory. Total gastrectomy or en-bloc resection of adjacent organs is not advised. Recurrent disease may be managed with repeated non-radical surgical resection or targeted therapies such as imatinib [17].

21. **What moles should be removed?**

Any mole that is asymmetric, increases in size, has an irregular border, changes color (either darker or lighter), has color that is not uniform, itches, or ulcerates should be removed for histologic examination.

22. **What is a Spitz nevus and how is this different from a Spitzoid melanoma?**

Spitz nevus is a benign tumor characterized by large neoplastic melanocytes with no metastatic potential. It is most frequently diagnosed in children and adolescents and found in the head and neck area. Spitz nevi are often nonpigmented or poorly pigmented when compared to other benign nevi. Histologically, Spitz nevi are composed of spindle cells, epithelioid cells, or a mixture of both. Nuclear atypia can be seen in Spitz nevi, which makes the histologic distinction from Spitzoid melanoma difficult. Spitzoid melanoma is a malignant tumor that may bear striking resemblance to Spitz nevi. However, Spitzoid melanoma also contains malignant features including irregular architecture and variations in cell type resulting in overall lesional asymmetry, presence of mitotic activity at the deep dermal border, atypical mitotic figures, central epidermal flattening or ulceration, presence of dermal nodules, and inflammatory infiltrate beneath areas of dermal invasion. Nevertheless, the pathologic distinction can be difficult [18].

23. **What surgical margins should be utilized in the wide local excision of pediatric melanoma? When should a sentinel lymph node biopsy be performed?**

The following margin guidelines are used in both adult and pediatric patients, when possible. However, in very young patients or in cosmetically sensitive areas such as the face, margins greater than 1 cm may not be practically feasible. The decision to choose a smaller than recommended margin should be discussed with the multidisciplinary oncology team. Involvement of a plastic surgeon for reconstruction or eventual skin grafting should also be strongly considered in young patients when goal margins exceed 1 cm [19].

Tumor thickness	Recommended margins
In situ	0.5–1 cm
≤1.0 mm	1 cm
>1.0–2 mm	1–2 cm
>2.0–4 mm	2 cm
>4 mm	2 cm

A sentinel lymph node biopsy should be performed for all melanomas with a Breslow depth ≥ 1 mm.

For tumors with a Breslow depth < 1 mm, the following clinical and pathologic features are relative indications for sentinel lymph node biopsy because they have been associated with increased rates of nodal positivity: ulceration, younger age, increased mitotic rate (≥1 mitosis/mm^2), and presence of pathologic regression.

24. **When should a completion lymphadenectomy be performed for pediatric melanoma?**

The fundamental purpose of a sentinel lymph node biopsy is to accurately stage disease. If the sentinel node is negative, regional lymph node dissection is not indicated. Importantly, approximately 75% of patients with a positive sentinel node will not have additional lymph nodes that are positive for melanoma. The recently published Multicenter Selective Lymphadenectomy Trial (MSLT-II) trial conducted in adult patients compared completion lymph node dissection to observation for melanoma patients with positive sentinel nodes. This study showed that completion lymphadenectomy increased the rate of regional disease control, but not the melanoma-specific survival in patients with positive sentinel nodes [20].

Although this is an evolving area of understanding and prospective pediatric studies have not been conducted, currently, completion lymphadenectomy is not routinely recommended in pediatric melanoma patients who have positive sentinel lymph node biopsies.

Clinically positive nodes are a contraindication to sentinel lymph node biopsy. For patients who present with clinically positive nodes without radiologic evidence of distant metastases, wide excision of the primary site and lymph node dissection of the affected nodal basin is advised.

25. **What patients are at risk for the development of malignant peripheral nerve sheath tumors? How can a malignant peripheral nerve sheath tumor be differentiated from a neurofibroma?**

4% of patient with Neurofibromatosis 1 will develop malignant peripheral nerve sheath tumors (MPNST). MPNST can also arise sporadically. MRI and FDG PET/CT can be used to help differentiate between lesions which are likely benign neurofibromas versus MPNST. MRI characteristics that differentiate MPNST from neurofibromas include large tumors (>5 cm), fat plane infiltration, heterogeneous appearance, irregular margins, and surrounding edema. FDG-avidity on PET scan can be used in combination with the above MRI findings to differentiate between these two tumor types [10].

References

1. Gurria JP, Dasgupta R. Rhabdomyosarcoma and extraosseous Ewing sarcoma. Children (Basel). 2018;5(12).
2. Njere I, Smith LL, Thurairasa D, et al. Systematic review and meta-analysis of appendiceal carcinoid tumors in children. Pediatr Blood Cancer. 2018;65(8):e27069.
3. Messinger YH, Stewart DR, Priest JR, et al. Pleuropulmonary blastoma: a report on 350 central pathology-confirmed pleuropulmonary blastoma cases by the International Pleuropulmonary Blastoma Registry. Cancer. 2015;121(2):276–85.
4. Feinberg A, Hall NJ, Williams GM, et al. Can congenital pulmonary airway malformation be distinguished from Type I pleuropulmonary blastoma based on clinical and radiological features? J Pediatr Surg. 2016;51(1):33–7.
5. Bauer AJ, Stewart DR, Kamihara J, et al. DICER1 and associated conditions: identification of at-risk individuals and recommended surveillance strategies-response. Clin Cancer Res. 2019;25(5):1689–90.
6. Heaton TE, Davidoff AM. Surgical treatment of pulmonary metastases in pediatric solid tumors. Semin Pediatr Surg. 2016;25(5):311–7.
7. Osei H, Munoz-Abraham AS, Bates KS, et al. Laparoscopic division of median sacral artery and dissection of types III and IV sacrococcygeal teratomas to decrease intraoperative hemorrhagic complications: case series and review of the literature. J Laparoendosc Adv Surg Tech A. 2019;29(2):272–7.
8. Rintala R, Lahdenne P, Lindahl H, Siimes M, Heikinheimo M. Anorectal function in adults operated for a benign sacrococcygeal teratoma. J Pediatr Surg. 1993;28(9):1165–7.
9. Padilla BE, Vu L, Lee H, et al. Sacrococcygeal teratoma: late recurrence warrants long-term surveillance. Pediatr Surg Int. 2017;33(11):1189–94.

10. Childhood Soft Tissue Sarcoma Treatment (PDQ(R)): Health professional version. In: PDQ cancer information summaries. Bethesda (MD); 2002.
11. Dalton BG, Thomas PG, Sharp NE, et al. Inflammatory myofibroblastic tumors in children. J Pediatr Surg. 2016;51(4):541–4.
12. Shamberger RC, LaQuaglia MP, Gebhardt MC, et al. Ewing sarcoma/primitive neuroectodermal tumor of the chest wall: impact of initial versus delayed resection on tumor margins, survival, and use of radiation therapy. Ann Surg 2003;238(4):563–7; discussion 567–8.
13. Bedetti B, Wiebe K, Ranft A, et al. Local control in Ewing sarcoma of the chest wall: results of the EURO-EWING 99 trial. Ann Surg Oncol. 2015;22(9):2853–9.
14. Fernandez-Pineda I, Daw NC, McCarville B, et al. Patients with osteosarcoma with a single pulmonary nodule on computed tomography: a single-institution experience. J Pediatr Surg. 2012;47(6):1250–4.
15. Hayes-Jordan A, LaQuaglia MP, Modak S. Management of desmoplastic small round cell tumor. Semin Pediatr Surg. 2016;25(5):299–304.
16. Subbiah V, Lamhamedi-Cherradi SE, Cuglievan B, et al. Multimodality treatment of desmoplastic small round cell tumor: chemotherapy and complete cytoreductive surgery improve patient survival. Clin Cancer Res. 2018;24(19):4865–73.
17. Weldon CB, Madenci AL, Boikos SA, et al. Surgical management of wild-type gastrointestinal stromal tumors: a report from the National Institutes of Health Pediatric and Wildtype GIST Clinic. J Clin Oncol. 2017;35(5):523–8.
18. Menezes FD, Mooi WJ. Spitz tumors of the skin. Surg Pathol Clin. 2017;10(2):281–98.
19. Coit DG, Thompson JA, Albertini MR, et al. Cutaneous Melanoma, Version 2.2019, NCCN clinical practice guidelines in oncology. J Natl Compr Canc Netw. 2019;17(4):367–402.
20. Faries MB, Thompson JF, Cochran AJ, et al. Completion dissection or observation for sentinel-node metastasis in melanoma. N Engl J Med. 2017;376(23):2211–22.

Chapter 66
Pediatric Radiology

Abdullah Alshabanat, Ailish Coblentz, and Alan Daneman

Abstract This chapter illustrates the most common neonatal and pediatric surgical conditions evaluated by the pediatric radiologist. Clinical vignettes are presented and the relevant imaging modalities are discussed to reflect on the surgical – radiologic correlation of each condition. The chapter ranges from cases of neonates and infants with chest masses or upper or lower intestinal obstruction, to emergency cases of children with acute abdominal pain or malignancies.

Keywords Abdominal ultrasound · MRI scan · Meckel scan

1. **What is the most likely diagnosis in a 6 year-old boy with right lower quadrant pain, fever and rebound tenderness?**

Acute appendicitis (Fig. 66.1). Acute appendicitis is the most common cause for abdominal pain in children presenting to the emergency department. Graded-compression US has excellent specificity and is free of radiation. Findings of a non-compressible enlarged appendix with transverse diameter greater than 6 mm is worrisome for acute appendicitis. Additional findings of increased flow in the wall with color Doppler, periappendiceal fluid, and increased echogenicity of the omental fat raises the likelihood. CT scan with intravenous contrast is usually used in cases with negative/ equivocal US findings and persistent clinical suspicion. It may also be used to evaluate for complications of acute appendicitis, such as perforation and abscess formation. At many institutions, MRI is now being utilized as an alternative to CT scan in equivocal cases.

A. Alshabanat · A. Coblentz · A. Daneman (✉)
Department of Diagnostic Imaging, Hospital for Sick Children and Department of Medical Imaging, University of Toronto, Toronto, Canada
e-mail: alan.daneman@utoronto.ca

M. Lacher et al. (eds.), *Pearls and Tricks in Pediatric Surgery*,
https://doi.org/10.1007/978-3-030-51067-1_66

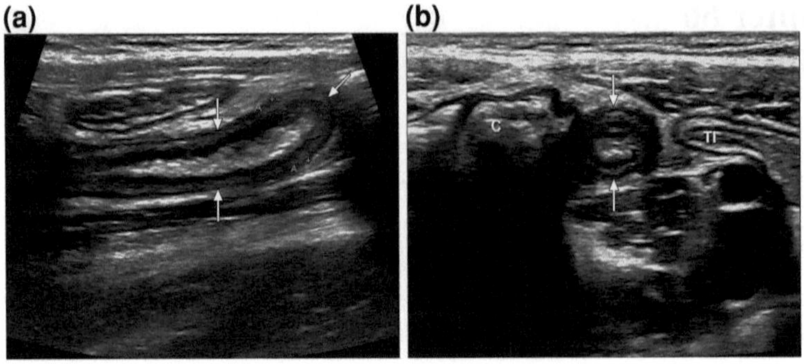

Fig. 66.1 Right lower quadrant ultrasound. **a** Longitudinal and **b** transverse scans show a thickened and distended appendix (arrows) interposed between the normal cecum **c** and terminal ileum (TI). There is increased echogenicity of the surrounding fat, compatible with edema. The electronic cursors in (A) show the appendix is dilated to above 6 mm and was non-compressible

2. **What diagnosis maybe found on ultrasound in a 2 years old girl with 1-day history of colicky abdominal pain and blood per rectum?**

Intussusception (Fig. 66.2). An intussusception occurs when the intussusceptum (proximal bowel) invaginates into a more distal bowel segment (intussuscipiens). It is considered one of the most common abdominal emergencies in the pediatric age group, occurring most commonly between 3 and 24 months of age. True lead points are almost always present in patients younger than 3 months of age. However, a lead point is observed in only 10% of cases overall, inclusive of all ages. The diagnosis is made by ultrasonography, with sensitivity and specificity approaching 100%.

The treatment choice depends on the type of intussusception. In the majority of cases, small bowel intussusceptions may be monitored and will reduce spontaneously without surgical intervention. Uncomplicated ileocolic intussusceptions without evidence of necrosis or a complex lead point can often be reduced by air enema, which has a success rate of 80–95%.

Recent literature has shown that the presence of an inner fatty core in the intussusception, lesion diameter greater than 2.2 cm, and the presence of lymph nodes in the lesion may allow reliable differentiation between ileocolic and small-bowel intussusceptions (3).

Air enema reduction under fluoroscopic guidance is considered to be the standard of care in most pediatric centers, replacing the previously used hydrostatic reduction using barium.

3. **What is the differential diagnosis in 2-day-old neonate with emesis, abdominal distention and failure to pass meconium?**

Lower intestinal obstruction (Fig. 66.3). Lower intestinal obstruction is not an uncommon neonatal entity, especially in pediatric hospitals and referral centers. It is also considered among the most common surgical emergencies in the neonatal period.

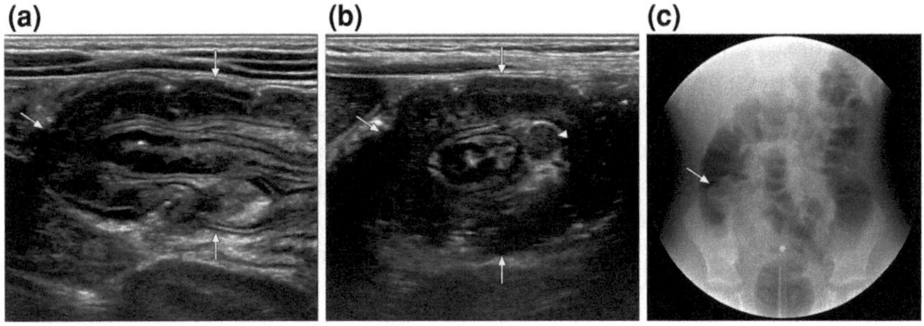

Fig. 66.2 Ultrasound of the abdomen shows a mass (arrows) in the right upper quadrant which represents an intussusception. The longitudinal appearance **a** of the intussusception is often described as 'kidney-like' and the transverse view **b** as 'target-like'. The transverse view nicely depicts a lymph node (arrowhead) within the intussusception. Air contrast enema on the same patient **c** shows a rounded, soft tissue mass (arrow) in the cecum in the right lower quadrant, representing the ileocolic intussusception. This eventually reduced completely with the air enema technique

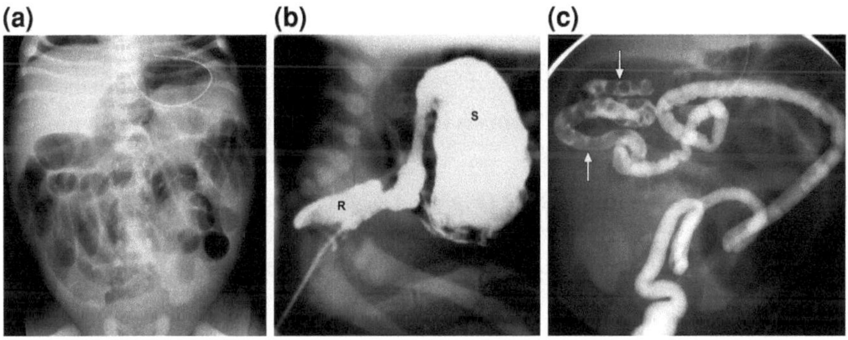

Fig. 66.3 Examples of low bowel obstruction. **a** Anteriorposterior view of the abdomen shows multiple dilated loops of bowel, in a pattern consistent with a lower bowel obstruction. **b** Subsequent contrast enema revealed this patient to have Hirschsprung disease. Note the abnormally distended sigmoid colon (S) as compared to the narrower rectum (R). **c** Contrast enema in a different patient shows a small calibre (micro) colon. Multiple filling defects are present in the terminal ileum (arrows), compatible with meconium ileus. This patient was subsequently confirmed to have cystic fibrosis

An obstruction is considered lower GI when the level of the obstruction occurs distal to the jejunum (i.e. involves the ileum or colon). Accuracy in diagnosis is important in order to provide appropriate treatment and decrease mortality rate. Neonates with obstructions are usually first evaluated with abdominal X-ray to determine whether the obstruction is proximal or distal. In cases of distal obstruction, a contrast enema (CE) examination is often the next step. This frequently provides a specific diagnosis and may be therapeutic.

A rectosigmoid diameter ratio of less than 1 is classic for Hirschprung disease. A sawtooth pattern of the distal rectal mucosa may also be observed, representing irregular contractions secondary to aganglionosis.

Functional immaturity of the colon is another cause of lower intestinal obstruction. Infants of diabetic mothers and infants of mothers who receive magnesium sulfate as treatment for preeclampsia are at increased risk. The X-ray findings of this entity are nonspecific, usually showing a pattern of distal bowel obstruction. CE will typically show a small distal colon with a normal rectosigmoid ratio. This should not be mistaken for diffuse microcolon.

Microcolon is defined as a small caliber colon with normal length and anatomic location. It is the result of disuse, and develops when meconium does not pass through the colon during in utero development. It is therefore the main finding in cases of distal small bowel obstruction, such as meconium ileus and ileal atresia.

Contrast reflux into the distal small bowel loop outlining multiple filling defects may be seen with meconium ileus. In 90% of cases, the patient will have cystic fibrosis. Therapeutic enemas may be performed using a hyperosmotic contrast agent. This causes water to shift into the bowel, helping to evacuate the sticky meconium.

Complications of distal small bowel obstruction include segmental volvulus, necrosis and perforation.

https://www.ajronline.org/doi/10.2214/AJR.17.19378.

4. **What is the most likely diagnosis in preterm 28 week GA boy with abdominal distention and sepsis?**

Necrotizing enterocolitis (NEC) (Fig. 66.4). NEC is a common acute abdominal condition in preterm infants. Early diagnosis and management is associated with decreased morbidity and mortality. Usually infants present with NEC in the first or second week of life, however, the time of presentation varies with gestational age and birth weight.

X-ray is typically the first line modality for diagnosing NEC, and the findings usually correlate with the clinical presentation. The earliest finding may simply be dilated gas-filled loops of bowel. The most reliable finding is the presence of intramural gas (pneumatosis intestinalis). Portal venous gas and intraperitoneal free air are usually late findings.

Ultrasound may demonstrate thinning of the bowel wall, decreased peristalsis, and hypoperfusion on color Doppler evaluation. Somewhat counterintuitively, sometimes the bowel wall may be abnormally thickened, or show increased perfusion! The presence of echogenic intraabdominal fluid or formed collections predict an unfavorable outcome.

https://link.springer.com/article/10.1007/s00247-013-2725-y

https://pubs.rsna.org/doi/full/10.1148/rg.272055098.

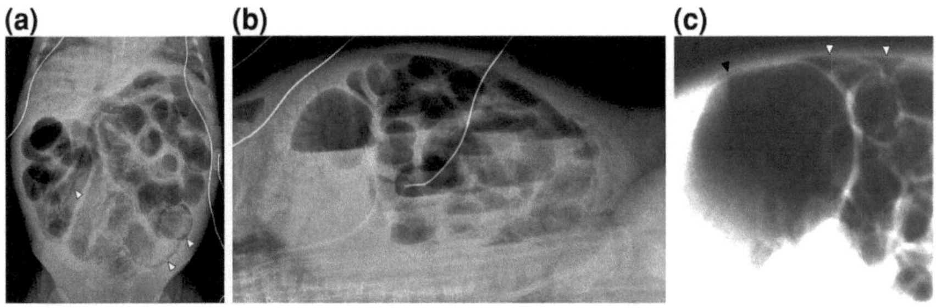

Fig. 66.4 Anteroposterior (**a**) and lateral radiographs (**b**) in a premature infant suspected to have NEC. Note the intramural gas in keeping with extensive intramural gas (arrowheads). Serpiginous gas overlying the liver represents portal venous gas. The lateral view with a horizontal x-ray beam is essential for assessing for free air when there is concern for perforation. **c** In another patient the lateral shoot-through view shows very small quantities of free intraperitoneal gas which appear either as triangles (white arrowheads) or are linear in shape (black arrowhead)

5. **What may be the diagnosis in a 5-week-old child with abdominal pain and bilious emesis?**

Malrotation with midgut volvulus (Fig. 66.5). Congenital rotational anomalies lead to abnormal positioning of the bowel within the peritoneal cavity, secondary to incomplete or absent embryologic bowel rotation. Resultant abnormal fixation of the bowel and the presence of mesenteric bands may lead to midgut volvulus, obstruction and subsequent bowel necrosis.

In non-rotation, the small bowel loops are positioned within the right aspect of the abdomen, and the colon is on the left. This abnormal positioning can be demonstrated with both upper and lower GI studies. In non-rotation, there is a broad mesenteric root, which leads to a low risk of midgut volvulus.

The diagnosis of malrotation may be made by UGI when an abnormal course of the duodenum is observed. Normally, the duodenum should take a retroperitoneal course, and the duodenojejuncal junction should be located to the left of the spine. If either of these features is absent, concern should be raised for malrotation.

An associated midgut volvulus is diagnosed when there is a corkscrew configuration of the duodenum. Ultrasound may be used to help diagnose midgut volvulus by assessing the relationship of the SMA/SMV, and attempting to demonstrate the course of the third part of the duodenum. Demonstration of the whirlpool sign, defined by clockwise swirling of the mesenteric vessels, is virtually diagnostic of midgut volvulus.

https://pubs.rsna.org/doi/10.1148/rg.265055167

https://www.ajronline.org/doi/10.2214/AJR.17.19378.

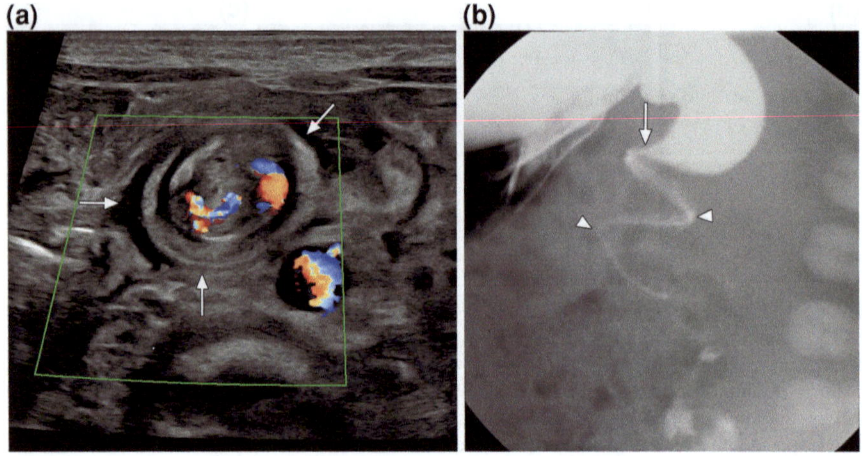

Fig. 66.5 Abdominal ultrasound and upper GI study in a patient with midgut volvulus. Abdominal ultrasound **a** depicts the 'whirlpool sign' of a volvulus (arrows). There is a round soft tissue mass (the volved bowel and mesentery) with swirling of the mesenteric vessels. **b** Upper GI study in the same patient shows a beak sign (arrow) in the duodenum at the site of obstruction followed by the corkscrew configuration (arrowheads) of the duodenum and proximal jejunum within the volvulus. These are characteristic signs of a volvulus

6. **What may be seen by abdominal ultrasound in a 4 week old boy with projectile, non-bilious emesis?**

Hypertrophic pyloric stenosis (HPS) (Fig. 66.6). Idiopathic hypertrophy of the pyloric muscle leads to thickening and elongation of the pyloric channel. Eventually, this results in progressive gastric outlet obstruction. While very common in infants 2–12 weeks old, HPS only rarely occurs at less than a week, or older than three months. While variable between institutions, commonly accepted sonographic criteria for HPS are:

- Pyloric muscle single wall thickness > 3 mm
- Pyloric channel length > 15 mm

Sonography for pyloric stenosis is a dynamic examination. Failure of the pylorus to show passage of gastric contents, or to change during the examination are strong ancillary findings. Gastric distension and retrograde peristalsis may also be demonstrated. If performed, upper GI examination shows minimal barium passing through the narrowed pylorus.

π **The Pi rule**: The pylorus should be no more than 3 mm thick, and 14 mm long.

7. **What may be the diagnosis in a 6-year-old boy with painless hematochezia?**

Meckel diverticulum (Fig. 66.7), which can be diagnosed by a Meckel scan using Tc-99 m pertechnetate. Although often present in the general population and

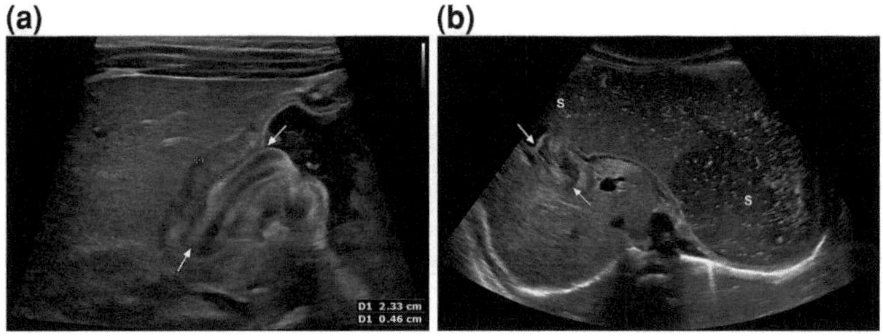

Fig. 66.6 Ultrasound of pyloric stenosis. **a** Note the 2.3 cm elongated and curved pyloric channel (arrows) with thickened muscle walls, measuring up to 0.5 cm between the electronic cursors. **b** Transverse image of the same patient, showing the markedly distended and fluid filled stomach (S). The thickened pylorus is displaced posteriorly in this image (arrows)

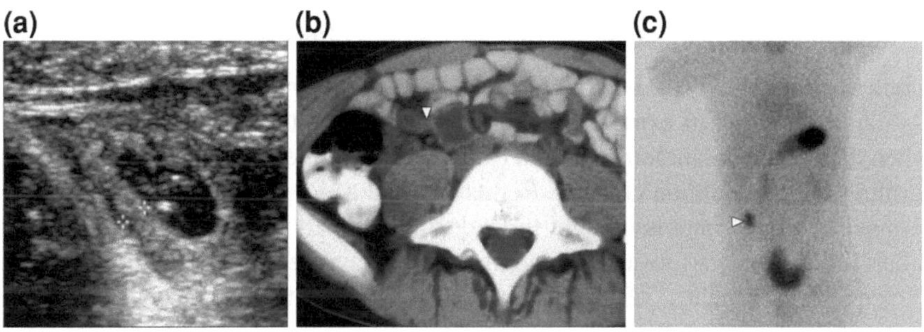

Fig. 66.7 Ultrasound, CT and 99mTc pertechnetate Meckel's scan. **a** Ultrasound shows a thick-walled (between electronic cursors), tear drop shaped cystic structure in the right lower quadrant. **b** Subsequently performed CT revealed this to be connected to a loop of adjacent ileum (arrowhead). **c** Confirmatory Meckel's scan shows intense activity in the right lower quadrant due to gastric mucosa in the Meckels diverticulum (arrowhead). Images acquired earlier in the study showed this activity to appear at the same time as the normal gastric mucosa. The kidneys can be faintly seen as pertechnetate is excreted through the renal system into the urinary bladder, which shows concentrated activity

asymptomatic, Meckel diverticula can cause symptoms in a few ways. Young children may present with intussusception, in which the diverticulum inverts and acts as a lead point. Older children may present with bleeding due to ectopic gastric mucosa, or infection within the diverticulum (Meckel's diverticulitis). Fortunately, it is estimated that 65% of symptomatic Meckel diverticula contain ectopic gastric mucosa. Pertechnetate, the radiotracer used in the Meckel scan, accumulates in mucous cells in the stomach as well as in ectopic gastric mucosa within the diverticulum. This is typically seen as faint early activity in the diverticulum, at the same time as the stomach. The activity typically becomes more intense with time. If the patient is actively bleeding during the scan, the radiotracer may appear to move downstream inside the lumen of the bowel. Of note, if there is a high clinical suspicion, a repeat study may be warranted. Half of those originally negative scans are positive on the second study.

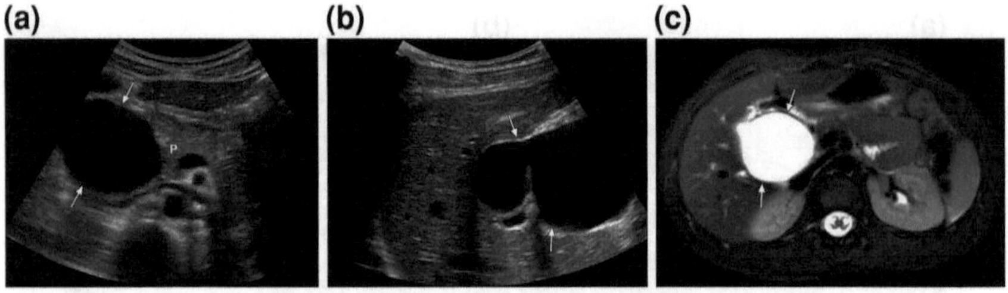

Fig. 66.8 Transverse **a** and longitudinal **c** images from a right upper quadrant ultrasound show massive cystic dilatation of the common bile duct (arrows) extending inferiorly to the level of the pancreatic head (P) and duodenum. No pancreatic ductal dilatation was seen. **c** Axial T2 image from an MRCP verified the presence of this Type 1 choledochal cyst (arrows)

8. **An abdominal ultrasound is obtained in a 6-year-old child with progressive jaundice and right upper quadrant pain. What is the diagnosis? What additional studies may be obtained to support the diagnosis?**

Choledochal cyst, Type I (Fig. 66.8). A choledochal cyst is a localized cystic dilatation of the intra- or extrahepatic biliary system. One theory is that this develops when there is an anomalous junction of the common bile duct and pancreatic duct, forming a long common channel. Reflux of pancreatic enzymes into the common channel and bile ducts is thought to lead to inflammation, stenosis, and upstream biliary dilatation. Various classification systems have been proposed to categorize choledochal anomalies, of which the Todani classification into 5 types, is most common:

Type 1: Solitary fusiform or cystic dilation of the extrahepatic bile duct (most common, representing 80–90% of cases)
Type 2: True diverticulum arising from the CBD
Type 3: Dilation of the intraduodenal segment of the extrahepatic duct (choledochocele)
Type 4: Multiple biliary cysts, of the extrahepatic, or intra- AND extrahepatic biliary tree
Type 5: Intrahepatic biliary cysts ONLY (a.k.a. Caroli disease)

Historically, hepato-iminodiacetic acid (HIDA) nuclear medicine scans were used to demonstrate communication of the cyst with the biliary tree, however they yield little additional anatomic information. Magnetic resonance cholangiopancreatography (MRCP) nicely delineates the cystic dilatation and its relationship with the hepatobiliary tree. The use of hepatobiliary-specific contrast agents (which are excreted into the biliary system) can prove communication of the cyst with biliary tree.

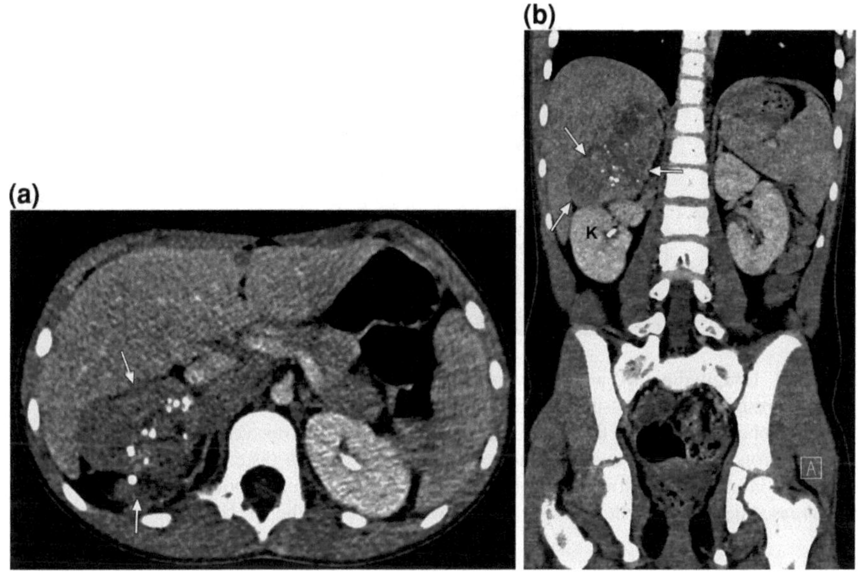

Fig. 66.9 **a** Axial abdominal CT image shows a heavily calcified mass (arrows) in the right suprarenal fossa. **b** The coronal plane best depicts the mass effect on the right kidney (K), which is displaced inferiorly by this right adrenal neuroblastoma

9. **What is the most likely diagnosis in a 2-year-old boy with a palpable mass and calcifications on abdominal radiograph? What nuclear medicine study may be helpful?**

Neuroblastoma (Fig. 66.9). While ultrasound is an excellent first line modality for assessing a palpable abdominal mass in a child, cross-sectional imaging is mandatory for tumor characterization and delineating anatomic extent. MR is increasingly used over CT due to the lack of ionizing radiation, and its ability to detect intraspinal tumor extension. High quality imaging is mandatory, as the current staging system for neuroblastoma uses 'image-defined risk factors' (IDRFs) for pre-treatment risk classification. These IDRFs are based on surgical risk factors that would impact resection, surgical complications and outcome. MIBG scintigraphy is a nuclear medicine study that can be used to evaluate for bone metastases. MIBG is related to norepinephrine and is taken up by catecholamine-producing tumors and metastases.

10. **What non-abdominal diagnosis should be included in the differential of a child with fever, diffuse abdominal pain and guarding?**

Basilar pneumonia with diaphragmatic irritation (**Fig. 66.10**). In children, pneumonia is the most frequent extra-abdominal cause for acute abdominal pain. The symptoms may be severe enough to overshadow the respiratory ones, leading clinicians to focus their attention below the diaphragm. This can result in delayed

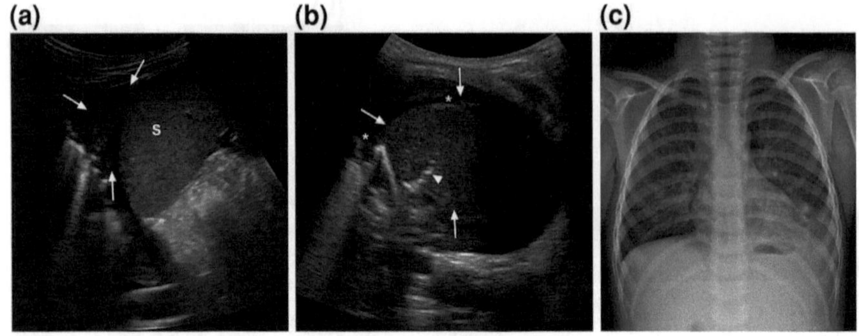

Fig. 66.10 Longitudinal (**a**) and transverse (**b**) sonographic images of the left upper quadrant in a patient presenting with a "surgical" abdomen. A wedge of dense consolidation (arrows) in the left lower lobe is seen above the spleen (S) and diaphragm. The transverse image shows an echogenic air bronchogram (arrowhead) and a small pleural effusion (asterisk). Frontal chest radiograph (**c**) confirms the left lower lobe pneumonia and pleural effusion both of which contribute to the increased density in the left lower zone and which obscures the left hemidiaphragm

diagnosis and initiation of appropriate treatment. In our case, the patient was seen in the emergency department and evaluated surgically and by abdominal ultrasound to exclude appendicitis. Fortunately, the basilar pneumonia was captured on the acute abdominal radiographic series. The important teaching point of this case is to ensure that a chest radiograph is included with all pediatric acute abdominal series. Simple views of the lung bases on an abdominal film are inadequate for diagnosis, in part due to the different technique by which abdominal and chest radiographs are acquired.

11. **A 3-year-old boy presents with acute scrotal pain. What radiologic study should you order?**

Ultrasonography with color Doppler (Fig. 66.11). Ultrasound with color Doppler allows differentiation of testicular torsion from the more common pediatric condition of torsion of the testicular (or epididymal) appendage. In testicular torsion, spontaneous or traumatic twisting of the spermatic cord within the scrotum may lead to vascular occlusion and eventual parenchymal infarction. Ultrasound may depict an enlarged testis with decreased or absent blood flow, and/or twisting of the spermatic cord. Emergent diagnosis is imperative, as surgical salvage rates are 80–100% within 6 h of pain onset, and effectively 0% after 12 h. Time is testicle!

12. **What is the differential for a prenatally-diagnosed chest mass in a neonate?**

Congenital diaphragmatic hernia, congenital pulmonary airway malformation (CPAM), diaphragmatic eventration, congenital lobar overinflation (CLO), bronchopulmonary sequestration (Fig. 66.12).

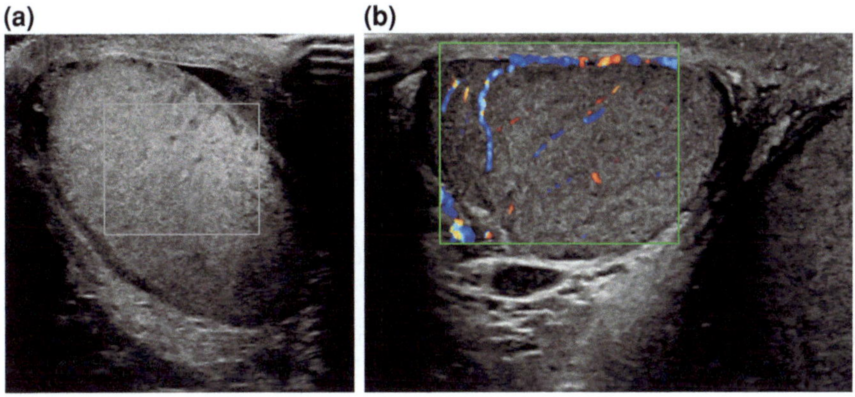

Fig. 66.11 Transverse sonogram of the symptomatic left (**a**) and asymptomatic right (**b**) testes. The images show an enlarged left testicle (**a**) with swelling of the scrotal wall and a small reactive hydrocele. There is heterogeneity of the parenchyma, concerning for developing necrosis. Doppler sonographic evaluation shows a lack of blood flow, in keeping with testicular torsion. (**b**) Comparative image of the right side shows the presence of blood flow in a normal-appearing testicle

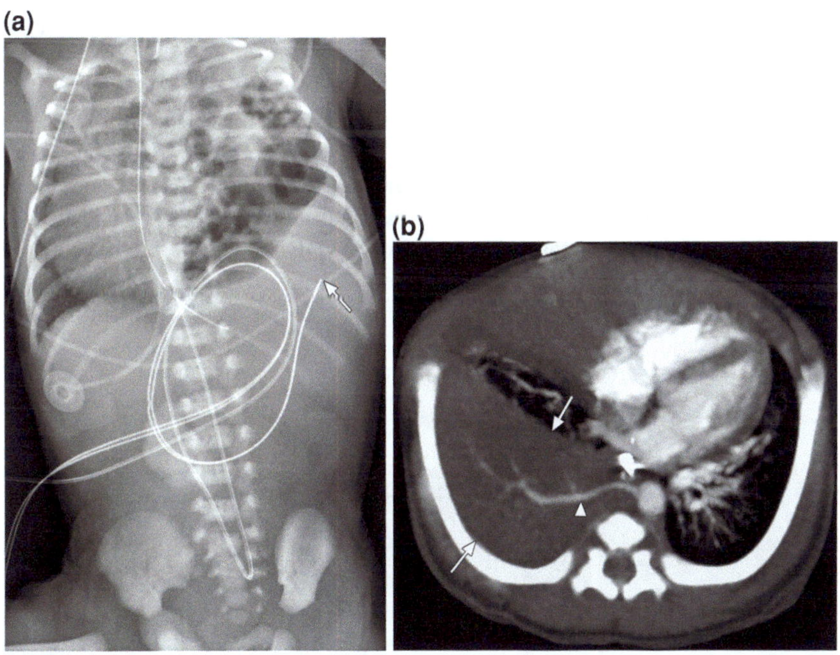

Fig. 66.12 Frontal chest radiograph (**a**) and axial CT chest (**b**) in two different neonates with prenatally diagnosed chest masses. Patient A has a large left congenital diaphragmatic hernia, with multiple intrathoracic loops of bowel, and rightward mediastinal shift. Note how the umbilical venous catheter (arrow) courses up into the liver, which is also contained within the hernia. A small amount of portal venous gas in the left lobe of the liver is related to the umbilical venous catheter insertion. The patient in (B) has a mass in the lower part of the right hemi-thorax which is consistent with a pulmonary sequestration (arrows). A large feeding artery (arrowhead) to the sequestration arises from the aorta

There are many congenital causes for a thoracic mass. In diaphragmatic hernia, the abdominal contents herniate into the chest via a congenital diaphragmatic defect, which is most commonly left-sided and posterior (Bochdalek). Fetal US and MRI may be used to guide prognosis, which is most related to the severity of pulmonary hypoplasia. Postnatally, chest imaging other than conventional radiography is rarely necessary. The other differentials will typically require a chest CT for further evaluation.

13. **What may be the cause of pain in a 6 year old girl with progressive left lower quadrant pain?**

Ovarian torsion (Fig. 66.13). Ovarian torsion is a gynecological emergency that my lead to loss of the ovary if not treated. While usually associated with a cyst or tumor, isolated ovarian torsion is also seen. Torsion initially obstructs the low-pressure venous vasculature, leading to ovarian congestion and enlargement. Later obstruction of the arterial flow results in ischemia and infarction.

Ultrasound will show asymmetric enlargement of the affected ovary as compared to the contralateral side. The follicles may be peripherally displaced.Color Doppler ultrasound is used to assess the presence of arterial and venous flow within the ovary. However, the presence of flow does not completely exclude torsion. Ultrasound can also show whether there is an associated ovarian cyst/tumor, which may aid in surgical planning.

MRI is superior to ultrasound in diagnosing ovarian torsion. As on ultrasound, findings include enlargement of the ovary with peripheral follicles, and abnormal edematous or hemorrhagic signal intensity due to infarction. The ovary may be displaced within the pelvis and the twisted pedicle may sometimes be seen. Gadolinium administration will result in an absent or abnormal pattern of enhancement. If there is an associated lead point, MRI is helpful in characterizing the mass. The most common lesion associated with a torsed ovary is a physiologic follicular or corpus luteal cyst. The most common tumor associated with a torsed ovary is a dermoid.

Read More: https://www.ajronline.org/doi/10.2214/AJR.10.7293.

(a) (b) (c)

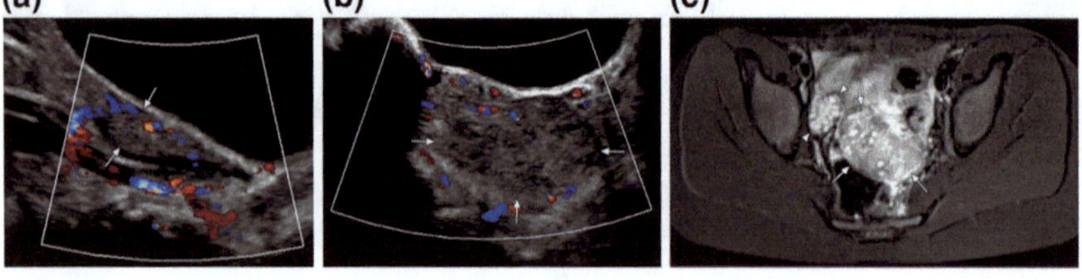

Fig. 66.13 Sonographic images of the right (**a**) and left (**b**) ovaries in a young female presenting with left lower quadrant pain. The right ovary (arrowheads) in **a** is normal in size, echogencity and flow. In **b** the left ovary (arrows) is enlarged and edematous, with poorly visualized follicles. It has markedly diminished blood flow compared to the normal right side. **c** A pelvic MRI shows characteristic features of ovarian torsion. The left ovary (arrows) is enlarged, edematous and extends abnormally medially. The smaller right ovary (arrowheads) is normal. Following contrast administration, the left ovary showed profoundly diminished enhancement compared to the right

Chapter 67
Transplantation in Children

Michael Berger

Abstract Liver transplant is the only cure for end stage liver disease, regardless of its ethiology. Further, in children, liver transplantation can be a cure for many other diseases independent of liver failure, such as unresectable malignant liver tumors or metabolic disease. Despite the complexity involved when performing a pediatric liver transplantation, in experienced centers it sustains excellent survival rates and is now considered standard therapy. Similarly, kidney transplantation is a cure of end stage renal disease and can prevent the need for hemodialysis in affected children. Outcomes are excellent. Small bowel transplantation can be a potential cure for short gut syndrome. Unfortunately, despite many advances in the field of pediatric transplantation, small bowel transplantation still carries many risks and pitfalls. Also, compared to the liver and kidneys, there are much fewer graft options available. Consequently, it is offered only in few specialized centers throughout the world and results are heterogeneous.

Keyword Pediatric liver transplantation · End stage liver failure · Hepatoblastoma · Biliary atresia · Technical variant graft · SPLIT liver transplant · MELD score · PELD score · kidney transplantation · Small bowel transplantation

1. **Who performed the first kidney transplant? What about the liver?**

The first successful solid organ transplant in the world was a kidney transplant. Dr. Joseph Murray performed the operation in Boston on December 23, 1954. The donor and recipient were identical twins, which is how Murray circumvented the need for immunosuppression, which was not invented yet. In 1963, Thomas Starzl

M. Berger (✉)
Pediatric Surgeon, Hepatobiliary Surgeon, Abdominal Organ Transplant Surgeon, Dr. von Hauner Children's Hospital, Munich University Hospital, Ludwig-Maximilians-University, Lindwurmstr, 4, 80337 Munich, Germany
e-mail: michael.berger@med.uni-muenchen.de

M. Lacher et al. (eds.), *Pearls and Tricks in Pediatric Surgery*,
https://doi.org/10.1007/978-3-030-51067-1_67

in Colorado for the first time ever intended a liver transplant. The recipient was a child with biliary atresia. The child died during the operation due to uncontrollable hemorrhage. Several attempts on adults followed, all of which were unsuccessful and the patients died. In 1967, he successfully transplanted a 19-month old girl with hepatoblastoma. The child recovered well from the operation and lived for 400 days before dying from tumor recurrence.

2. **What are common indications for a liver transplant in children?**

In this order: biliary atresia (>50%), fulminant hepatic failure, liver tumors, metabolic disease, Alagille syndrome, others.

3. **What are common contraindications for liver transplant in children?**

Absolute contraindications for liver transplantation in children are extrahepatic disease (in case of liver malignancy) that is not amenable to chemotherapy or surgical resection, progressive terminal non-hepatic disease, uncontrolled sepsis, and irreversible neurological injury. Relative contraindications must be evaluated on an individual case basis and include controlled acute systemic infections, chronic infections such as HIV, advanced hepatic encephalopathy, inflow obstruction due to portal vein thrombosis that extends throughout the mesenteric venous system, and significant psychosocial problems that make post-transplant compliance doubtful.

4. **Which diseases can be treated with liver transplant?**

In principle, any disease that produces end stage liver disease (ESLD)—warranted that there are no contraindications as described above—can be treated with liver transplant.

5. **How does the allocation system work for a pediatric transplant?**

This depends heavily on the organ to be transplanted. Also, the exact allocation system differs from country to country throughout the world. In general, however, all allocations systems throughout the developed world have some things in common. For the liver, generally speaking, allocation is based on the likelihood of a potential recipient to die while on the waiting list (see MELD score below) rather than waiting time on the waiting list. This is very different compared to kidney transplantation, were waiting time that accumulated on the waiting list is the most important factor for receiving an organ.

6. **Are children favored on the waiting list?**

Again, it all depends on the specific country, but in general in most developed countries in the world children are favored on the waiting list one way or another. This preference has very obvious reasons. The impact of spending 5 years on hemodialysis during early childhood has a much higher emotional morbidity than spending the same 5 years on the hemodialysis during one's fifties.

7. **What is the MELD score?**

The MELD score (MELD = Model of End Stage Liver Disease) is a scoring system and relies on the patient's values for serum bilirubin, serum creatinine, and the international normalized ratio for prothrombin time (INR) and is calculated as:

MELD = 3.78 × ln[serum bilirubin (mg/dL)] + 11.2 × ln[INR] + 9.57 × ln[serum creatinine (mg/dL)] + 6.43.

The score predicts the likelihood for any given patient with ESLD to die while awaiting liver transplant. The score is fairly accurate and is used through the world for the allocation of organs for liver transplantation. For children, it is much less acurate.

8. **What is the PELD score?**

The PELD score (Pediatric End-Stage Liver Disease) is the intention of the equivalent of the MELD score for patients < 12 years old. However, for children both the MELD and PELD score have less impact than in the adult world because exception points are frequently added depending on the nature of the pediatric disease. This listing above MELD/PELD has the goal to get children to transplant as quickly as possible.

9. **Which impact does sarcopenia have on patients undergoing liver transplantation?**

Sarcopenia, meaning the reduction of core muscle mass as a biomarker of severe nutrition independent of body weight, is a prognostic marker for poor outcome in children undergoing liver transplantation [1].

10. **Which graft options exist for donation for pediatric liver transplantation?**

A liver in a child can be transplanted either as a whole organ from a size matched donor (a child) or as a so-called technical variant graft. The latter refers to organs that are reduced in size and can stem from a deceased adult donor (either as an ex-situ SPLIT or an in-vivo SPLIT) or from a live donor hepatectomy. Typically, in true pediatric liver transplantation, which entails a recipient weight of < 20 kg, a left lateral segment (segment 2 and 3) is used.

11. **How does a liver transplant work from a technical standpoint?**

A pediatric liver transplant, especially if performed as a technical variant graft, is rather challenging and involves four defined phases: 1. Complete hepatectomy, 2. Anhepatic phase, 3. Implantation, and 4. Reperfusion. Depending on the details of the case, this will take 4–6 hours.

12. **What are typical ischemia times in liver transplantation?**

Ideally, ischemia times are kept as low as 6 hours. Everything under 10 hours is probably fine, everything above 12 hours is really suboptimal and may cause poor organ function or even primary non-function.

13. **What is a back table dissection?**

During the back table dissection, the organ is prepared for transplantation. This step is performed in the cold, meaning on ice. After thorough inspection of the organ for any flaws potentially inhibiting transplantation, excessive fat is removed, the vessels are dissected out and are freshened on their edges, and the bile duct is shortened. Also, in case of a technical variant graft, the splitting of the organ is carried out at this point. This part of the transplant is usually done in parallel while a second team is preforming the hepatectomy of the recipient native liver in order to save time. Therefore, an additional operating table with a separate sterile field and set of instruments is set up in the back of the room, hence the term *back table*.

14. **What is the most feared complication in liver transplantation?**

The most feared complication of liver transplantation is hepatic artery thrombosis (HAT) [2]. The risk is about 3–6% in adults and can be up to 10% in children. The smaller the child is, the greater is the risk for HAT. HAT usually results in organ loss unless detected and revised within the hour. Risk for HAT can be reduced by the use of systemic anticoagulation during and after the transplant (for example heparin) as well as meticulous technique [3].

15. **What are other common short-term complications of liver transplantation?**

Portal vein thrombosis causing poor graft function, outflow obstruction causing congestation of the graft, and bile leak causing bilioma. If managed appropriately and timely by an experienced center, different from HAT, these complications should not lead to graft loss.

16. **How immunogenic is the liver? How does that compare to other organs commonly transplanted, such as the kidney and the heart?**

The liver is, especially compared to kidney and heart, not very immunogenic. Hence, less immunosuppression is required following a liver transplant and rejection is more subtle.

17. **How important is blood type when allocating a donor and a recipient?**

Liver transplants in children can be carried out against blood type in children <1 year of age without additional risk and at ages 1–2 years with manageable risk. Above 2 years of age, transplanting against blood type increases the risk of rejection significantly [4]. This is not possible in kidney transplantation.

18. **How important is HLA typing when allocating a donor and a recipient?**

HLA typing plays no role in pediatric liver transplantation and is usually not assessed when evaluating a recipient. On the contrary, it is extremely relevant in kidney transplantation.

19. **Which immunosuppression regimen is used in pediatric transplantation?**

Following a liver transplant, typically children are started on steroids at the time of the operation. After initial high doses, steroids are tapered out over about 3 months. Tacrolimus is usually started on postoperative day one and is given for life. Therapeutic levels immediately after transplant are 12–16, but many different protocols exist. These levels can be adjusted to something closer to 10–12 during the first year after transplant and about half that in the subsequent years. Few children come off tacrolimus entirely and most take small amounts with levels of 3–7 for a lifetime. Following kidney transplantation, often basiliximab is added for additional protection against rejection on day 0 and day 4, but again, many different protocols exist.

20. **What are long-term complications of pediatric liver transplantation?**

Chronic rejection can occur slowly and over years, ultimately leading to fibrosis and loss or organ function. Apart from optimization of the immunosuppressive regimen, there is currently no way to prevent this from happening. Due to prolonged treatment with tacrolimus, renal insufficiency is a true problem often leading to end-stage renal disease.

21. **What is the overall prognosis of pediatric liver transplantation?**

	1-year graft survival (%)	5-year graft survival (%)	References
Liver	90	85	Cuenca et al., Semin Pediatr Surg (2017)
Kidney	95	93	Aoki et al., Int J Urol (2019)
Small bowel	90	80	Nayyar et al., Semin Pediatr Surg (2010)
Lung	87	49	Valappour et al. Am J Transplant (2013)

22. **What are some of the hazards living with a liver transplantation long-term?**

Living with a liver transplant is a lifelong commitment and follow-up never stops. Although the risk for rejection is highest in the first year of life, there is a lifelong risk for rejection. The second peak of risk for rejection is during puberty. These children often stop taking their immunosuppressive medicine in an act of rebellion, resulting in rejection. Further, although transplanted livers can easily last 25 years and longer, one must consider the possibility that a child will need a second or a third liver transplant as an adult.

23. **What is the most common indication for a kidney transplant in children?**

The most common indication for a kidney transplant in a child is obstructive uropathy, such as posterior urethral valves. Because affected children are often born with these conditions, significant damage to the kidneys already exists by the time children become available for treatment.

24. **What donor options exist for kidney transplantation?**

In most cases, organs can come from adult donors. These can either be cadaveric organs or live donors. There is no size match required, but recipients should be at least approximately 10 kg in order to receive a kidney transplant. Typically, live donors such as the parents are the preferred option for children. In good functioning transplant communities, up to 90% of kidneys transplanted in children stem from live donors [5]. Organs from live donors are preferable in children because transplantation can be planned in such a way that dialysis can be avoided. Also, they typically last longer.

25. **What are the technical steps in a kidney transplantation?**

In a standard kidney transplant, the right groin is opened with a semilunar incision from above the pubic symphysis to the right lower abdomen. After proper exposure, the donor renal artery is sown onto the right recipient iliac artery and the donor renal vein onto the right recipient iliac vein. In small children or on a third transplant when both left and right groins have been used, the abdomen is opened midline and the kidney is sown directly on the aorta and vena cava.

26. **Is it necessary to remove the native kidney?**

No, typically the diseased kidneys remain in situ, especially since they often have some remaining function and although they cannot concentrate, do can diurese. A notable exception is polycystic kidney disease. These kidneys often have little to no remaining function and often are so large that they limit the available space for kidney transplantation. Hence, they are sometimes removed prior to or at the time of transplant.

27. **What is the most common indication for a small bowel transplantation?**

The most common indication for a small bowel transplant is an extreme variant of short gut syndrome that results in failure to thrive and dependence on total parenteral nutrition (TPN). Typical conditions that can induce such significant short gut syndrome are loss of bowel from NEC, volvulus, gastroschisis, or intestinal atresia. Some functional disorders, such as total aganglionosis or intestinal pseudoobstruction can also lead to the need for a small bowel transplant.

28. **What triggers listing for small bowel transplantation?**

Typically, it is complications from TPN such as loss of all vascular access, progressive vascular thrombosis, life-threatening catheter infections, and TPN-related liver disease that mandate listing for small bowel transplant.

29. **Are there contraindications for bowel transplantation?**

Contraindications are systemic and untreated local infections (bacterial, fungal, viral), malignancies (other than the indications for multivisceral transplants), and severe cardiac, pulmonary, or neurologic disease that will prevent adequate quality of life. Additionally important for children, the recipient weight should be near 10 kg or above at the time of transplant.

30. **When do we offer isolated bowel versus combined liver-bowel versus multivisceral transplantation?**

Small bowel transplants alone usually go to children with intestinal failure that cannot be controlled by total parenteral nutrition and that only have mild to moderate liver dysfunction. Combined bowel-liver transplants are offered to patients with intestinal failure and irreversible liver failure due to total parenteral nutrition. Multivisceral transplants usually go to children with intra-abdominal tumors that are otherwise non-resectable.

31. **What are specific indications for lung transplantation ?**

This depends on the age of the recipient. In children <1 year of age, surfactant protein-B deficiency, congenital heart disease and idiopathic pulmonary arterial hypertension (IPAH) are the more common indications. For children aged 1–5 years, it is IPAH and idiopathic pulmonary fibrosis. For children above the age of 6 years, by far the most common indication is cystic fibrosis.

References

1. Lurz E, Patel H, Frimpong RG, Ricciuto A, Kehar M, Wales PW, et al. Sarcopenia in children with end-stage liver disease. J Pediatric Gastroenterol Nutr. 2018 Feb;66(2):222–6
2. Ma N, Song Z, Dong C, Sun C, Meng X, Zhang W, et al. Risk factors of hepatic artery thrombosis in pediatric deceased donor liver transplantation. PediatrSurg Int. Springer Berlin Heidelberg; 2019 Aug;35(8):853–9.
3. Heffron TG, Pillen T, Welch D, Smallwood GA, Redd D, Romero R. Hepatic artery thrombosis in pediatric liver transplantation. Transplant Proc. 2003 Jun;35(4):1447–8
4. Honda M, Sugawara Y, Kadohisa M, Shimata K, Sakisaka M, Yoshii D, et al. Long-term outcomes of ABO-incompatible pediatric living donor liver transplantation. Transplantation. 2018 Oct;102(10):1702–9
5. Aoki Y, Hamasaki Y, Satoh H, Matsui Z, Muramatsu M, Hamada R, et al. Long-term outcomes of pediatric kidney transplantation: a single-center experience over the past 34 years in Japan. Int J Urol. John Wiley & Sons, Ltd (10.1111); 2019 Dec 11;17:1324.

Are there contraindications for bowel transplantation?

[illegible]

[illegible]

[illegible]

What are specific indications for lung transplantation?

[illegible]

[illegible]

[illegible]

Chapter 68
The Neonatal Surgical Patient

Francesco Morini, Patrizia Bozza, and Pietro Bagolan

Abstract It is universally agreed that the child is not a small adult in terms of physiology, pathophysiology, pathology and response to surgical stress. Similarly, the neonate is not a small child. The neonate represents a unique surgical patient with specific characteristics depending on its immaturity, also due to preterm birth in some cases, and the type of disorders, usually congenital and complex. In this chapter, we introduce the characteristics the surgical neonate and will discuss the general aspects of its management.

Keywords Neonatal nutrition · Pain management · Perioperative antibiotic prophylaxis · Surgical neonate

1. **How can neonates be classified according to their level of maturation (gestational age) and development (weight)?**

A term, appropriate for gestational age infant is one born between 37 and 42 weeks of gestation with a birth weight greater than 2.500 gr (Table 68.1). Maturation and development are crucial factors influencing the infant outcome (Table 68.2).

2. **What are the features of small for gestational age (SGA) newborns?**

Newborns whose birth weight is below the 10th percentile are defined SGA. Placental, maternal, and/or fetal abnormalities may cause restricted intrauterine

F. Morini · P. Bagolan (✉)
Neonatal Surgery Unit, Department of Medical and Surgical Neonatology, Ospedale Pediatrico Bambino Gesù, IRCCS, Rome, Italy
e-mail: pietro.bagolan@opbg.net

P. Bozza
Department of Anesthesia and Critical Care, Ospedale Pediatrico Bambino Gesù, IRCCS, Rome, Italy

M. Lacher et al. (eds.), *Pearls and Tricks in Pediatric Surgery*,
https://doi.org/10.1007/978-3-030-51067-1_68

Table 68.1 Newborn classification by maturation and development (gestational age)

By maturation	Age at birth
Preterm Term Post-term	Before 37-week gestation period Between 37- and 42-week gestation period After 42-week gestation period
By development	**Birth weight**
Small for gestational age (SGA) Appropriate for gestational age Large for gestational age	Below 10th percentile Between 10 and 98th percentile Greater than 98th percentile

Table 68.2 Newborn clinical classification by birth weight

Classification	Birth weight (g)	% preterm births	Mortality versus term
Moderately low	2500–1501	82	×40
Very low	1500–1001	12	×200
Extremely low	<1000	6	×600

Table 68.3 Common conditions associated with intrauterine growth retardation

Age at delivery	Condition
Preterm	Placental insufficiency, discordant twinning, chronic maternal hypertension, intrauterine infection, toxemia
Term	Congenital anomalies, microcephaly
Post-term	Placental insufficiency

growth (Table 68.3). It is important to differentiate infants born small as a result of factors such as ethnicity, sex, and geography from those whose relatively low birth weight is a result of genetic or intrauterine abnormality.

3. **What are the physiological and anatomical factors that make the preterm infant vulnerable and what are the sequelae?**

   - Central nervous system immaturity: apnea, bradycardia, weak sucking reflex, increased risk of brain hemorrhage.
   - Pulmonary immaturity: surfactant deficiency, hyaline membrane disease, respiratory distress at birth.
   - Vascular immaturity and fragility: increased risk of intraventricular hemorrhage and retinopathy of prematurity.
   - Skin immaturity: underdeveloped stratum corneum with significant transepithelial water loss and complicated thermal regulation and fluid status management.
   - Gastrointestinal immaturity: inadequate absorption and risk of necrotizing enterocolitis.
   - Cardiovascular immaturity with patent ductus arteriosus or patent foramen ovale: potential persistent left-to-right shunting and cardiac failure.

4. **What are the differences between associations, syndromes and sequences?**

Associations are groups of malformations occurring together more often than expected by chance, and do not have evidence of a single unifying cause. Syndromes have more than one phenotypic feature and consist of malformations that occur together more than expected by chance, with a single unifying or presumed cause. Sequence is a consequence, result, or subsequent development of a disease (e.g. Pierre-Robin sequence: micrognatia causes glossoptosis that causes cleft palate).

Associations, syndromes and sequences are frequent in surgical neonates with a congenital anomaly. Therefore, a systematic screening of all organs and systems is required.

5. **How can fluid and electrolytes requirement be calculated in the newborn baby (Table 68.4)?**

   a. The basic maintenance requirement is the volume required to support growth and replace losses from renal excretion (renal water), skin, lungs, and stool. Invisible continuing water loss occurs from the lungs (respiratory water loss) and skin (transepithelial water loss) and constitutes insensible water loss (IWL). The insensible water loss for a full-term infant in a thermoneutral environment at 50% humidity is approximately 12 mL/kg per 24 hours (33% respiratory, 50% transepithelial).
   b. Dextrose infusion to maintain appropriate blood glucose levels. The fetus has limited capacity of gluconeogenesis and limited liver glycogen stores, rapidly depleted within 2 to 3 hours after birth. Also, the neonate has limited ability to synthesize glucose from fat or protein substrates.
   c. Electrolytes added in amounts to appropriately maintain homeostasis. Basic electrolyte and energy requirements are provided by NaCl (2–5 mEq/kg/day) with addition of potassium (2–3 mEq/kg/day) once urine production has been established. Calcium gluconate (1–2 g/L fluid) may be added, especially in preterm infants [1].

Table 68.4 Maintenance fluid requirements of neonates, usually as 10% dextrose (mL/kg/day)

Birth weight (g)	1–2 days of age (ml)	3–7 days of age (ml)	7–30 days of age (ml)
<750	100–250	150–300	120–180
750–1000	80–150	100–150	120–180
1000–1500	60–100	100–150	120–180
1500–2500	60–80	100–150	120–180
>2500	60–80	100–150	120–180

6. **What are the metabolic requirements for the surgical neonate?**

In the neonate, energy requirements are higher (higher growth rate and lower energy reserves). For enterally fed infants, the total energy requirement is 100–120 kcal/kg/day in term infants and 110–160 kcal/kg/day in preterm infants. In infants receiving total parenteral nutrition (TPN), energy requirements are slightly lower (80–100 kcal/kg/day), due to reduced energy losses. The neonate does not seem to have a significant metabolic response to surgery [2].

7. **Which are the nutritive options in the surgical neonate?**

Feeding should be through the enteral route whenever possible (less infectious risks, better immune response and entero-hepatic circulation of bile acids). Breast milk is the first choice as it contains several antimicrobial factors, antioxidant molecules and growth factors. If breast milk is not available or in case of nutrition through a jejunal tube, formulas tailored to the specific needs are available. Milk contains approximately 70 kcal every 100 ml. If enteral nutrition is not possible or contraindicated, and if fasting is predicted to last longer than 7 days, TPN should be provided (Table 68.5). If a central venous line cannot be obtained, peripheral PN with lower osmolarity (maximum 10–12.5% dextrose) and shorter duration (<2 weeks) can be provided. In addition to carbohydrates, lipides and aminoacids, TPN should contain electrolytes, minerals, vitamins, trace elements, and water. For vitamins and micronutrients, we suggest referring to specific NASPGHAN guidelines [3]. During PN, electrolytes, urea and creatinine, liver function tests, triglyceride levels, and trace elements should be monitored (once a week).

8. **When does a surgical neonate require central venous access?**

Central venous access is required for long-lasting therapies with hypertonic or irritating solutions, repeated blood sampling and invasive hemodynamic monitoring. Central venous access may be obtained shortly after birth through the umbilical vein (UV) (lasts less than 7 days), using peripherally inserted central lines (although only very thin catheters can be inserted and have a limited life: 30 days), or can be placed under ultrasound guidance or direct vision surgical venotomy in the internal jugular, the subclavian or the femoral vein. These last longer and may be larger and allow to draw blood, that is usually not possible with tiny peripherally inserted catheters.

Table 68.5 TPN components in neonates

TPN component	Purpose	Initial (g/kg/day)	Increase rate (g/kg/day)	Maximum (g/kg/day)
Carbohydrates	Energy (4 kcal/g)	7–8	1.5–4	17–22
Lipids	Energy (9 kcal/g)	1–2	0.5–1	3
Aminoacids	Protein turnover and tissue growth	2–3	1	3–4

9. **What are the risks related to central venous catheters?**

Short-term:
- Malfunction/displacement
- Infection
- Perforation and development of accidental hemorrhage
- Hemopericardium
- Cardiac arrythmias (if in the right atrium)
- Air embolus. In a spontaneously breathing baby, never open a catheter to the air (if the tip is above the diaphragm for UV catheters).

Long-term:
- Malfunction/displacement
- Infection
- Embolization and infarcts
- Thrombosis of hepatic vein (UV catheters)
- Liver necrosis (UV catheters)

10. **What are the goals of appropriate preoperative care** [4]**?**

a. Identifying, optimizing and managing coexisting clinical conditions
- Preoperative evaluations performed by the anesthesia team
- Full review of all systems

b. Preparing the patient for the specific operation: Informed consent

Except in the rare case where surgical intervention is necessary to prevent imminent death, informed consent in neonates requiring surgery mandates effective preoperative family education and counseling. Informed consent should disclose at least the following information:

- Surgeon understanding of the problem;
- Further measures to be taken to clarify the diagnosis, if indicated;
- Indication for emergency operation;
- Brief description of the procedure;
- Alternatives to treatment, including the option of doing nothing;
- Surgeon recommendation as to the best alternative;
- Benefits and risks of the proposed operation, compared with alternatives;
- Anticipated outcome

c. Preparing the family for the perioperative period.

11. **What are the aims of preoperative anesthesia assessment?**

- To obtain the clinical information for conducing the anesthesia
- To decide which examinations are indicated
- To give the risk assessment
- To obtain parents' informed consent
- To prescribe preoperative fasting
- To decide which anesthetic technique is best tailored to the patient's needs.

12. **Do surgical neonates need routine laboratory or instrumental testing?**

Infants scheduled for minor surgery, with silent medical history and/or negative physical examination, do not need particular pre-operative tests. In neonates undergoing major surgeries, preoperative tests are indicated, based on patient history and clinical examination performed during the preoperative evaluation.

13. **What is the definition and treatment of anemia in neonates?**

Anemia is a reduction of hemoglobin levels (or hematocrit) below 2SD normal values. Causes of anemia include reduced red blood cells production, increased destruction, and blood losses. Anemia may present with a variety of clinical manifestations including pallor, tachycardia, tachypnea or apnea, lethargy, poor feeding, increased oxygen requirements, poor growth, jaundice, and metabolic acidosis. As red blood cell transfusions are not exempt from risks, they should be limited to neonates with severe clinical manifestations. The majority of red blood cell transfusions to neonates are top-up transfusions of small volumes, typically 10–20 ml/kg over 4 hours (Table 68.6).

14. **What are the pre-operative fasting times in a surgical neonate?**

Two hours for clear liquids, four hours for breast milk, and 6 hours for infant formula.

15. **Why is gastric decompression in neonates undergoing surgery important** [4]?

Gastric distension carries the risk of regurgitation, aspiration and pneumonia, and may impair diaphragmatic excursion, with respiratory distress. In patients where ventilation is impaired for intestinal distention (intestinal atresia, congenital diaphragmatic hernia), or where intestinal distension impedes reduction of herniated intestine into the abdominal cavity (abdominal wall defects), gastric and intestinal distention may be prevented and/or alleviated by adequate orogastric decompression.

Tips for gastric decompression:

- Check the correct tube position in the stomach measuring the tube before insertion, noting the nature of the aspirate, and radiography (when required).
- Carefully tape the tube to avoid displacement.
- Use low continuous suction. If a single-lumen tube is used, intermittent aspiration is required.
- Use of gastrostomy tubes for postoperative gastric decompression may be considered, if present.

Table 68.6 Suggested transfusion thresholds

Gestational age (postnatal age)	Ventilated/cyanotic	Stable/off oxygen
<37 weeks (1st week)	12 g/dl	10 g/dl
<37 weeks (2nd week on)	10 g/dl	8 g/dl
>37 weeks	10 g/dl	7 g/dl

16. **What is the optimal temperature in a surgical neonate and how can it be maintained** [4]**?**

Neonates are susceptible to heat loss and have poor heat production competence. Hypothermia may increase the risk of intra-operative and post-operative complications, such as acidosis, bleeding, impaired immune function and delayed wound healing. Environmental temperature must be maintained near the thermoneutral zone appropriate for age: 32 °C-34°C in term infants, and 34 °C-35°C in low-birth-weight infants.

- The neonate environmental temperature is best controlled in an incubator
- Covering the head with an insulated hat can reduce heat loss (reducing cold stress by up to 15%)
- Use of insulating padding. Incubators themselves are plastic-walled containers that warm the infant by convection. Humidity can also be provided to the incubator environment, reducing evaporative heat loss.
- Radiant warmers provide open access to and visibility of infants who require frequent manipulation. However, they do not prevent heat loss by convection and often lead to higher evaporative water and heat losses. This evaporative heat loss may be reduced by plastic sheets.

In the operating room or radiology suite heat loss may be reduced by:

- Wrapping the head, extremities, and as much of the trunk as possible in clothing, plastic sheets, or aluminum foil.
- A plastic sheet beneath the infant may decrease humidity of the microenvironment
- Exposed intestine should be wrapped in plastic/warm gauzes.
- A heater system should be used during induction of anesthesia, preparation for operation, and at the termination of the operation.
- Solutions used for skin cleansing as well as intracorporeal irrigation should be warmed.

17. **Where should we operate on the preterm neonate?**

Disadvantages of surgery in the NICU.

- Unfamiliarity with the NICU environment. This entails ensuring that there is reliable availability of the necessary equipment, instruments, and disposables that surgeons and anesthesiologists will require.
- Restricted workable space for the surgical team, potentially limiting the ability to give quality care to the infant.
- Specific training to anesthesiologists on the NICU ventilators so that necessary adjustments can be made promptly as the patient's condition requires.

Benefits of surgery in the NICU.

- Infants can continue to receive their ongoing intensive care with minimal disruption and immediate return to the care of medical and nursing staff, once the procedure is completed.
- No exposure to the inherent risks of transport

– NICU surgery should be avoided where necessary bulky or overtly impractical ancillary equipment is necessary (intraoperative diagnostic imaging, laparoscopic, thoracoscopic, and endoscopic procedures, or where particular patient positioning is required). By contrast, some patients are currently operated on in the NICU: operations on ECMO, exploration and closure of postoperative sternotomies, ligation of PDAs and particularly ligation or partial occlusion of arterio-pulmonary shunts on extracorporeal circuits, need for high-frequency oscillatory ventilation.

18. **Describe antibiotic prophylaxis in the surgical neonate.**

In the surgical neonate, post-operative infectious complications contribute significantly to morbidity and mortality. Perioperative antibiotic prophylaxis (PAP) may reduce this burden. Appropriate antibiotic prophylaxis should cover the potential pathogens while reducing the risk of development of antibiotic resistant organisms. PAP is defined based on the type of surgery: **clean, clean-contaminated, contaminated** [5]. PAP is begun at anesthesia induction.

In Table 68.7 our Hospital's PAP.

Table 68.7 Antibiotic prophylaxis in neonatal surgery

Clean	**Prophylaxis**	
CVC/Broviac/Port	None	
Bronchoscopy		
Circumcision		
Inguinal hernia		
Neonatal testicular torsion		
Ovarian cyst		
Clean-contaminated		
Biliary tract/choledochal cyst	Cefazolin	1 dose
Congenital diaphragmatic hernia		
Gastroschisis/omphalocele		
Duodenal atresia		
Gastrostomy tube		
Nissen fundoplication		
Liver biopsy		
Head and neck surgery		
Contaminated		
Lung surgery	Cefazolin (lung/upper GI)	48–72 h
Esophageal atresia/	Cefoxitin + Gentamycin (lower GI)	
tracheo-esophageal fistula		
Jejunal/ileal atresia		
Hirschsprung disease pullthrough		
Ostomy closure		
Anorectoplasty		

19. **Which are the most common general post-operative complications in the neonate?**

Neonates have a unique response to surgery and may develop complications unrelated to the type of surgery they underwent. The newborn, especially if preterm, is particularly sensitive to pain and stress. Uncontrolled pain and stress may result in several adverse responses in circulatory, metabolic, immunologic, and hematic systems. In addition, the neurologically immature brain is most susceptible to long-term developmental effects. The immature central nervous system of the newborn is particularly susceptible to post-operative respiratory problems, predisposing to apnea, and is prone to depression following general anesthesia and administration of analgesics or sedatives. Moreover, residual effect of neuromuscular blocking agents may cause post-operative respiratory compromise. As a consequence, neonates need post-operative continuous monitoring of heart rate, respiration and oxygen saturation.

20. **What pharmacological post-operative pain management is available for the surgical neonate?**

Opioids provide the most effective therapy for moderate to severe pain. They produce both analgesia and sedation, have a wide therapeutic window, and attenuate the physiologic responses to stress. Among opioids, morphine and fentanyl are the most commonly used.

Paracetamol is frequently used in conjunction with other analgesics to decrease opioid use. Its main toxicity is liver damage; however, when given in appropriate doses, it is safe and effective.

Surgical stress response may also be effectively mitigated by regional anesthesia such as subarachnoid block (little use in neonates), lumbar/thoracic epidural analgesia, peripheral blocks, associated with a low risk of complications and a reduced need for intraoperative and post-operative opioid analgesics. Figure 68.1 shows a tiered approach to neonatal pain [6].

21. **How is post-operative pain assessed in a surgical neonate?**

In neonates, the management of pain must rely on behavioral and physiological markers.

<u>Behavioral indicators</u>: crying, facial activity, body language, complex behavioral responses. <u>Physiological indicators</u>: changes in heart and respiratory rate, blood pressure, oxygen saturation, vagal tone, palmar sweating, and plasma cortisol or catecholamine levels.

Currently the most used pain-assessment tools are:

- PIPP (Premature Infant Pain Profile), used in a gestational age of 28–40 weeks for procedural and postoperative pain;
- CRIES (Crying, Requires Oxygen Saturation, Increased Vital Signs, Expression, Sleeplessness), used in a gestational age of 32–36 weeks for postoperative pain;
- NIPS (Neonatal Infant Pain Scale), used in a gestational age of 28–38 weeks for procedural pain.

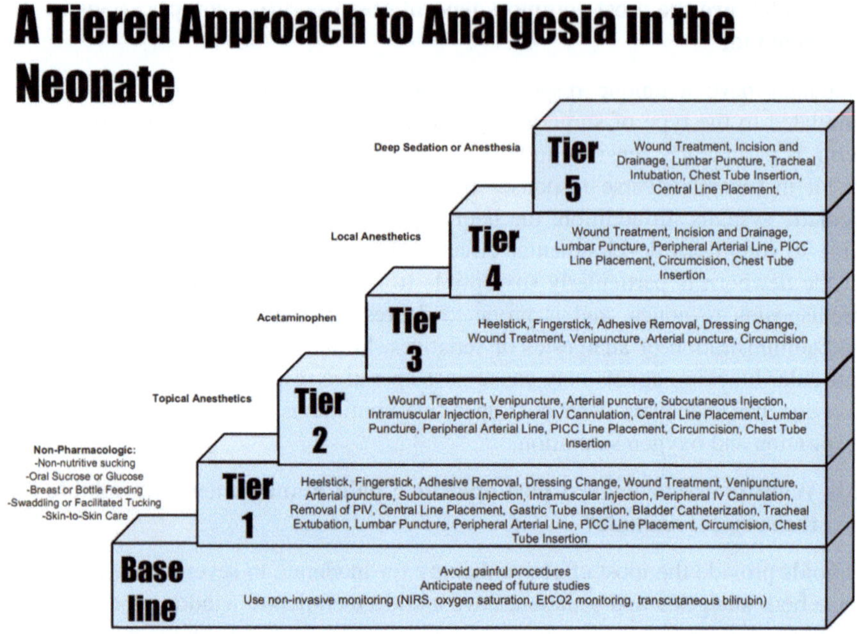

Fig. 68.1 A tiered approach to neonatal pain (from Witt N, Coynor S, Edwards C. et al. Curr Emerg Hosp Med Rep. 2016;4:1–10)

22. **What is the post-operative time to resume enteral feeding?**

It depends on the disease leading to the operation and the surgical procedure. In general, after a surgical procedure not involving the digestive system and in case of an operation not causing a postoperative ileus, the rule is two hours for clear liquids and three hours for milk and solid food. In case of abdominal surgery, small-volume feeding may be resumed when gastric aspirate or drainage is below 20 ml/kg/day and there is evidence of bowel function and should be increased gradually (1–2 ml/hour/day). Tolerance should be assessed controlling the amount of gastric aspirate/residual, the stoma/stool output, and abdominal girth.

References

1. D'Haringue AE, Byrne WJ. Nutrition in the newborn. In: Schaffer and Avery's Diseases of the Newborn, pp. 709–725. HW Taeusch, et al. Eeds. W.B. Saunders, Philadelphia, USA, 1991
2. Pierro A, Eaton S. Metabolism and nutrition in the surgical neonate. Semi Pediatr Surg. 2008;17:276–84.
3. https://www.naspghan.org/files/documents/pdfs/Parenteral%20Nutrition%20Slide%20Set.pdf.

4. Bruzoni M, Albanese CT. Perioperative Management of the Neonatal Patient. In: Surgical Care of Major Newborn Malformations, pp 1–32. Dolgin SE, Hamner CE Eds. World Scientific Publishing Co. Pte. Ltd. Singapore, 2012
5. National Collaborating Centre for Women's and Children's Health (UK). Surgical Site Infection: Prevention and Treatment of Surgical Site Infection. London: RCOG Press; 2008 Oct. (NICE Clinical Guidelines, No. 74.) Available from: https://www.ncbi.nlm.nih.gov/books/NBK53731/
6. Witt N, Coynor S, Edwards C, et al. A Guide to pain assessment and management in the neonate. Curr Emerg Hosp Med Rep. 2016;4:1–10.

Chapter 69
Pediatric Endocrine Diseases

Jason D. Fraser

Abstract Pediatric endocrine diseases are uncommon however knowledge of the most commonly encountered endocrine disorders is necessary for pediatric surgical practice. This chapter will review the most common non-tumorpediatric endocrine diseases with a focus on the thyroid gland, parathyroid glands, and adrenal glands.

Keyword Endocrine · Goiter · Thyroid gland · Hyperthyroidism · Parathyroid gland · Hyperparathyroidism · Adrenal gland

1. **What is the embryology of the thyroid gland?**

The thyroid gland arises as a thickening of the endoderm of the pharynx. It then descends anterior to the hyoid bone with the thyroglossal duct to rest in the lower neck. The thyroglossal duct then retracts in the 5th week to form the foramen cecum. A portion of the thyroid originates from the 4th and 5th pharyngeal pouches which form the parafollicular C cells (which make calcitonin) [1].

2. **What is a goiter?**

A goiter is a thyroid gland that is abnormally enlarged. Endemic goiter is due to dietary iodine deficiency. Simple goiter refers to an enlarged thyroid gland without a known cause (eg iodine deficiency or mass).

3. **What is Hashimoto disease?**

Chronic lymphocytic (Hashimoto) thyroiditis is the most common cause of acquired hypothyroidism in pediatric patients.Workup includes TSH, free T4,

J. D. Fraser (✉)
Associate Professor, University of Missouri, Children's Mercy Kansas City, Kansas CityKansas City, MO, USA
e-mail: jdfraser@cmh.edu

M. Lacher et al. (eds.), *Pearls and Tricks in Pediatric Surgery*,
https://doi.org/10.1007/978-3-030-51067-1_69

antithyroid peroxidase antibodies (TPO), and antithyrolobulin antibodies. It resolves in up to 1/3 of patients so can be managed expectantly [2].

4. **What is the most common cause of hyperthyroidism in children?**

Graves disease is the most common cause of hyperthyroidism in children. It is diagnosed with a high T4 and T3 and a very low TSH. It is caused by TSH receptor antibodies.

5. **What is the treatment of Graves disease?**

Treatment includes antithyroid medication (methimazole), radioactive iodine ablation, and/or thyroidectomy (if not responsive to medical therapies or unable to take the medication or undergo radiation).

6. **What causes congenital hypothyroidism?**

Congenital hypothyroidism is caused by either malformation of the thyroid or inability of a normal thyroid gland to produce thyroid hormone.

7. **What is the embryology of the parathyroid glands?**

The parathyroid glands begin to form during the 5th week of gestation from the 3rd (inferior glands and thymus) and 4th (superior glands) pharyngeal pouches [1, 3]. Knowledge of this embryology is important during parathyroidectomy as the inferior parathyroid glands may be located within the thymus or other aberrant locations.

8. **What is the primary function of the parathyroid glands?**

The parathyroid glands maintain calcium hemostasis by releasing parathyroid hormone (PTH) which activates osteoclasts to break down bone and release calcium. It also increases renal and gastrointestinal calcium absorption [4].

9. **What are the different endocrine neoplasia syndromes?**

There are three different multiple endocrine neoplasia syndromes, each with its own characteristic set of associated diseases. MEN 1: hyperparathyroidism (due to four gland hyperplasia), pancreatic tumors, and pituitary tumors. MEN 2a: medullary thyroid cancer, pheochromocytoma, and parathyroid hyperplasia. MEN 2b: medullary thyroid cancer, pheochromocytoma, neuromas, and marfanoid body habitus.

10. **What are the common presenting signs and symptoms of hyperparathyroidism?**

Hperparathyroidism can present with hypercalcemia, kidney stones, mood disturbances (depression), constipation.

11. **What are the different types of hyperparathyroidism?**

There are three different types. Primary hyperparathyroidism occurs when a parathyroid gland (adenoma) or all four parathyroid glands (diffuse) produce an inappropriate amount of PTH due to lose of regulation. Surgical excision is usually curative. Secondary hyperparathyroidism is caused by renal insufficiency resulting in decreased GI calcium absorption which results in increased PTH production. Treatment is usually medical. Tertiary hyperparathyroidism occurs from long term hypocalcemia with a resultant PTH by the parathyroid gland that persists even after correction of the underlying problem (renal transplant). This is due to hyperplasia of all four parathyroid glands and usually requires (near) total parathyroidectomy with auto-transplantation.

12. **What is the initial laboratory workup for hyperparathyroidism?**

The workup consists of basic metabolic panel including calcium, serum PTH level, 24-hours urine calcium, and serum 25-OH-vitamin D.

13. **What imaging should be done to localize the cause of primary hyperparathyroidism?**

Sestamibi scintigrapy with single proton emission computed tomography (SPECT) is the best method for preoperative localization of a parathyroid adenoma. Ultrasound is also highly sensitive but is operator dependent [5].

14. **What is the utility of intraoperative PTH levels in parathyroid surgery?**

Using rapid PTH assays allows the surgeon to check a baseline level prior to excision of a suspected parathyroid adenoma. Due to the short half-life of PTH, levels are able to be checked at regular intervals (5,10,15 min) to monitor for a decline in PTH indicating removal of the affected gland(s). This is indicated by a fall of PTH level of more than 50% from baseline or return to normal. (5) This allows the surgeon to target the operation, perform a smaller incision, and not explore other non-affected areas of the neck.

15. **How is bilateral adrenal hyperplasia causing hyperaldosteronism diagnosed?**

When hyperaldosteronism is diagnosed axial imaging (CT or MRI) is done to look for adrenal mass. When none is found bilateral adrenal venous sampling can be performed or scintography with NP-59. A functional adrenal adenoma is treated with surgical excision, but bilateral adrenal hyperplasia is treated with spironolactone.

References

1. Policeni BA, Smoker WR, Reede DL. Anatomy and embryology of the thyroid and parathyroid glands. Semin Ultrasound CT MR. 2012;33:104–14.
2. Feingold SB, Smith J, Houtz J, et al. Prevalence and functional significance of thyrotropin receptor blocking antibodies in children and adolescents with chronic lymphocytic thyroiditis. J Clin Endocrinol Metab. 2009;94:4742–8.

3. Fancy T, Gallagher D 3rd, Hornig JD. Surgical anatomy of the thyroid and parathyroid glands. Otolaryngol Clin North Am. 2010;43:221–7.
4. Alemayehu H, Fraser JD. Endocrine Disorders and Tumors. In *Ashcraft's Pediatric Surgery*. 7th Edition. Holcomb GW III, Murphy JP, St. Peter SD Eds. 2019. Elsevier. Philadelphia, PA
5. Lew JI, Solorzano CC. Surgical management of primary hyperparathyroidism: state of the art. Surg Clin North Am. 2009;89:1205–25.

Chapter 70
Pediatric Anesthesia

Nan Gai and Jason Maynes

Abstract The pediatric population possesses unique anatomical, physiological and pharmacological challenges that add distinct risks to their peri-operative care. These challenges are exacerbated in the neonatal and infant groups, where rapid developmental changes can further complicate care decisions and outcomes. For anesthetic management, thermoregulation, fasting times, fluid administration and pain treatment are specific areas where pediatric patients (especially neonates and infants) differ considerably from adults, leading to the potential for significant post-operative complications. While adverse peri-operative events occur with the same relative frequency, the type and etiology differ profoundly between adults and children. For the pediatric surgeon, careful attention to NPO times, early administration of dextrose-containing fluid, the use of multimodal (opiate nominal) pain treatment modalities and attention to thermoregulation will help to ensure better patient outcomes.

Keywords Anesthesia · Sedation · Pain · Opiate · Peri-operative · Outcomes

1. **Why are neonates at an increased risk of perioperative hypothermia compared to adults?**

The lowering of core body temperature primarily occurs via two mechanisms: redistribution of heat from the core to the extremities (heat movement) and radiation (actual heat loss). Children have larger surface area:weight ratios than adults, making heat redistribution and loss occur more quickly and to a larger overall

N. Gai · J. Maynes (✉)
Anesthesia and Pain Medicine, The Hospital for Sick Children, 555 University Avenue, Toronto M5G 1X8, Canada
e-mail: jason.maynes@sickkids.ca

N. Gai
e-mail: nan.gai@sickkids.ca

M. Lacher et al. (eds.), *Pearls and Tricks in Pediatric Surgery*,
https://doi.org/10.1007/978-3-030-51067-1_70

magnitude. Neonates have the largest surface area:weight ratio, making them the most susceptible.

2. **What are the potential complications of perioperative hypothermia?**

Perioperative hypothermia increases the risk of coagulopathy and the incidence of surgical site infections (SSI), prolongs anesthesia emergence, and significantly alters drug pharmacokinetics and pharmacodynamics. The World Health Organization recommends the use of warming devices to reduce the incidence of SSI [1]. Profound hypothermia is associated with cardiac arrhythmias.

3. **What methods can prevent hypothermia or warm a pediatric surgical patient?**

Intra- and peri-operative hypothermia can be prevented or treated by: (1) warming the operating room (to at least 26 °C), (2) the use of warming blankets and/or underbody devices, (3) administering warmed fluid (intravenous and in the surgical field), and (4) minimizing skin exposure.

4. **What are the standard preoperative fasting guidelines in children?**

To minimize the risk of aspiration in non-emergent cases, children should be fasted prior to the induction of anesthesia. It is safe to give children clear fluids up to 2 hours, breast milk up to 4 hours, other milk or light meals up to 6 hours, and fatty meals up to 8 hours prior to induction of anesthesia,[3]. Recent pediatric studies have suggested that clear fluids up to 1 hour prior to induction may be safe.

5. **How frequent are significant critical events in children undergoing anesthesia or in the immediate peri-operative period?**

The incidence of peri-operative severe critical events is best reported at 5.2%[4]. Severe critical events include laryngospasm, bronchospasm, pulmonary aspiration, drug error, anaphylaxis, cardiovascular instability, neurological damage, perioperative cardiac arrest, and stridor. The incidence of respiratory critical events was reported at 3.1%.

6. **What are major risk-factors for severe critical events in children undergoing anesthesia?**

Major risk factors for severe critical events include young age, medical history and co-morbidities (i.e. history of reactive airways, recent upper respiratory tract infection), and physical status (i.e. history of prematurity, snoring).

7. **What are the risks of anesthesia on neurodevelopmental outcomes?**

Human studies have not shown a clear link between anesthetic exposure and neurodevelopment. The general anaesthesia or awake-regional anaesthesia in infancy (GAS) [5] trial did not identify altered neurodevelopmental outcome in children exposed to general anesthesia as an infant, compared to an awake-regional technique. No study has addressed the risk of repeated anesthetics.

8. **Are children at increased risk of complications from regional anesthesia?**

Pediatric regional anesthesia is comparably safe to adult practice [6]. This is the case despite the standard of placing blocks under general anesthesia in children. Reported serious complication rates are less than 4 in 10,000, with transient nerve deficit being the most common.

9. **Why do neonates and young infants require admission to the hospital for otherwise ambulatory procedures?**

Neonates and young infants are at an increased risk of post-operative apnea, most significantly in the first 30-days of life. Although institution specific, typically term infants up to a post-conceptual age (PCA) of 46–52 weeks require at least 12 hours of monitoring. Ex-premature infants are at even greater risk of apnea post-anesthesia, requiring monitoring up to 55–60 weeks PCA.

10. **Succinylcholine is a fast-acting depolarizing muscle relaxant described as part of a classic rapid sequence induction technique to minimize the risk of aspiration. What are contraindications to the use of succinylcholine?**

Contraindications to succinylcholine include: a history or familial risk of malignant hyperthermia, known pseudocholinesterase deficiency, neuromuscular disorders, skeletal muscle myopathies, existing hyperkalemia, and conditions that predispose the patient to succinylcholine-induced potassium release (post-significant burn injury, major trauma, acute upper motor neuron injury, extensive denervation of muscle or deconditioning (i.e. ICU patient).

11. **What are the perioperative risks associated with a recent respiratory tract infection?**

A recent or active upper respiratory tract infection increases the perioperative risk of laryngospasm, bronchospasm, desaturation events, severe coughing, and breath-holding. The risk of peri-operative complications remains for four to six weeks after resolution of symptoms.

12. **What is laryngospasm?**

Laryngospasm is a reflex closure of the vocal cords that can occur after general anesthesia or sedation. It is caused by stimulation that occurs during an inadequate plane of anesthesia for the level of stimulation. Signs of upper airway obstruction not relieved by repositioning or an oral airway is highly suspicious for laryngospasm. Treatment is a jaw thrust, increased sedation, and muscle relaxation (i.e. succinylcholine).

13. **Which pharmacologic agents used in a common anesthetic can cause respiratory depression?**

Most sedatives (i.e. benzodiazepines), hypnotics (i.e. propofol) and opiates (i.e. morphine) can induce respiratory depression. Benzodiazepines and opiates are less potent depressants on their own, but synergize with other agents to more significantly affect the respiratory drive. Sedatives and hypnotics with less effect include ketamine and dexmedetomidine.

14. **Which anesthetic agents also have analgesic properties?**

Ketamine has well-established analgesic properties. Dexmedetomidine and inhaled nitrous oxide can also be used for their analgesic properties. Hypnotic and sedatives like propofol and the benzodiazepines do not demonstrate analgesic properties.

15. **Which is the only anesthetic agent thus far shown to be protective against neuronal apoptosis?**

Dexmedetomidine has been shown to be neuroprotective in animal models of stroke and ischemia–reperfusion. Other benefits of dexmedetomidine over other anesthetic and analgesic agents include the absence of respiratory depression and protection against emergence agitation.

16. **How can the hourly fluid requirements for children be calculated on a per weight basis?**

The 4/2/1 rule can be used to estimate the maintenance fluid rate (4 mL/kg/h for the first 10 kg of a child's weight, plus 2 mL/kg/h for the second 10 kg, plus 1 mL/kg/h for the remainder of the child's weight). This does not include ongoing losses (i.e. evaporative loss from open wounds) or states that increase baseline requirements (i.e. fever). A more accurate assessment can be obtained by taking daily maintenance fluid required to be 2 L/m^2 surface area/day to determine an hourly administration rate.

17. **Which patients require perioperative dextrose supplementation to prevent hypoglycemia?**

Patients at an increased risk for perioperative hypoglycaemia include neonates and infants, those receiving hyperalimentation, and those with endocrine disorders [7]. Due to decreased liver stores, very young patients are at risk of perioperative hypoglycaemia. Neonates should receive an isotonic dextrose-containing solution, with glucose administered at 4–8 mg/kg/min. Patients receiving total parenteral nutrition should either have it continued or receive glucose-containing solutions. Otherwise healthy children do not require routine dextrose supplementation, except with prolonged periods of NPO.

18. **How should postoperative pain be managed in patients undergoing pyloromyotomy?**

Patients with pyloric stenosis are at increased risk of postoperative apnea, in addition to pre-existing apnea risk given their typically young age. The analgesic plan for such patients should therefore minimize any respiratory depressants such as opioids. A multi-modal opioid-sparing approach including infiltration of local anesthetic and acetaminophen is well tolerated (equivalently for open and laparoscopic approaches).

19. **Are there potential consequences of spinal or epidural anesthesia in neonates?**

Spinal anesthesia is an alternative to general anesthesia for procedures below the umbilicus. This technique can also avoid concerning respiratory complications related to induction of general anesthesia. Because neonates have an immature sympathetic nervous system, a spinal anesthetic causes no or minimal hypotension. There is no evidence that neonates have any increased risk of complications from a spinal anesthetic, but do require a lower dose of the local anesthetic.

20. **What are the benefits of regional anesthesia for treating pain in children?**

Regional anesthesia is effective as an analgesic technique, and can minimize or eliminate the need for opioids, minimizing many potential side effects of opioid use. Nerve blockade can prevent the cellular changes that can lead to chronic pain. Other reported benefits include improved respiratory function, earlier return of bowel function, and earlier ambulation.

21. **What are regional anesthetic techniques that could be considered for the following procedures?**

    a. Laparotomy
    b. Thoracotomy
    c. Inguinal hernia
    d. Circumcision

        a. Low thoracic epidural, transversus abdominis plane block for lower incisions, rectus sheath block for higher incisions, or paravertebral block.
        b. High-mid thoracic epidural, serratus anterior plane, erector spinae plane, intercostal nerve, or paravertebral block.
        c. Inguinal (Ilioinguinal and iliohypogastric nerve), or caudal block.
        d. Penile, pudendal, or caudal block.

References

1. World Health Association. Global guidelines for the prevention of surgical site infection. J Hosp Infect. 2016:184. doi:10.1016/j.jhin.2016.12.016
2. Smith I, Kranke P, Murat I, et al. Perioperative fasting in adults and children. Eur J Anaesthesiol. 2011;28(8):556–69. https://doi.org/10.1097/EJA.0b013e3283495ba1.
3. Practice Guidelines for Preoperative Fasting and the Use of Pharmacologic Agents to Reduce the Risk of Pulmonary Aspiration: Application to Healthy Patients Undergoing Elective Procedures. Anesthesiology. 2011;114(3):495–511. doi:10.1097/ALN.0b013e3181fcbfd9
4. Habre W, Disma N, Virag K, et al. Incidence of severe critical events in paediatric anaesthesia (APRICOT): a prospective multicentre observational study in 261 hospitals in Europe. Lancet Respir Med. 2017;5(5):412–25. https://doi.org/10.1016/S2213-2600(17)30116-9.
5. McCann ME, Berde C, Soriano S, et al. Neurodevelopmental outcome at 5 years of age after general anaesthesia or awake-regional anaesthesia in infancy (GAS): an international,

multicentre, randomised, controlled equivalence trial. Lancet. 2019;393(10172):664–77. https://doi.org/10.1016/S0140-6736(18)32485-1.
6. Walker BJ, Long JB, Sathyamoorthy M, et al. Complications in pediatric regional anesthesia. Anesthesiology. 2018;129(4):721–32. https://doi.org/10.1097/ALN.0000000000002372.
7. Bailey AG, Mcnaull PP, Jooste E, Tuchman JB. Perioperative crystalloid and colloid fluid management in children: where are we and how did we get here? Anesth Analg. 2010;110(2):375–90. https://doi.org/10.1213/ANE.0b013e3181b6b3b5.

Chapter 71
Fetal Surgery

Seyed Arshia Arshad and KuoJen Tsao

Abstract Antenatal surgical intervention, also known as maternal-fetal surgery, is one of the more recently expanding areas in the field of pediatric surgery. With a stalemate in the advances of post-natal interventions for conditions such as congenital diaphragmatic hernia (CDH), twin-twin transfusion syndrome (TTTS), congenital pulmonary malformations, myelomeningocele, and others, surgeons have looked to the antenatal period for opportunities for early intervention. Traditionally, maternal-fetal surgery was limited to conditions which portended antenatal or neonatal demise. However, with the advancement of surgical technology and our understanding of these conditions, as well as minimizing the maternal risks, antenatal surgery has evolved to ameliorate post-natal morbidity.

Keywords Maternal–Fetal Surgery ·
Congenital Diaphragmatic Hernia (CDH) ·
Fetoscopic Endoluminal Tracheal Occlusion (FETO) ·
Ex utero Intrapartum Treatment (EXIT) ·
Twin-Twin Transfusion Syndrome (TTTS) ·
Selective Fetoscopic Laser Ablation (SFLP) ·
Congenital Pulmonary Airway Malformation (CPAM) ·
Myelomeningocele (MMC) Repair

S. A. Arshad · K. Tsao (✉)
Department of Pediatric Surgery, McGovern Medical School at The University of Texas Health Science Center at Houston (UTHealth), Houston, TX, USA
e-mail: KuoJen.Tsao@uth.tmc.edu

M. Lacher et al. (eds.), *Pearls and Tricks in Pediatric Surgery*,
https://doi.org/10.1007/978-3-030-51067-1_71

Questions

1. **What is maternal-fetal surgery**?

Surgical interventions performed on a fetus, ie: during the antenatal period, by way of ultrasound guided needle-based, fetoscopic, or open hysterotomy techniques.

2. **Who performs maternal-fetal surgery**?

   a. A multi-disciplinary team including a core of maternal fetal medicine, obstetrics, pediatric surgery, neonatology, adult and neonatal anesthesiology, as well as operation-specific specialists such as pediatric cardiology, pediatric otolaryngology, pediatric cardiothoracic surgery, and pediatric neurosurgery.
   b. Since surgery is being performed on the mother and fetus simultaneously, there are often multiple operating teams (each team employing anesthesiologists, surgeons, circulating nurses and scrub techs). There are additional teams and operating rooms on standby depending on the type of surgery and viability of the fetus.

3. **When was the first maternal-fetal surgery performed**?

First performed by Dr. Michal Harrison at the University of California in San Francisco in 1981. His team performed an *in utero* vesicostomy for a fetus with congenital hydronephrosis secondary to posterior urethral valves[1].

4. **What are the most common procedures performed in maternal-fetal surgery? What are the indications for these procedures?**

   a. Needle-based

      i. Umbilical cord coagulation (by radiofrequency ablation (RFA), bipolar or interstitial laser)

         1. Twin Reversed Arterial Perfusion (TRAP)
         2. Selective Fetal Intrauterine Growth Restriction (sIUGR)

      ii. Single-needle thoracentesis, thoracoamniotic shunt

         1. Congenital Pulmonary Airway Malformation (CPAM)
         2. Bronchopulmonary Sequestration (BPS) (Rare requirement)
         3. Congenital Lobar Emphysema (CLE) (Rare requirement)
         4. Bronchogenic Cysts (Rare requirement)

   b. Fetoscopic

      i. Selective Fetoscopic Laser Ablation (SFLP)

         1. Twin-to-Twin Transfusion Syndrome (TTTS)
         2. Twin Anemia Polycythemia Sequence (TAPS)

3. Selective Fetal Intrauterine Growth Restriction (sIUGR)

ii. Release of amniotic bands
iii. Fetoscopic Endoluminal Tracheal Occlusion (FETO)—experimental

1. Congenital Diaphragmatic Hernia (CDH)

iv. Myelomeningocele (MMC)—experimental

c. Open hysterotomy

i. Myelomeningocele (MMC) Repair
ii. Sacrococcygeal Teratoma (SCT) Resection
iii. Treatment of Fetal lung lesions

d. Ex Utero Intrapartum Treatment (EXIT) Procedures

i. EXIT-to-airway: Congenital High Airway Obstruction Syndrome (CHAOS), severe micrognathia, obstructing mass, retained tracheal balloon (from FETO)
ii. EXIT-to-Resection: large head, neck, thoracic (Congenital Pulmonary Airway Malformation (CPAM)), or mediastinal mass
iii. EXIT-to-ECMO: Cardiothoracic anomaly or severe CDH—Very rare
iv. EXIT-to-Separation: Conjoined twins—Very Rare

5. **What is the rate of maternal risk associated with maternal–fetal interventions?**

Overall complication rate of 6.2% in fetoscopic surgeries and 20.9% open fetal surgeries. Serious complication rate of 1.7% in fetoscopic surgeries and 4.5% in open fetal surgeries (From meta-analysis of 166 studies) [2]. The complication rates are dependent on the exact method employed.

6. **What is the fetal intervention for severe CDH?**

Fetoscopic Endoluminal Tracheal Occlusion (FETO); this is currently in clinical trials.

7. **How is Lung-to-head ratio (LHR) obtained?**

The area of the lung contralateral to the diaphragmatic defect divided by the head circumference. These measurements are obtained by ultrasound and only valid from gestational age 22–28 weeks [3]. These measurements are dependent on the time during gestation they were obtained, therefore the observed to expected lung-to-head ratio (o/e LHR) is more often used throughout the gestation [4].

8. **What findings on prenatal ultrasound portend a poor outcome**?

Lower o/e LHR, increasing percentage of intrathoracic liver, decreasing total fetal lung volume [3].

9. **What are the selection criteria for which patient should undergo Fetoscopic Endoluminal Tracheal Occlusion (FETO)?**

   a. Still undergoing clinical trials. Different centers use different criteria (some use o/e LHR while others use LHR with or without position of the liver)
   b. The largest ongoing study is the Tracheal Occlusion To Accelerate Lung Growth (TOTAL) Trial [5]:

      i. Moderate risk: o/e LHR of 25–34.9% regardless of liver position OR o/e LHR of 35–44.9% with liver in the chest measured at the latest at 32 weeks and 5 days
      ii. Severe risk: o/e LHR < 25% measured at the latest at 29 weeks and 5 days

10. **When is the tracheal occlusion device in Fetoscopic Endoluminal Tracheal Occlusion (FETO) placed? Removed? Why?**

    a. Placement: 27 0/7 – 29 5/7 weeks' gestation [6]
    b. Removal: 34 0/7 and 34 6/7 weeks [6]
    c. Prenatal removal allows for maturation of type 2 pneumocytes and surfactant production and has been associated with improved neonatal outcomes [7].

11. **How does FETO improve CDH patient survival?**

Theorized to be secondary to the accumulation of fluid produced by the lung, now trapped within the lung, increases the intrapulmonary pressure and therefore stimulating pulmonary hyperplasia/growth [6].

12. **How is FETO performed?**

    a. Under ultrasound guidance the fetus is positioned so that the oropharynx can be accessed through the upper half of the uterus. A 10Fr trocar is inserted through the abdominal wall and uterus and a 1.2mm fetoscope is advanced to perform fetoscopy. Using a combination of ultrasound and fetoscopic visualization, the fetoscope is advanced through the fetal oropharynx making use of the tongue and uvula as anatomic landmarks. The fetoscope is advanced into the trachea to the level of the carina to confirm positioning. A preloaded balloon is advanced through the second working channel of the scope and is inflated and deployed in the trachea [6].
    b. The balloon can be removed by fetoscopy, ultrasound-guided puncture, or if emergent during EXIT procedure [6].

13. **What is an EXIT procedure? What are the goals in an EXIT procedure?**

    a. EXIT: Ex Utero Intrapartum Treatment
    b. To establish airway and/or cardiopulmonary stability (intubation, tracheostomy, neck mass resection with tracheostomy)

14. **How is an EXIT procedure performed?**

While maintaining uterine relaxation, and placental support, a planned partial delivery of the fetus is performed through a hysterotomy. The lower body is kept within the amniotic sac to maintain uterine volume (to prevent premature contraction) and prevent heat loss. This partial delivery allows for establishing neonatal cardiopulmonary support and access for interventions as described above in question 5 [8].

15. **What is the major risk to a mother during an EXIT procedure?**

The major risk to the mother during an EXIT procedure is uterine hemorrhage. Average estimated blood loss is >1 L. The risk of uterine hemorrhage is greater than that for standard cesarean section secondary to prolonged uterine relaxation, larger hysterotomy, and higher likelihood of placental abruption and laceration [8].

16. **What type of multigestational pregnancies are prone to fetal syndromes? What are these syndromes?**

    a. Monochorionic pregnancy (single shared placenta) [9]
    b. Twin-Twin Transfusion Syndrome (TTTS), Twin Reversed Arterial Perfusion (TRAP) sequence, Twin Anemia Polycythemia Sequence (TAPS), and selective Fetal Intrauterine Growth Restriction (sIUGR)

17. **What is the pathophysiology of these syndromes in multigestational pregnancies?**

Between fetuses in a monochorionic (single placenta) gestation, there exists vascular communications across the shared placenta. If there is unequal placental sharing or unbalanced flow of blood between the fetuses, these syndromes can occur [9, 10].

18. **What is the selection criteria for a patient who should undergo SFLP for TTTS?**

    a. Quintero Stage II and greater TTTS. There is currently a clinical trial evaluating use in Stage I [11].
    b. The Quintero staging system describes the severity of TTTS; in summary [10]:

        i. I: Bladder visualized in both fetuses and no fetal distress
        ii. II: Bladder not visualized in donor after 60 min; Donor considered to have severe oligohydramnios/anhydramnios.
        iii. III: Critically abnormal doppler study: Absent or reversed umbilical artery end-diastolic flow, reversal of ductus venosus a-wave, or pulsatile umbilical vein flow.
        iv. IV: Ascites or hydrops in either twin
        v. V: Death of either twin.

19. **How is selective fetoscopic laser ablation (SFLP) performed?**

Similar to FETO, after proper anesthesia, a port is placed under ultrasound guidance through the maternal abdominal wall, myometrium, and into the amniotic sac. The port has 3 operating channels (one for the fetoscope, a fluid exchange port, and one for the laser diode). Mapping of the placental surface vasculature is then performed (each vessel is followed to its cord insertion site to ensure it is not a paired vessel). The laser fiber is utilized for ablation. "Solominzation" (ablating a thin line of placental tissue along the entire length of the vascular equator) is then performed to reduce the chance of recannulation. An amnioreduction is then performed [12].

20. **What are some limitations of selective fetoscopic laser ablation (SFLP) ?**

There may be missed anastomoses (vascular connections), deep vessels unable to be visualized, and treated vessels that can recannulize.

21. **What are the risks associated with fetalpulmonary lesions, such as CPAM?**

External compression, pulmonary hypoplasia, vena caval compression, heart failure, hydrops fetalis [13]

22. **What are the indications for fetal intervention for CPAM?s**

For microcystic CPAM not responsive to maternal corticosteroids, large macrocystic lesions not responsive to shunting/drainage, and evidence of impending fetal demise (ie: heart failure on echocardiography) [13]

23. **The criteria to qualify for open MMC repair is based on? What are the criteria?**

    a. The Management of Myelomeningocele Study (MOMS) [14]

        i. Inclusion criteria: Singleton pregnancy, MMC no higher than T1 or lower than S1, hindbrain herniation, gestation age of 19 weeks 0/7 days to 25 weeks 6/7 days, normal karyotype, maternal age > 18
        ii. Exclusion criteria: fetal anomaly unrelated to MMC, severe kyphosis, risk of preterm birth (ie: short cervix or history of preterm birth), placental abruption, BMI $\geq$ 35, placenta previa, contraindications to surgery (ie: previous hysterotomy in location where hysterotomy will be required for MMC repair).

24. **What are the benefits of prenatal Myelomeningocele (MMC) repair (as compared to post-natal repair)?**

    a. Theorized to decrease trauma to an exposed cord (by providing coverage prior to birth) [14]

b. Studies have shown less hindbrain herniation (64% in prenatal repairs, compared to 96% in postnatal repairs at 12 months), decreased severity of herniation, decreased need for ventriculoperitoneal (VP) shunt placement (72% compared to 93%), improved motor function (37.9% had 1 or more anatomic levels of improvement by motor function as compared to what would be expected for the level of defect vs. 19.5%) [14]

References

1. Harrison MR, Golbus MS, Filly RA, et al. Fetal surgery for congenital hydronephrosis. N Engl J Med. 1982;306(10):591–3. https://doi.org/10.1056/NEJM198203113061006.
2. Sacco A, Van der Veeken L, Bagshaw E, et al. Maternal complications following open and fetoscopic fetal surgery: a systematic review and meta-analysis. Prenat Diagn. 2019;39(4):251–68. https://doi.org/10.1002/pd.5421.
3. Oluyomi-Obi T, Kuret V, Puligandla P, et al. Antenatal predictors of outcome in prenatally diagnosed congenital diaphragmatic hernia (CDH). J Pediatr Surg. 2017;52(5):881–8. https://doi.org/10.1016/j.jpedsurg.2016.12.008.
4. Jani J, Nicolaides KH, Keller RL, et al. Observed to expected lung area to head circumference ratio in the prediction of survival in fetuses with isolated diaphragmatic hernia. Ultrasound Obstet Gynecol. 2007;30(1):67–71. https://doi.org/10.1002/uog.4052.
5. Home—TOTALtrial. https://totaltrial.eu. Accessed July 31, 2019.
6. Deprest J, Nicolaides K, Done' E, et al. Technical aspects of fetal endoscopic tracheal occlusion for congenital diaphragmatic hernia. J Pediatr Surg. 2011;46(1):22–32. https://doi.org/10.1016/j.jpedsurg.2010.10.008.
7. Flageole H, Evrard VA, Piedboeuf B, Laberge JM, Lerut TE, Deprest JA. The plug-unplug sequence: an important step to achieve type II pneumocyte maturation in the fetal lamb model. J Pediatr Surg. 1998;33(2):299–303. https://doi.org/10.1016/s0022-3468(98)90451-1.
8. Moldenhauer JS. Ex Utero Intrapartum Therapy. Semin Pediatr Surg. 2013;22(1):44–9. https://doi.org/10.1053/j.sempedsurg.2012.10.008.
9. Lewi L, Jani J, Blickstein I, et al. The outcome of monochorionic diamniotic twin gestations in the era of invasive fetal therapy: a prospective cohort study. Am J Obstet Gynecol. 2008;199(5):514.e1-514.e8. https://doi.org/10.1016/j.ajog.2008.03.050.
10. Quintero RA, Ishii K, Chmait RH, Bornick PW, Allen MH, Kontopoulos EV. Sequential selective laser photocoagulation of communicating vessels in twin-twin transfusion syndrome. J Matern Neonatal Med. 2007;20(10):763–8. https://doi.org/10.1080/14767050701591827.
11. Ville Y. Randomized Controlled Trial Comparing a Conservative Management and Laser Surgery (TTTS1). https://clinicaltrials.gov/ct2/show/NCT01220011. Published 2013. Accessed July 31, 2019.
12. Quintero RA, Morales WJ, Mendoza G, et al. Selective photocoagulation of placental vessels in twin-twin transfusion syndrome: evolution of a surgical technique. Obstet Gynecol Surv. 1998;53(12 Suppl):S97–103. https://www.ncbi.nlm.nih.gov/pubmed/9870237. Accessed July 31, 2019.
13. Khalek N, Johnson MP. Management of prenatally diagnosed lung lesions. Semin Pediatr Surg. 2013;22(1):24–9. https://doi.org/10.1053/j.sempedsurg.2012.10.005.
14. Adzick NS, Thom EA, Spong CY, et al. A Randomized Trial of Prenatal versus Postnatal Repair of Myelomeningocele. N Engl J Med. 2011;364(11):993–1004. https://doi.org/10.1056/NEJMoa1014379.

Chapter 72
How to Become a Pediatric Surgeon?

Sara Mahler and Oliver J. Muenster

Abstract As thc titlc of this chapter already suggests, in this chapter the path of how become a pediatric surgeon is described and important question on this issue are answered. These questions are all dealing with the process and the structure of pediatric surgery training and the requirements which are necessary to become a pediatric surgeon. In preparation of this book chapter, we performed an online survey about the organization and structure of pediatric surgery training around the world. The survey was sent to all official national admissions departments and organizations of pediatric surgery. Thus, data from 28 different countries were compiled. They serve as the basis of some of the questions and answers below. Our survey and this chapter intend to present an international overview of the training modalities in pediatric surgery to the readership.

Keywords Pediatric surgery · Training · Requirements · Organization · Applying

72.1 Introduction

In preparation of this book chapter we performed an online survey about the organization and structure of pediatric surgery training around the world. The survey was sent to all official national admissions departments and organizations of pediatric surgery. Thus, data from 28 different countries were compiled. They serve as the basis of some of the questions and answers below. The intention of

S. Mahler · O. J. Muensterer (✉)
Department of Pediatric Surgery, University Medical Center of the Johannes Gutenberg University Mainz, Langenbeckstrasse 1, 55131 Mainz, Germany
e-mail: oliver.muensterer@unimedizin-mainz.de

S. Mahler
e-mail: sara.mahler@unimedizin-mainz.de

M. Lacher et al. (eds.), *Pearls and Tricks in Pediatric Surgery*,
https://doi.org/10.1007/978-3-030-51067-1_72

our survey and this chapter is to present an international overview of the training modalities in pediatric surgery to the readership.

1. **What is a pediatric surgeon?**

A pediatric surgeon is a specialist in the operative treatment of children. Some pediatric surgeons also manage congenital anomalies in fetuses before birth, and some also care for adults with specific congenital anomalies when an appropriate adult specialist is not available. However, a pediatric surgeon covers much more than just the operative treatment of children: They are involved in the prenatal, postnatal, pre- and postoperative management of children. As specialists, they are responsible for finding the diagnosis and for the decision on the necessity for operations in children. The spectrum of pediatric surgery is wide and includes a variety of different subspecialties. The scope may differ from country to country, and among practitioners.

2. **How long does it take to become a pediatric surgeon?**

The path to becoming a pediatric surgeon in most places takes at least 5 years or more in specialty training. Depending on the country, it might be necessary to train in general surgery first, before commencing pediatric surgery. Nevertheless, pediatric surgery is recognized as its own specialty in most countries all over the world. In almost all of these countries, a final exam must be completed successfully before becoming certified and beginning self-responsible practice.

3. **What kind of operations/procedures are performed by pediatric surgeons?**

Pediatric surgery is a very versatile specialty. One of the most important fields in pediatric surgery is the management and treatment of children with congenital malformations, such as esophageal atresia, congenital diaphragmatic hernia, anorectal malformations, bowel atresia, gastroschisis and omphalocele, but pediatric surgeons cover many more indications and procedures in children: Other types of neonatal surgery, thoracic surgery, oncological surgery, the management of multiple trauma, transplant surgery, hepatobiliary surgery, plastic and reconstructive surgery, management of burns, some neurosurgery, management of child abuse, vascular birth marks, as well as general pediatric surgery such as appendicitis or intussusception, surgery of hernias, gastro-esophageal reflux disease, and many more.

Pediatric surgeons not only perform operations but are inherently involved in the management of the child with surgical disease as well. In this function, pediatric surgeons often attend their patients from the intrauterine period until adulthood. In specific situations and cases, they are the only ones who have the perspective to overlook the complex situation of a patient and coordinate between different physicians that cooperate in treating a particular patient, up into adulthood.

4. **What is the training like to be a pediatric surgeon?**

The training curriculum in pediatric surgery depends on the country in which you live and practice [1]. Several countries require experience of at least 5 years or more in general surgery or even a full certification in general surgery (for example United States, Canada, United Kingdom, Uzbekistan, Belgium, Netherlands). Other countries (for example Egypt, Russia, Ukraine, Syria, Germany, Pakistan, South Africa) do not require obligatory experience in general surgery, but in most of them, a certain experience in another specialty is necessary for applying.
After finishing all formal training requirements (most countries require a defined number of operations per trainee), a final exit examination (mostly oral and written) must be completed successfully before receiving certification.
Over the last decades, an increasing number of training programs have been established in the United States and elsewhere [2]. This is in part because working rules in the United States and Europe has made call coverage possible only with an increasing number of trainees. There is some concern that the number of index cases by each trainee will thus decrease in the future, and indeed, a recent analysis has highlighted this trend [3, 4]. There are certain challenges that young pediatric surgery trainees, and females face in particular that can be reviewed in depth in the quoted references [5, 6].

5. **When should you apply for pediatric surgery training?**

To answer this question, young applicants should keep in mind that requirements may vary with location and change with time. Therefore, it is important that candidates inform themselves at their respective certification agency in due time. For example, in some countries like Spain, a formal selection exam is held to select young trainees for postgraduate training, whereas others select their applicants throughout interviews at the individual institutions in combination with references and letters of recommendation. The preparation for this process can be quite time-consuming. Because in most countries pediatric surgery is highly competitive, it is useful to start the process of gathering information and making contact to persons in the field as soon as the decision to become a pediatric surgeon has been made. Furthermore, it is probably a good idea to think about possible alternatives or about options for bridging the time until acceptance into a training program, which may take as long as 1–2 years.

6. **What requirements are necessary? (examples by country)**

   - Graduation from medical school (as the only formal prerequisite):

     Spain, Germany, Russia, Uzbekistan*, Ukraine, Austria, North Macedonia.

   - Fully accreditation in general surgery:

     India, Japan, Ghana, Kenya, USA, Canada, Belgium*, Netherlands*

– Expert interviews and/ or formal selection examination:

UK, USA, Liberia.

Some countries require recertification after a certain amount of time (for example, every 10 years in the United States) or some form of continuous medical education.

*= countries without recognition of pediatric surgery as an independent specialty

Most other countries require experience in other specialties, most often 2-3 years in general surgery and sometimes a defined time in pediatrics or pediatric intensive care.

7. **Who should write letters of recommendation?**

Letters of recommendation are usually written by the head of the department where you are known, have worked, trained or performed elective rotations during your time in medical school or postgraduate training. Also, research mentors are good resources for letters of recommendation. The format of letters varies considerably. In Germany, for example, it is custom that the candidates themselves provide the letters of recommendation openly along with their application. In other countries, such as the United States, the letters are sent directly from the author to the institution that you applied to. Standard letters will cover how long the author knows you, your experience at that department, your strengths, your weaknesses, and your social skills. It usually wraps up by a perspective of how the author expects you to perform in the new environment or concludes with personal wishes. As a rule, the more strong letters of recommendation you can supply, the better your chances. However, some programs have limits of their number, and then the potentially strongest letters should be selected and solicited.

8. **Does previous research and/or clinical experience affect my chance of acceptance?**

Yes, without a doubt, both previous research and/or clinical experience remains a great advantage when applying for a program in pediatric surgery. Even if the department or institution in which you gained your experience is not strictly related to the field of pediatric surgery, it will improve your chances by characterizing your background. You should ask for letters of recommendation from any research or clinical mentor you encounter during your career.
One study showed that doing a bridging pediatric surgical subspecialty fellowship such as research, intensive care, extra corporeal life support (ECMO), or minimal invasive surgery (MIS) actually helped candidates obtain a pediatric surgical training position [2].

9. **Is research an obligatory part of the training in pediatric surgery?**

Although research is mostly not obligatory in most pediatric surgery training curricula around the world, it has become a voluntary part of training to bridge waiting periods until acceptance, or to boost one´s chances of being selected. In our survey, at least 8 out of 28 countries named research an obligatory part in the training schedule. Most academical centers offer a certain amount of time to focus on research, in the form of so-called research fellowships.

10. **How many active pediatric surgeons currently work per capita in different countries?**

The density of pediatric surgeons shows wide variation. Currently, in Germany 640 accredited pediatric surgeons take care of a population of about 82 million (about 1 pediatric surgeon per 128,000 inhabitants). According to our survey, the numbers differ widely, spanning from roundabout 10 pediatric surgeons per country, for example in Ireland, Pakistan and Syria up (less than 1 pediatric surgeon for half a million inhabitants) to 200-300 in Spain, Italy and Greece, for example. Overall, there seems to be a high variability in pediatric surgeon density worldwide, with a significant shortage in countries that are poor or have a high birth rate [3].

11. **What qualities are programs looking for in an applicant?**

Working with children is challenging and requires special character traits. As a pediatric surgeon, you need a high degree of empathy and patience, a great amount of manual skills, you should be willing to work hard and be ready to spend a lot of time in the hospital, along with a strong interest to learn.

12. **Do most of the Pediatric Surgeons work in academic or nonacademic centers?**

In the recent literature, European children have an average of a pediatric surgery center for every 177,000 children. Quite a high number of these centers are academic or are affiliated with an academic center [4]. On the website of the "Deutsche Gesellschaft für Kinderchirurgie", the German pediatric surgeon's association, 31 out of 88 centers for pediatric surgery in Germany academic and therefore located at a university medical centers (35%) [4, 6].

13. **Are there standardized diplomas in Pediatric Surgery?**

Most countries issue a certificate of completion of pediatric surgical specialty training after meeting the respective specific requirements. The American Board of Surgery (ABS) certifies candidates within the United States and Canada but does not certify any outside candidates. The European Board of pediatric Surgery (EBPS) established a 2-part examination process that can be taken by candidates from Europe and other countries beyond. It affords the title "Fellow of the European Board of pediatric surgery" (FEBPS) upon successful completion. While it serves as a benchmark for quality and competency, it is currently recognized legally only by few countries. Most also require obtaining a national certificate as well. In the European Union however, all pediatric surgery diplomas are recognized mutually among nations. In our survey, select other international diplomas were recognized in only about half of the responding countries.

References

1. Driller C, Holschneider AM. Training in pediatric surgery—a comparison of 24 countries in Europe and other countries around the world. Eur J Pediatr Surg. 2003;13(2):73–80.
2. Derderian SC, Benge MJ, Karrer FM, Acker SN, Roach JP. Filling the gap: objective data to guide pediatric surgery applicants who do not match on the first attempt. J Pediatr Surg. 2019.
3. Lalchandani P, Dunn JC. Global comparison of pediatric surgery workforce and training. J Pediatr Surg. 2015;50(7):1180–3.
4. Parigi GB, Czauderna P, Rolle U, Zachariou Z. European census on pediatric surgery. Eur J Pediatr Surg. 2018;28(3):227–37.
5. Optimal resources for children's surgical care. Executive Summary. World J Surg. 2019;43(4):978–80.
6. Deutsche Gesellschaft für Kinderchirurgie e.V. (DGKCH). https://www.dgkch.de/.

Chapter 73
Evidence Based Medicine Concepts/Clinical Research

Peter C. Minneci and Katherine J. Deans

Abstract Clinical research provides evidence to help guide patient care. Evidence based medicine is using the best available clinical research to guide treatment decisions. This chapter provides an overview of concepts related to clinical research and evidence-based medicine relevant to pediatric surgery.

Keywords Clinical research · Evidence-based medicine · Clinical trial · Randomized trial · Pragmatic trial · Levels of evidence

1. **What is evidenced-based medicine?**

Evidence-based medicine is the use of the best available evidence from research to make treatment decisions for the care of individual patients. It integrates clinical experience and patient values with the best available research to answer clinical questions.

2. **What is clinical research, outcomes research, and comparative effectiveness research (CER)?**

Clinical research is any investigation that looks at a disease process and reports characteristics about the disease or outcomes. Outcomes research focuses on

P. C. Minneci (✉) · K. J. Deans
Professor of Surgery and Pediatrics, The Ohio State University College of Medicine, Columbus, USA
e-mail: Peter.minneci@nationwidechildrens.org

P. C. Minneci · K. J. Deans
Center for Surgical Outcomes Research, Abigail Wexner Research Institute and Department of Surgery, Nationwide Children's Hospital, 611 Livingston Ave, FOB 3A.3, Columbus, OH, USA

M. Lacher et al. (eds.), *Pearls and Tricks in Pediatric Surgery*,
https://doi.org/10.1007/978-3-030-51067-1_73

studying outcomes from a disease. CER compares specific treatments for a disease to determine differences in outcomes.

3. **What are case series and their strengths and weaknesses?**

Case series are retrospective reviews of institutional experiences and they make up a large portion of the pediatric surgical literature as many of the diseases we treat are rare and not amenable to prospective trials. These studies have inherent biases as they are retrospective and usually represent either a single surgeon/center experience with limited generalizability.

4. **What are case-control studies and their strengths and weaknesses?**

Case-control studies represent retrospective comparative research that compares the effectiveness of two treatments on outcomes. These studies are oftentimes the only available comparative data for disease treatments. These studies are subject to selection bias and limited generalizability.

5. **What is health services research (HSR)?**

HSR examines access, costs, quality, delivery, organization, financing, and outcomes of healthcare. HSR can include descriptive studies of cohorts of with a specific disease; longitudinal natural history studies, resource utilization studies, studies of practice variation across institutions; benchmarking studies comparing rates of specific procedures, outcomes, or complications across institutions; or comparative effectiveness studies.

6. **What are the strengths and weaknesses of administrative database studies?** [1]

Administrative databases are aggregated healthcare billing records from payers or healthcare providers across hospitals, regions, or states. Advantages include their large size, greater generalizability, and potential use for longitudinal analysis (with specific datasets). Limitations include lack of clinical granularity due to poor specificity of ICD-9, ICD-10, and CPT coding and varying levels of reliability with different rates of misclassification of variables and missing data.

7. **What are clinical registries?** [2]

Clinical registries contain data on patients with specific diagnoses or procedures. Registries vary in their data collection methods and elements, accessibility to researchers at non-participating institutions, and cross-sectional versus longitudinal design.

8. **What are prospective observational studies?**

Prospective observational studies follow specific patient populations over time with specific inclusion criteria and collection of defined clinical and outcome variables. These studies are less biased but are limited to establishing associations between variables or treatments and outcomes.

9. **What is a clinical trial?** [3]

According to the National Institutes of Health, a clinical trial is a research study in which human subjects are prospectively assigned to one or more interventions to evaluate the effects of those interventions on health-related biomedical or behavioral outcomes. They test a pre-specified hypothesis in specified number of patients to have sufficient statistical power to detect the proposed treatment difference.

10. **What are the phases of clinical trials evaluating a new treatment or intervention?** [3]

Phase I trials test a potential therapy for the first time in humans to establish its safety, determine a safe dosage range, and identify side effects. Phase II trials more comprehensively evaluate a treatment's safety and begin to establish efficacy. Phase III trials attempt to confirm a treatment's efficacy against the current standard treatments, monitor for adverse effects, and establish effectiveness if large enough. Phase IV trials are performed after a treatment has received FDA approval; they evaluate long-term side effects and establish effectiveness of treatments in clinical practice outside the controlled trial setting.

11. **What are the key components of a clinical trial?** [3]

A specific study question; well-defined patient population with specific inclusion and exclusion criteria; clearly defined treatment groups with a single intervention group and a single control group; a specified method of treatment allocation (e.g. randomization, cluster randomization, patient choice); primary and secondary outcomes defined a priori with a power analysis and sample size estimation based on the primary outcome; and a pre-specified analytic plan.

12. **What type of control group should a clinical trial have?** [3]

The control group should reflect the best accepted "standard of care". Placebo controls should be used if there is no accepted standard treatment in clinical practice; this allows for blinding. An active control group is when control patients receive the standard of care. In many surgical trials, a placebo (sham operation) is impossible, and the study group allocation may have to be unblinded.

13. **How does the definition of the study population affect a clinical trial?** [3]

A study population in a trial can be either homogeneous or heterogeneous. More homogenous populations have less variability on covariates and allow for smaller sample sizes to detect a treatment effect. However, homogeneity may limit the generalizability of the results. A more heterogeneous study population will facilitate generalizability but will require a larger sample size to detect a treatment effect.

14. **What is the difference between internal and external validity?**

Internal validity relates to how well a study controls for confounding such that inferences from the results about causal relationships are valid. External validity is the validity of generalizing the conclusions outside the context of the study. Stringent RCTs with homogeneous populations have high internal validity but may have limited external validity.

15. **What is the difference between an "efficacy" and an "effectiveness" trial?** [3]

Efficacy trials, also referred to as "explanatory" trials, are designed to test causal research hypotheses; they determine the effects of a treatment under ideal circumstances in relatively homogeneous patient populations. Effectiveness trials, also referred to as pragmatic trials, aim to generate results that can be used by clinicians to choose between treatments; they determine the effects of a treatment in conditions similar to usual care.

16. **What is a pragmatic trial?** [4]

Pragmatic clinical trials attempt to establish the relative effectiveness of two treatment strategies with the goal of generating results that can be implemented into every day practice in a diverse patient population. Their study protocols should be reflective of usual care and have broad inclusion criteria to enroll a representative patient population.

17. **What is a randomized controlled trial (RCT)?** [3]

The traditional "gold" standard of clinical evidence is the RCT which directly tests a treatment against a "control" and assigns treatment group using randomization.

18. **What are the major advantages of a RCT?**

Randomization can control for selection bias and the design allows for a direct causal link to be drawn between an intervention and changes in the primary outcome.

19. **What are the disadvantages of a RCT?**

RCTs require significant financial resources, may not be feasible for rare conditions, and may have limited generalizability of the results depending on the inclusion/exclusion criteria and what percentage of the eligible population enrolls. RCTs with homogeneous study populations or that enroll a minority of eligible patients may have limited external validity.

20. **What is a systematic review and meta-analysis?** [5]

Systematic reviews are literature reviews that report on the effectiveness of a therapy for a specific disease across available studies. These reviews can assess the consistency of the treatment effects across studies, evaluate why different trials had varying results, and when appropriate, meta-analysis can combine the results of the individual studies to provide an overall estimate of the treatment effect.

21. **What is an expert consensus guideline?**

A consensus guideline is typically developed by a group of national and international experts who review and grade the available literature and make varying levels of treatment recommendations based on the strength of evidence to support the recommendation.

22. **What are the levels of clinical evidence?**

There are multiple classification systems for the hierarchy of levels of evidence for each study type. Below is the system used by the Journal of Pediatric Surgery for treatment studies: Level I: RCT with adequate power and >80% follow-up; Level II: lesser quality/smaller RCTs, prospective comparative study; level III: case–control study, retrospective comparative study; Level IV: case series without comparison group; Level V: expert opinion.

23. **What is quality improvement (QI) and how does it differ from research?**

Research is an investigation to test a hypothesis to address a knowledge gap, whereas QI is a process of incorporating practices or interventions with established benefits in previous research into clinical care. QI aims to improve adoption of evidence-based "best practices" to reduce care variation and improve outcomes.

References

1. Harbaugh CM, Cooper JN. Administrative databases. Semin Pediatr Surg. 2018;27(6):353–60.
2. Hebal F, Hu YY, Raval MV. Research using clinical registries in children's surgical care. Semin Pediatr Surg. 2018;27(6):345–52.
3. Minneci PC, Deans KJ. Clinical trials. Semin Pediatr Surg. 2018;27(6):332–7.
4. Weinfurt K. What is a pragmatic clinical trial: definition of a pragmatic clinical trial. In: Rethinking clinical trials: a living textbook of pragmatic clinical trials. Bethesda, MD. NIH Health Care Systems Research Collaboratory. https://rethinkingclinicaltrials.org/chapters/pragmatic-clinical-trial/what-is-a-pragmatic-clinical-trial-2/. Updated November 30, 2018. 10.28929/090
5. Baird R. Systematic reviews and meta-analytic techniques. Semin Pediatr Surg. 2018;27(6):338–44.

Chapter 74
Short Bowel Syndrome

Annika Mutanen and Mikko P. Pakarinen

Abstract Pediatric short bowel syndrome (SBS) is an increasingly encountered complex and devastating condition in which the remaining intestine is unable to absorb adequate amounts of fluid and nutrients leading to intestinal failure and need for long-term parenteral support (PS). The goal of SBS treatment is to ascertain normal growth and development while pursuing enteral autonomy (weaning off PS) with individualized treatment strategies. Children with SBS are at risk for multiple complications such as intestinal failure associated liver disease (IFALD), recurrent septic episodes, central line complications, intestinal bacterial overgrowth, metabolic bone disease, impaired renal function, failure to thrive and increased mortality.

Keywords Adaptation · Bianchi · Central line · Intestinal failure · Intestinal transplantation · Liver disease · Parenteral nutrition · Sepsis · STEP

1. **What is short bowel syndrome?**

Short bowel syndrome (SBS) is defined as reduction of functional gut mass or length below the minimal amount necessary for adequate digestion and absorption to satisfy nutrient and fluid requirements for maintenance of normal growth and development in children.

2. **How is SBS classified?**

SBS is the most common cause for pediatric intestinal failure and results from surgical bowel resection for congenital or acquired gastrointestinal diseases or

A. Mutanen · M. P. Pakarinen (✉)
Children's Hospital, Stenbackinkatu 11, PL 281, 00029 HUS Helsinki, PL, Finland
e-mail: mikko.pakarinen@hus.fi

A. Mutanen
e-mail: annika.mutanen@hus.fi

M. Lacher et al. (eds.), *Pearls and Tricks in Pediatric Surgery*,
https://doi.org/10.1007/978-3-030-51067-1_74

congenitally short intestine. In addition, intestinal failure can be caused by disorders of gastrointestinal motility (e.g. intestinal pseudo-obstruction) and congenital enterocyte disorders (e.g. microvillus inclusion disease, tufting enteropathy, and others).

From functional point of view, SBS may be classified based on the remaining bowel anatomy: type (1) end-jejunostomy, type (2) jejuno-colic anastomosis after small bowel and partial colon resection, and type (3) jejuno-ileocolic anastomosis after small bowel resection with intact colon and some ileum preserved. Type 3 anatomy carries the best prognosis, followed by type 2 and type 1.

3. **What is the etiology of SBS?**

The most common underlying etiology of short bowel syndrome is necrotizing enterocolitis followed by volvulus, small bowel atresia, gastroschisis and total/near total aganglionosis (Hirschsprung disease). Approximately, 20% of pediatric short bowel syndrome develops after the neonatal period when volvulus and trauma are the leading etiologies while Crohn's disease and malignancies are less frequent.

4. **What is the incidence of pediatric SBS?**

According to a population-based study, the incidence of SBS is 24.5/100 000 live births [1]. The incidence of SBS is higher in premature and low birth weight infants as the incidence is 0.7% (7 per 1000) in very low birth weight infants and 1.1% (11 per 1000) among extremely low birth weight infants [2].

5. **What is the normal length of neonatal bowel?**

Neonatal bowel length depends on the gestational age. A term baby has approximately 200 cm of small bowel and 40–50 cm of colon while a baby born at 25 weeks of gestation has 70 cm of small bowel and 22 cm of colon.

6. **How much bowel grows in utero?**

During the last trimester, the small bowel and colon will double in length. Hence, outcome of a 25-week gestation baby with 30 cm of residual small bowel may be very different from a term baby with 30 cm of residual small bowel, because of greater potential of the bowel to grow in length as the premature baby matures.

7. **How much bowel grows after birth?**

The small and large bowel grow substantially after birth, since in a term baby the length of small bowel is approximately 200 cm and the length of colon is 40–50 cm compared to 450 cm of small bowel and 150 cm of colon in an adult.

8. **What bowel length is considered too short?**

In addition to the absolute length, the length of residual bowel should be also evaluated as percentage of expected for a particular age to account for the gestational age and growth potential of the remaining bowel. In general, <40 cm or 25% of remaining small intestine associates with a severe intestinal failure.

9. **Why does it matter which part of the bowel is remaining?**

The probability of weaning off PS is dependent on length, anatomy and functional state of the remaining bowel. Of patients with $>50\%$ of expected small bowel remaining, nearly all will wean off PS in 1–2 years regardless of how much colon is remaining. In patients with $<50\%$ of small bowel remaining, the colon has much more important role in approving absorption and chances for weaning off PS. Some patients with even less than 10% of expected small bowel length may be able to wean off PS in several years if they have $>50\%$ of colon remaining [3].
Even a short part of preserved ileum, ileocecal valve and colon improve function of the remaining bowel in short bowel patients in several ways. The remaining ileum is able to absorb water against concentration gradient, conjugated bile acids and vitamin B_{12}. In addition, the ileum is a major source of entero-endocrine hormones such as glucagon like peptide 1 and 2 and peptide YY, which promote intestinal absorptive function in multiple ways. Preserved colon absorbs significant amounts of water and electrolytes and increases intestinal energy salvage by metabolizing carbohydrates to short chain fatty acids. The ileocecal valve slows small intestinal transit and prevents colonization of the small intestine by colonic micro-organisms.

10. **What is meant by intestinal adaptation?**

After partial small intestinal resection, the process of intestinal adaptation is a compensatory process in the remaining bowel which undergoes structural and functional chances that gradually increase its absorptive capacity. Histologic hallmarks of adaptation are increased villus height and crypt depth, which are accompanied with macroscopic bowel lengthening and dilatation. Adaptation is promoted by several factors including enteral nutrition, intestinal microbiota, and mechanical factors. Of them oral feeding is the most crucial stimulus for intestinal adaptation.

11. **How long can adaptation continue?**

The most active period of adaptation takes place two years after intestinal resection, but it continues for more than five years and even longer [3].

12. **Are there pharmacological treatments for short bowel syndrome?**

Antisecretory agents (e.g. H_2 receptor blockers, Proton-pump inhibitors) may be used to reduce gastric hypersecretion and anti-motility agents (e.g. loperamide) to reduce rapid intestinal transit. Severe intestinal bacterial overgrowth may be treated with (cyclic) enteral antibiotics, although unnecessary use of antibiotics should be avoided to maintain healthy intestinal microbiota. Adaptation, including increased absorption of fluid and nutrients as well as mucosal growth, may be promoted with glucagon-like peptide 2 analogues.

13. **Are there any surgical options to enhance adaptation?**

Autologous reconstructive surgery in patients with SBS fall into several categories [4, 5]. These operations are designed to.

(1) Recruit the entire remaining intestine by closing diverting enterostomies and repairing strictures, blind loops or enteroenteric fistulas.
(2) Improve intestinal motility and function of dilated small intestinal loops by performing tapering enteroplasty, longitudinal intestinal lengthening and tailoring (LILT or Bianchi) or serial transverse enteroplasty (STEP). Length of the remaining small intestine also increases after LILT and STEP.
(3) Slow intestinal transit in the absence of bowel dilatation by segmental reversal of small bowel or isoperistaltic colonic interposition.
(4) Increase mucosal surface area by controlled tissue expansion followed by STEP or LILT.

14. **What is the STEP procedure?**

Serial transverse enteroplasty (STEP) was first described by Kim in 2003. In this procedure, intestinal tapering and lengthening is accomplished without any loss of surface area and with minimal mesenterial dissection.

15. **Who is a candidate for the STEP procedure?**

STEP procedure may be considered for a SBS patient with imaging proved segmental bowel dilatation with poor peristalsis and symptomatic bacterial overgrowth who is unable to wean of PS. Dilatation of more than 3.5–4 cm is considered the lower limit for efficient STEP procedure [5].

16. **What are key steps of the STEP procedure?**

In the STEP procedure, the luminal channel is narrowed by firing a series of staples from alternating and opposite directions perpendicular to the long axis of the bowel in a zig-zag pattern without interfering with the blood supply of the bowel. Small openings are created in the mesenterium at each point of stapler application. The distance between the stapler firings is guided by the pursued bowel diameter depending on age and size of the patient. After the STEP, the length of the operated bowel segment increases proportionally to the degree of the dilatation even more than 100% [4, 5].

17. **What is the Bianchi procedure?**

The longitudinal intestinal lengthening and tailoring (LILT or Bianchi) procedure was first described by Bianchi in 1980. In this procedure, intestinal tapering and lengthening is accomplished without loss of surface area. When completed, the Bianchi procedure results in a loop of bowel that is twice the length and half of the diameter of the original.

18. **Who is a candidate for Bianchi procedure?**

Bianchi procedure may be considered for a SBS patient with severe (>5 cm) segmental bowel dilatation and symptomatic bacterial overgrowth who is unable to wean of PS [5].

19. **What are key steps of Bianchi procedure?**

In the Bianchi procedure, an avascular plane is created longitudinally along the mesenteric border of a dilated loop of bowel. The bowel is then split lengthwise, taking care to allocate alternating blood vessels to each side to avoid bowel necrosis. Each side of the bowel is then tubularized and then anastomosed end-to-end in isoperistaltic fashion [4, 5].

20. **What are the main complications of short bowel syndrome?**

IFALD, recurrent septic episodes, central line complications, intestinal bacterial overgrowth, metabolic bone disease, impaired renal function, impaired neurocognitive development and failure to thrive are common complications related to SBS [6].

21. **What are the principles of nutritional therapy for short bowel syndrome?**

Meticulously parenterally administered fluid, electrolyte, and nutritional therapy together with oral feeds, is the mainstay of the treatment of SBS. In SBS, parenteral nutrition is life-saving and is used to secure electrolyte, fluid and energy balance as long as adaptation allows weaning off PS. The amount of PS is adjusted based on patient growth and weight. Prompt initiation of oral feeds, preferentially with fresh breast milk, after bowel resection improve chances of weaning off PS [7]. The amount of oral feeds are adjusted based on intestinal secretions and stool consistency. Supplemental parenteral nutrition in addition to oral feeds is continued as long as intestinal absorption alone cannot provide normal growth.

22. **How parenteral nutrition is given?**

Long-term PS is given to a tunneled single-lumen central venous catheter. Choice of access often depends on the size and age of the patient as well as institutional strategies. Peripherally inserted central catheter lines are suitable for very small neonates as they are easy to insert and remove. Subcutaneously inserted ports require a needle puncture of the skin and should be avoided. To minimize patient morbidity, including IFALD, and to improve quality of life, PS infusion time is minimized and infused over night when possible.

23. **What are the common complications related to long-term parenteral nutrition?**

Prolonged parenteral nutrition is associated with several complications, including IFALD, central line associated bloodstream infections, mechanical catheter complications (breakage or thrombosis), and metabolic bone disease [6].

24. **What is catheter related blood stream infection (CLABSI)?**

Catheter related blood stream infection (CLABSI) is a serious complication of PS. The diagnosis is typically made by signs and symptoms of sepsis, possibly infected central line site and positive blood cultures without evidence of other infection sources. The most common causative organisms are staphylococci, enterococci and candida species.

25. **What is the incidence of CLABSI?**

Incidence of CLABSI in SBS patients on long-term PS ranges between 0.2 to 2.3 per 1000 catheter days [6].

26. **How is CLABSI treated?**

The first line treatment is intravenous antimicrobial therapy, which is adjusted based on blood culture results. Catheter removal is necessary if no clinical response to antibiotics is achieved or whenever CLABSI is caused by fungi.

27. **Can CLABSI be prevented?**

The risk of CLABSI can be reduced by meticulous and aseptic central line management and infusion technique, use of ethanol or taurolidine locks, subcutaneous port rather than tunneled catheter, and avoidance of unnecessary line access [6].

28. **What is intestinal failure associated liver disease (IFALD)?**

One of the most significant complications of short bowel syndrome is a unique type of liver injury referred to as intestinal failure associated liver disease (IFALD) without efficient medical therapy currently available. IFALD results from combined consequences of compromised intestinal function and parenteral nutrition. Liver histology features inflammation and cholestasis with variable progression of fibrosis and steatosis, associated with increased biochemical markers of cholestasis and liver injury, while generally accepted diagnostic criteria for IFALD are still missing. Depending on the definition, IFALD affects 30–100% of SBS patients, but only a small proportion of patients develop a progressive form of the disease [6].

29. **Can IFALD be prevented?**

The etiology of IFALD is multifactorial and risk factors include long-term PS, parenteral plant sterols present in all parenteral vegetable oil lipid preparations, recurrent septic episodes secondary to central lines or intestinal bacterial overgrowth, prematurity and lack of enteral nutrition. Strategies to prevent IFALD include early introduction of enteral feeds, use of modern intravenous lipid preparations (fish oil-based lipids, SMOF lipids), cycling of PS, use of lipid-free PS infusion days and efficient prevention and treatment of septic episodes [7].

30. **What is bacterial overgrowth?**

Intestinal bacterial overgrowth is a common finding in patients with SBS and is related to impaired intestinal motility, abnormal bowel dilatation, resection of the ileocecal valve and force feeding. Symptoms of bacterial overgrowth include vomiting, increased intestinal secretions, abdominal distension and pain, bacterial translocation induced sepsis and D-lactic acidosis [7]. Intestinal bacterial overgrowth or dysbiosis severely interferes with intestinal adaptation and absorptive function.

31. **What is the treatment for bacterial overgrowth?**

Severe bacterial overgrowth may be treated empirically with short cyclic courses of enteral antibiotics (e.g. metronidatzole, ciprofloxacin). Bacterial overgrowth associated with dilated loops should be treated surgically using tapering and lengthening procedures [7].

32. **What is short bowel syndrome related metabolic bone disease?**

Patients with SBS and long-term PS are at significant risk for metabolic bone disease characterized by incomplete mineralization of osteoid and consequent disturbances ranging from osteopenia to severe bone disease with pathologic fractures [6].

33. **How common is short bowel syndrome related metabolic bone disease?**

The prevalence of metabolic bone disease is up to 80% and it is associated with long-term PS, short residual small bowel length, increasing age, and insufficient calcium and vitamin D supplementation [6].

34. **What is short bowel syndrome related kidney disease?**

The pathophysiology of SBS related kidney disease is multifactorial and is related to chronic dehydration and electrolyte imbalances due to malabsorptive intestinal losses, recurrent sepsis, nephrocalcinosis, and nephrotoxic medications [6].

35. **How common is short bowel syndrome related kidney disease?**

Depending of the definition, impaired kidney function is reported in 29% to 100% of pediatric SBS patients. All SBS patients on long-term PS require regular monitoring of kidney function [6].

36. **What are indications for intestinal transplantation?**

Children with SBS who have failed intestinal rehabilitation and have developed life-threatening complications (severe and progressive IFALD, loss of central venous access, recurrent catheter-related sepsis episodes, recurrent blowouts of severe dehydration or metabolic abnormalities), intestinal transplantation may be considered. In the absence of significant liver dysfunction, isolated intestinal transplantation is the procedure of choice. In case of advanced liver disease, especially with severe portal hypertension, combined liver-intestine transplant is considered. As current 5-year survival after intestinal transplantation (60%) is less than that of long-term PS (90%), poor quality of life is not currently considered to justify listing for transplantation as a single criterion [4].

37. **What is the effect of short bowel syndrome on quality of life?**

Self-reported quality of life seems to be similar to that of healthy population in children with home PS despite the problems with SBS, including life-style, frequent hospitalizations and dietary restrictions, and they can maintain a positive outlook and cope with illness-related demands. In contrast, parental stress seems to be significantly increased and parent reported quality of life decreased with parents of children with SBS [6].

References

1. Wales PW, de Silva N, Kim J, Lecce L, To T, Moore A. Neonatal short bowel syndrome: population-based estimates of incidence and mortality rates. J Pediatr Surg. 2004;39:690–5.
2. Cole CR, Hansen NI, Higgins RD, Ziegler TR, Stoll BJ. Very low birth weight preterm infants with surgical short bowel syndrome: incidence, morbidity and mortality, and growth outcomes at 18 to 22 months. Pediatrics. 2008;122:e573–82.
3. Belza C, Fitzgerald K, de Silva N, Avitzur Y, Steinberg K, Courtney-Martin G, et al. Predicting intestinal adaptation in pediatric intestinal failure: a retrospective cohort study. Ann Surg. 2019;269:988–93.
4. Iyer KR. Surgical management of short bowel syndrome. JPEN J Parenter Enteral Nutr. 2014;38:53S-59S.
5. Pakarinen MP. Autologous intestinal reconstruction surgery as part of comprehensive management of intestinal failure. Pediatr Surg Int. 2015;31:453–63.
6. Mutanen A, Wales P. Etiology and prognosis of pediatric short bowel syndrome. Semin Pediatr Surg. 2018;27:209–17.
7. Duggan CP, Jaksic T. Pediatric intestinal failure. N Engl J Med. 2017;17:666–75.

Chapter 75
Evidence in Minimally Invasive Surgery

Rim Kiblawi, Benno Ure, and Jens Dingemann

Abstract The term "Minimally Invasive Surgery" or "MIS" refers to operations performed through small incisions in the abdomen ("laparo-scopy"), in the chest ("thoraco-scopy"), or in the retroperitoneum ("retroperitoneo-scopy"). Compared to adult surgery, the evolution of MIS in infants and newborns was delayed due to obstacles such as the limited working-space, the unique physiology of the newborn organism and the limited availability of suitable instruments. However, in the following years, the enthusiasm of the international pediatric surgical community in MIS led to an increasing number of publications describing new procedures, showing safety and feasibility.

Keywords Minimally Invasive Surgery (MIS) · Laparoscopy · Thoracoscopy · Video Assisted Thoracoscopic Surgery (VATS) · Evidence based medicine

In recent years, the aim of academic studies has shifted to a critical evaluation of additional measurable outcomes. This led to an increasing number of prospective randomized trials, delivering the highest level of evidence possible. This chapter aims to give an overview about the highest available evidence of pediatric MIS. Examples for evidence based advantages and disadvantages of several laparoscopic and thoracoscopic procedures will be given.

1. **Which are the advantages of laparoscopy compared to laparotomy?**

Obvious advantages compared to the corresponding open procedure are better cosmetic result, less operative trauma and lower postoperative pain levels. Moreover, better intraoperative visualization and surgical precision due to optical magnification. Some authors assume less postoperative adhesions and shorter hospital stay.

R. Kiblawi (✉) · B. Ure · J. Dingemann
Center of Pediatric Surgery, Hannover Medical School and Bult Children's Hospital, Hannover, Germany
e-mail: kiblawi.rim@mh-hannover.de

M. Lacher et al. (eds.), *Pearls and Tricks in Pediatric Surgery*,
https://doi.org/10.1007/978-3-030-51067-1_75

2. **Which are the advantages of thoracoscopy compared to thoracotomy?**

Regardless of the specific procedure performed, thoracoscopy does not require transection of the thoracic wall muscles (m. latissimus and m. serratus) and re-approximation of ribs as in thoracotomy. This prevents musculoskeletal sequelae such as chest asymmetry and scoliosis [1].

3. **Which are the challenges and difficulties in newborns?**

The restricted space of the neonatal abdominal and thoracic cavity demands fine movements. Operative time is more important than in older children, due to the potential risk of longer capnoperitoneum. Abdominal distension may cause increased vagal tone and bradycardia. CO_2 absorption in newborns is higher inducing acidosis and decreased cerebral perfusion. The abdominal pressure of capnoperitoneum usually creates transient anuria. Evaporative cooling caused by dry gas may consume a large fraction of infant's metabolic rate.

4. **Which instruments are used?**

Compared to adult surgery instruments and ports are usually 10, 5 or 3 mm diameters. Additional specific pediatric instruments may be needed, like the pylorus-spreader.

5. **What is evidence-based medicine and how is evidence classified?** [2–5]

Evidence-based medicine is defined as the conscientious, explicit and judicious use of current best evidence in making decisions about the care of individual patients.

According to the Oxford Center for Evidence-Based Medicine (CEBM), evidence may be graded in 5 levels (1–5), resulting in 4 grades of recommendation (A–D), (Tables 75.1 and 75.2). One of the cornerstones of evidence-based medicine has always been the recommendation to use the current best evidence to make a decision for or against a certain treatment.

In the following, the best level of evidence available for different types of pediatric MIS-procedures will be given. We chose only studies providing at least Level 3 evidence.

75.1 Laparoscopy

75.1.1 Abdominal Surgery [2–4]

6. **Which types of laparoscopic fundoplication do you know?**

Nissen (360°), Toupet (270° posterior), Thal (270° anterior) and Dor (180° anterior) may all be performed laparoscopically.

Table 75.1 Levels of evidence (**modified from** www.CEBM.net)

Level 1a	Meta-analysis with homogeneity of Randomized control trials (RCT)
Level 1b	Individual RCT with narrow Confidence Interval
Level 2a	Meta-analysis with homogeneity of cohort studies
Level 2b	Individual cohort study (including low-quality RCT, <80% follow-up)
Level 3a	Meta-analysis with homogeneity of case–control studies
Level 3b	Individual case–control studies
Level 4	Case series (and poor quality cohort and case–control studies)
Level 5	Expert opinion without explicit critical appraisal

Table 75.2 Grades of recommendation (modified from www.CEBM.net)

Grade A	Consistent level 1 studies support the recommendation
Grade B	Consistent level 2 or 3 studies or extrapolation from level 1 studies support the recommendation
Grade C	Level 4 studies or extrapolation from level 2 or 3 studies support the recommendation
Grade D	Level 5 evidence or troublingly inconsistent or inconclusive studies or any level support the recommendation

7. **Which are the advantages of laparoscopic fundoplication compared to open?**

Level 1a/Grade A (meta-analysis of 7 RCT)

Laparoscopic compared to open Nissen fundoplication was associated with higher recurrence rates, but same rates of mortality, reoperations and complications (wound infection/hernia, food impaction, gastrostomy dislocation, airway complications).

8. **Which disadvantages and advantages are attributable to laparoscopic Nissen compared to Thal?**

Level 1b/Grade A (RCT)

Laparoscopic Nissen was associated with a lower recurrence rate than laparoscopic Thal fundoplication, but significantly higher rate of severe dysphagia.

9. **Which is the main complication described for laparoscopic pyloromyotomy?**

Level 1a/Grade A (meta-analysis of 5 RCT)

Laparoscopic pyloromyotomy was associated with shorter postoperative time to full feed and better cosmesis, but with a higher rate of incomplete pyloromyotomy compared to the open technique.

10. **Are there any disadvantages of laparoscopic duodenal atresia repair compared to the open approach?**

Level 3a/Grade B (meta-analysis of 3 case-control studies)

No differences in time to oral feeds, length of stay and anastomotic complications between laparoscopic and open technique were reported. However, longer operative time was reported for laparoscopic duodenal atresia repair.

11. **Which risks are attributable to laparoscopic Kasai portoenterostomy compared to the open procedure?**

Level 2b/Grade B (cohort study)

In 2011 a prospective non randomized trial comparing laparoscopic to open Kasai has been early stopped due to the significantly higher rate of liver transplantation after laparoscopic Kasai at 6- and 24-months follow-up [6].

12. **May resection of choledochal cyst be performed laparoscopically?**

Level 3a/Grade B (meta-analysis of 7 case-control studies)

Although laparoscopic resection of choledochal cyst was associated with longer operative time in comparison with the open procedure, it has been shown to be a feasible and safe alternative. The advantages were shorter hospital stay, time to feed, less intraoperative bleeding and lower rate of bowel obstruction or stenosis.

13. **Which are the advantages of laparoscopic Ladd´s procedure compared to the open approach?**

Level 3a/Grade B (meta-analysis of 6 case-control studies)

It was described shorter time to full feeds, hospital stay and less readmission rate for MIS approach. However, laparoscopic Ladd's procedure seems to associate with a higher risk of post-operative volvulus.

14. **List different techniques of laparoscopic appendectomy.**

Laparoscopic appendectomy is commonly performed using a three-port technique. Single Incision Laparoscopic Surgery (SILS) or Trans-Umbilical Laparoscopic Assisted Appendectomy (TULAA) are also feasible options.

15. **Which are the advantages of laparoscopic appendectomy compared to open appendectomy?**

Level 1a/Grade A (meta-analysis of 7 RCT)

No differences were found regarding wound infections, intrabdominal abscess and postoperative ileus but laparoscopic appendectomy allowed earlier return to normal activity.

16. **Name a possible downside of SILS appendectomy.**

Level 1b/Grade A (RCT)
SILS appendectomy was associated with increased pain level compared to multiple ports appendectomy. No differences were found regarding length of hospital stay and complication rate.

17. **When to consider laparoscopy for ano-rectal malformation?**

There is an ongoing debate regarding the indication for laparoscopically assisted ano-rectal pull-through (LAARP) or posterior-sagittal anorectoplasty (PSARP). LAARP has been described for recto-bladderneck, selected recto-prostatic, recto-vaginal fistula and anorectal agenesis.

18. **How does LAARP influence the bowel function in comparison to PSARP?**

Level 1b/Grade A (RCT)

No differences were found regarding incontinence, fecal staining and squeezing force, but better improvement in anal canal resting pressure at the anorectal manometry and a reduced length of hospital stay for LAARP comparing to PSARP.

75.1.2 Urology [2, 4]

19. **Which are the advantages of laparoscopic pyeloplasty?**

Level 1b/Grade A (RCT)

Laparoscopic pyeloplasty was associated with shorter hospital stay, similar success rate but longer operative time compared to open procedure.

20. **Why would you suggest laparoscopic inguinal hernia repair?**

Level 1a/Grade A (meta-analysis of 5 RCT)

Laparoscopic repair was associated with shorter operative time for bilateral hernia, lower rates of iatrogenic ascent of the testis, atrophy, hydrocele and wound infection, but similar recurrence rates compared to the open approach.

21. **What is the role of laparoscopy in undescended testis?**

Laparoscopy is being used for diagnostic and therapeutic procedures in non-palpable testes.

22. **Which are the advantages of laparoscopic orchidopexy?**

Level 1b/Grade A (RCT)

Laparoscopic orchidopexy (second stage Fowler Stephens for high abdominal testis and primary orchidopexy for low abdominal testis) was associated with shorter operative time, hospital stay and return to the normal activities compared to the respective open procedure. However, no differences were found regarding atrophy, recurrence and success rates.

23. **Is laparoscopy a valid option for varicocelectomy?**

Level 1b/Grade A (RCT)

Yes. Laparoscopic Palomo procedure was associated with less wound complications and tissue edema, shorter operative time and hospitalization compared to the open approach. No significant differences were found in terms of recurrence rate and postoperative hydrocele.

75.2 Thoracoscopy[4, 5]

24. **What are pathophysiological concerns of thoracoscopy in newborn?**

Level 1b/Grade A (RCT)

A pilot RCT has demonstrated that thoracoscopic repair of congenital diaphragmatic hernia (CDH) may be associated with prolonged and severe intraoperative hypercapnia and acidosis, compared with open surgery. This was not associated with changes in arterial oxygenation.

Level 2b/Grade B (cohort study)

A following prospective study showed that thoracoscopic esophageal atresia (EA) repair was associated with a reversible hypercapnia and acidosis. However, no variation of cerebral oxygenation was found.

25. **Is the outcome of thoracoscopic EA repair unfavorable compared to open?**

Level 3a/Grade B (2 meta-analyses of case-control studies)

No. Thoracoscopic EA repair was associated with a similar complication rates, anastomotic leaks and strictures but longer operative time. Advantages of the thoracoscopic approach were shorter times to extubation and first enteral feeding resulting in shorter hospital stay.

26. **Which are the advantages of thoracoscopic lung resection?**

Level 3a/Grade B (2 meta-analyses of case-control studies)

Thoracoscopic versus open lung resection for congenital pulmonary malformation was associated with shorter duration of chest drain and hospital stay, but longer operative times.

27. **What is the impact of thoracoscopic repair of congenital diaphragmatic hernia?**

Level 3a/Grade B (2 meta-analyses of case-control studies)

Thoracoscopic repair of CDH was associated with shorter duration of postoperative ventilation, lesser need of narcotics, faster enteral feeding and shorter hospitalization. However, it must be considered that usually cardiorespiratory stable patients with smaller defects are selected for thoracoscopic repair, bearing a potential selection bias. Conversely, thoracoscopic CDH repair was associated with increased risk of recurrence.

References

1. Lawal TA, Gosemann JH, Kuebler JF, Glüer S, Ure BM. Thoracoscopy versus thoracotomy improves midterm musculoskeletal status and cosmesis in infants and children. Ann Thorac Surg. 2009;87(1):224–8.
2. Dingemann J, Ure BM. Systematic review of level 1 evidence for laparoscopic pediatric surgery: do our procedures comply with the requirements of evidence-based medicine? Eur J Pediatr Surg. 2013;23:474–9.
3. Lacher M, Kuebler JF, Dingemann J, Ure BM. Minimal invasive surgery in the newborn: current status and evidence. Semin Pediatr Surg. 2014;23(05):249–56.
4. Schukfeh N, Kuebler JF, Dingemann J, Ure BM. Thirty years of minimally invasive surgery in children: analysis of meta-analyses. Eur J Pediatr Surg. (2019).
5. Dingemann C, Ure BM, Dingemann J. Thoracoscopic procedures in pediatric surgery: what is the evidence? Eur J Pediatr Surg. 2014;24:14–9.
6. Ure BM, Kuebler JF, Schukfeh N, Engelmann C, Dingemann J, Petersen C. Survival with the native liver after laparoscopic versus conventional kasai portoenterostomy in infants with biliary atresia: a prospective trial. Ann Surg. 2011;253(4):826–30.

Index

A
Abdominal trauma, 287, 376, 393–395, 397
Abdominal ultrasound, 173, 265, 267, 270, 290, 333, 470, 472, 474
Acute pancreatitis, 268, 288–291
Acute scrotum, 351–353
Adaptation, 9, 316, 529–531, 533
Adhesions, 31, 159, 172, 199, 341, 365, 399, 535
Adhesive small bowel obstruction, 31, 33, 155–160, 176, 197
Adrenal gland, 92, 425, 426, 497
Advanced Burn Life Support, 416, 419
Aganlionosis, 211
Airway, 4, 48, 54, 59, 64, 67, 69–75, 77–87, 89–92, 103, 182, 295, 298, 302–304, 374, 416, 453, 457, 474, 502, 503, 508–510, 537
Anal fissure, 247, 249–251
Androgen insensitivity syndrome, 364, 368, 370, 371
Anemia, 221, 228, 281, 284, 362, 426, 433, 439, 441, 446, 490, 508, 511
Annular pancreas, 162, 287, 288
Anorectal disease, 247
Anorectal malformation, 38, 133, 155, 170, 212, 233–237, 239, 241, 243, 244, 258, 516
Appendectomy, 156, 157, 176, 195, 197–199, 205, 456, 457, 538, 539
Appendiceal carcinoid, 455–457
Appendicitis, 117, 155, 156, 176, 192, 195–199, 205, 230, 465, 474, 516
Appendicostomy, 217
Applying, 417, 421, 517, 518
Atresia, 2, 35–38, 42, 45, 84, 87, 96, 126, 127, 133, 155, 161–166, 170, 173, 180, 212, 234–236, 241, 257, 258, 275, 277, 288, 319, 362, 363, 468, 478, 482, 490, 516, 528, 538
Auerbach plexus, 151

B
Bianchi, 530, 531
Biliary atresia, 162, 257, 275, 277, 478
Bilious emesis, 128, 165, 169, 171, 173, 207, 212, 469, 470
Biological agents, 219
Birth defect, 61, 86
Bites, 401, 403, 405, 406
Bladder exstrophy, 131, 133, 136, 368
Blunt liver injury, 394, 395, 397
Blunt splenic injury, 394, 395
Blunt trauma, 375, 391, 393, 401, 406
Bochdalek hernia, 26
Body, 7, 23, 38, 53–55, 57, 60, 69–75, 96, 99, 104, 125, 137, 152, 155, 192, 223, 240, 277, 279, 281, 289, 293, 314, 341, 355, 371, 374, 379, 385, 387, 403, 410, 415, 416, 418–420, 423, 457, 459, 479, 493, 498, 501, 502, 511
Botulinum toxin, 216, 217, 251, 313, 316
Bowel management, 233, 243
Branchial arch anomalies, 311
Branchial cleft anomalies, 299, 305–311
Branchial cleft cysts, 295–297, 299, 302, 309
Branchial clef remnants, 306, 308–311
Branchial fistula, 310
Branchial sinus, 310, 311

M. Lacher et al. (eds.), *Pearls and Tricks in Pediatric Surgery*,
https://doi.org/10.1007/978-3-030-51067-1

Branchio-Oto-Renal syndrome (BOR), 311
Bronchogenic cyst, 59, 60, 64, 89, 91, 508
Bronchopulmonary sequestration, 59, 60, 64, 474, 508
Bulking agents, 336, 338
Burn, 49, 50, 72, 110, 377, 384, 415–423, 503, 516
Button battery, 50, 53–56, 72

C
Caustic ingestion, 47–51, 391
Caustic injury, 47–50
Caustic strictures, 49, 50
Central line, 135, 488, 527, 531, 532
Cervical cysts, 305
Cervical lymphadenitis, 297, 299
Cervical spine injury, 374, 379, 381, 383, 385, 410
Chance fracture, 394, 410, 411
Chest wall deformities, 13, 23
Children, 1–4, 7–11, 33, 42–44, 47, 48, 51, 53, 54, 57, 63, 64, 66, 67, 69–75, 77, 78, 80–83, 85, 86, 89, 90, 92, 93, 106, 115–117, 120, 121, 131, 133, 134, 140, 142–144, 155–160, 166, 169, 177, 183, 185–189, 195–199, 201, 202, 211–213, 216, 217, 219–224, 227–231, 234, 239, 243, 248–254, 259, 262, 266, 269, 271, 272, 275–277, 279, 281–285, 287, 289, 290, 292, 293, 295, 296, 301–303, 312, 315, 317, 320, 321, 325, 327–329, 331–336, 338, 339, 348, 349, 351, 352, 354, 359, 361, 365, 373–377, 379–385, 387–391, 394–398, 401–405, 410, 412, 413, 416, 418–423, 425, 428, 431–434, 436–442, 445, 447, 450, 453, 455, 457, 458, 460, 461, 465, 471, 473, 477–483, 498, 501–505, 516, 519, 527, 533, 534, 536
Choking, 42, 70, 71, 75
Cholangiogram, 258, 261, 274
Cholangitis, 221, 257, 261, 265, 267–270, 273, 322
Cholecystitis, 197, 267, 271–273
Choledochal cyst, 162, 265–270, 288, 289, 472, 538
Choledocholithiasis, 267, 271–273, 289
Cholelithiasis, 272
Chronic pancreatitis, 290, 291
Circumcision, 142, 328, 339–344, 505
Clinical research, 521
Clinical trial, 107, 434, 509–511, 523, 524
Cloaca, 132, 148, 233, 241, 243
Cloacal exstrophy, 131, 133, 244
Colitis, 219, 220, 222, 224, 228
Colonic atresia, 162, 165, 166
Colonic motility, 208, 216, 217
Compartment syndrome, 33, 128, 314, 404, 405, 414
Complication, 7, 9, 10, 19, 23, 32, 35, 39–41, 43–45, 50, 53, 55, 57, 62–64, 71, 73, 75, 86, 92, 93, 99, 103, 110, 111, 113, 118–121, 127, 134, 136, 139, 159, 169–171, 176, 179–181, 193, 195, 198, 199, 214, 223, 224, 247, 249, 251, 257, 261, 265, 267–270, 273, 277, 278, 283, 285, 290, 291, 295, 298, 303, 304, 308–311, 317, 333, 338, 362, 369, 388, 396, 414, 428, 434, 436, 447, 465, 468, 473, 480–482, 491–493, 501–503, 505, 509, 522, 527, 531–533, 537–540
Congenital, 7, 9, 13, 14, 25–28, 35, 36, 38, 40–42, 59, 60, 63, 77–79, 84, 86, 87, 95, 97, 101, 103–105, 113, 121, 125, 129, 131, 135, 147, 161–164, 170, 186, 191, 192, 212, 236, 258, 265, 266, 269, 284, 287–289, 295, 299, 305, 306, 308, 311–317, 321, 322, 325, 341, 342, 345, 347, 348, 368, 369, 434, 457, 469, 474–476, 483, 485–487, 490, 498, 507–509, 516, 527, 528, 540, 541
Congenital adrenal hyperplasia, 236, 368–371
Congenital anomaly, 9, 35, 36, 42, 77, 125, 212, 258, 287, 288, 347, 486, 487, 516
Congenital defect, 41
Congenital Diaphragmatic Hernia (CDH), 25–33, 60, 170, 474, 475, 490, 507, 509, 510, 516, 540, 541
Congenital Hyperinsulinism (CHI), 287–289
Congenital Pulmonary Airway Malformation (CPAM), 59–63, 457, 474, 508, 509, 512
Congenital tracheal stenosis, 78, 86
Contrast enema, 161, 165, 166, 181, 182, 187, 201, 204, 207–209, 212, 215, 216, 467
Corrosive ingestion, 47
Crohn's disease, 197, 219, 220, 222–224, 252, 254, 528

Cryptorchidism, 128, 142, 143
Cyst excision, 268–270
Cystic fibrosis, 67, 164, 179, 209, 272, 467, 468, 483

D
Dehydration, 7, 10, 127, 180, 181, 213, 271, 533
Desmoid-type fibromatoses, 455, 459
Diagnosis, 14, 15, 19, 20, 23, 28, 29, 31, 35, 37, 38, 41, 43, 47, 59, 66, 69, 73, 83, 85, 86, 89, 91, 92, 97, 101, 110, 116, 117, 122, 133, 139, 140, 143, 156, 161, 163, 165, 166, 171, 173, 174, 176, 186, 187, 192, 201, 203, 205, 209, 212, 213, 215, 216, 219–221, 224, 227–231, 240–242, 249, 252, 260, 261, 263, 265–268, 274, 284, 287, 289, 293, 295, 296, 299, 303, 309, 313, 315, 316, 321, 325, 331, 333, 351–353, 359, 362, 364, 365, 368, 370, 371, 388, 390, 391, 397, 404, 415, 425–428, 432–436, 439, 440, 456, 458, 465–470, 472–474, 489, 532
DICER1 syndrome, 455, 457, 458
DiGeorge Anomaly, 311
Disorders of sex development, 367–372
Distal intestinal obstruction syndrome, 181, 182
Distal obstruction, 161, 467
Duodenal atresia, 2, 133, 162, 163, 173, 234, 538
Duodenoduodenostomy, 163, 288
Dynamic compression system, 20
Dyskinesia, 274
Dyspnea, 48, 90, 289, 303, 310, 426

E
Eagle-Barrett syndrome, 139
Ectopic pregnancy, 199, 359, 361, 362, 364
Ectopic ureter, 321, 325, 329
Embryology, 26, 140, 147, 169, 309, 497, 498
Empyema, 65–67
Encopresis, 215, 217, 239, 249, 251, 426
Endocrine, 290–293, 342, 367, 443, 444, 497, 498, 504
Endocrine tumors, 293, 443, 444
Endoscopy, 47, 48, 55, 79, 80, 229, 230, 276, 279, 305, 310, 311
End stage liver failure, 262
Enema reduction, 204, 205, 466
Energy, 2, 7, 9, 10, 62, 375, 390, 487, 488, 529, 531
Enterocolitis, 2, 9, 122, 155, 185, 211, 213–215, 468, 486, 528
Epididymitis, 351, 353, 354
Epigastric, 42, 48, 113, 115, 121, 122, 152, 293
Epispadias, 131–135, 345, 347
Esophageal atresia, 35–40, 42, 45, 84, 162, 234, 258, 288, 516
Esophageal foreign body, 53–55, 57
Esophageal injury, 47, 49, 50, 391
Esophageal strictures, 47, 50
Esophagitis, 42–44, 49
Evaluation, 1–4, 19, 28, 48, 51, 78–81, 102, 127, 162, 166, 187, 207, 209, 216, 222, 227, 236, 243, 262, 276, 305, 308, 315, 327, 342, 368–371, 373, 375, 377, 380, 385, 393, 394, 401, 451, 456, 468, 475, 476, 489, 490, 535
Evidence based medicine, 521, 536
Extracorporeal Membrane Oxygenation (ECMO), 25, 30–33, 492, 509, 518
Ex Utero Intrapartum Treatment (EXIT), 61, 87, 90, 509–511

F
Failed medical management, 216
Fertility, 137, 144, 199, 354, 365, 367, 370, 371, 452
Fetal, 25, 27, 28, 35, 59–61, 90, 96, 126, 148, 191, 207, 241, 326, 328, 360, 368, 369, 452, 476, 507–512
Fetoscopic Endoluminal Tracheal Occlusion (FETO), 28, 29, 509, 510, 512
Fibromatosis coli, 314
First branchial anomaly, 306, 308
Fistulae-in-ano, 247
Fixation, 170–172, 302, 353, 360, 412–414, 469
Foley balloon extraction, 54, 55
Follow-up, 9, 14, 15, 19, 33, 49, 197, 207, 209, 223, 252, 254, 265, 270, 285, 338, 459, 481, 525, 537, 538
Fontan, 98, 99
Foreign, 23, 53–55, 57, 69–75, 155, 192, 403
Functional constipation, 211, 216, 217
Fundoplication, 33, 40, 43–45, 536, 537

G

Gallbladder, 147, 162, 180, 183, 261, 268, 271–274, 284, 293
Gastritis, 42, 228
Gastroesophageal reflux disease, 39–45, 82, 182
Gastrointestinal bleeding, 227–231, 262, 276
Gastrointestinal tract, 7, 55, 147, 148, 161, 179, 180, 220, 244
Gastroschisis, 42, 125–129, 165, 166, 170, 482, 516, 528
Germ cell tumors, 89, 91, 361, 449–451, 453
Glasgow coma scale, 376, 379–384
Goiter, 3, 497
Goldenhar's Syndrome, 311, 312

H

Haemorrhoid, 247
Heart, 17, 27, 28, 30, 35, 36, 38, 60, 89, 95–98, 134, 144, 164, 170, 186, 237, 288, 375, 388, 389, 441, 480, 483, 493, 512
Hedgehog-signaling, 441
Hemangioma, 103, 104, 202, 249, 284, 437, 438, 441
Hematemesis, 48, 228, 229
Hematochezia, 42, 228, 229, 248, 470
Hemolytic anemia, 281
Hepatico-duodenostomy, 265, 269
Hepatico-jejunostomy, 265, 269
Hepatoblastoma, 437–441, 458, 478
Hernia, 3, 25–27, 31, 32, 42, 44, 45, 60, 110, 111, 113, 115–118, 120–123, 128, 133, 134, 155, 158, 170, 171, 176, 192, 261, 262, 351–353, 474–476, 490, 505, 507, 509, 516, 537, 539–541
Hernia repair, 31, 111, 113, 116, 118, 120, 123, 133, 539, 541
Hirschsprung disease, 44, 155, 166, 211–216, 445, 467, 528
Hydrocele, 115–117, 351, 352, 451, 475, 539, 540
Hydrocolpos, 241, 242
Hydrometrocolpos, 359, 362
Hydronephrosis, 140, 197, 239, 241, 242, 319–321, 325–329, 332, 362, 508
Hydrostatic reduction, 466
Hyperparathyroidism, 443, 444, 498, 499
Hyperthyroidism, 498
Hypospadias, 341, 342, 345–347, 354

I

Ileocolic, 201–204, 466, 467, 528
Image Defined Risk Factors (IDRF), 425–428, 473
Immune thrombocytopenia purpura, 282, 283
Incarceration, 111, 113, 116, 117, 120
Incisional, 119, 122, 123, 176, 297
Inflammatory bowel disease, 219–224, 228, 250–254, 365
Inflammatory myofibroblastic tumor, 455, 460
Intestinal atresia, 126, 155, 163, 170, 173, 180, 212, 482, 490
Intestinal failure, 128, 272, 483, 527–529, 532
Intestinal obstruction, 9, 118, 128, 155, 161, 162, 171, 179, 181, 192, 204, 211, 214, 230, 465, 466, 468
Intestinal transplantation, 533
Intussusception, 2, 44, 155, 159, 170, 173, 177, 192, 201–205, 466, 467, 471, 516

J

Jejunal atresia, 162, 258

K

Kasai portoenterostomy, 257, 258, 260–263, 538
Kidney cancer, 434
Krickenbeck classification, 234

L

Ladd's procedure, 135, 169, 175, 176, 261, 538
Laryngeal cleft, 37, 78, 84–86
Laryngomalacia, 78–80
Levels of evidence, 43, 525, 535–537
Liver disease, 128, 275, 276, 278, 461, 477–479, 482, 527, 532, 533
Liver resection, 438, 441
Liver surgery, 269, 479, 480
Liver transplantation, 257, 269, 276, 440, 441, 477–481, 538
Liver tumors, 437–439, 441, 477, 478
Lobar emphysema, 59, 508
Lund and Browder diagrams, 418
Lung malformation, 59–63, 87
Lung-to-Head Ratio (LHR), 25, 28, 509, 510
Lymphoma, 89–92, 199, 202, 284, 296, 299, 436

M

Magnetic resonance enterography, 219, 222, 254
Malignant peripheral nerve sheath tumor, 455, 463
Malone, 217, 244
Malrotation, 31, 128, 133, 155, 156, 162–164, 169–177, 212, 261, 288, 469
Maternal diabetes, 208, 258
Maternal-fetal surgery, 508
Mayer-Rokitansky-Kuster-Hauser syndrome, 368
Meatal stenosis, 341, 345
Meckel scan, 192, 193, 229, 230, 470, 471
Meckel's diverticulum, 148, 191–193, 202, 229, 230
Meconium ileus, 155, 179–181, 212, 467, 468
Mediastinum, 60, 72, 89–92, 310, 388, 390, 427, 453
Meissner plexus, 151
MELD score, 478, 479
Melena, 42, 228, 229
Meso-rex-bypass, 276–279
Midgut volvulus, 155, 169–177, 469, 470
Minimally Invasive Surgery (MIS), 33, 428, 535, 536, 538
Mixed gonadal dysgenesis, 368, 370, 371
MRI scan, 381, 383, 433
Multicystic dysplastic kidney, 319–321
Multilocular cystic nephroma, 319–321
MYCN, 425, 427
Myelomeningocele (MMC) repair, 512

N

National Emergency X-radiography Utilization Study (NEXUS), 375, 383
Neck cysts &masses, 295–297, 299, 302, 304, 306, 308, 510
Necrotizing enterocolitis, 2, 9, 122, 127, 155, 185–189, 468, 469, 482, 486, 528
Neonatal nutrition, 488
Neonatal surgical emergency, 466
Nephroblastoma, 431
Nephron-sparing surgery, 435, 436
Neuroblastoma, 90, 92, 425–429, 433, 438, 458, 473
Neurogenic tumors, 89, 91
Nissen fundoplication, 44, 45, 537
Non-operative management, 157–159, 181, 320, 393–398, 412
Non-perforated, 195–197, 199

O

Omphalitis, 109
Omphalocele, 42, 125–129, 132, 134, 135, 170, 244, 516
Omphalomesenteric duct, 110, 148, 191, 192
Opiate, 501, 503
Orchidopexy, 118, 354, 355, 539
Organization, 8, 65, 367, 428, 502, 515, 522
Osteotomy, 22, 134–136, 244
Ovarian cysts, 197, 359–361, 476
Ovarian torsion, 197, 359, 360, 365, 476
Ovarian tumors, 361, 452, 476

P

Pain, 17, 31, 42, 48, 50, 53, 63, 72, 90, 118, 122, 152, 156, 159, 171, 177, 182, 192, 196, 201, 203, 205, 220, 222, 224, 228, 242, 248, 249, 251, 271, 272, 274, 283, 284, 289–291, 293, 295, 296, 310, 329, 333, 351–353, 356, 359, 361, 362, 364, 365, 376, 377, 381, 384, 385, 388, 394, 395, 403, 404, 411, 413–417, 419–422, 426, 433, 439, 446, 449, 453, 465, 466, 469, 472–474, 476, 493, 501, 504, 505, 533, 535, 539
Pain management, 493
Palliation, 95, 98
Pancreas divisum, 287, 288
Pancreatic injury, 398, 399
Pancreatic insufficiency, 179, 181, 183
Pancreaticobiliary malunion, 287, 288
Pancreatic tumors, 287, 291–293, 498
Pancreatobiliary maljunction, 266
Parapneumonic effusion, 65, 66
Parathyroid gland, 306, 312, 497–499
Peanut, 74, 298
Pectus carinatum, 13, 14, 19, 20, 22, 23
Pectus excavatum, 5, 13–15, 17, 19, 23, 33
Pediatric, 1, 7, 13, 41, 53, 55, 57, 59, 61, 63, 64, 67, 73, 78, 80–82, 90, 95, 101, 113, 117, 120–123, 139, 147, 156–158, 160, 173, 179, 187, 192, 196, 211, 219–224, 227–231, 233, 247, 254, 259, 262, 271, 272, 295, 296, 298, 302, 306, 314, 325, 331, 332, 334, 339, 341, 359, 367, 373–377, 379–381, 384, 385, 387, 391, 393–396, 402, 409, 415–423, 425, 431, 434, 436, 438, 441, 443, 455–458, 461–463, 465, 466, 474, 477–481, 497, 501–503, 507, 508,

515–519, 522, 525, 527, 528, 533, 535, 536
Pediatric brain trauma, 379
Pediatric cancer, 431, 432, 450
Pediatric liver transplant, 441, 479
Pediatric liver transplantation, 477, 479–481
Pediatric melanoma, 455, 462, 463
Pediatric oncology, 436
Pediatric surgery, 61, 507, 508, 515–519, 521, 525
Pediatric trauma, 373–375, 377, 391
PELD score, 479
Pelvic apophyseal fractures, 412
Pelvic inflammatory disease, 359, 361, 364, 365
Penetrating trauma, 388, 395, 401
Perforated, 155, 156, 176, 195, 196, 198, 199
Perioperative antibiotic prophylaxis, 492
Perirectal abscess, 251, 252, 254
Phimosis, 340–344
Physical therapy, 313–316, 411
Physiology, 42, 95, 115, 147, 215, 271, 485, 535
Pierre Robin sequence, 311, 312
Pleuropulmonary blastoma, 3, 63, 455, 457
Pneumatic reduction, 204
Polycystic kidney disease, 319, 321, 482
Portal hypertension, 229, 248, 259, 261, 262, 275–277, 284, 322, 533
Posterior urethral valves, 141, 325, 327, 328, 482, 508
Post-splenectomy sepsis, 281, 284, 285
Pragmatic trial, 524
Premalignant condition, 265
Prenatal diagnosis, 28, 37
Prevention, 42, 49, 75, 189, 261, 532
Prune belly syndrome, 139, 142

R

Randomized trial, 66, 403, 535, 538
Rectal prolapse, 134, 179, 183, 239, 248, 249
Rectourethral fistula, 233, 234, 237
Rectovestibular fistula, 233, 234, 236, 239, 240
Recurrent bowel obstruction, 159
Renal injury, 397, 398, 405
Rex-shunt, 276, 278
Rhabdomyosarcoma, 437, 455–458

S

Sacrococcygeal teratoma, 455, 458, 459, 509
Sedation, 29, 62, 73, 157, 267, 303, 382, 406, 421, 459, 493, 503
Selective Fetoscopic Laser Ablation (SFLP), 508, 511, 512
Sepsis, 32, 157, 173, 185, 188, 189, 249, 270, 272, 281, 284, 285, 420, 468, 478, 532, 533
Serial Transverse Enteroplasty (STEP), 530
Short bowel syndrome, 127, 176, 527–534
Shoulder dislocation pulseless, 411
Shunt, 96–99, 116, 121, 276–279, 388, 492, 508
Sickle cell disease, 4, 197, 272, 283, 348
SIOPEL, 439, 441
Sirolimus, 105, 107
Sistrunk procedure, 298, 299, 301, 303
Small bowel obstruction, 31, 33, 155, 156, 159, 176, 197, 199, 224, 468
Soave cuff, 215
Sodium, 9, 10, 106, 160, 214
Soft tissue injuries, 375, 401–403
Spherocytosis, 272, 282–284
Spinal Cord Injury Without Radiographic Abnormality (SCIWORA), 374, 385, 410
Splenectomy, 276, 281–285, 399
Splenic injury, 282, 394, 395, 397
SPLIT liver transplant, 479
Sternocleidomastoid, 296, 302, 309, 314, 316, 317
Stoma, 9, 122, 159, 181, 189, 236, 237, 244, 260, 494
Subglottic stenosis, 78, 81–83
Supracondylar fracture, 411, 412
Surgery, 2, 4, 7, 9, 10, 17, 22, 31–33, 45, 55, 57, 61, 63, 80, 82, 86, 89, 90, 93, 97, 106, 110, 118, 120, 122, 134, 137, 144, 156, 159, 160, 175–177, 181, 182, 186, 188, 193, 197–199, 201, 213, 224, 227, 229, 230, 234, 239, 249, 259, 262, 265, 266, 268, 269, 276–279, 283, 297, 303, 304, 329, 336, 338, 352, 360, 361, 367, 377, 395, 399, 411, 412, 416, 418, 421, 422, 426, 428, 431, 434, 435, 438, 440, 448–453, 455, 458, 461, 488–494, 499, 507–509, 512,

515–519, 521, 525, 530, 535, 536, 538, 540
Surgical neonate, 485, 487, 488, 490–493

T

Technical variant graft, 479, 480
Testicular torsion, 197, 353, 474, 475
Testicular tumors, 351, 449, 451
Thermal injury, 374, 416, 419, 420
Thoracoscopy, 25, 31, 66, 89, 399, 460, 536, 540
Thymoma, 89, 90, 92
Thyroglossal duct remnants, 295, 296, 298, 299, 301–304, 306, 497
Thyroid gland, 299, 301, 497, 498
Tibial fractures, 413, 414
Torticollis, 296, 313–317, 384
Tracheobronchial, 69–75, 86, 390
Tracheobronchomalacia, 78, 83, 84
Tracheoesophageal fistula, 35–37, 44, 48, 50, 57
Training, 134, 135, 217, 459, 491, 515–519
Transient lower esophageal sphincter relaxations, 42, 44
Transplant surgery, 516
Treacher Collins Syndrome, 311
Treatment, 2, 10, 17, 20, 22, 23, 28, 31, 41–44, 56, 61, 63, 71, 73, 75, 81, 83, 84, 86, 87, 95, 97, 103, 104, 131, 147, 157, 159, 161, 163, 177, 179, 181–183, 185, 188, 189, 193, 195–198, 211, 213, 222, 223, 227–230, 236, 240, 248, 250, 252, 260, 262, 268, 272–277, 289–291, 293, 297, 303, 305, 308, 311, 313–316, 321, 329, 331, 335, 336, 338, 343–345, 353, 354, 356, 360, 362, 365, 369, 371, 382, 383, 388–391, 393, 395, 399, 406, 409, 412, 415, 417, 426–428, 431, 433, 434, 436, 437, 439, 440, 443, 446, 447, 449, 452, 453, 456, 458–461, 466–468, 473, 474, 481, 482, 489, 490, 498, 499, 501, 503, 509, 510, 516, 521–525, 527, 529, 531–533, 536
Tumor surgery, 440
Twin-Twin Transfusion Syndrome (TTTS), 507, 511

U

Ulcer, 42, 43, 49, 107, 221, 228, 362, 446
Ulcerative colitis, 219, 220, 222, 224
Umbilical hernia, 110, 111
Undescended testicle, 139, 354
Urachus, 109, 110, 141
Ureteral reimplantation, 331, 336–338
Ureterocele, 321, 325, 329
Ureteropelvic junction obstruction, 325
Urinary Tract Infection (UTI), 136, 139, 142, 144, 197, 237, 320, 328, 331–333, 335, 336, 338, 341, 353, 354

V

VACTERL, 36, 37, 234, 241, 242, 368
Vacuum bell, 14, 17
Vaginal agenesis, 359, 363, 364, 368, 370, 371
Varicocele, 351, 355, 356, 433
Vascular malformation, 101, 102, 105–107, 296
Vesicoureteral Reflux (VUR), 131, 136, 141, 142, 144, 239, 320, 327, 331–336, 338, 347
Video Assisted Thoracoscopic Surgery (VATS), 66, 67
Vitelline duct, 109, 148, 155, 191, 192, 230
Vocal cord palsy, 78, 83
Voiding Cystourethrogram (VCUG), 110, 144, 239, 244, 320, 327, 328, 331–334, 338

W

Wilms tumor, 320, 431–433, 458

MIX
Papier aus verantwortungsvollen Quellen
Paper from responsible sources
FSC® C105338

If you have any concerns about our products,
you can contact us on
ProductSafety@springernature.com

In case Publisher is established outside the EU,
the EU authorized representative is:
Springer Nature Customer Service Center GmbH
Europaplatz 3, 69115 Heidelberg, Germany

Printed by Libri Plureos GmbH
in Hamburg, Germany